The Third Histamine Receptor

Selective Ligands as
Potential Therapeutic Agents in
CNS Disorders

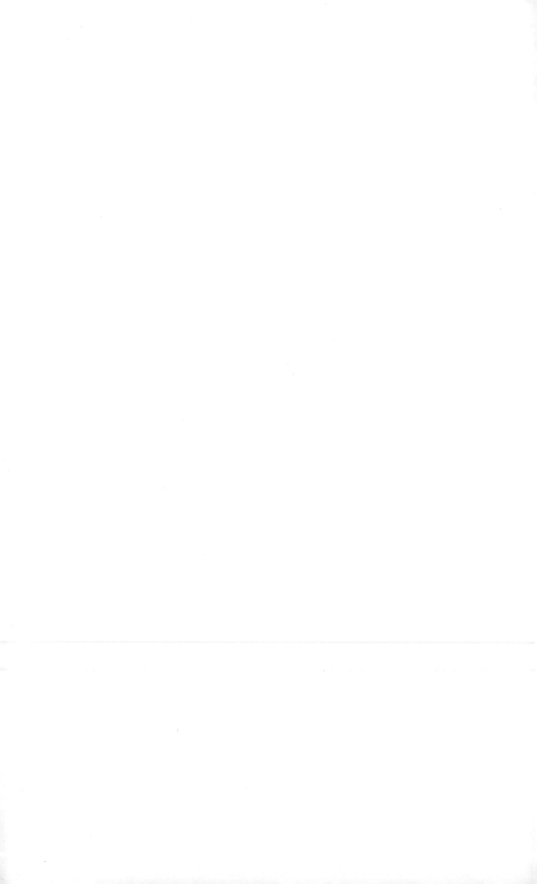

The Third Histamine Receptor

Selective Ligands as
Potential Therapeutic Agents in
CNS Disorders

Editor

Divya Vohora

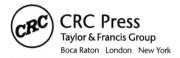

CRC Press
Taylor & Francis Group
Boca Raton   London   New York

CRC Press is an imprint of the
Taylor & Francis Group, an **informa** business

CRC Press
Taylor & Francis Group
6000 Broken Sound Parkway NW, Suite 300
Boca Raton, FL 33487-2742

© 2009 by Taylor & Francis Group, LLC
CRC Press is an imprint of Taylor & Francis Group, an Informa business

First issued in paperback 2019

No claim to original U.S. Government works

ISBN-13: 978-0-367-45251-3 (pbk)
ISBN-13: 978-1-4200-5392-0 (hbk)

Library of Congress Cataloging-in-Publication Data

The third histamine receptor : selective ligands as potential therapeutic agents in CNS
  disorders / edited by Divya Vohora.
    p. ; cm.
  Includes bibliographical references and index.
  ISBN-13: 978-1-4200-5392-0 (hardcover : alk. paper)
  ISBN-10: 1-4200-5392-2 (hardcover : alk. paper)
  1. Histamine--Receptors. 2. Central nervous system--Diseases--Chemotherapy. 3.
Antihistamines. I. Vohora, Divya.
  [DNLM: 1. Histamine H3 Antagonists--therapeutic use. 2. Central Nervous System
Diseases--drug therapy. 3. Receptors, Histamine H3--metabolism. QV 157 T445 2009]

QP801.H5T53 2009
612.8'2--dc22   2008019288

Visit the Taylor & Francis Web site at
http://www.taylorandfrancis.com

and the CRC Press Web site at
http://www.crcpress.com

Contents

Preface vii
Editor ix
Contributors xi

SECTION A   Introduction

Chapter 1 H_3 Receptor Target: Past, Present, and Future
Perspectives from Worldwide H_3 Experts 3

*Divya Vohora, Andrew D. Medhurst, Nicholas I. Carruthers,
and Sylvain Celanire*

Chapter 2   Third Histamine Receptor: From Discovery
to Clinics, Long-Lasting Love Story at INSERM
and Bioprojet 13

Jean-Charles Schwartz

Chapter 3   Histamine as Neurotransmitter 31

Oliver Selbach and Helmut L. Haas

SECTION B   The Third Histamine Receptor

Chapter 4   Phylogeny, Gene Structure, Expression, and Signaling 83

*Pertti Panula, CongYu Jin, Kaj Karlstedt,
and Remko A. Bakker*

Chapter 5   Drug Discovery: From Hits to Clinical Candidates......................... 103

Sylvain Celanire, Florence Lebon, and Holger Stark

Chapter 6   Peripheral Actions and Therapeutic Potential
in Periphery 167

Gabriella Coruzzi and Maristella Adami

SECTION C   *Therapeutic Potential in Central Nervous System Disorders*

Chapter 7   Cognitive Functions, Attention-Deficit Hyperactivity Disorders, and Alzheimer's Disease 213

Maria Beatrice Passani, Patrizio Blandina, Kaitlin E. Browman, and Gerard B. Fox

Chapter 8   Sleep Disorders.. 241

Jonathan E. Shelton, Timothy W. Lovenberg, and Christine Dugovic

Chapter 9   Obesity 277

Timothy A. Esbenshade, Michael E. Brune, and Marina I. Strakhova

Chapter 10   Epilepsy 305

Divya Vohora and Krishna K. Pillai

Chapter 11   Schizophrenia.. 329

Kaitlin E. Browman, Min Zhang, Gerard B. Fox, and Lynne E. Rueter

Chapter 12   Other Central Nervous System Diseases and Disorders 355

Paul L. Chazot and Fiona C. Shenton

Index   371

Preface

The third histamine receptor, identified in 1983, generated widespread interest as a potential target for its extensive role in the central nervous system (CNS). The first book on this subject, edited by Leurs and Timmerman, was available in 1998. However, many advances have taken place since then. Molecular advances in the past few years followed by cloning of human H_3 receptors and development of a large number of selective and nonimidazole H_3 receptor antagonists with pharmacological evidence in a number of different therapeutic conditions raise the hope for having an H_3 receptor-related drug to hit the market soon. In this book, an attempt has been made to bring together worldwide scientists actively involved in the H_3 field both from academia and from pharmaceutical industry including medicinal and computational chemists, biologists, and pharmacologists. This book aims to provide a single source of information from the identification and localization of H_3 receptor to the development of novel ligands incorporating preclinical and more recent clinical studies, indicating the earliest possible stage of development of these ligands. It is a blend of almost all the therapeutic activities being explored for these ligands with literature from studies using cutting-edge research techniques as well as patent literature.

The format is organized to provide the readers with the introduction of the field starting with the expert opinion in the light of knowledge available with discussion on the pitfalls and key issues related to H_3 receptor research. One of the key features of this section is that it incorporates suggestions from leading International experts in the field. It is hoped that these suggestions would provide directions for future research for scientists involved in drug development. The introductory section continues with the history of the field by one of the pioneers of the field, the discoverers of histamine H_3 receptor, Professor J. C. Schwartz from Bioprojet, France, and a general overview of histamine as a neurotransmitter in the brain by a very eminent scientist, Professor H. L. Haas from Heinrich-Heine University, Düsseldorf, Germany. This is followed by a chapter on H_3 receptor phylogeny, gene structure, and signaling. The selective ligands developed so far by different research groups along with details of the stages of development are discussed in the next chapter. A separate chapter is devoted to the peripheral actions of H_3 receptors and the therapeutic potential of these ligands in the periphery. Subsequent chapters describe various CNS disorders in which H_3 receptors are known to have a major role including cognitive functions, attention-deficit hyperactivity disorder, Alzheimer's disease, sleep disorders, obesity, epilepsy, schizophrenia, depression, nociception, and neurodegeneration. Each chapter addresses issues relevant to drug development.

Hopefully this book will be a valuable source of information for researchers entering the field of histamine research and will provide a comprehensive resource for those already in this field. This book is expected to generate interest among the scientific community and is intended to benefit both academic and industrial researchers from various disciplines including physiologists, biochemists, pharma-cologists, and others.

I am indebted to all the contributors (30 eminent scientists from 14 organizations located in 9 countries), who accepted my request and enabled the publication of this book. Special thanks are due to Professors Schwartz and Haas, who, despite being busy, squeezed their schedules and agreed to submit their valuable contributions. Dr. Sylvain Celanire, leader of the histamine H_3 project at the UCB Center for CNS innovation, Belgium, helped in this venture in many ways. I appreciate the time and effort he invested, and I express my gratitude for the same. Thanks and regards are due to Professor Pillai, Head of the Department of Pharmacology, Jamia Hamdard, New Delhi, who introduced me to this field of H_3 receptors way back in 1998. I thank my husband and my daughter for their love and support.

Editor

Dr. Divya Vohora (Shangari) received her masters in 1997 and doctorate in 2001 in pharmacology from Jamia Hamdard, New Delhi, where she joined as a faculty member in 1999 and is currently working as a reader in the Department of Pharmacology. Her research interests include pharmacology of the central nervous system with particular emphasis on epilepsy, cognitive functions, neurodegenerative diseases, and 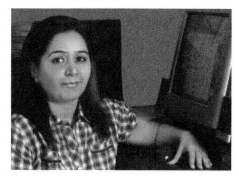 histamine. She developed interest in the H_3 receptor field in 1998 when she investigated the role of brain histamine and H_3 receptor ligands in modulating both experimental seizures and action of antiepileptic drugs. She has worked as a principal investigator in many funded research projects and has received grants from All India Council for Technical Education (AICTE), Indian Council of Medical Research (ICMR), University Grants Commission (UGC), Council of Scientific and Industrial Research (CSIR), and Department of Science and Technology (DST), Government of India. She has supervised eight masters and three doctoral theses and has received awards of national distinction including Career Award for Young Teachers, Fast Track Award for Young Scientists, and Chandra Kanta Dandiya Prize in pharmacology. She has authored more than 60 papers in national and international journals with more than 100 citations.

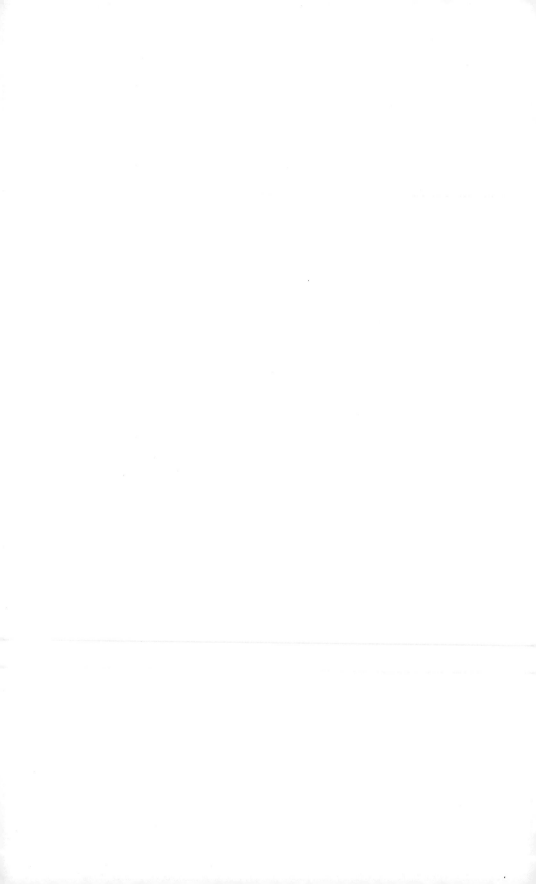

Contributors

Maristella Adami
Department of Human Anatomy,
  Pharmacology, and Forensic Medicine
University of Parma
Parma, Italy

Remko A. Bakker
Department of Medicinal Chemistry,
  Leiden/Amsterdam Center for
  Drug Research
VU University Amsterdam
Amsterdam, The Netherlands

Patrizio Blandina
Department of Clinical and
  Preclinical Pharmacology
University of Florence
Florence, Italy

Kaitlin E. Browman
Global Pharmaceutical Research
  and Development
Abbott Laboratories
Abbott Park, Illinois

Michael E. Brune
Global Pharmaceutical Research
  and Development
Abbott Laboratories
Abbott Park, Illinois

Nicholas I. Carruthers
Pharmaceutical Research and
  Development
Johnson & Johnson
San Diego, California

Sylvain Celanire
Global Chemistry
UCB
Braine L'Alleud, Belgium

Paul L. Chazot
Centre for Integrative Neuroscience
School of Biological and
  Biomedical Sciences
Durham University
Durham, United Kingdom

Gabriella Coruzzi
Department of Human Anatomy,
  Pharmacology, and Forensic Medicine
University of Parma
Parma, Italy

Christine Dugovic
Pharmaceutical Research
  and Development
Johnson & Johnson
San Diego, California

Timothy A. Esbenshade
Global Pharmaceutical Research
  and Development
Abbott Laboratories
Abbott Park, Illinois

Gerard B. Fox
Global Pharmaceutical Research
  and Development
Abbott Laboratories
Abbott Park, Illinois

Helmut L. Haas
Institute of Neurophysiology
Heinrich-Heine University
Düsseldorf, Germany

CongYu Jin
Institute of Biomedicine/Anatomy
University of Helsinki
Helsinki, Finland

Kaj Karlstedt
Department of Biology
Abo Akademi University
Turku, Finland

Florence Lebon
Global Chemistry
UCB
Braine L'Alleud, Belgium

Timothy W. Lovenberg
Pharmaceutical Research
  and Development
Johnson & Johnson
San Diego, California

Andrew D. Medhurst
Neurology and GI Centre of Excellence
  for Drug Discovery
GlaxoSmithKline
Essex, United Kingdom

Pertti Panula
Institute of Biomedicine/Anatomy
University of Helsinki
Helsinki, Finland

Maria Beatrice Passani
Department of Clinical and
  Preclinical Pharmacology
University of Florence
Florence, Italy

Krishna K. Pillai
Department of Pharmacology
Jamia Hamdard
New Delhi, India

Lynne E. Rueter
Global Pharmaceutical Research
  and Development
Abbott Laboratories
Abbott Park, Illinois

Jean-Charles Schwartz
Bioprojet Biotech
Saint-Grégoire, France

Oliver Selbach
Institute of Neurophysiology
Heinrich-Heine University
Düsseldorf, Germany

Jonathan E. Shelton
Pharmaceutical Research
  and Development
Johnson & Johnson
San Diego, California

Fiona C. Shenton
School of Biological and
  Biomedical Sciences
Durham University
Durham, United Kingdom

Holger Stark
Institute of Pharmaceutical Chemistry
Johann Wolfgang Goethe University
Frankfurt, Germany

Marina I. Strakhova
Global Pharmaceutical Research
  and Development
Abbott Laboratories
Abbott Park, Illinois

Divya Vohora
Department of Pharmacology
Jamia Hamdard
New Delhi, India

Min Zhang
Global Pharmaceutical Research
  and Development
Abbott Laboratories
Abbott Park, Illinois

Section A

Introduction

1 H_3 Receptor Target: Past, Present, and Future Perspectives from Worldwide H_3 Experts

Divya Vohora, Andrew D. Medhurst,
Nicholas I. Carruthers, and Sylvain Celanire

CONTENTS

Introduction...3
Questionnaire to the Experts 4
Expert Opinion 6
Summary...8
Acknowledgments... 11
References 11

INTRODUCTION

Ever since the work of Schwartz et al. [1], histamine has been recognized to function as a neurotransmitter and modulator in the central nervous system (CNS). Neuroanatomical, neurochemical, and electrophysiological evidences have highlighted that histamine is an important regulator of sleep/wake states as well as emotional/cognitive states including arousal and alertness. Indeed, histamine is released in the brain from a discrete group of highly localized posterior hypothalamic neurons that project their nerve endings to many critical brain regions. As an example, the multiple interconnections between histaminergic and cholinergic synapses have led to the hypothesis that the depolarization of cholinergic neurons by histamine plays an important role relative to cognitive deficits. Thus, as an autoreceptor and heteroreceptor on nonhistaminergic neurons, the histamine H_3 receptor (H_3R) subtype represents a unique and key modulatory site for drug development targeting CNS disorders.

Since the discovery of the H_3R in the 1980s, we have witnessed unprecedented efforts by both academic groups and pharmaceutical companies worldwide, leading to impressive medicinal chemistry efforts to deliver clinical drug candidates. The drug discovery process around H_3 ligands has not been an easy task. Since the discontinuation of Gliatech's GT2331 candidate, both public and private institutions have developed numerous screening assays across many disciplines (biology, pharmacology, drug metabolism and pharmacokinetics DMPK, formulation, toxicology, safety, etc.) as well as radiolabeled ligands to identify potential issues within their own chemical series. Many companies faced numerous challenges in the identification of highly potent and selective H_3 antagonist series with an adequate pharmacokinetic/pharmacodynamic profile, brain penetration, or more importantly, free from any toxicity and cardiovascular liabilities. Furthermore, the development of new hybrid compounds such as the recent dual H_3-SSRI ligands by Johnson & Johnson, may be of great interest as an alternative treatment of depressive state in which cognition is also impaired.

A number of scientific publications, posters, oral communications, and patent applications [2] have highlighted that the H_3 community has never been so close to the clinical proof of concept in human of H_3 antagonists/inverse agonists for the treatment of CNS disorders. To date, three candidates have reached phase I clinical trials; for the treatment of dementia (GSK189254, GSK239512), cognitive deficit in schizophrenia (BF-2.649, GSK189254), and neuropathic pain (GSK189254). Two phase II clinical trials are still ongoing with JNJ17216498 and GSK189254 for the treatment of narcolepsy. Despite a conflicting rationale regarding the role of histamine H_3R in the pathophysiology of epilepsy, BF-2.649 showed positive results in phase II studies. The H_3 research community is now awaiting results of these clinical phases to define the potential benefit of such drugs for the symptomatic treatment of severe CNS diseases.

Scientists from all over the world, passionate about the histamine field, have been strongly committed to this book dedicated to the histamine H_3R (Figure 1.1). From the identification and localization of the H_3R to the clinical studies of innovative ligands, through the preclinical proof of concept in animal models of CNS disorders (attention/cognition, narcolepsy, sleep/wakefulness, obesity, schizophrenia, and epilepsy), medicinal and computational chemists, biologists, and pharmacologists have provided an outstanding scientific contribution to the drug discovery research in this field.

QUESTIONNAIRE TO THE EXPERTS

We decided to send a questionnaire to the experts of histamine H_3R field in the pharma industry and asked them to address some of the key issues in the area according to the following questions:

- What is the main progress and breakthrough in terms of chemistry, biology, and pharmacology of the ligands discovered so far since the H_3R identification in the 1980s?
- What were the successes/pitfalls that scientists faced in H_3R-related drug research?
- Why an H_3R-related drug has not been introduced so far? What were the main challenges that faced and what are the challenges likely to be faced by scientists in the near future?

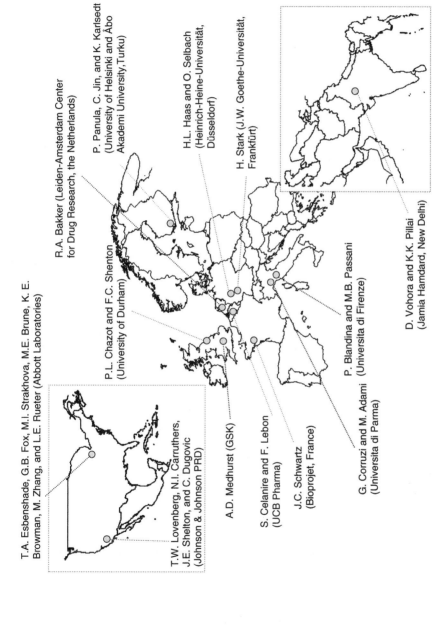

FIGURE 1.1 Worldwide contributing authors to the present book.

- Is there still some chemical space unexplored in this strong competitive field maintained by both academic and pharmaceutical companies?
- What are the main potential therapeutic indications of H_3R agonist and antagonist/inverse agonist?
- What are your suggestions/advice for researchers in this field?

EXPERT OPINION

ANDREW D. MEDHURST

Andrew D. Medhurst obtained his BSc (hons) in pharmacology at King's College, London in 1989. He joined SmithKline Beecham in 1990, where he started work on *in vitro* characterization of 5-HT_{1D} and 5-HT_4 receptor pharmacology. In 1995, he shifted emphasis onto molecular biology, and in particular gene expression studies, using novel techniques such as differential display and quantitative TaqMan reverse transcriptase–polymerase chain reaction (RT–PCR). Andy gained his PhD in molecular pharmacology in 2000 for his work on tachykinin NK_3 receptors and the characterization of novel nonpeptide NK_3 antagonists. In 2001, he developed an interest in the H_3R field and went on to become biology leader for the H_3 antagonist program at GlaxoSmithKline (GSK). Andy currently leads a neuropharmacology group at GSK in Essex, U.K., working on a number of different symptomatic and disease-modifying targets for neurodegenerative disorders.

There are currently a number of H_3R antagonists being evaluated in ongoing clinical studies for various disease indications (www.clinicaltrials.gov), making it a very exciting period in the history of the H_3R. Since the identification of functional H_3Rs more than 20 years ago [3], a number of key breakthroughs have contributed to this progression of H_3 antagonists into humans. For example, the discovery of highly selective H_3 agonists (e.g., R-α-methylhistamine) and antagonists (e.g., thioperamide) back in the late 1980s allowed a more precise characterization of H_3R pharmacology [4]. Several subsequent studies with a number of H_3R ligands have been key in defining the therapeutic potential of targeting the H_3R with selective molecules. These studies included the localization of H_3Rs in the CNS, the identification of neurotransmitters modulated by the H_3R *in vivo*, and the demonstration of efficacious effects with H_3 antagonists in animal models of cognition and sleep/wake behavior [5,6].

Despite the initial discovery of H_3 antagonists 20 years ago, significant progress into clinical studies, particularly in patients, was hampered due to development issues such as cytochrome P450 liability related to imidazole-based structures [7]. In the late 1990s, two major breakthroughs occurred to reignite the H_3 field. First, the human H_3R was cloned [8], allowing the detailed investigation of H_3 pharmacology in a homogenous system and the initiation of several high-throughput screening efforts. Second, nonimidazole-based antagonists were discovered, providing the opportunity to circumvent the suboptimal properties of first-generation imidazole-based H_3 antagonists [7]. Since then, huge and diverse patent activity has occurred in the nonimidazole H_3 antagonist area, with some exemplified compounds reaching clinical studies [2].

Another key development was the identification and understanding of species differences in H_3R pharmacology observed following the cloning of the rat receptor [9]. This enabled further understanding of how some compounds interact differently at the molecular level with human and rat receptors and aided subsequent identification of compounds with equivalent or greater affinity for human compared with rodent H$_3$Rs.

There have also been a number of interesting phenomena identified that complicate a clear understanding of the H$_3$R, including the existence of constitutive receptor activity, protean ligands, receptor dimers, diverse signaling pathways, and numerous splice variants/isoforms [7]. However, the significance of these exciting findings, particularly in terms of how they may influence *in vivo* responses to compounds preclinically, and their possible relevance to the potential future clinical application of H$_3$ antagonists, will require considerable further investigation.

Another recent challenge has emerged following the observation that some H$_3$ antagonists including thioperamide exhibit potent activity at the H$_4$ receptor [10]. Because numerous studies have utilized thioperamide in the past, interpretation of historical data becomes more difficult, particularly in models where immune cells expressing H$_4$ receptors could be involved. However, many of the recently described nonimidazole H$_3$ antagonists lack H$_4$ activity, thus providing more selective tools for the future [2].

There is great interest in the potential use of H$_3$ antagonists in a diverse number of therapeutic disease areas including narcolepsy, excessive daytime sleepiness, cognitive dysfunction (in Alzheimer's disease, other dementias, and schizophrenia), neuropathic pain, attention-deficit hyperactivity disorder (ADHD) and obesity [6,7]. Given the proven pedigree of other members of the histamine receptor family as successful therapeutic targets, it is hoped that modulation of H$_3$R function may also yield useful therapies for a number of disease conditions in the not too distant future. The challenge will be to identify which patient populations are likely to benefit most from therapeutic efficacy coupled with minimal side effects.

NICHOLAS I. CARRUTHERS

In 1999, Nicholas I. Carruthers joined the Johnson & Johnson Pharmaceutical Research & Development L.L.C. in San Diego as chemistry team leader for neuroscience. Among his roles in the neuroscience team, he is responsible for programs aimed at exploiting many targets identified by his biology counterparts. Before joining Johnson & Johnson, Dr. Carruthers was at Schering-Plough where he was primarily involved in the allergy and immunology area. He began his industrial career at Hoechst in the United Kingdom in the area of anti-infective research. Dr. Carruthers obtained his PhD in 1980 from Heriot-Watt University, Edinburgh, Scotland, which was followed by a NATO Research Fellowship at the University of California, Berkeley. He has more than 60 published papers to his credit, in excess of 100 patents and patent applications and was elected a Fellow of the Royal Society of Chemistry in 1997.

The histamine H$_3$R was first characterized, in 1983, as a presynaptic autoreceptor controlling histamine release in the brain [3] using existing H$_1$ and H$_2$ antagonists as probes in a classical pharmacological approach. Subsequently it was shown to presynaptically inhibit the release of other monoamines and acetylcholine on nonhistaminergic neurons. The early phase of research was bolstered by the discovery of both a potent and selective agonist, (*R*)-α-methylhistamine (RAMH), and an antagonist, thioperamide [4]. The pharmacological evaluation of these and related histamine (imidazole)-based structures, together with autoradiographic studies confirmed extensive receptor localization and provided the basis for predicting the therapeutic utility of H_3 ligands. Two compounds from these imidazole-based ligands were reported to be evaluated in man. The RAMH prodrug, BP2-94 [11], and GT-2331 (Gliatech Inc, Press Release, May 24, 2000) were reportedly evaluated for pneumoallergic disorders and ADHD, respectively.

In the early 1990s, advances in molecular biology led to the cloning of the H_1 and H_2 receptors. However, cloning of the H_3R proved more difficult than anticipated due to the lack of homology between the two previously cloned receptors but was finally cloned in 1999 [8]. The cloning of rat, mouse, and other species followed shortly thereafter permitting an understanding of pharmacological differences between species and reinforcing the importance of selecting the appropriate species for screening. This in turn has led to a refinement in the description of H_3 ligands (agonists, inverse agonists, antagonists, and protean agonists), and in some instances a revision of their functional behavior [12]. Indeed, at this juncture it was discovered that GT-2331 behaved as a partial agonist at the human receptor [13]. Nonetheless, these discoveries prompted a renaissance in the H_3 field, allowing pharmaceutical companies in particular to apply high-throughput screening techniques to identify new templates for medicinal chemistry. Before 1999, medicinal chemists from both academia and industry had used the natural ligand as a basis for drug design and produced a range of imidazole-containing structures. Although these compounds were useful for gaining insight into the possible therapeutic applications of histamine H_3 ligands, the presence of an imidazole moiety greatly limited brain penetration and also introduced the potential for cytochrome P450 interactions. One of the first approaches to obtain nonimidazole ligands, arising from collaboration between several academic laboratories [14], identified cyclic aliphatic amines as imidazole replacements. Ironically, in the same time frame, similar structures were obtained through high-throughput screening of corporate compound databases [12]. The availability of small molecule nonimidazole-based structures gave medicinal chemists the ability to design drug-like molecules and evaluate their potential in a range of conditions: in the CNS on sleep/wake disorders (narcolepsy), ADHD, and cognition; metabolic disorders (obesity); neuropathic pain; and allergic rhinitis.

With several companies now acknowledging advanced clinical evaluation of H_3 antagonists, the therapeutic potential for histamine H_3R ligands to treat human disease(s) may soon be realized.

SUMMARY

H_3R has indeed come a long way from its first identification by J. C. Schwartz and his group at INSERM in 1983 [3]. Autoradiographic studies confirming highest densities of these receptors in basal ganglia, hippocampus, cortical and striatal areas of brain, and the autoreceptor/heteroreceptor function of these receptors to modulate not just histamine but many other neurotransmitters prompted researchers to investigate their potential in various disorders of the CNS. The interest in the H_3R field increased after first identification of selective ligands thioperamide and RAMH in 1987 [4]. Since then, the interest continued to rise with a tremendous rise in the number of publications in the Pubmed (>300 in the past 5 years itself as depicted

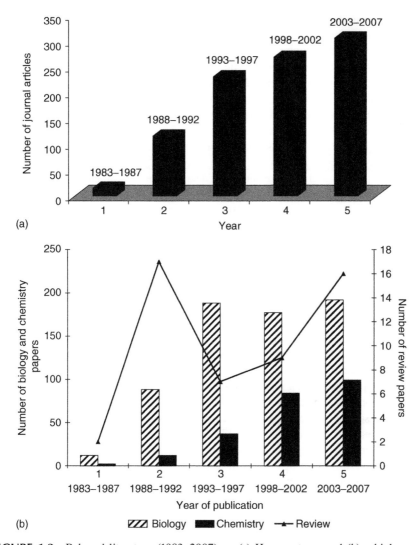

FIGURE 1.2 Pubmed literature (1983–2007) on (a) H$_3$ receptors and (b) a biology and chemistry perspective as well as review papers on H$_3$ receptors.

in Figures 1.2a and 1.2b) as well as the patent applications appearing at a rapid pace (Chapter 5, Figures 5.1 and 5.2), and it can be anticipated that this will continue during the coming years. The successful cloning of this receptor in 1999 by T. Lovenberg and his group at Johnson & Johnson [8] led to the classification of H$_3$R as G-protein-coupled receptor and discovery of several signal transduction pathways modulated by human H$_3$Rs and thus enabled our understanding of these receptors in various pathophysiological conditions. A high constitutive activity of this receptor (ability to transfer signals even without activation by an agonist) coupled with the fact that its ligands displayed protean agonism (ability to produce different responses from full agonism to inverse agonism) as well as a lot of pharmacological heterogeneity found among various species and the human receptors complicated the H_3R pharmacology [15]. Detection of various receptor isoforms (>20) having different signal transduction mechanisms further added to the complexities [16].

The H_3R ligands discovered earlier were imidazole-based with a number of drawbacks to be clinically useful drugs, such as cytochrome P450 inhibition, low affinity for human H_3Rs, lack of selectivity (affinity for H_4 receptors as well), low brain penetration, and toxic effects such as hepatotoxicity reported with thioperamide and some other compounds. Various nonimidazole H_3R ligands were then developed by efforts of various pharmaceutical companies and academic research groups. Many of these were more selective (devoid of H_4 activity) and had better pharmacokinetic profile and CNS penetration. The preclinical evidence of antagonists/inverse agonists of these receptors in various CNS disorders including narcolepsy, cognitive disorders, dementias, ADHD, Alzheimer's disease, schizophrenia, epilepsy, neuropathic pain, and obesity has given the impetus for the launch of a number of clinical trials, some showing encouraging results whereas for some the results are very eagerly awaited [2]. The first compound to enter clinical trial was GT-2331 for ADHD, but its development was later halted (Figure 5.39 in Chapter 5 shows the various H_3R ligands in various phases of clinical development). Although a lot of potential for these compounds in obesity was suggested in preclinical studies and a number of compounds were developed by Abbott for this indication, these compounds could not undergo clinical evaluation due to the problems of either contradictory data or adverse cardiovascular and genotoxic effects (see Chapter 9 for details). Nevertheless, results on obesity are encouraging, and a new chemical series with better safety profile is being investigated.

Studies on antagonists/inverse agonists in animal models of various CNS disorders offered some or the other advantage over the drugs those are currently available for such indications. For instance, JNJ-17216498 and GSK-189254, currently in phase II for narcolepsy as provigilant drugs, have shown, in preclinical studies, an advantage over other waking drugs either in terms of a lack of appetite-suppressant and locomotion-enhancing effects or in terms of offering a unique mechanism with no liabilities associated with DA release (also see Chapter 8). Similarly, in epilepsy models, H_3 antagonists/inverse agonists have beneficial effects as also being procognitive and provigilant and offer an edge over other drugs in view of the sedative and cognitive effects associated with currently available antiepileptic drugs (AEDs). In addition to effects on preclinical models, one such compound (BF 2.649) exhibited encouraging results in pharmacoresistant epilepsy in epileptic patients (phase II trial) (Chapter 10). The drug is also in phase I trial for treating cognitive deficits in schizophrenic patients. This is interesting as H_3 antagonists/inverse agonists have shown antipsychotic-like effects in schizophrenic animal models (Chapter 11). However, there have also been instances where a particular H_3 antagonist/inverse agonist efficacious in one particular indication lacks efficacy in the other. For example, JNJ-5207852 promotes wakefulness but lacks effects on obesity models, whereas some antiobesity H_3 antagonists are not effective in cognition models (Chapter 9). This questions the attribution of a particular indication to the H_3R class as a whole. At the same time, it offers benefit in terms of selective pharmacological activity associated with a compound and thus lesser potential for adverse effects due to its other indication.

Although H_3Rs are mainly located in CNS, they are also detected in peripheral tissues in amounts lower than that in CNS. There is evidence from preclinical studies that these receptors may have a potential therapeutic role in gastrointestinal (GI) disorders, asthma, nasal congestion, and myocardial ischemia. Although the latter appeared to be a very promising indication from preclinical studies, there is limited availability of human data to substantiate the claims made in preclinical studies. Some preliminary studies indicated a possible use of H_3R agonists as anti-inflammatory agents, but there are no confirmatory studies available. As mentioned in Chapter 6, if any such role is confirmed, we may see a novel class of gastrosparing nonsteroidal anti-inflammatory drugs (NSAIDs), but this being too optimistic at this stage.

Interesting combinations were studied as promising strategies. This was either to synergize the therapeutic effects based on a common target altered by them or to minimize the adverse effects. For instance, dual H_3/H_1 antagonist and dual H_3/leukotriene (LT) antagonist for nasal decongestion, dual H_3/M_2 antagonist for Alzheimer's disease, and recently dual H_3/SSRI for augmenting antidepressant effect as also for combating side effect fatigue of antidepressant treatment regime.

Preclinical data are promising and suggest a tremendous potential of H_3R-related drugs in various diseases. However, we must remember that data on chronic studies are meager, and many of the therapeutic conditions in which H_3Rs play a role are chronic diseases requiring long-term treatment. The therapeutic applications for agonists/antagonists/inverse agonists of these receptors, thus, require further validation and clinical evaluation. Nevertheless, clinical trials are underway in a number of conditions including ADHD, Alzheimer's disease, narcolepsy, neuropathic pain, and schizophrenia and the results being awaited with much interest. Hopefully, we may see a novel class of drugs for disorders of the CNS that have so far been largely refractory to pharmacotherapy.

ACKNOWLEDGMENTS

We gratefully thank Professors Helmut Hass (University of Dusseldorf), Henk Timmerman and Rob Leurs (LACDR, The Netherlands), Jean-Charles Schwartz (Bioprojet, France), Jean-Michel Arrang (INSERM, France), Walter Schunack (University of Berlin, Germany), Dr. Karin Rimvall (Novo Nordisk, Denmark), and late Dr. Arthur Hancock (Abbott Labs, United States) for their strong commitment to the histamine H_3 field, and passionate members of the European Histamine Research Society (EHRS).

REFERENCES

1. Schwartz, J. C., Barbin, G., Garbarg, B. M., Pollard, H., Rose, C. and Verdiere, M. 1976. Neurochemical evidence for histamine acting as a transmitter in mammalian brain. *Adv Biochem Psychopharmacol* 15:111–126.
2. Celanire, S., Wijtmans, M., Talaga, P. et al. 2005. Keynote review: Histamine H_3 receptor antagonists reach out for the clinic. *Drug Disc Today* 10:1613–1627.
3. Arrang, J. M., Garbarg, M. and Schwartz, J. C. 1983. Auto-inhibition of brain histamine release mediated by a novel class (H_3) of histamine receptor. *Nature* 302:832–837.

4. Arrang, J. M., Garbarg, M., Lancelot, J. C. et al. 1987. Highly potent and selective ligands for histamine H_3-receptors. *Nature* 327:117–123.

5. Alguacil, L. F. and Perez-Garcia, C. 2003. Histamine H_3 receptor: A potential drug target for the treatment of central nervous system disorders. *Curr Drug Targets CNS Neurol Disord* 2:303–313.

6. Passani, M. B., Lin, J. S., Hancock, A., Crochet, S. and Blandina, P. 2004. The histamine H_3 receptor as a novel therapeutic target for cognitive and sleep disorders. *Trends Pharmacol Sci* 25:618–625.

7. Leurs, R., Bakker, R. A., Timmerman, H. and de Esch, I. J. 2005. The histamine H_3 receptor: From gene cloning to H_3 receptor drugs. *Nat Rev Drug Discov* 4:107–120.

8. Lovenberg, T. W., Roland, B. L., Wilson, S. J. et al. 1999. Cloning and functional expression of the human histamine H_3 receptor. *Mol Pharmacol* 55:1101–1107.

9. Lovenberg, T. W., Pyati, J., Chang, H., Wilson, S. J. and Erlander, M. G. 2000. Cloning of rat histamine H_3 receptor reveals distinct species pharmacological profiles. *J Pharmacol Exp Ther* 293:771–778.

10. Hough, L. B. 2001. Genomics meets histamine receptors: New subtypes, new receptors. *Mol Pharmacol* 59:415–419.

11. Krause, M., Stark, H. and Schunack, W. 1998. Medicinal chemistry of histamine H_3 receptor agonists. In: *The Histamine H_3 Receptors*, eds. R. Leurs and H. Timmerman, pp. 175–196, Elsevier, Amsterdam.

12. Letavic, M. A., Barbier, A. J., Dvorak, C. A. and Carruthers, N. I. 2006. Recent medicinal chemistry of the histamine H_3 receptor. *Prog Med Chem* 44:181–206.

13. Esbenshade, T. A., Krueger, K., Denny, L. I., Miller, T., Kang, C. H., Witte, D., Yao, B., Black, L., Bennani, Y. L., Decker, M., Pan, J. B., Fox, G. and Hancock, A. 2001. Complex pharmacological effects of GT-2331. *Soc Neurosci Abstr* 27:378.

14. Ganellin, C. R., Leurquin, F., Piripitsi, A., Arrang, J. M., Garbarg, M., Ligneau, X., Schunack, W. and Schwartz, J. C. 1998. Synthesis of potent non-imidazole histamine H_3 receptor antagonists. *Arch Pharm* 331:395–404.

15. Arrang, J. M., Morisset, S. and Gbahou, F. 2007. Constitutive activity of the histamine H_3 receptor. *Trends Pharmacol Sci* 28:350–357.

16. Hancock, A. A. 2006. The challenge of drug discovery of a GPCR target: Analysis of preclinical pharmacology of histamine H3 antagonists/inverse agonists. *Biochem Pharmacol* 71:1103–1113.

2 Third Histamine Receptor: From Discovery to Clinics, Long-Lasting Love Story at INSERM and Bioprojet

Jean-Charles Schwartz

CONTENTS

Histamine Autoreceptors Discovered and Identified
as Non-H1 and Non-H2 Receptors 14
Development of the First Selective Ligands for the H3 Receptor 16
Novel H3-Receptor Ligands: A Long and Difficult
Journey to a Drug Candidate 18
From Antagonists to Inverse Agonists and Protean Ligands 20
H3-Receptor Inverse Agonists Enhance Wakefulness and Cognition 22
Antinarcoleptic Efficacy of Tiprolisant, an H3-Receptor
Inverse Agonist: From Mice to Humans 23
Tiprolisant in ADHD: Again from Mice to Patients 24
Are H3-Receptor Inverse Agonists Useful in Epilepsy? 25
Are H3-Receptor Ligands Useful in Schizophrenia? 26
This Is Not a Conclusion! 27
References 28

I have been fascinated by the physiology of histamine since the beginning of my scientific career and, more specifically, uncovering the function of this amine in the brain has been my aim and that of several of my coworkers during the past 40 years. Because I personally like to read *science stories* and believe that such stories might, occasionally, be useful to young scientists, I have written here a short and partial account of my lifelong love story with a mysterious substance which was, for a long time, considered essentially a dangerous one, for which protection against its detrimental effects in airways or stomach was searched by many talented medicinal chemists.

The existence of a third histamine receptor was discovered at our Parisian laboratory of INSERM (the French National Institute of Health and Medical Research) by the beginning of the 1980s, rather than earlier, because it is only at this time that both conceptual and experimental tools had been made available through our own previous efforts together with those of others during the few preceding years.

By the mid-1970s, we had demonstrated that histamine was to be added to the growing list of novel cerebral neurotransmitters [1,2], at a time when most neuroscientists admitted that only acetylcholine and catecholamines were playing such a role. In agreement, with Monique Garbarg et al. [3], we had shown that electrolytic lesions of the Medial Forebrain Bundle elicited dramatic decreases, in the telencephalon, in the level of L-histidine decarboxylase, the histamine-synthesizing enzyme (that we had characterized in rat brain a few years ago with Christiane Rose, a young technician, and Christiane Lampart, a young internist [4]). Since we had previously shown that the enzyme was present in isolated nerve-endings, we interpreted the lesion studies as reflecting the anterograde degeneration of a major histaminergic neuronal bundle emanating from an area posterior to the lateral hypothalamic area and projecting in a diffuse manner to the whole telencephalon, a disposition which was largely confirmed, several years later, when histochemical methods were developed by Takehiko Watanabe and Panula. In addition, with Helene Pollard and Serge Bischoff, we had identified the mechanisms of brain histamine inactivation through methylation followed by deamination [5] and, with Michel Baudry and Marie-Pascale Martres, shown the presence of the two classes of receptors, H1 and H2, in brain mediating the effects of histamine in peripheral tissues [6]; at about the same time, Helmut Haas had characterized the H2 receptor (H2R) electrophysiologically.

In other words, at the beginning of the 1980s, after nearly a decade of efforts, almost the whole machinery of histaminergic neuronal transmission had been uncovered, and, conceptually, the time had come to assess whether, as mentioned earlier about catecholaminergic neurons, histaminergic neurons were endowed with autoreceptors.

HISTAMINE AUTORECEPTORS DISCOVERED AND IDENTIFIED AS NON-H1 AND NON-H2 RECEPTORS

Autoreceptors, that is, receptors expressed on neuronal cell bodies or terminals and inhibiting catecholamine release or synthesis, had become, at the beginning of the 1980s, a field of intense research. Such receptors were often and conveniently studied by labeling the endogenous neurotransmitter stores of noradrenaline or dopamine neurons using corresponding radioactive amines uptake in brain slices or synaptosomes through their high-affinity transport systems. When the analogy between catecholaminergic and histaminergic neurons had become apparent, it was tempting to assess whether autoreceptors were also present on the latter.

There had been attempts in several laboratories to perform release experiments following incubation of brain preparations with highly radiolabeled histamine, but data obtained through this approach were hardly interpretable. On our side we avoided this approach, knowing from previous studies that high-affinity transport systems for histamine could not be evidenced in either brain slices or synaptosomes. However, we had put a lot of efforts earlier to develop a method to label endogenous stores of histamine selectively through the incubation of the cerebral preparations by the 3H-aminoacid precursor. Schwartz et al. [5], to succeed, had painstakingly developed ion-exchange chromatography methods on small columns, first to purify 3H-histidine (by eliminating a preformed H3-histamine contamination present in the commercial samples and thereby reducing a background noise), then to isolate small amounts of synthesized H3-histamine (present only in L-histidine decarboxylase-containing cells) from a huge excess of 3H-histidine (actively uptaken in all cells). As is often the case in research, the development of an original experimental tool paves the way for new findings. Here, this rather *tricky* methodology had already allowed characterizing the histamine-release process in potassium-depolarized brain slices, showing, for instance, the calcium dependency of the process [7].

In 1982, Jean-Michel Arrang, a young pharmacist without any experience in research, joined our laboratory to prepare a science doctorate (PhD). In such cases, my philosophy is to propose a novel and, therefore, rather risky topic for the newcomer to have a chance to not only show his capacities but, at the same time, to limit the risks by providing already developed methodologies and allowing him to collaborate with an experienced researcher. In this case, the topic that we proposed to Jean-Michel was the search of presynaptic receptors on histaminergic neurons using brain slices and the 3H-labeling procedure using the precursor aminoacid, a robust method currently applied in the laboratory. He was also introduced to neuropharmacology by Monique Garbarg, an experienced researcher, who looked after him and also collaborated in some experiments. Slices from rat cerebral cortex were selected for initial studies because we already knew from deafferentation studies [8] that this area contains exclusively terminals from histaminergic neurons, and it represents an abundant source of tissue, allowing to prepare large numbers of slices from a single brain. Because we had in mind to conduct conveniently large numbers of parallel incubations (necessary to construct dose–response curves, the *golden rule* in traditional pharmacology), we deliberately selected a very simple device. It consisted of common test tubes in which slice batches were distributed, oxygenated superficially at the beginning and depolarized by addition of potassium ions. At this time, this procedure was considered less *fashionable* than superfusion of the slices and electrical depolarization.

Quite rapidly, Jean-Michel showed our simplified process to work reliably and reproducibly, and he discovered that addition of nonradioactive histamine in the medium reduced the amount of 3H-histamine released by the depolarizing stimulus. Initially, we were not sure that this reduction resulted from a receptor-mediated effect rather than a kind of isotopic dilution effect. However, it soon became clear that the histamine-induced braking effect on its own release could be blocked competitively by known histamine antagonists and mimicked by histamine analogs; this implied the involvement of a presynaptic receptor. Was this receptor one of the two already defined at this time?

From the beautiful work performed a few years earlier by Jim Black, Robin Ganellin, and their colleagues, we had in hands the necessary tools to answer this question, that is, a series of compounds acting more or less selectively at either the

H1 receptor (H1R) or the H2R, each of them being characterized by its apparent affinity constant. From their dose–response curves, we derived apparent dissociation constants of antagonists (using the Schild plot analysis) and the relative potencies of agonists. Using these classical pharmacology tools carefully, it became clear that we were dealing with a non-H1R, non-H2R: for instance, the effect of histamine was hardly affected by mepyramine at micromolar concentrations (whereas the drug displays nanomolar affinity at the H1R) and impromidine, a potent H2R agonist, behaved as a rather potent antagonist in our model, two examples among many others that fortified our conviction that we had discovered a novel histamine receptor.

We sent a letter to *Nature* telling this story and proposing to call H3 receptor this novel entity. We felt that our experimental demonstration, performed in the pure style of the classical British pharmacology, on a topic, that of histamine, illustrated by the names of great British pharmacologists (Sir Henry Dale, Sir James Black, and Heinz Schild) had to be published in this prestigious British journal. The manuscript was well received by the referees, except one (that we soon identified by the nature of his semantic criticisms!) who mainly objected about naming the novel receptor H3 rather than H2B. But we resisted strongly to this unfounded suggestion and convinced the *Nature*'s editor that it did not reflect a purely scientific rationale; this was confirmed when the cloning of the H3 receptor showed its poor aminoacid sequence analogy with the H2R.

This letter [9] was the birth declaration of the third histamine receptor subtype.

DEVELOPMENT OF THE FIRST SELECTIVE LIGANDS FOR THE H3 RECEPTOR

Identifying a novel receptor was considered a major achievement in the before cloning (BC) years of pharmacology, and the histamine H3 receptor was among the very last ones to be identified through traditional pharmacological approaches. However, for various reasons we were not fully satisfied at this point. First, evaluating the physiological implications of the receptor *in vivo* required the use of selective agonists and antagonists that were not available. Second, working in a famous Parisian psychiatric hospital (where schizophrenic patients had received a neuroleptic drug, chlorpromazine, for the first time in history), I was struck by the poverty of the psychiatric pharmacopoeia, contrasting with the importance of therapeutic needs as well as the large variety of potential drug targets in brain, and I was extremely motivated to contribute improvements in this matter. Colleagues generally considered, at this time, that designing a novel pharmacological tool or, even more, developing a novel class of drug was neither a *fashionable* nor an easy task to be performed in an academic environment. I was convinced of the contrary, since we had successfully and rather easily designed during the preceding years, in an academic environment, a novel drug class: the *enkephalinase* inhibitors, starting from the discovery of the biological target in our laboratory. In collaboration with Jeanne-Marie Lecomte, a pharmacist with a strong industrial experience in large companies, we had even started to develop such a drug (Tiorfan®, now used by millions of patients) and created the pharmaceutical start-up Bioprojet for this purpose.

For these reasons, we decided to embark on a medicinal chemistry H3 project in a purely academic environment. However, although we had in hands a model to test new molecules on the novel target, we had neither the know-how nor the facilities to prepare such molecules in the laboratory. At this time, I participated with Jeanne-Marie in a dopamine symposium that took place in Beerse, in Paul Janssen's laboratory, during which one of his collaborators showed 3D formulas of neuroleptics and discussed their analogy with the structure of dopamine. This gave me the very straightforward idea that we could, in a parallel way, imagine obtaining an H3-receptor antagonist, starting from the structure of histamine, maintaining its imidazole ring, and replacing the ethylamine chain by a piperidine residue. We submitted the idea to Max Robba, a professor of medicinal chemistry at the University of Caen, in Normandy, that we both knew because he had given pharmacochemistry courses to both of us at the Parisian Faculty of Pharmacy, and, even more, Jeanne-Marie had prepared her PhD in his laboratory. Max accepted enthusiastically to collaborate on this project; Bioprojet provided him a salary for a technician who started to synthesize molecules according to the line imagined in Beerse, and these molecules were tested on brain slices of rat against histamine at our INSERM laboratory. After no more than a few dozen molecules prepared and tested in this way, structure–activity relationships had become quite clear, and we obtained thioperamide, a compound displaying low nanomolar affinity as a competitive antagonist, as revealed by Schild plot analysis. Thioperamide was not only the first selective H3-receptor ligand *in vitro*, but we rapidly showed that, given systemically in low dosage to rats, it also enhanced markedly the turnover of histamine in brain as measured by pulse-labeling the endogenous pool with 3H-histidine, a very reliable technique that we had developed a few years before. We were quite excited by this result because we realized that we had designed the first drug able to activate histaminergic neurons in brain, that is, an important tool to characterize their functional role, a tool that was lacking at this time.

In 1984, I organized, with Robin Ganellin (the *father*, together with Jim Black, of Tagamet®, the first H2R antagonist), an international symposium on histamine in the honor of Heinz Schild, who had just passed away. At this occasion, I discussed with Robin my intention to design a selective H3-receptor agonist, although I was not willing to collaborate with him on this project despite the warm sympathy I had for him and the admiration I had for his skills and achievements in medicinal chemistry; at this time, he was the director of the Smith Kline and French research center at Welwyn's Garden, and I wanted to collaborate exclusively with academics (as an external advisor I had witnessed how easily an original project could be killed for nonscientific reasons within a multinational pharmaceutical company). Very friendly, Robin told me that the person I should contact was Walter Schunack, an excellent German medicinal chemist who, for many years, had focused his activity on imidazole derivatives acting on the H1R and H2R. The occasion to meet Walter was the Histamine Symposium, which took place in Jouy-en-Josas, near Paris, on the campus of a famous commercial high school, and we started discussing the project in front of a poster, continuing under the candles of the *Galerie des Glaces* of the Versailles Castle where we had managed to organize a private visit and a big dinner for all symposium attendees. I discovered in Walter a dynamic and pleasant person; the prejudices I had against Germans (I am a survivor of the Holocaust) immediately vanished at his contact, and we started a collaboration that lasted over two decades and progressively transformed itself into a solid friendship.

The main ingredients for a successful collaboration such as original project, complementary skills, and pleasant human relationships were present in our understatement, and, quite rapidly, we identified with the R-isomer of α-methylhistamine prepared in Walter's laboratory, a stereospecific, highly potent, and selective ligand of the H3 receptor. Again we showed that the H3-receptor agonist was active *in vivo*: it decreased histamine turnover in brain, an effect that could be blocked by thioperamide. Furthermore, we had R-α-methylhistamine synthesized in triturated form with high specific radioactivity and showed that it could be used to selectively label the H3 receptor in cerebral membranes for drug-binding studies or, even more importantly, in autoradiographic studies that revealed its widespread distribution in brain.

Finally, as we also characterized the first partial agonist, we had designed prototypes for all classes of ligands for the H3 receptor, thereby completely confirming its existence as a novel pharmacological entity.

We submitted the whole story to *Nature*, and the journal accepted, without any reservation, to publish the manuscript as a full article [10]. Along the years, this article became a highly cited one because it provided several useful tools to study the physiology of histaminergic systems in brain, to characterize the presence of H3 receptors in human brain slices, to identify it as a G-protein-coupled receptor [11] and, at a later date, to *deorphanize* it by Lovenberg and colleagues.

NOVEL H3-RECEPTOR LIGANDS: A LONG AND DIFFICULT JOURNEY TO A DRUG CANDIDATE

Thioperamide and R-α-methylhistamine, both compounds displaying a good selectivity profile and acceptable potency *in vivo* could have represented good candidates for drug development, and, at Bioprojet, Jeanne-Marie and myself were absolutely convinced that we could undertake such development. We were reinforced in our rather bold conviction by our current success in developing, entirely by ourselves, Tiorfan as the first member of an innovative class of drug in gastroenterology.

The following years showed us that the life of drug developers is not always, as we say in French, "paved of roses."

Thioperamide rather rapidly showed its hepatotoxicity in rats, a deceiving observation that we could have, probably, anticipated from the presence of a thioamide group in its structure that had been introduced for synthesis commodity. On its side, R-α-methylhistamine, which displays acceptable pharmacokinetics in rodents, revealed its unacceptably short half-life in medical students, that is, healthy human volunteers. Hence these two failures led us to interrupt the development of both compounds, which, nevertheless, continued their long and successful lives as prototypic pharmacological tools (more than 600 and nearly 300 Pubmed citations for thioperamide and R-α-methylhistamine, respectively, during their first 20 years of existence).

Considering the number of interesting animal observations that were performed by us or published by others, in both cases using these two compounds (that we largely provided to the scientific community), we were strongly convinced that H3-receptor ligands constituted a potentially important novel drug class, particularly the antagonists as awakening and procognitive agents. And we decided to continue our search for drug candidates.

To be more effective on this matter, we organized a real European research network comprising the medicinal chemistry laboratories of Walter Schunack and Robin Ganellin, my neuropharmacological INSERM unit, and the pharmaceutical start-up Bioprojet directed by Jeanne-Marie Lecomte. Walter had just moved to well-equipped laboratories at the Free University of Berlin, where several hard-working and talented pharmacochemists were preparing for their PhD, including Holger Stark who has remained on the topic until now and is the *father* of many hundreds of compounds. Robin had left SKF to occupy a prestigious SKF professorship in medicinal chemistry at University College London, and this move greatly facilitated our collaboration; he was working mainly with postdocs from an amazing variety of national origins, all solidly supervised by Basil Tertiuk, an old and deeply experienced technician who had worked with him for several decades. At our laboratory, the previous team was reinforced by the arrival of Xavier Ligneau, a young biological engineer, who undertook the systematic trial of compounds. The task of Bioprojet, a company without laboratory, was to provide some salaries and financial contribution, to take patents in the name of inventors, to perform the various steps of pharmaceutical development through CROs, for example, toxicity and clinical trials and, importantly, to provide expertise on clinical and pharmaceutical aspects of the research (at a later date, performance became better with Bioprojet's acquisition of a research center, in Britanny, with a large number of skilled scientists joining the company).

The collaboration was formalized by written agreements between the parties, including the relevant academic authorities, and went on smoothly and pleasantly along the years. Information and data were distributed immediately among participants and programs agreed during meetings taking place, often in Paris or, sometimes, at an international conference, during which researchers made formal presentations and informal discussions followed. These meetings were useful not only for the advancement of the program but also to teach the participants, namely, the youngest ones, ways of thinking belonging to disciplines outside their own domain of activity: drug design is obviously a multidisciplinary venture. I am very grateful to my colleagues for these so pleasant and intellectually enriching years of friendly collaboration.

The collaboration was so fruitful that several thousands of original compounds were synthesized and tested *in vitro* and, very often, *in vivo*, particularly when we developed a radioimmunological test to assess conveniently the activity of histaminergic neurons by measuring *tele*-methylhistamine (*t*-MeHA) levels in the brain of a mouse. Along the years, five very active compounds at low oral doses were selected for development but had to be abandoned, one after the other, due to animal toxicity problems, generally consisting in metabolic disorders apparently independent from the H3 activity. Thereafter, our screening procedure comprised the assessment of cholesterol and glucose levels in blood, and we identified an extremely potent compound, ciproxifan, which was apparently devoid of this drawback [12]. In addition, to our delight, ciproxifan appeared as an antiobesity drug in chronically treated rats that drastically lost body weight, but the delight was of short duration since we discovered that they had lens opacification, which probably prevented these poor blind rats to find their food.

Taking into account these difficulties, we felt that we had to move out from the series of imidazole derivatives to which all our compounds belonged. More specifically, Robin and his team focused on this challenge in a very rational way: he retained the nonimidazole part of one of our potent antagonists and branched it systematically to various nitrogen-containing residues. This strategy fully succeeded, a lead in which the imidazole residue was replaced by a piperidine ring being identified and the affinity being progressively improved, namely, through the efforts of Walter Schunack, Holger Stark, and their colleagues in Berlin [13]. In Paris, some of the compounds of this new series were found to be extremely potent *in vivo*, even when administered by oral route. Our British and German medicinal chemistry colleagues may have together performed a major achievement in their discipline, which is, in some sense, witnessed by the fact that the large majority of the thousands of compounds thereafter synthesized in drug companies have been obtained using the same *recipe*, that is, a similar scaffold.

A first compound, BF2.649 (now named tiprolisant according to a proposal from the WHO), was selected for the development, which, so far, seems to fulfill our expectations: it is entering phase III clinical trials in 2008 with several potential therapeutic indications having already been validated.

FROM ANTAGONISTS TO INVERSE AGONISTS AND PROTEAN LIGANDS

From the careful studies of Jean-Michel and Xavier with brain slices or, even, synaptosomes, it had become clear that a number of our antagonists not only blocked completely the inhibitory effects of agonists on 3H-histamine release but also facilitated this release over the basal level. One explanation could have been that these compounds were relieving the *brake* exerted by endogenous histamine released under these circumstances. But another explanation could have been that the H3 autoreceptor was constitutively active, that is, was exerting a brake on the release system, even in the absence of histamine or agonist. This question was not settled until Lovenberg et al. [14] (see Chapter 8) cloned the H3 receptor and use identified *neutral antagonists* in our chemical library.

In fact we had made serious efforts to clone the receptor since the introduction of molecular biology techniques in our laboratory. Our efforts of homology cloning were based on our initial observation that binding of agonists to the H3 receptor was regulated by guanyl nucleotides, strongly suggesting that this receptor belonged to the superfamily of heptahelical receptors, like the two other histamine receptor subtypes. In fact our *fishing expeditions* with degenerated probes allowed us to discover the 5-HT6 and 5-HT7 receptor, but not the H3 receptor. The latter was beautifully identified by Lovenberg and colleagues among *orphan* heptahelical receptors, after expression and characterization of its pharmacological profile. Its sequence is far enough from those of H1R or H2R to explain how it had escaped our valuable efforts of homology cloning.

The disclosure of the sequence of the human H3 receptor has allowed many drug companies that had not contributed before to more easily enter the field, as it is shown by the large number of patents, which appeared thereafter. On our side, we could derive the sequences of the receptor in several species and, using site-directed mutagenesis, show that the marked pharmacological differences between the human and the rat receptors, at least regarding some compounds, were attributable to only two amino acids in the whole sequence [15].

In addition, we identified some splice variants of the H3 receptor mRNAs, but we decided not to invest more time on this type of heterogeneity, which we had discovered several years earlier in the case of the dopamine D2 receptor but whose biological significance had (and has still) remained largely elusive [16,17].

More importantly, we found that the H3 receptor was endowed with large constitutive activity. Finding that, using artificial cell systems in which the receptor is overexpressed, is certainly trivial, since this has been reported with many members of the superfamily and might be regarded as a kind of artifact of little physiological relevance. But, quite interestingly, we discovered that only this receptor, among a number of others, displayed constitutive activity when tested in native form, in cerebral membranes. Furthermore, using proxyfan, a neutral antagonist (i.e., a compound able to block the effect of agonists but not to reverse the receptor constitutive activity), which we had identified in our chemical library, we showed that only reversal of the constitutive activity (by inverse agonists) can enhance transmitter release from histaminergic terminals [18]. This observation is of high potential importance for therapeutic applications inasmuch as it suggests that inverse agonists, in contrast with neutral antagonists, may have different intrinsic activities and, thereby exert different effects (or, at least, different maximal effects) *in vivo*. In agreement with these theoretical views, we have observed that diverse inverse agonists display different degrees of intrinsic activity [19].

More recently, we observed that proxyfan should be, in fact, considered as a *protean* ligand (from the name of Proteus, a marine divinity from Greek mythology, having the power to metamorphose himself), maybe the first example of such a pharmacological curiosity, although the existence of such entities had been predicted on theoretical grounds. In agreement, a single compound, proxyfan, was shown to act on the H3 receptor as a partial agonist, a full agonist, a neutral antagonist, a partial or full inverse agonist, depending on the test system on which it is evaluated. Needless to say, it is difficult to predict the therapeutic utility of complex compounds of this type.

Interestingly, tiprolisant was shown to display high intrinsic activity as an inverse agonist and, probably as a consequence, to potently activate histaminergic neurons in brain [19]. With this drug, showing an acceptable safety profile in animal toxicity studies, we have been able to confirm, among humans, the positive role of histaminergic neurons in arousal and cognition and, in a series of *proof-of-concept* studies, determine potential therapeutic indications of H3-receptor inverse agonists.

H3-RECEPTOR INVERSE AGONISTS ENHANCE WAKEFULNESS AND COGNITION

As early as the mid-1970s, we proposed that the main function of histaminergic neurons is the maintenance of wakefulness, a proposal-based only, at this time, on their anatomical disposition, their silencing by sedative drugs, the waking action of intraventricular administration of histamine, and the sleep-inducing effects of *anti-histamines*, that is, H1-receptor antagonists crossing the blood–brain barrier [2].

By the mid-1980s, Michel Jouvet, a famous expert in sleep research, having discovered the *paradoxical sleep*, now more often called REM sleep, and the role of monoaminergic systems in states of vigilance, decided to focus his attention on histaminergic neurons that were neglected by most *sleepologists*. He proposed the subject to a young Chinese MD, Jian-Sheng Lin who had recently joined his reputed research laboratory in Lyons. Michel was not familiar with the available pharma-cological tools to manipulate histaminergic neurotransmission, and he introduced me to Lin, asking me to advise him in this respect. I accepted with pleasure and excitation, since I was, for a long time, convinced of the importance of the topic, but nobody in my laboratory had any know-how in experimental sleep studies and, in addition, I admired the achievements and the warm personality of Michel Jouvet. For about 10 years, Lin worked hard to prepare a huge and magnificent PhD thesis, using various neurobiological approaches to definitively establish histamine as a major waking neurotransmitter. I followed with interest his pharmacological studies in the cat, simply pointing to him the *cleanest* drugs to modify histamine metabolism or actions. All data he obtained could be interpreted as going in the same direction but a drug-enhancing histaminergic neuron activity was lacking to complete the beauti-ful pharmacological demonstration.

When we designed thioperamide, such a drug became available and we provided it to Lin who found, as could have been expected, that it induced a prolonged arousal in his cats; instead of spending the whole day in a succession of short periods of sleep and wakefulness (like all cats around the world!), the electronencephalogram (EEG) and electromyogram (EMG) recordings showed that they remained awake for hours [20]. Such observation was repeated by Lin, first in cats, then in mice, with all other H3-receptor inverse agonists that we provided him with, including ciproxifan [12] and tiprolisant [19,21], and by others using various other drugs of the same class; the effect is blocked by mepyramine, an H1-receptor antagonist, thus leaving little doubt about the involvement of endogenous histamine released under these circumstances.

The waking action with this class of drugs has two remarkable features, which suggested their high interest for therapeutic applications. First, it is not accompa-nied, as is the case, for example, amphetamines, by any behavioral excitation: cats are aroused but remain calm; rodents do not display any locomotor activation. Sec-ond, the prolonged waking effect is accompanied, in cats as in mice, by a shift of the power distribution pattern of the cortical EEG in favor of the highest frequency rhythms, which are known to accompany cognitive activities such as attention or learning. This is consistent with many observations, made in several laboratories and various models, of enhanced attention, for example, the effect of ciproxifan on the five-choice test in rats [12] or facilitated learning, for example, the effect of thioper-amide or tiprolisant on the two-trial object-recognition test in mice [19].

All clinical data, obtained so far with tiprolisant, indicate that these observations on cats and mice can be safely extrapolated to humans. In agreement, a similar shift in EEG power patterns toward fast rhythms was observed in healthy volunteers, particularly at the end of the day, when vigilance tends to decline; also the same subjects performed significantly better in the critical flicker fusion test, showing thereby an improved attention (in preparation).

In patients with excessive daytime sleepiness (EDS) of various etiologies, for example, in obstructive sleep apnea, narcolepsy, or Parkinson's disease, tiprolisant markedly improved the symptomatology and was generally well tolerated; the most common side effect was nocturnal insomnia attributable to overdosage. These proof-of-concept observations, performed on groups of ~25 patients, remain to be confirmed in larger studies, but their statistically significant and convergent results leave little doubt about the interest of this class of drugs in the treatment of pathologies where EDS is a major incapacitating symptom.

In addition, the procognitive (namely, the proattentional) potential of H3-receptor inverse agonists, now evidenced not only in rodents but also in healthy human volunteers, is obviously encouraging for exploring their therapeutic utility in diseases in which cognitive deficits represent the major symptomatology. Double-blind controlled studies with tiprolisant in dementias are currently ongoing, and their outcome is waited with high interest.

ANTINARCOLEPTIC EFFICACY OF TIPROLISANT, AN H3-RECEPTOR INVERSE AGONIST: FROM MICE TO HUMANS

Narcolepsy is a rare disabling sleep disorder characterized by EDS and abnormal REM sleep manifestations including cataplexy (sudden loss of muscle tone triggered by strong emotions), sleep paralysis, hypnagogic hallucinations, and sleep onset REM (SOREM) periods.

Deficient hypocretin/orexin transmission appears to be at the origin of narcolepsy. Hypocretins are excitatory peptides released by neurons from the lateral hypothalamus with widespread projections, namely, to aminergic neurons, for example, histaminergic or noradrenergic neurons. As hypocretin neurons promote wakefulness, treatment by orexins would be desirable in narcolepsy but, as it is often the case with peptides, is not practically feasible for bioavailability reasons.

We reasoned that the lack of orexins could be circumvented by activating histaminergic neurons pharmacologically, that is, using tiprolisant, an inverse agonist at the H3 receptor assuming that these neurons are not defective and can still be activated in the disease. We first tested this hypothesis throughout a reliable animal model of narcolepsy, the orexin (–/–) mouse, which displays all the major symptoms of the disease.

Unexpectedly, we found that the baseline activity of these neurons was not significantly reduced in the brain of *orexin homozygote* knockout (KO) mice, and the same was true for noradrenergic and serotonin neuron activity. Furthermore, tiprolisant was able to enhance indices of histamine and noradrenaline release to approximately the same extent in *orexin* KO as in their wild-type (WT) counterparts, suggesting that the two ascending waking systems can still be stimulated in this valuable animal model of narcolepsy.

In these *narcoleptic* mice, tiprolisant enhanced wakefulness approximately to the same extent as modafinil—an inhibitor of dopamine uptake currently used to treat EDS in narcoleptic patients but which does not affect cataplexy. However, in contrast with modafinil, which did not affect the occurrence of SOREM episodes that is regarded as an equivalent to the cataplectic episodes in humans, such episodes were significantly reduced by tiprolisant.

Obviously, these results were highly encouraging to proceed to clinical trials.

A pilot trial with a simple design, the first clinical trial with any H3-receptor inverse agonist, was undertaken to assess the potential of tiprolisant in alleviating EDS in narcoleptic patients.

It was a comparative, placebo-controlled, single-blind study, where 22 patients received placebo on the first week and the drug in single dosage; for safety reasons, they were allowed to continue their anticataplectic treatments with antidepressant drugs, which did not allow to assess the effect of tiprolisant on cataplexy.

This phase II study was able to demonstrate a statistically and clinically significant improvement of EDS in comparison to placebo. All the measures of EDS studied were consistent with this improvement: the Epworth somnolence scale was diminished, the number and the duration of diurnal somnolence and sleep episodes were reduced drastically [22].

In a second proof-of-concept trial in narcoleptic patients, not only the reduction of EDS was confirmed, but a reduced number of cataplectic episodes were also observed, in agreement with data obtained in orexin KO mice (Y. Dauvilliers, personal communication).

In summary, both preclinical and clinical data indicate that H3-receptor inverse agonists constitute a novel, effective, and well-tolerated treatment in narcolepsy, but these results from small-size studies need, obviously, to be confirmed in larger populations, using a double-blind design.

TIPROLISANT IN ADHD: AGAIN FROM MICE TO PATIENTS

One possible model for attention-deficit hyperactivity disorders (ADHD) is the mouse with knocked out dopamine transporter (DAT). Although it is not clearly established whether the human pathology is anyhow related to DAT, the mouse in which this essential component of the dopaminergic synapse is absent displays some of the characteristics of the patients: it is hyperactive, it has attentional/learning deficits, and its locomotor hyperactivity is paradoxically counteracted by amphetamines, a recognized treatment of the disease.

This interesting model was established in the laboratory of Marc Caron by Bruno Giros, a former PhD student in my laboratory, in which he has introduced molecular biology techniques and contributed to the discovery of the dopamine D3 receptor and the two isoforms of the D2 receptor. Coming back from his postdoctoral stay at Duke University, he has established his own successful research group in Paris where, with coworkers, they still raise and play with the DAT-KO mice.

Bruno immediately accepted my proposal of studying the effect of tiprolisant on his hyperactive mice. The experiment was a great success: the spontaneous and very marked locomotor hyperactivity of these animals was almost completely abolished, a remarkable effect since, in contrast to amphetamines, the drug neither modifies locomotor activity nor striatal dopamine release in control animals. Another remarkable effect was the procognitive effect in the DAT-KO mice exemplified by a significant improvement in their learning deficit revealed by an improved performance in the Morris swimming pool.

The extension of these studies to adult ADHD was started in Brussels at Erasmus hospital by an old friend, Julien Mendlewicz, and his young and enthusiastic colleague, Pierre Oswald; and a single-blind proof-of-concept study on about 20 patients, analyzed through two distinct ADHD rating scales, essentially confirmed the expectations born with the results of the mice study (in preparation).

Years ago, a clinical trial in adult ADHD with an H3-receptor ligand seems to have been performed by a company called Gliatech, which thereafter disappeared without publishing the results. One can guess that they were probably negative, but, afterward, the compound was shown to behave as a partial agonist, which may reinforce the conviction that inverse agonists may be preferable for a number of indications.

Theoretically, H3-receptor inverse agonists should be more safe than the amphetamines currently used in ADHD, being devoid of the cardiovascular side effects and drug abuse or psychotogenic potential of the latter.

ARE H3-RECEPTOR INVERSE AGONISTS USEFUL IN EPILEPSY?

The role of brain histamine in convulsive disorders has been evoked for a long time, mainly starting from the observations of seizures as a side effect of H1 antihistamines crossing the blood–brain barrier. Another indication is that treatments enhancing brain histamine levels, for example, administration of L-histidine (the histamine precursor), metoprine (an inhibitor of histamine degradation), or exogenous histamine itself, tend to protect rodents from convulsions, whereas inhibition of histamine synthesis is proconvulsant.

However, it has remained unclear whether blockade of H3 receptors could represent a mechanism for a new class of antiepileptic drugs.

Indeed blockade of H3 autoreceptors enhance histamine release from histaminergic neurons in brain and could, thereby, protect from convulsions but H3-receptor antagonists/inverse agonists may have other actions through H3 receptors located on other classes of neurons. Therefore, it is not easy to predict what would be the final outcome of H3-receptor blockade on convulsions, and there are conflicting reports in the literature.

To settle this question, we asked Dr. Depaulis—belonging to a reputed group in Strasbourg expert in rodent seizures—to study tiprolisant on some of their models. This group is particularly known for having developed a rat genetic model of human epilepsy (particularly of *absence* epilepsy in children and adults), the Genetic Absence Epilepsy, Rat from Strasbourg (GAERS). On this animal model, tiprolisant diminished the number and duration of spike-and-wave discharges by up to 77%, that is, characteristic EEG changes of the disorder.

In addition, in intrahippocampal kainate-induced epilepsy in mice, a model of pharmacoresistant epilepsy in humans, the same drug reduced significantly the frequency of discharges. Interestingly, these changes occurred without any significant modification of the interictal EEG profiles, which exclude a nonspecific sedative effect.

Encouraged by these preclinical data, we have started studies in a series of human epileptic subjects prone to photosensitive seizures and remaining so despite their treatment with various current antiepileptic drugs. Tiprolisant was found to dose-dependently suppress EEG changes (or at least enhanced their threshold) preceding convulsions that were experimentally triggered by repetitive photic stimulation.

Taken together, these observations suggest that the antiepileptic potential of this drug class deserves further attention.

ARE H3-RECEPTOR LIGANDS USEFUL IN SCHIZOPHRENIA?

Although the role of histaminergic neurons in schizophrenia and in the effects of antipsychotic drugs has been less studied than those of other aminergic neurons, the topic deserves attention [21].

In agreement, histamine neuron activity seems to be enhanced in both rodent models of schizophrenia (changes elicited by dopamine-releasing or glutamate-blocking drugs) and the human disease. Methamphetamine markedly increases histamine neuron activity, a response resulting from the stimulation of histaminergic neurons by endogenous dopamine selectively activating D2 receptors. In rats or mice receiving methamphetamine repeatedly and showing locomotor sensitization, the basal activity of histaminergic neurons is persistently enhanced. Phencyclidine (PCP), a nonselective *psychotogenic* NMDA receptor antagonist, significantly enhances t-MeHA levels in various regions of mouse's brain, an action mimicked by MK-801, another NMDA open-channel blocker. Jack Peter Green, a pioneer in brain histamine research, having painstakingly devised gas-chromatographic methods to measure histamine metabolites in human CSF, found that levels of t-MeHA are significantly elevated in patients with chronic schizophrenia, whereas others found H1-receptor-mediated responses and H1-receptor binding reduced in these patients' brain, possibly reflecting a down-regulation of the receptor consequent to overstimulation by endogenous histamine.

In addition, antipsychotic drugs affect histaminergic neurotransmission in various ways: (i) a large number of APDs are potent H1-receptor antagonists, a feature which confers them sedative and pro-obesity side effects; (ii) typical APDs tend to inhibit histaminergic neuron activity, whereas atypical APDs have opposite effects as a result of their 5-HT_{2A} antagonism.

The preceding information suggested the interest of testing agents affecting selectively histaminergic neurotransmission in psychotic states. So far, only the negative effects of H1-receptor antagonists of the first generation, that is, the brain-penetrating *antihistamines*, were assessed.

A number of recent observations with tiprolisant have strengthened the view that H3-receptor inverse agonists may have therapeutic utility in schizophrenia [21].

First, tiprolisant shows some efficacy in various *models* of schizophrenia. For instance, it partially reduces the hyperlocomotor and stereotypic behaviors of direct or indirect dopaminergic agonists, as do, with higher potencies, the antipsychotic drugs; the hyperlocomotor activity of dizocilpine is also partially reversed, indicating that the drug affects the dopamine–NMDA imbalances. The mechanism of these actions, although not well understood, is not related to the blockade of dopaminergic receptors. Interestingly enough, Aude Burban and Jean-Michel Arrang have also recently shown that the drug almost completely reverses the deficit of prepulse inhibition (PPI) of the acoustic startle response induced by apomorphine in mice; the low dosage of tiprolisant that was required, together with similar effects on gating deficit reported by the Abbott group with another compound, indicates that this is a drug class effect. Reversal of PPI inhibition is probably one of the best predictors of antipsychotic potential for nondopaminergic drug candidates, inasmuch as it explores a sensorimotor gating deficit, which is considered as a cardinal sign of schizophrenia. Second, drugs showing, such as H3-receptor inverse agonists, a large spectrum of procognitive efficacy are actively explored for improvement of the cognitive deficits in remaining of the schizophrenic patients, even treated with antipsychotic drugs of the second generation.

Finally, our studies in healthy volunteers support the notion that association of tiprolisant with antipsychotic drugs might compensate the pro-obesity potential of those in which it clearly appears now to be related with blockade of H1 receptors in brain. In agreement, olanzapine, an extremely potent H1-receptor antagonist, elicited a clear-cut antisatiety effect in a group of healthy volunteers, evidenced with an adequate self-rating scale, which was completely abolished when it was associated with tiprolisant: presumably, the histamine release elicited by the latter in brain had competitively displaced olanzapine from the H1 receptor. It should be underlined that these antisatiation effects of a large number of antipsychotics are likely at the origin of the development of the *metabolic syndrome*, a major side effect, as well as a major obstacle to compliance.

Hence, we strongly believe that, for diverse and complementary reasons, the H3-receptor inverse agonists deserve further attention in schizophrenia.

THIS IS NOT A CONCLUSION!

When, about 40 years ago, with a few young students, we started to study, in a small and poorly equipped laboratory, the metabolism of histamine in brain, the dream we shared was to be able, one day, to disclose the mysterious role of this amine in brain and use this knowledge to provide new types of drugs to cure patients with neuropsychiatric disorders.

Although very few scientists were interested in the topic at that time, it is rewarding to note how much the situation has changed today; the topic drawing the efforts of a growing number of academic and industrial scientists is testified by the present volume. All their efforts have progressively allowed to draw a more and more precise picture of the role of the histaminergic neuronal system in higher brain functions.

With the first proof-of-concept clinical trials with H3-receptor inverse agonists, it has already become clear that a novel and therapeutically useful class of neuropsychiatric drugs is born.

The challenge of the 1960s has been largely met. But the chapter will only be closed, our initial challenge met and a true conclusion written, when a large number of patients will benefit from these promising agents, hopefully in near future.

REFERENCES

1. Schwartz, J.-C. 1975. Histamine as a transmitter in brain. *Life Sci* 17:503–517.
2. Schwartz, J.-C. 1977. Histaminergic mechanisms in brain. *Annu Rev Pharmacol Toxicol* 17:325–339.
3. Garbarg, M., Barbin, G., Feger, J., and Schwartz, J.-C. 1974. Histaminergic pathway in rat brain evidenced by lesions of the medial forebrain bundle. *Science* 186:833–835.
4. Schwartz, J.-C., Lampart, C., and Rose, C. 1970. Properties and regional distribution of histidine decarboxylase in rat brain. *J Neurochem* 17:1527–1534.
5. Schwartz, J.-C., Pollard, H., Bischoff, S., Rehault, M.C., and Verdière-Sahuké, M. 1971. Catabolism of 3H-histamine in the rat brain after intracisternal administration. *Eur J Pharmacol* 16:326–335.
6. Baudry, M., Martres, M.-P., and Schwartz, J.-C. 1975. H1 and H2 receptors in histamine-induced accumulation of cyclic AMP in guinea pig brain slices. *Nature* 253:362–364.
7. Verdière, M., Rose, C., and Schwartz, J.-C. 1975. Synthesis and release of histamine studied on slices of rat hypothalamus. *Eur J Pharmacol* 34:157–168.
8. Barbin, G., Hirsch, J.C., Garbarg, M., and Schwartz, J.-C. 1975. Decrease in histamine content and decarboxylase activities in an isolated area of the cerebral cortex of the cat. *Brain Res* 92:170–174.
9. Arrang, J.-M., Garbarg, M., and Schwartz, J.-C. 1983. Auto-inhibition of brain histamine release mediated by a novel class (H3) of histamine receptor. *Nature* 302:832–837.
10. Arrang, J.-M., Garbarg, M., Lancelot, J.-C. et al. 1987. Highly potent and selective ligands for histamine H3 receptors. *Nature* 327:117–123.
11. Arrang, J.-M., Roy, J., Morgat, J.-L., Schunack, W., and Schwartz, J.-C. 1990. Histamine H3 binding sites in rat brain membranes: modulation by guanyl nucleotides and divalent cations. *Eur J Pharmacol* 188:219–227.
12. Ligneau, X., Lin, J.S., Vanni-Mercier, G. et al. 1998. Neurochemical and behavioral effects of ciproxifan, a potent histamine H3-receptor antagonist. *J Pharmacol Exp Ther* 287:658–666.
13. Ganellin, C.R., Leurquin, F., Piripitsi, A. et al. 1998. Synthesis of potent non-imidazole histamine H3-receptor antagonists. *Arch Pharm* 331:395–404.
14. Lovenberg, T.W., Roland, B.L., Wilson, S.J., et al., 1999. Cloning and functional expression of the human histamine H3 receptor. *Mol Pharmacol* 55:1101–1107.
15. Ligneau, X., Morisset, S., Tardivel-Lacombe, J. et al. 2000. Distinct pharmacology of rat and human histamine H3 receptors: role of two aminoacids in the third transmembrane domain. *Br J Pharmacol*, 131:1247–1250.
16. Morisset, S., Sasse, A., Gbahou, F. et al. 2001. The rat H3 receptor: gene organization and multiple isoforms. *Biochem Biophys Res Commun* 280:75–80.
17. Giros, B., Sokoloff, P., Martres, M.-P. et al. 1989. Alternative splicing directs the expression of two D2 dopamine receptor isoforms. *Nature* 342:923–926.
18. Morisset, S., Rouleau, A., Ligneau, X. et al. 2000. High constitutive activity of native H3 receptors regulates histamine neurons in brain. *Nature* 408:860–864.
19. Ligneau, X., Perrin, D., Landais, L. et al. 2007. BF2.649, a nonimidazole inverse agonist/antagonist at the human histamine H3 receptor. Preclinical pharmacology. *J Pharmacol Exp Ther* 320:365–370.

20. Lin, J.S., Sakai, K., Vanni-Mercier, G. et al. 1990. Involvement of histaminergic neurons in arousal mechanims demonstrated with H3-receptor ligands in the cat. *Brain Res* 523:325–330.
21. Ligneau, X., Landais, L., Perrin, D. et al. 2007. Brain histamine and schizophrenia: potential therapeutic applications of H3-receptor inverse agonists studied with BF2.649. *Biochem Pharmacol* 73:1215–1224.
22. Lin, J.S., Dauvilliers, Y., Arnulf, I. et al. 2008. An inverse agonist of the histamine H(3) receptor improves wakefulness in narcolepsy: studies in orexin(−/−) mice and patients. *Neurobiol Dis* (in press).

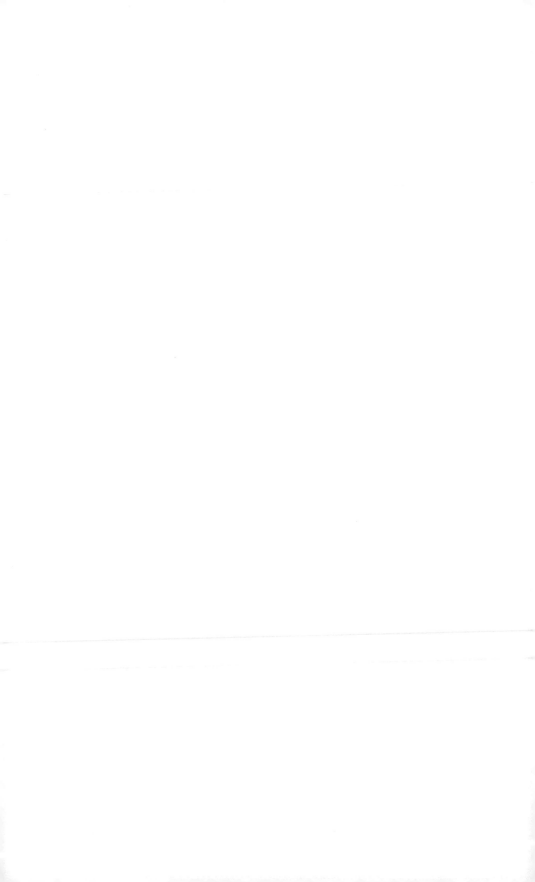

3 Histamine as Neurotransmitter

Oliver Selbach and Helmut L. Haas

CONTENTS

Introduction 31
    Histamine Metabolism in the Brain 32
    Histamine Neurons: Location and Morphology 34
    Histamine Neurons: Physiology 35
    Histamine Neurons: Inputs 38
    Histaminergic Pathways 42
    Histamine Receptors 43
        Ionotropic Receptors 43
        Polyamine-Binding Site of NMDA Receptors 43
        Metabotropic Receptors 43
    Histaminergic Actions 48
        Spinal Cord and Brainstem 48
        Hypothalamus 50
        Thalamus 51
        Basal Ganglia 51
        Hippocampus 52
        Cortex 53
        Synaptic Plasticity 53
        Glia 54
    Histamine and Behavior 54
        Sleep–Waking Regulation 54
        Body Weight and Appetite Control
            (Energy Metabolism and Feeding Rhythms) 56
        Thermoregulation 56
        Learning and Memory 56
Histamine Pathophysiology and Disease 58
Conclusion 59
References 59

INTRODUCTION

Henry Dale and Laidlaw [1] discovered the biological actions of histamine 100 years ago: the contraction of intestinal smooth muscles and vasodilatation. Ten years later, the effect on acid secretion in the stomach was published [2]. Feldberg [3] found that histamine release from mast cells causes bronchial constriction during anaphylactic shock. Kwiatkowski [4] detected histamine in the brain, and White [5] demonstrated its synthesis and catabolism. Antihistamines [6] have been used for allergy for the past 70 years, and their sedative side effects lead to the suggestion that histamine is a *waking substance* [7]. Major advances in the biochemistry of the histaminergic system in the brain came from Jean-Charles Schwartz and his group [8,9] in Paris who also located the histaminergic neurons and their projections pretty well through lesion experiments. The histaminergic system was long neglected in comparison with the catecholamine and the serotonin systems due to its late precise morphological characterization. Reasons for the general neglect at this time are, first, the competition of the other aminergic systems, which had become visible and could be exactly located in the brain through fluorescent histochemistry in the 1960s; and second, there was no evidence for involvement in a major neuropsychiatric disease. Electrophysiological recordings on central neurons as well as the study of behavior during central infusion of histamine supported the role of histamine as a transmitter in the brain, and Jack Peter Green [10] with his group at Mt. Sinai in New York was a major advocate of this role over decades. Sir James Black et al. [11] and his group identified the second histamine receptor and revolutionized the treatment of stomach ulcers. The H2 receptor (H2R) is also abundant in the central nervous system, and central actions were soon detected [12]. The groups of Hiroshi Wada in Osaka and Pertti Panula in Washington brought a breakthrough for the histaminergic system with the immunohistochemical localization of the histaminergic neurons in the tuberomamillary nucleus (TMN) in the posterior hypothalamus and its wide projections using antibodies against histidine-decarboxylase (HDC) [13] or histamine [14]. It was the group of Schwartz again, who identified the H3-autoreceptors that control the activity of histaminergic neurons: histamine synthesis, release, and electrophysiology [15]. The most recent addition is the H4R whose presence and function in the nervous system seem to be minimal. The histaminergic system in the brain is now recognized as the major waking center of the brain with implications in many basic homoeostatic functions [16]. More details on the history of histamine research is available in Ref. 17 and on the homepage of the European Histamine Research Society (EHRS).

HISTAMINE METABOLISM IN THE BRAIN

Histamine in histaminergic neurons is synthesized from histidine through decarboxylation by HDC (EC 2.1.1.22; Figure 3.1), a pyridoxal $5'$-phosphate-(PLP)-dependent enzyme [18] highly conserved throughout the animal kingdom [19,20]. Restricted and cell-specific expression of HDC in peripheral tissues is controlled at both transcriptional [21] and posttranslational levels. The rate of histamine synthesis, in contrast to that of other biogenic amines, is determined by the bioavailability of histidine, an amino acid taken up into the cerebrospinal fluid and neurons through L-amino acid transporters. HDC activity can be inhibited by alpha-fluoromethylhistidine (α-FMH), a suicide substrate leading to a marked depression of histamine levels [22].

Histamine is stored in neuronal somata and axon varicosities [23–25], where it is carried into vesicles by exchange of two protons through the vesicular monoamine

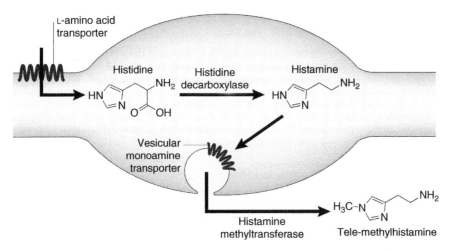

FIGURE 3.1 Histamine synthesis and metabolism. Histidine is taken up in the varicosity and decarboxylated; histamine is transported into a vesicle, released, and methylated. (Modified from Haas, H.L., Panula, P., *Nat. Rev. Neurosci.*, 4, 121–130, 2003. Copyright Macmillan Magazines Ltd.)

transporter (VMAT)-2 (Figure 3.1) and released on arrival of action potentials [26]. The level of histamine in brain tissue is to some extent lower than that of other biogenic amines, but its turnover is considerably faster (in the order of minutes) and varies with functional state [27,28]. Brain histamine levels exhibit profound circadian rhythms in accordance with the firing of histamine neurons during waking [29]. Histamine levels in the preoptic/anterior hypothalamus follow the sleep stages: wakefulness > non-rapid eye movement (REM) sleep > REM sleep [30]. A direct correlation between histamine levels in the hypothalamus and behavioral state was determined by electroencephalography [31]. Synthesis and the release of histamine are controlled by H3-autoreceptor-mediated feedback [15,32,33]. The release of histamine is also modulated by transmitters affecting histamine neuron firing and release from varicosities bearing inhibitory M1-muscarinic, α2-adrenergic, and peptidergic receptors [31,34–36].

Histamine in the brain is inactivated in the extracellular space by methylation through neuronal histamine N-methyltransferase (HNMT; EC 2.1.1.8; Figure 3.1) [37]. Histamine methylation requires S-adenosyl-methionine as the methyl donor [38,39]. HNMT is also found in the walls of blood vessels where bloodborne histamine and histamine released from mast cells are methylated and inactivated [40]. Tele-methylhistamine in the brain undergoes oxidative deamination through a monoamine oxidase (MAO)-B to t-methyl-imidazoleacetic acid [39,41]. Histamine hardly passes the blood–brain barrier. The main histamine-degrading enzyme in peripheral tissues (gut, connective tissues) and invertebrates is diamine oxidase (DAO), which directly converts histamine into imidazoleacetic acid. DAO activity in the brain is negligible under basal conditions but when HNMT is inhibited, it may represent a salvage pathway for the production of imidazoleacetic acid, an effective $GABA_A$ receptor agonist [42,43].

The brains of most species investigated contain variable numbers of mast cells, which release histamine and can contribute substantially to brain histamine content. Mast cells in circumventricular organs, meninges, hypophysis, pineal gland, area postrema, median eminence, hypothalamus, and along blood vessels in the gray matter contain a pool of histamine that turns over much more slowly than neuronal histamine [44,45]. Mast cells can rapidly enter the brain, particularly during the development and under pathological conditions associated with increased demand for neural circuit plasticity. Their number varies greatly between species, regions, time of the year and day, age, sex, and behavioral state [46].

HISTAMINE NEURONS: LOCATION AND MORPHOLOGY

A histaminergic system in rat brain arises transiently, ~2 weeks after gestation (E13), in the midbrain at the location of adult serotonergic neurons [47–49]. One week later (E20), the transient histaminergic system disappears, and the first histamine-immunreactive neurons are found in the caudal tuberal diencephalon forming the TMN. The hypothalamic histamine system reaches an adult state 2 weeks postnatally (P14). The functional significance of the transient histamine system is unknown.

Interestingly, in the most primitive vertebrate, the lamprey, it is preserved in adulthood, whereas in all other adult vertebrates (fish, turtle, frogs, rodents, and primates), the location of histaminergic neurons is restricted to the posterior hypothalamus. In the zebrafish, histamine is solely found in the brain [50]. This allows a pharmacologic analysis of endogenous histaminergic function *in vivo* simply by adding drugs to the aquarium water [51,52].

The vertebrate histaminergic nucleus is located in the posterior hypothalamus (Figures 3.2 and 3.3) [53]. Ericson subdivided this nucleus for the rat in a ventral group around the mamillary bodies close to the surface of the brain (TMV), a medial group around the mamillary recess (TMM), and a diffuse part [54]. A further subdivision of the TMV in a rostral and caudal and the TMM in a dorsal and ventral part is proposed by Wada's group [55,56]. The subdivisions are bridged by scattered neurons, indicating that a continuous cell group became dispersed during the development [13]. Tracing studies have so far revealed no topological organization, but there is evidence for heterogeneity within the histaminergic neuron population [57–59]. The TMN in the mouse brain is less compact and contains fewer and smaller neurons than in the rat [60]. The histaminergic neurons in the guinea pig are more widely distributed than in the rat and the mouse extending in the supramamillary nucleus [61,62]. In the tree shrew [63] and cat [64,65], the nucleus is rather more compact and located mainly in the ventrolateral part of the posterior hypothalamus.

The human brain contains about 64,000 neurons in and around the TMN, a size similar to the noradrenergic locus coeruleus. A well-organized network of varicose histaminergic fibers is seen in the cortex [66]. In the rodent hypothalamus, the dendrites of TMN neurons make close contact to the brain surface, whereas in the human posterior hypothalamus, varicose axons accumulate in this location. Four subgroups of the histaminergic nucleus include a major ventral part corresponding to the classical TMN, a medial part extending to the supramamillary nucleus, a caudal

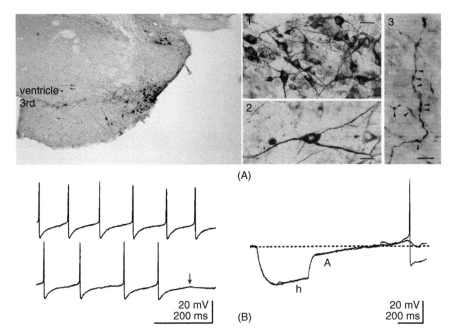

(A)

(B)

FIGURE 3.2 Histaminergic neurons of the TMN. (A) *Left*: slice from posterior hypothalamus, stained with histamine-antibody (From Parmentier, R., Lin, J.S., Lyon, A.). *Right*: histaminergic neurons in organotypic culture stained with antibody against HDC. (1) Median TMN group, calibration bar 50 µm; (2) isolated neuron (25 µm); (3) histaminergic varicose fiber in the hippocampal CA1 area (grown in coculture, 5 weeks), calibration bar 10 µm. (Modified from Diewald, L., Heimrich, B., Busselberg, D., Watanabe, T., Haas, H.L., *Eur. J. Neurosci.*, 9, 2406–2413, 1997.) (B) Electrophysiological properties. *Left*: spontaneous firing of histamine neuron in a hypothalamic slice. Arrow indicates an occasional miss of action potential, unmasking a depolarizing prepotential. *Right*: response to hyperpolarizing current injection. h—Hyperpolarization activated inward rectification due to Ih current and A—slow return to membrane potential due to A-current.

paramamillary, and a minor lateral area. Thus, the histaminergic neurons occupy a comparatively larger part of the posterior hypothalamus [67].

The rat TMN displays an intense immunohistochemical reaction toward adenosine deaminase [68]. The number of stained cells indicates that a smaller population of nonhistaminergic neurons is also positive. The function of adenosine deaminase located in the cytosol or the outer membrane of these neurons is unknown. A number of cotransmitters or their synthetic enzymes are expressed within TMN neurons [69,70]: GAD 65/67 implies a GABAergic phenotype, but no evidence of GABA release from TMN neurons is available. TMN subpopulations express also galanin, enkephalins, thyrotropin releasing-harmone (TRH), and substance P with some variation between species.

HISTAMINE NEURONS: PHYSIOLOGY

Histaminergic neurons resemble the other aminergic neuron populations in many respects. They fire slowly at 1–4 Hz in the absence of synaptic activation [71,72],

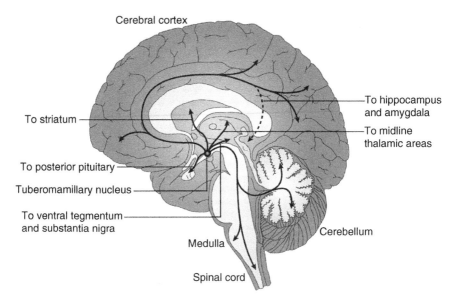

FIGURE 3.3 The histaminergic system in the human brain. The histaminergic fibers emanating from the TMN project to and arborize in the whole central nervous system. (Modified from Haas, H.L., Panula, P., *Nat. Rev. Neurosci.*, 4, 121–130, 2003. Copyright Macmillan Magazines Ltd.)

even in isolated neurons [73]. In behaving animals (cats, rats, and mice), the firing pattern is variable during waking, depending on the arousal state, and missing during sleep [60,74–76] (Figure 3.4) (for review, see Ref. 77). Recordings from identified TMN neurons revealed a membrane potential of about −50 mV and a broad action potential (up to 2 ms midamplitude duration at 35°C) with a significant contribution from Ca^{2+} channels followed by a deep (15–20 mV) afterhyperpolarization. Two opposing membrane conductances give the TMN neurons a typical electrophysiological appearance (Figure 3.2). The response to a hyperpolarizing current injection deviates from a capacitive behavior through activation of a depolarizing current of the h-type [78]. HCN3 and HCN1 are predominantly found in the rat; the current is not modified by cyclic nucleotides. The involvement of Ih in the TMN pacemaker cycle is questionable as blocking Ih through Cs ions does not affect the firing rate, and the half maximal activation occurs at about −100 mV [79,80], whereas the afterhyperpolarization takes the membrane potential from −75 to −80 mV [81]. This afterhyperpolarization is sufficient to remove inactivation of the fast outward current ($I_A$fast, 4-aminopyridine sensitive) [82] that delays the return to firing threshold and thus slows the firing. A further inactivating K-current ($I_A$slow), which is not blocked by 4-aminopyridine and requires long-lasting hyperpolarizations for removal of inactivation, is unlikely to affect spontaneous firing. A recent detailed analysis of the A-type current in mouse TMN revealed a subthreshold activation of I_A by fast ramps that imitated the spontaneous depolarizations during pacemaking [83].

A noninactivating Na^+ current has been identified in TMN neurons [73,80,81,84]. This current likely flows continuously even at −70 mV and is sufficient to drive

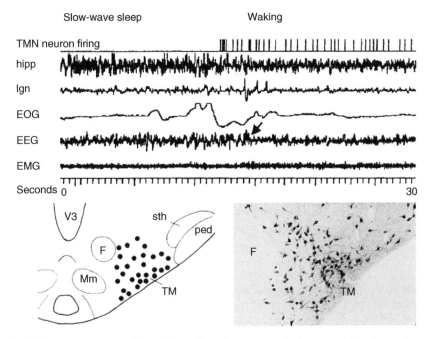

FIGURE 3.4 Tuberomamillary histaminergic neurons during transition from sleep to waking. Polygraphic recording from freely behaving cat, waking up at arrow in electroencephalogram (EEG). (Tuberomamillary [histaminergic] wake-on neuron single-unit firing; hipp, hippocampal EEG; lgn, lateral geniculate nucleus EEG; EOG, electrooculogram; EEG, neocortical EEG; V3, third ventricle; sth, subthalamic nucleus; ped, pedunculum; F, fornix; and Mm, corpus mamillare) (Modified from Lin, J.-S., *Sleep Med. Rev.*, 4(5), 471–503, 2000).

spontaneous firing. Taddese and Bean [85] were able to assess the role of this sodium current in pacemaking by using the cells' own pacemaking cycle as a voltage command. They suggested that the persistent sodium current originates from subthreshold gating of the same sodium channels that underlie the phasic sodium current. None of these intrinsic currents has been found to respond to transmitters or other endogenous neuroactive substances.

Ca^{2+}-dependent depolarizing potentials contribute to the repetitive firing of TMN neurons. These prepotentials are evident when Na^+-dependent action potentials fail and persist under tetrodotoxin (TTX). Ba^{2+} converts them into full-blown action potentials. Reduction by Ni^{2+} indicates a low threshold type of Ca^{2+} current. The histamine release from dendrites and the autoreceptor-mediated negative feedback are likely to be achieved through these Ca^{2+} currents [80] (Figures 3.5 and 3.6). Five types of such Ca^{2+} currents have been characterized pharmacologically in TMN neurons, including N- and P-type currents, which were sensitive to histamine H3R activation [86]. At the onset of spontaneous firing *in vitro*, a large increase of intracellular Ca^{2+} level has been measured [87].

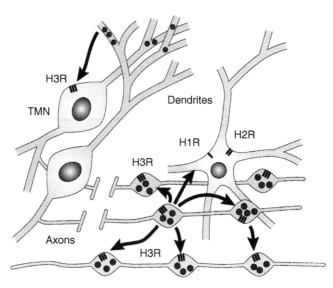

FIGURE 3.5 Histaminergic neurons and targets. H3R on TMN somata and varicosities from both TMN neurons (autoreceptor) and other neurons (heteroreceptor). (Modified from Haas, H.L., Panula, P., *Nat. Rev. Neurosci.*, 4, 121–130, 2003. Copyright Macmillan Magazines Ltd.)

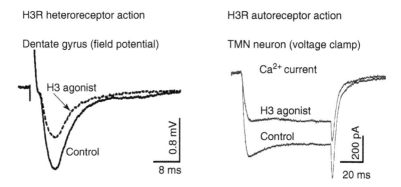

FIGURE 3.6 Histamine H3R actions on heteroreceptor and autoreceptor in hippocampus and hypothalamus. Glutamatergic field potential in dentate gyrus and Ca^{2+} current in histaminergic neuron are reduced. (Modified from Haas, H.L., Panula, P., *Nat. Rev. Neurosci.*, 4, 121–130, 2003. Copyright Macmillan Magazines Ltd.)

Histamine Neurons: Inputs

The histaminergic neurons receive innervation from the preoptic area of the hypothlamus, the septum, the prefrontal cortex, the subiculum, and the dorsal tegmentum [88,89]—regions that are targets of TMN projections. Stimulation of the preoptic area and the anterolateral hypothalamus can evoke synaptic potentials in TMN neurons, suggesting afferents releasing GABA and glutamate [90]. Aminergic and petidergic fibers innervate the TMN neurons and form functional inputs [91–97].

Glutamate released from afferent fibers excites TMN neurons, which carry both alpha-amino-3-hydroxy-5-methyl-4-isoxazolepropionic acid (AMPA) and N-methyl-$_D$-aspartate (NMDA) receptors [90]. Electrical stimulation of lateral preoptic and hypothalamic areas can evoke glutamatergic excitatory potentials in TMN neurons [90]. Spontaneous excitatory postsynaptic potentials or miniature excitatory postsynaptic currents (mEPSCs) have not been observed in TMN neurons. AMPA receptors are composed of four subtypes, GluR1–4. GluR2 mRNA is most frequently found, followed by GluR1 and GluR4, with the flip splice variant prevailing over flop and GluR3 missing. The presence of GluR2 is responsible for Ca^{2+} impermeability of TMN AMPA receptors. Expression of GluR4 flop correlates with the fastest desensitization of glutamate-evoked responses and is coordinated with the expression of a K^+-dependent Na^+/Ca^{2+}-exchanger (NCKX2, single-cell reverse transcriptase polymerase chain reaction [RT-PCR] data), thus providing faster integration and more precise timing of synaptic signals in neurons with this AMPAR subtype [98]. Three of four AMPA receptor subunit pre-mRNAs undergo editing by adenosine deaminases acting on RNA (ADAR1-3). In TMN neurons, editing determines desensitization properties [99].

The presence of glycinergic fibers in the posterior hypothalamus is uncertain, but glycine inhibits a subpopulation of histaminergic neurons, which exhibit different sensitivities to glycine according to neuron size [100]. In smaller (>20 μm) HDC mRNA-positive neurons, glycine responses are small or absent. The osmolyte taurine, which can reach relevant concentrations in the extracellular space, gates strychnine-sensitive glycine receptors and $GABA_A$ receptors ($GABA_A$Rs). Taurine efficacy at $GABA_A$R is independent of $GABA_A$R composition and taurine will thus, in contrast to GABA, equally inhibit (and protect from overexcitation) a large range of neurons.

GABAergic innervation deriving from mostly hypothalamic sources is essential for the sleep–waking regulation, especially the input from the ventralateral preoptic hypothalamus (VLPO) area that fires high during sleep [89,101–103]. TMN $GABA_A$Rs are heterogeneous; three groups with different GABA sensitivities show differential expression of the γ-subunit of the ionotropic GABA receptor [59]. The sedative component of general anesthetics (e.g., propofol) [104] is attributed to actions on GABAergic afferents to the TM nucleus, with one key to this action being the low expression of the $GABA_A$R ε-subunit [105]. Histamine neuron firing correlates with consciousness: in narcoleptic patients, when a sudden onset of REM-sleep paralysis occurs out of the waking state (cataplexy), histaminergic neurons remain active, creating a conscious dream state, such as hallucinations, that is experienced. The GABAergic inputs to the TMN are under feedback control of $GABA_B$Rs: no postsynaptic $GABA_B$R-mediated effects but $GABA_A$R-mediated synaptic potentials are strongly suppressed by baclofen, a $GABA_B$R agonist [106].

Acetylcholine excites TMN neurons through nicotinic α7-type acetylcholine receptors [107,108]. These bungarotoxin-sensitive receptors represent a sensor for the central waking actions of nicotine. Choline has been put forward as the natural ligand in TMN [87,109]. Modulation of histamine-release through muscarinic M1 or M3 heteroreceptors *in vivo* [33] occurs presumably on histaminergic axons.

Catecholaminergic adrenergic and dopaminergic inputs reach the TMN from the noradrenergic cell groups including the locus coeruleus, and dopamine neurons in the midbrain and hypothalamus. Noradrenaline does not affect histaminergic neurons directly but effectively controls GABAergic input through α2-adrenoreceptors mediating an inhibition of inhibitory postsynaptic currents (IPSCs): evoked GABAergic excitatory postsynaptic potentials (EPSPs) are reduced by noradrenaline and clonidine but not isoproterenol, whereas exogenously applied GABA responses remain unaffected [93]. Dopamine excites histamine neurons through D2 receptor activation [110].

Histaminergic neurons of the rat are excited by serotonin through activation of Na^+–Ca^{2+} exchange (NCX) [94,96,111]. This electrogenic transporter exchanges three Na^+ ions for one Ca^{2+} ion, resulting in a depolarization and excitation in the absence of conductance change. Serotonin 2C receptors undergo posttranscriptional gene modifications, and the editing status can predict psychiatric disease [112]. Unedited and edited points on mRNA species generate 14 different isoforms of the $5\text{-}HT_{2C}R$. None of the five editing sites (A–E) depends on the known ADAR enzymes in TMN neurons, which are always edited at A and variably edited at B–D sites; formation of the fully edited $5\text{-}HT_{2C}Rs$, which are less responsive to agonists, is prevented; editing of C and D sites is negatively correlated [99].

Ionotropic and metabotropic purine receptors mediate excitation of histaminergic neurons. Synaptic release of nucleotides or nucleosides onto histamine neurons has not been shown but may be relevant for homoeostatic sleep regulation. ATP-induced inward currents in neurons from the tuberomamillary region were first reported by Furukawa et al. [113]. ATP evokes fast non-desensitizing inward currents in TMN neurons. Single-cell RT-PCR and pharmacological analysis revealed $P2X_2$ receptors as the major receptor type that occurs in all TMN neurons [114]; five further types are expressed rarely. Zinc modulates $P2X_2$ receptors [115]. ATP, ADP, UTP, and 2meSATP excite TMN neurons through metabotropic receptors; P2Y1 and P2Y4 are prevailing [116], which undergo a developmental downregulation. Immunohistochemistry demonstrated neuronal and glial localizations of P2Y1 receptors [116].

ATP is extra- and intracellularly broken down into adenosine; adenosine that inhibits many neurons and synaptic transmissions has no effect on TMN firing or TMN inputs. The TMN displays a very strong expression of adenosine deaminase, which has led to the suggestion that it may also use adenosine as a transmitter. So far such a role of adenosine is elusive, there is no evidence for synaptic release of this nucleoside, but it is sedative through adenosine A1 receptors. Histaminergic neurons are insensitive to adenosine [116]. A2A receptors have also been implicated in sleep regulation through the enhancement of the GABAergic inhibition of histamine neurons [117,118]. Adenosine A1 and A2 selective agonists in the lateral preoptic area induced waking and sleep, respectively, by inhibiting the GABAergic neurons that project to the TMN through A1 receptors and exciting them through A2A receptors. Extracellular adenosine accumulation also causes sleep [119,120]. Adenosine accumulates during wakefulness and is considered an endogenous sleep pressure substance [121–123]; it prevents overexcitation and neurotoxicity and acts as an endogenous antiepileptic [124].

Galanin is coexpressed in histaminergic neurons of rodents [70,101,125,126] not in the human TMN [127] and in the GABAergic inputs to them [102]. Galanin inhibits TMN neuron firing [128] and has been shown to act on TMN axon autoreceptors [34].

It may thus contribute to both intrinsic feedback inhibition and extrinsic inhibition from the VLPO. Moreover, galanin exerts orexigenic, antiepileptic, sleep-propensing, and neurotrophic actions.

Orexin/hypocretin-containing neurons are located in the lateral hypothalamus and perifornical area, close to the histamine neurons, with which they intermingle partially and form a functional entity. Degeneration of hypocretin neurons is the cause of most cases of narcolepsy, with excessive daytime sleepiness and cataplexy [129,130]. Hypocretin neurons maintain wakefulness, particularly in the context of metabolic challenges, and function like a flip-flop switch that prevents frequent transitions among behavioral states [131]. Both hypocretins (1 and 2, also known as orexin A and B) excite histamine neurons through the hypocretin-2 receptor and activation of NCX [94–97]. This action is secondary to a rise in intracellular Ca^{2+} that probably comes from both extra- and intracellular sources. Hypocretin neurons also express dynorphin that contributes to the excitation of histaminergic neurons by suppressing inhibitory GABAergic inputs [92]. TMN neurons *in vivo* remain active during cataplexy in narcoleptic hypocretin-2 receptor-deficient dogs [76], and both the effects of hypocretin on vigilance [132] and food intake [133] require H1 receptor (H1R) activation. In contrast to various other knockout (KO) mice, H1R-KO have lower hypocretin levels [134].

Despite morphological and functional evidence for an interaction of histamine neurons with corticotrophin-releasing hormone (CRH) and TRH with respect to glucagon like peptide-1 and leptin effects on food intake [135,136], direct actions of these food-related peptides on TMN neurons are largely unknown. Leptin, the hormone from fat that controls food intake and body weight, has no obvious effect on TMN neurons, but the latter are secondary targets and mediators of leptin actions in the brain [137]. Neuropeptide Y (NPY)-containing fibers are found close to histaminergic neurons [138], and NPY indirectly affects histamine release [139]. The appetite stimulating stomach-derived ghrelin inhibits a potassium channel (Kir3) in cultured TMN neurons [140]. TRH reduces food intake [136] and sleeping time in rats and counteracts excessive sleepiness in canine narcolepsy [141]. The majority of the TMN neurons are excited by TRH [142], likely conveyed also through inputs from the dorsomedial hypothalamus (DMH) [143].

Nociceptin (orphanin FQ) is expressed in the arcuate nucleus and occurs in many fibers near histaminergic somata in the TMN region. It hyperpolarizes TMN neurons by activating an inwardly rectifying K^+ conductance. Morphine excites TMN neurons through disinhibition, by inhibiting GABAergic neurons [97]. The κ-agonist dynorphin has no direct postsynaptic effect but gates GABAergic inputs to the TMN [92]. Substance P-immunoreactive (SP-IR) terminals make synaptic contacts with the somata, somatic spines, and dendrites of histaminergic neurons [144].

A number of additional paracrine, nutritional, metabolic, and hormone like signals impinge on histaminergic neurons. TMN neurons of the E4 and E5 subgroup in the tuberomamillary region are activated by insulin-induced hypoglycemia [57]. Estrogen receptor expression in the human TMN varies in relation to metabolic activity, sex, aging, and Alzheimer's disease [145]. Prostaglandin E2 activates the TMN through the EP4 receptor to induce wakefulness in rats [146]. Endocannabinoids increase histamine release selectively in the TMN through CB1R [58]. The involvement of histamine H1Rs in hypoxic ventilatory responses during light and dark periods suggest that the tuberomamillary histaminergic neurons are involved in CO_2-mediated arousal [147,148], synergistically or convergent with hypocretin neurons [149].

HISTAMINERGIC PATHWAYS

Antibodies against histamine stain the histaminergic fibers better than antibodies against HDC, although both HDC and histamine are present in TMN somata and axon varicosities. Similar projection patterns of histaminergic neurons are found in several species, but there are significant quantitative differences with regard to the innervation density of the target regions. Axons with multifold arborization reach the entire central nervous system through two ascending and one descending bundle [13,14,23,62,150] (Figures 3.3 and 3.5). One ascending pathway travels at the ventral surface of the median eminence to the hypothalamus, the diagonal band, the septum and the olfactory bulb, hippocampus, and cortex, and the other leaves the TMN dorsally and runs along the third ventricle to thalamus, basal ganglia, hippocampus, amygdala, and cortex. The descending path goes with the medial longitudinal fasciculus to the brain stem and spinal cord. There seems to be no topological correlation between the location of TMN somata and their projections. Tracing studies have shown that many histaminergic fibers cross in the suprachiasmatic and supramamillary decussations, and many neurons branch into more than one pathway [54,151,152].

The hypothalamus houses the highest density of histaminergic fibers, with some bundles passing through and most parts of this structure receiving a dense innervation. The anterior periventricular, retrochiasmatic, supraoptic decussation, and latero-basal regions display the highest histamine immunoreactivity; dense networks of histaminergic fibers are found in the medial preoptic, periventricular, supraoptic, and suprachiasmatic nuclei. A medium density is found in the paraventricular, dorsomedial, ventromedial, and arcuate nuclei. In the posterior hypothalamus, histaminergic fibers often make close contact to the brain surface.

The nuclei of the diagonal band and the septum receive a strong histaminergic innervation. A dense fiber network passes through and innervates the supramamillary nucleus that contains glutamatergic neurons projecting to cortical areas. The ventral tegmentum and the dopaminergic nuclei (substantia nigra and ventral tegmental area [VTA]) receive significant histaminergic input. This is true also for the tectum with a particularly interesting basket like innervation pattern of the mesencephalic trigeminal nucleus. Some neurons in the pontine central grey also display immunoreactive terminal-like structures [151], and the mesencephalic reticular areas giving rise to the ascending reticular activating system and the aminergic nuclei (the noradrenergic locus coeruleus and the serotonergic raphe nuclei) are moderately innervated. Histaminergic fibers descend further to the spinal cord [153].

The area surrounding the glomeruli in the olfactory bulb and the olfactory nuclei receive a moderate innervation. The fiber density in the striatum varies; moderate densities are observed in anterior parts of the dorsal striatum and in the nucleus accumbens. The periventricular and the posterolateral thalamic nuclei receive a moderate innervation too: paraventricular nucleus, medial habenula, and medial geniculate nucleus. Lower densities are seen in further thalamic nuclei, including lateral habenula and lateral geniculate nucleus (LGN). Most neocortical and allocortical areas contain moderately dense or sparse histaminergic fibers. Histaminergic fibers enter the hippocampus through both an anterior and a posterior pathway and reach a moderate density in the basal parts of cornu ammonis, subiculum, and dentate gyrus. The amygdala also receive histaminergic inputs of moderate fiber densities.

HISTAMINE RECEPTORS

Ionotropic Receptors

Histamine activates chloride conductances in the thalamus [154] and hypothalamus [155]. This effect is blocked in the supraoptic nucleus by picrotoxin and H2R antagonists, whereas in thalamic interneurons, it is also mediated by an H2-like receptor but not picrotoxin sensitive. Histaminergic ionotropic receptors seem to play a minor role in the vertebrate brain in contrast to molluscs and arthropods where they are a major target for histamine in the retina [156].

Polyamine-Binding Site of NMDA Receptors

Histamine directly facilitates NMDA receptors and enhances excitatory transmission [157,158] (Figure 3.7). This action is occluded by spermidine [158] and pH sensitive [159,160], indicating an action antagonistic to the known NMDA receptor depression by protons. In a slightly acidified environment (pH 7.0), but not at pH 7.4, the histamine enhances the late NMDA-component of extra- and intracellularly registered excitatory postsynaptic potentials (EPSPs) in hippocampal slices. Such pH shifts occur physiologically during metabolic challenges accompanying intense neuronal firing and burst discharges, or under pathological conditions during hypoxia, hypoglycemia, ischemia, or epilepsy. The histamine-dependent potentiation of NMDA currents is selective for the NR1/NR2B variety of the NMDA receptor [161], which plays a decisive role in long-term potentiation (LTP) induction. It is not mediated by known histamine receptors but mimicked by the histamine metabolite 1-methylhistamine. The direct action of the diamine histamine on the polyamine site of the NMDA receptor is in keeping with the cross-reaction of histamine–spermidine in the early attempts of histamine fluorescence histology [10]. A second-messenger-mediated modulation of ionotropic receptors is known for several transmitters: facilitation of NMDA receptors through protein kinase C (PKC) and a reduction of the Mg^{2+} block have been described as a result of H1R activation [162].

Metabotropic Receptors

Four metabotropic histamine receptor types (H1R–H4R) have been cloned so far. H1R–H3R are expressed in abundance in the brain, and the H4R occurs mainly in peripheral tissues [163]. All metabotropic histamine receptors (H1R–H4R) belong to the rhodopsinlike family of G-protein-coupled receptors (GPCR) [39,164,165]. Each receptor consists of seven large transmembrane-spanning elements with prototypic domains determining agonist binding specificity and activation [166,167], G-protein coupling and constitutive activity [168,169], as well as covalent modifications, homo- and heterodimerization, trafficking, and membrane anchoring implicated in receptor sensitization and desensitization [170].

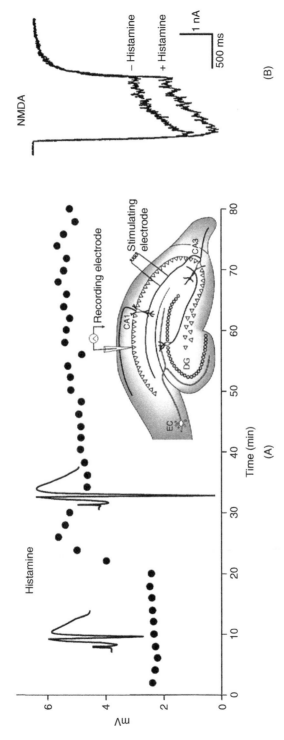

FIGURE 3.7 Histamine and synaptic plasticity. (A) Histamine evokes a LTP (without high frequency stimulation) of population spikes shown before and after histamine perfusion for 5 min. This effect is prevented by an H2R antagonist given with histamine but not after the potentiation is installed. (B) Histamine potentiates NMDA current by acting on the polyamine site. (Modified from Haas, H.L., Panula, P., *Nat. Rev. Neurosci.*, 4, 121–130, 2003. Copyright Macmillan Magazines Ltd.)

H1 Receptors

The gene encoding the human H1R is located on chromosomes 2p25, 3p14–21 [171,172]. With site-directed mutagenesis and molecular modeling [173], Leurs et al. [165] characterized important steps in the activation of the human histamine H1R involving specific residues that are conserved among rhodopsinlike GPCRs. The signaling of H1R [174] is prototypic for and convergent with that of other $G\alpha_{q/11}$-protein-coupled receptors [94,95,111,175–177]. It includes activation of phospholipase C (PLC) promoting inositoltrisphosphate-dependent (IP3R) release of Ca^{2+} from intracellular stores and diacylglycerol (DAG)-sensitive activation of PKC, which facilitates capacitive Ca^{2+} entry through voltage-dependent calcium channels (VDCC), cation channels of the transient receptor potential channel family (TRPC) [111,177], and stimulation of an NCX [94,95]. Other effector pathways of H1R include production of arachidonic acid, nitric oxide (NO), and cyclic guanosine-monophosphate (cGMP) [174] through pertussis toxin-sensitive Gi/Go-protein-mediated activation of phospholipase A2 (PLA2), $[Ca^{2+}]i$-dependent NO synthases, and NO-dependent guanylate cyclases (GC), respectively. Importantly, H1R-activate AMP-kinase, a checkpoint in the control of energy metabolism [178], and nuclear factor-kappaB (NF-κB) [179], a key transcription factor controlling readout of immunity- and plasticity-related genes.

Histamine through H1R excites neurons in most brain regions, including brainstem [75,180], hypothalamus, thalamus [181,182] (Figure 3.8), amygdala [183], septum [184,185], hippocampus [175,186], olfactory bulb [187], and cortex [188]. Ca^{2+}-dependent activation of K^+ channels by H1R decreases cell excitability and inhibits firing of hippocampal pyramidal neurons [175]. In glia cells [189], the activation of these channels relies on PLC activation and IP3-mediated release of Ca^{2+} from internal stores.

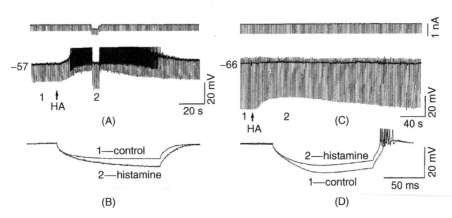

FIGURE 3.8 Histamine actions in thalamic relay neurons (slices from LGN). (A) Histamine causes an H1R-mediated depolarization. Manual clamp, 2, in (A) and (B) reveals an apparent conductance decrease (block of a leak current). (C) Small H2R-mediated depolarization associated with a substantial increase in apparent membrane conductance at hyperpolarized membrane potentials. (From McCormick, D.A., Williamson, A., *J. Neurosci.*, 11(10), 3188–3199, 1991. With permission.)

H1Rs are found throughout the whole body and nervous system with considerable variations among species. H1R density does not always match that of the less variable histaminergic innervation, and kainate-induced neuronal lesions using [3H]mepyramine binding indicate that a major portion of H1R is associated with nonneuronal elements such as glia, blood cells, and vessels. In human brain, the highest 3H-mepyramine binding is found in the cerebral cortex and the infralimbic structures [190]. With the availability of appropriate positron emission tomography (PET) tracers [191], H1R distribution and occupancy in humans have been mapped using functional imaging techniques [192]. In neuropsychiatric disorders, such as Alzheimer's disease, schizophrenia, depression, as well as in aging people, a lowered H1R binding was found [193].

Loss of H1R function in KO mice produces immunological [194], metabolic [195], and behavioral state abnormalities [196] similar to those observed in HDC-KO animals [60]. Most of the H1R antihistamines stabilize the receptor in its inactive state (inverse agonism) [166,167,172] and are well known for their sedative properties [75,188,196,197]. Many antidepressants or antipsychotics also bind to H1R, and this has been attributed to adverse side effects on body weight [178,198].

H2 Receptors

The gene encoding the human H2R, which is a 40-kD 359 amino acid peptide, is located on chromosome 5q35.5 and exhibits strong sequence homology (83–95% identity) with that in guinea pig, mouse, rat, and dog [199,200]. H2Rs exhibit constitutive activity [169] and inverse agonism of H2R antagonists accounts for upregulation of spontaneously active H2R, which may underlie the development of tolerance after prolonged clinical use [201]. The absence of histamine downregulates the expression of H2R but not that of H1Rs [202]. The C-terminus of the H2R plays a role in agonist-induced internalization [170], and fluorescent histamine receptor ligands may allow a close examination of these phenomena.

H2Rs are widely distributed in the rodent brain in approximate agreement with histaminergic innervation, indicating that H2R mediate a larger number of postsynaptic actions of histamine [203,204]. Colocalizations of H1R and H2R in some areas are in keeping with synergistic interactions between these receptor subtypes [175,205,206]. Dense labeling of H2R is found in the limbic areas including basal ganglia, amygdala, hippocampus, and cortex.

H2Rs signal through Gsα-proteins to increase intracellular cAMP [176,206,207], which activates protein kinase A (PKA) and the transcription factor CREB, all of which play key roles in neuronal physiology, plasticity, and survival. Independent from either cAMP or Ca^{2+} levels, H2Rs also mediate inhibition of PLA2 and thus release arachidonic acid, which likely account for the opposing physiological responses elicited by H1R and H2R in many tissues [207]. Cyclic AMP can directly interact with hyperpolarization-activated cation current (Ih, HCN2) shifting its activation curve to more positive levels and promoting depolarization in thalamic [181] (Figure 3.8) and hippocampal neurons [208]. Histamine through H2R and cAMP/PKA signaling, convergent with other aminergic and peptidergic signals, blocks a Ca^{2+}-activated potassium conductance (small K) responsible for the accommodation of firing and a long-lasting (seconds) afterhyperpolarization following action potentials [209,210] (Figure 3.9). Moreover, H2R- and PKA-dependent phosphorylation of

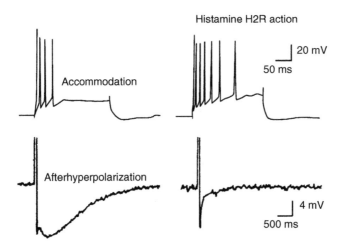

FIGURE 3.9 Histamine actions through H2R and cyclic AMP in hippocampus. Block of the accommodation of firing (human CA1 pyramidal cell) and the long-lasting afterhyperpolarization (dentate granule cell). A Ca^{2+}-dependent K^+ current (small K) is responsible for these phenomena. (Modified from Haas, H.L., Panula, P., *Nat. Rev. Neurosci.*, 4, 121–130, 2003. Copyright Macmillan Magazines Ltd.)

Kv3.2-containing potassium channels modulates hippocampal interneuron fast spiking [211]. Collectively, H2R activation sets neurons in a state of readiness to respond [209,210] and produces long-term increases in neuronal excitability [175] that may be operational during memory consolidation (Figures 3.7, 3.9, and 3.10).

Mice deficient in H2R function exhibit selective cognitive deficits along with an impairment in hippocampal LTP [212], an abnormal nociception [213], and an enhanced susceptibility to experimental allergic encephalomyelitis [214]. H2R antagonists are widely prescribed for stomach ulcers and seem to have antitumor activity [215]. Some antidepressants also have H2R antagonistic properties [216] and a few reports suggested efficacy of H2R antagonists in schizophrenia [217].

H3 Receptors
The H3R was discovered in 1983 by J.-C. Schwartz and coworkers in Paris [15]. Lovenberg et al. [218] reported its cloning in 1999. The expression of H3R is largely confined to the nervous system and is characterized by a high degree of molecular and functional heterogeneity achieved through differential transcriptional and posttranscriptional processing (splice-variants) [165]. Unique properties including constitutive activity *in vivo* [219,220] and recruitment of plasticity-related signal transduction pathways, including mitogen activated protein kinase (MAPK) and Akt/GSK3 signaling [221], currently, make the H3R the most prominent target for histaminergic drug development [165]. As an autoreceptor on somata, dendrites, and axons of TMN neurons, H3R activation inhibits cell firing [81], histamine synthesis [222], and release from varicosities [223]. As presynaptic heteroreceptors, H3Rs abundantly control outflow of various other transmitters, including biogenic amines [224], acetylcholine [225,226], glutamate [227,228], GABA [229], and peptidergic

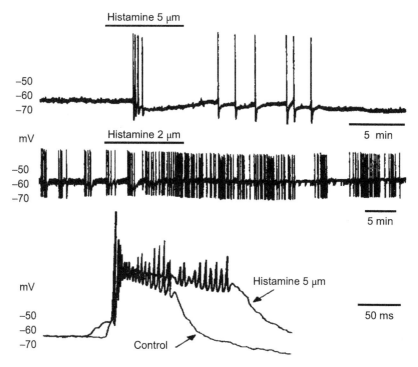

FIGURE 3.10   Effect of histamine in the hippocampal CA3 region. Histamine induces (upper trace) or increases (middle trace) burst activity. Burst frequency (middle trace) and duration (lower trace) are enhanced. Each horizontal stroke in the upper two traces corresponds to a burst as shown below. Such burst activity is conducted to the CA1 area where it can act as a perfect trigger for synaptic plasticity.

systems [230]. Loss of H3R function in KO mice is associated with behavioral state abnormalities, reduced locomotion, and a metabolic syndrome with hyperphagia, late-onset obesity, hyperinsulinemia, and leptinemia [231]. In keeping with data from genetic linkage studies, H3R-KO also exhibit increased severity and progression of neuroinflammatory diseases [232].

H4 Receptors
The recently cloned H4R exhibits molecular homology and pharmacology similar to H3Rs [233] but is expressed mainly in peripheral cells and tissues such as blood, spleen, lung, liver, and gut; it may be present in some parts of the brain, as well. 4-Methylhistamine is a selective agonist at the H4R.

HISTAMINERGIC ACTIONS

Spinal Cord and Brainstem

Histaminergic fibers in the spinal cord coming from the TMN are extensive in higher mammalian species [153]. Microionophoretic experiments revealed mostly inhibitory actions of histamine in the spinal cord and brain stem of the cat [234,235]. A recent study combining whole-cell recording in spinal (preganglionic) sympathetic neurons with single-cell RT-PCR revealed mRNA expression for H1R and an H1R-mediated depolarization through block of a K^+ conductance [236]. Histamine excites most of the neurons in the area postrema [237], a chemoreceptive circumventricular organ in the medulla oblongata implicated with nausea, emesis, and motion sickness.

Cholinergic nuclei in the brainstem, the basal forebrain, and the septum receive a strong histaminergic innervation [151]. Histamine in the cholinergic lateral dorsal tegmentum leads to increased vigilance and electroencephalogram (EEG) desynchronization [75]. Cholinergic neurons in the pons and basal forebrain are depolarized [238]. Histamine increases ACh release in the cortex [239] and the ventral striatum [240], whereas H3 heteroreceptor activation has opposite (depressant) effects on acetylcholine release [226,227]. Cholinergic neurons in the medial septum project to the hippocampus where they evoke θ-activity. They are excited by histamine (H1R) [184,185]. The cholinergic afferents involved in cortical activation and wakefulness are controlled by the histaminergic system [181,241]. The excitatory action of histamine on the cholinergic neurons is not counterbalanced by an excitatory cholinergic effect of comparable power and duration on histamine neurons: they respond only very briefly to fast desensitizing nicotinic receptor activation [108].

Noradrenergic neurons of the locus coeruleus are excited through H1R and H2R activation. Single-cell RT-PCR revealed the same percentages for the expression of these receptors [180]. Noradrenaline release from axon varicosities is reduced in brain slices [224]. As histaminergic neurons are disinhibited through a presynaptic action of noradrenaline (α2-receptors) [93], the two systems mutually excite one another at the somatic level.

Serotonergic neurons of the dorsal raphe are directly excited by histamine convergent with other arousal systems [177]. H1R activation causes an inward current through the opening of a mixed cation channel [177] of the TRPC family [111]. The firing of serotonergic dorsal raphe neurons can be depressed by microionophoretic histamine through H2R activation [242]. H3Rs constraint serotonin release [243].

Dopamine release in the striatum is under the control of H3R [244], suggesting the presence of H3R in dopaminergic axons. The substantia nigra pars reticulata receives moderate to dense histaminergic innervation [151] but GABAergic inhibition directly from the striatum. H3R activation reduces GABA and serotonin release [243] in this pathway. The GABAergic neurons are excited through H1Rs in both the substantia nigra and the ventral tegmentum of the rat, whereas the dopaminergic neurons in these structures are not directly affected [245] but indirectly inhibited by histamine. In a study on mouse slices, both H1R and H2R were found to be involved in the histaminergic excitation of the inhibitory projection neurons; H3R activation inhibited these neurons [182].

Neurons in trigeminal nuclei express H1R and H3R [246] and exhibit reciprocal excitatory relationships with histaminergic TMN neurons. Mastication and feeding are potent activators of the brain histamine system [247]. Oral sensations, in turn, conveyed through sensory and gustatory afferents of the trigeminal and facial nerve, respectively, provide glutamatergic excitatory input to the brain promoting cortical activation and arousal. Histamine actions on the trigemino-vascular system [248–250] control blood–brain barrier permeability [232] and aseptic neurogenic inflammations underlying vascular headaches [251].

Microionophoretic experiments revealed H1R-mediated excitation and H2R-mediated inhibition of firing in the vestibular nuclei [252]. Depolarization by histamine through H2R activation was seen in the medial vestibular nucleus. In the rat, a similar excitation was found in slices of the medial vestibular nucleus, displaying both H1R and H2R components [253]. Stimulation of the vestibular nerve causes histamine release in the brain stem and the hypothalamus [254]. Histamine receptors are found in the cochlea [255], and histamine can affect microcirculation and microphonic compound action potentials. Interestingly, the vestibular hair cells are also sensitive to histamine [255], causing influx and intracellular release of Ca^{2+}, which is needed for glutamate exocytosis. Purkinje cells, granule cells, and nucleus interpositus neurons exhibit H1R- and H2R-mediated excitatory responses to histamine bath perfusion in slices from rats [256].

Hypothalamus

Early work using histamine injections in the hypothalamus has revealed actions on feeding, drinking, and body temperature [257]. The central warm receptor is located in the medial preoptic area, whereas the detection of *cold* relies on peripheral receptors. Preoptic neurons, including warm-sensitive neurons, are mostly excited through H1R activation [258].

Histaminergic neurons innervating the suprachiasmatic nucleus (SCN) shift the circadian clock similar to light [259]. Histaminergic excitation of SCN neurons is mediated by H1R, inhibition by H2R [260], which are highly expressed in the SCN [261]. Histamine released from histaminergic fibers in the SCN seems to be taken up into SCN neurons and rereleased to participate in the histamine-mediated effects on the circadian system in concert with direct histaminergic inputs [262].

Endogenous histamine induces c-fos expression in both the supraoptic and the paraventricular nuclei [263,264] and histamine injections in the supraoptic region evoke antidiuresis [265,266]. Supraoptic neurons containing the antidiuretic hormone are depolarized by histamine, which prolongs depolarizing afterpotentials that promote the phasic bursts [267–269] underlying pulsatile antidiuretic hormone (ADH) release from axonal endings in the neurohypophysis [270,271]. The excitation was demonstrated not only by local application but also by stimulation of the TMN, through synaptic contact with supraoptic nucleus (SON) neurons [272]. The H1R-mediated excitation of SON has been attributed to several mechanisms: block of a K^+ conductance, intracellular IP3-mediated Ca^{2+} release, activation of a Ca^{2+}-dependent cationic current, and an NCX [269,270]. Single TMN stimuli elicit EPSPs in vasopressinergic SON neurons, whereas prolonged stimulation blocks non-NMDAR-dependent excitatory synaptic currents and results in a marked H1R-dependent increase of interneuronal coupling mediated through NO and cGMP-signaling cascades [273]. Supraoptic oxytocin neurons respond to TM stimulation with fast chloride-dependent IPSPs mediated by an ionotropic receptor that is sensitive to H2-antagonists. Furthermore, gap junctions between these neuroendocrine cells play an important role in synchronizing their action. Histamine as well as TMN stimulation reduced, through H2R activation, the coupling between them [155,274].

Suckling increases histamine and oxytocin concentrations in the paraventricular nucleus (PVN). H1R or H2R blockade prevents the increase in oxytocin release.

Histaminergic activation is necessary for oxytocin release in the PVN and systemically during parturition and lactation [272,275]. Oxytocin neurons are inhibited through H2R possibly suppressing untimely release of oxytocin, and this effect is overcome by the H1R-mediated excitation during parturition [276].

Neurons in the ventromedial hypothalamus (VMH) contain the liberating or inhibiting hormones for hormone release from the hypophysis, the peptides growth hormone-releasing hormone (GHRH), prolactin-releasing hormone (PRH), TRH, CRH, gonadotrophin-releasing hormone (GnRH), and dopamine (prolactin-inhibiting hormone, PIH). The histaminergic neurons densely innervate these regions and participate in the regulation of pituitary hormone secretion through both H1 and H2R [277]. The histamine-induced secretion of ACTH, beta-endorphin, and prolactin seems to be mediated through activation of hypothalamic ADH, oxytocin, and CRH neurons. Stress-induced corticosterone release is modulated by histamine [277,278]. Release of the anabolic hormones, growth harmone (GH) and thyroid-stimulating harmone (TSH), is inhibited through exogenous (icv) and endogenous histamine, presumably through an action on TRH- and GHRH-containing neurons at the hypothalamic level [279]. Early ionophoretic studies reported H1R-mediated excitation and H2R-mediated depression of firing [280,281]. An H1R-mediated excitation was found in arcuate nucleus neurons [282]. The perifornical area and lateral hypothalamus contains the orexin/hypocretin neurons that activate and orchestrate the aminergic wake-promoting nuclei. Although there is a strong mutual innervation between this nucleus and the TMN, an electrophysiological action has only been seen in one direction so far: hypocretins excite histaminergic neurons [95], but histamine seems to be ineffective on hypocretin neurons *in vitro* [283].

Thalamus

The relay neurons in the LGN are gatekeepers of cortical activation. When firing in a bursting mode at membrane potentials below −60 mV, no sensory information can pass to the cortex, at a slightly more depolarized level; however, they fire continuously and the gate is open [181,284]. Among other transmitters, this depolarization is promoted by histamine through combined activation of both H1Rs and H2Rs [181], which blocks a potassium current and enhances a hyperpolarization-dependent Ih (HCN2) cation current (Figure 3.8). Furthermore, GABAergic perigeniculate neurons are inhibited by histamine opening chloride channels, presumably an ionotropic action on an H2-like receptor [154].

Basal Ganglia

In the substantia nigra pars compacta and in the cortex, H3R mRNAs are present indicating H3 heteroreceptors on the major inputs to the striatum. No such signal is found in the ventral tegmental area [285]. In addition to neuronal sources, biochemical experiments have indicated histamine actions derived from type II mast cells in the neostriatum [286]. Microionophoretic experiments revealed excitatory actions of histamine on medium spiny neurons (MSN) in anesthetized rats [287]. We have not seen histamine effects on membrane potentials or conductances in intracellular recordings from MSN in slices but found a significant H3R-mediated reduction of glutamatergic transmission and synaptic plasticity evoked by cortical stimulation [227]. This action is severely compromised in an animal model of hepatic encephalopathy along with abnormalities in behavioral measures of basal ganglia output function, indicating significance for disease [288]. The dopaminergic nigrostriatal input that controls glutamatergic excitation (and drive of MSN) is regulated by histamine H3 heteroreceptors [244].

The spontaneously active giant interneurons from the striatum are excited through H1R (and H2R) blocking a potassium conductance [289,290] in accordance with histaminergic modulation of acetylcholine release in the striatum [291]. Local injection of histamine directly in the nucleus accumbens causes a transient H3R-mediated suppression of locomotion followed by an H1R-mediated hyperactivity. This histamine-induced hyperactivity can be increased by chronic intra-accumbens administration of a TRH analog [292] and suggests cooperation between histamine and TRH signaling in arousal and behavioral activity control.

Anatomical and functional data indicate a role for histamine in consolidation of amygdala-dependent fear memory [293–296] and epileptic kindling [297,298]. Intracellular and field potential recordings in rat brain slices [299] revealed bidirectional effects of histamine on excitatory synaptic transmission in the basolateral amygdala.

Hippocampus

The hippocampus receives two histaminergic fiber bundles through the fornix and a caudal route. The input pathway to the dentate gyrus from the entorhinal cortex is suppressed by H3R activation *in vitro* [300] (Figure 3.6) and *in vivo* [186]. Stimulation of the TM during exploratory behavior also inhibits this transmission through H3R activation [301].

The principal neurons in the hippocampus, CA1 pyramidal cells, and dentate granule cells are directly excited by postsynaptic H2R activation [209,302]. Intracellular recordings revealed a depolarization caused through a shift in the activation of the Ih current and a block of the Ca^{2+}-dependent K^+ channel responsible for a slow and long-lasting afterhyperpolarization (sAHP) and the accommodation of firing in response to depolarizing stimuli [209]. This effect is also seen in hippocampal pyramidal cells after stimulation of the histaminergic neurons in organotypic cocultures of posterior hypothalamus and hippocampus [25]. Thus, even in the absence of depolarization, the response to a given excitatory stimulus in a neuron residing in quiet readiness can be much potentiated by histamine. Other amines that are positively coupled to adenylyl cyclase produce similar actions—serotonin through 5-HT2, noradrenaline through β-receptors, and dopamine through D1 receptors. Dopamine at low concentration has the opposite effect; it enhances the afterhyperpolarization and the accommodation of firing [209], probably through D2R and negative coupling to adenylyl cyclase. Other neuroactive substances using this signaling pathway like the endogenous antiepileptic and sleep pressure factor adenosine [124] (A1R) and GABA (B-receptor) exert such an action, as well [303].

The histamine effects on PKA signaling, ion channel function, and neuronal excitability have been analyzed in synaptic isolation (low Ca^{2+}, high Mg^{2+}) [175]. Histamine has bidirectional effects on pyramidal cell firing in the CA1 region, an initial and short-lasting depression (H1R) followed by a long-lasting (>2 h) excitation (H2R). This excitation was less effective than a coincident activation of both H1R and H2R [164,175,189]. In addition, histamine causes a long-lasting enhancement of synaptically evoked population spikes in the CA1 and CA3 regions through H2R activation [304] (Figure 3.7). A postsynaptic effect of H2R in CA3 enhances the response to glutamate released at the mossy fiber synapse [305]. CA3 pyramidal cells synchronize themselves and discharge in bursts (Figure 3.10), which can be recorded as sharp waves in the EEG. This is an important effect in light of the decisive role of CA3 synchronization in synaptic plasticity and memory trace formation [306].

Deafferentation of histaminergic afferents leads to an overexcitable hippocampus (own unpublished observation), and H1R antagonists are epileptogenic [307]. Loss of direct (H1R-mediated) inhibitory actions on pyramidal cells and the reduction of excitatory drive in dentate granule cells may account for the proconvulsant effects of antihistaminics. Furthermore, histamine strongly excites inhibitory interneurons [82,305,308]. In patch-clamp recordings, another interesting action was observed: the maximum firing rate of the interneurons was curtailed by H2R-mediated phosphorylation of an identified potassium channel, Kv3.2 [211]. Icv-injected pyrilamine (H1R antagonist) increases the occurrence of sharp wave-related ripples in freely moving rats [309], whereas intraperitoneal injection of zolantidine, an H2R antagonist that reaches the brain, reduces the occurrence of these high frequency oscillations [310] implicated in memory consolidation [306].

Cortex

Ionophoretic local application of histamine demonstrated functional histaminergic projections to the cortex [268]. Depressant actions of histamine were blocked by the H2R antagonist metiamide [12,311,312]. Intracellular recordings from human cortex revealed H2R-mediated excitatory actions through block of $gK^+(Ca^{2+})$ [181,241], as described in the hippocampus of several species including man [16]. Furthermore, H1R-mediated excitation of principal cortical neurons has been identified as the target of the sedative antihistaminics [188]. A perforated patch-clamp study in olfactory bulb slices from newborn rabbits has revealed outward and inward currents in interneurons through H1R and H2R, respectively, whereas no changes were observed in the principal mitral cells [187]. Both these currents reversed at the potassium equilibrium. GABAergic interneurons in the olfactory bulb represent a cell population that is continuously replaced by adult stem cells throughout life [313].

Synaptic Plasticity

LTP and long-term depression (LTD) are persistent increases or decreases of excitatory synaptic transmission, which are considered cellular correlates of learned behaviors and memory trace formation. Many forms of synaptic plasticity involve NMDA receptors, intracellular Ca^{2+} increases and proteinkinases such as CaMKII, PKC, and PKA. NMDA receptors become coincidence detectors through a voltage-dependent block by Mg^{2+} ions. This block is reduced through H1Rs, and PKC facilitates NMDA receptor activation [162]. Two further mechanisms promote synaptic plasticity through H1R signaling: the release of Ca^{2+} from the endoplasmatic reticulum by IP3 and the synergism with H2R-coupled cAMP/PKA signaling [164,175]. The latter can by itself evoke and promote LTP and LTP-like phenomena independent of NMDAR [175,304,314]. NMDA-receptor-mediated currents can be directly potentiated through their polyamine-binding site by histamine [157,158] (see section Histamine Receptors).

The block of Ca^{2+}-dependent K^+ channels by histamine (H2R) increases the number of action potentials fired by a given stimulus and facilitates further Ca^{2+} influx (Figure 3.9). Thus, the synchronous burst discharges of selected pyramidal cell populations in the CA3-region that appear as sharp waves in field recordings are robustly potentiated by histamine [305,315] and represent a natural trigger for LTP [316,317] (Figure 3.10). The H3R-mediated reduction of glutamatergic transmission in the dentate gyrus (Figure 3.6) and in the corticostriatal pathway lasts up to several hours [186,227,300]. In rats carrying a portacaval shunt, a model for liver disease and hepatic encephalopathy, this form of synaptic plasticity is absent [288].

Collectively, the molecular and mechanistic signatures of histamine actions in the hippocampus point to a decisive role in the gating of synchronous network activity and synaptic plasticity [318]. Like memory formation, this requires coactivation of kinases, including PKC and PKA, and protein synthesis, all of which can be brought about by histamine through coincident activation of H1R, H2R, and NMDARs [175,317,319].

Glia

Glia cells express H1R and H2R, and H1R activation increases intracellular Ca^{2+} through IP3 signaling [320,321]. Astrocytes can release glutamate in response to neuronally released transmitters, including histamine through H1R activation [322]. Histamine promotes release of neurotrophins and cytokines from astrocytes in cultures [323] and ATP in hypothalamic slices [116]. Histamine effects on glia may play a role in astrocytic energy metabolism, glycogenolysis, electrolyte balance, and transmitter clearance. Studies of pial vessels and cultured endothelium reveal increased permeability of the blood–brain barrier [324]. Strategically positioned to contact, the cerebrospinal fluid histaminergic TMN neurons may sense and provide guidance cues, for example, for migration of neuronal and glial progeny. In fact, expression of HDC, H1R, and H2R in neuroepithelial tissue during development [325] and stress [326] suggests that the cerebrospinal fluid is part of a histaminergic signaling pathway in the developing and challenged brain.

HISTAMINE AND BEHAVIOR

Sleep–Waking Regulation

Some victims of the influenza epidemic of 1918 suffered from hypersomnia *encephalitis lethargica* associated with lesion in the posterior hypothalamus. Another group of victims who suffered from insomnia displayed lesions in the anterior hypothalamus/preoptic area [327]. The hypersomnia group had lost the histaminergic and the hypocretinergic neurons, whereas the insomnia group had lost the GABAergic neurons that inhibit these waking centers during sleep. Likewise, localized injections of muscimol, a long-acting $GABA_A$ agonist in the anterior hypothalamus evoke waking and hyperactivity in cats, whereas injection in the rostral and middle parts of the posterior hypothalamus (the location of the histaminergic nucleus) produce a pronounced increase in slow-wave sleep (SWS) [77,328].

Histaminergic afferents are essential for maintenance of cortical activation, independent of the brain stem reticular formation [77]. Histamine maintains wakefulness through direct projections of the TM nucleus to the thalamus and cortex, and indirectly through activation of other ascending arousal systems, mainly cholinergic [238,329] and aminergic nuclei [177,180,245] (for review, see Refs 16, 77, and 294). Cholinergic neurons in the pedunculopontine nucleus, basal forebrain, and septum project to the thalamus, hippocampus, and cortex, respectively; all receive excitatory histaminergic input [185,238]. The relay neurons in the LGN are depolarized and shifted to the regular firing mode, which allows sensory information to pass to perception and consciousness. At a more hyperpolarized state, the relay neurons produce rhythmic bursts coincident with delta waves in the EEG during sleep [181].

The role of histamine as a waking substance was recognized through the sedative effects of H1 antihistamines [7], which readily pass the blood–brain barrier [192]. H1 antihistamines cause an increase in cortical slow waves that is indistinguishable by power spectral analysis from that seen during SWS [77,328]. The H1R is generally made responsible for the waking actions of histamine as well as for that of orexins/hypocretins [95,132,134].

Histaminergic neuron activity is reduced by H3R activation and increased by block of H3R; the former causes sleep, the latter wakefulness in cats [330] and rodents [331–334]. In H1R-KO mice, the sleep–waking pattern shows subtle changes, and the waking response to H3R antagonists is abolished [195]. H2R block by zolantidine, a blood–brain barrier penetrating antagonist, does not affect the sleep–wake cycle but icv ranitidine (H2-antagonist) increases SWS in the cat [75,77,335]. The specific H3R antagonist ciproxifan induces waking in both H2R-KO and wild-type (WT) mice [334]. The maintenance of vigilance and attention is likely also supported by the long-lasting potentiating effect of H2R activation on excitability of many cortical neurons. The HDC blocker, α-FMH, markedly reduces histamine levels, decreases waking, and increases SWS with no changes in REM sleep in the cat [328] and the rodents [60].

A number of studies have shown c-fos activation of the TMN during waking [77,102,104,336–338]. Histamine release and turnover was found to be increased during the activity period (darkness) in rats [339], and the daily cycle of histamine release has also been demonstrated by microdialysis in freely moving animals [340]. In monkeys the histamine level correlates with individual waking periods [341]. Histaminergic neurons fire exclusively during wakefulness (Figures 3.2 and 3.4) in cats [77,336], dogs [76,342], and rodents [74]. They stop firing during drowsy states before sleep and resume activity only at a high level of vigilance after waking up [74]. Similar firing patterns have also been recorded in the TMN and adjacent areas of freely moving rats [343]. The exclusive firing of TMN during waking contrasts with the activity of REM-ON cholinergic neurons. During cataplexy, a cardinal symptom of narcolepsy, muscle tone is lost but not consciousness [342]. Noradrenergic and serotonergic neurons in the locus coeruleus and the dorsal raphe

[329,344,345] stop firing under this condition, whereas histamine neurons continue to discharge [76].

Body Weight and Appetite Control
(Energy Metabolism and Feeding Rhythms)

Brain histamine has a well-established role in energy metabolism and feeding rhythm control [247,346,347]. Increasing central histamine suppresses food intake. Vice versa, α-FMH or H1R antagonists increase food intake [348]. The preferential site of histamine-mediated suppression of food intake in the mammalian brain is the VMH, a prominent satiety center. A number of other neuroendocrine and peptidergic pathways converge on the central histamine system to regulate food intake and energy balance through H1R activation. This includes orexigenic actions of orexins/hypocretins [133], and anorexigenic effects of leptin [137,349], CRH, and TRH [135,136]. Mastication activates histamine neurons [247], and histaminergic mechanisms in the mesencephalic trigeminal nucleus affect food intake [350]. Turnover of neuronal histamine in the Me5 is elevated during early phases of feeding followed by that in the VMH at later stages, which is abolished by gastric distension. Mastication-induced activation of histaminergic neurons in turn suppresses food intake through H1Rs in the PVN and the VMH.

Thermoregulation

The autonomic responses that regulate heat conservation and production in mammals are controlled by the PVN and DMH and the nucleus raphe pallidus. Neurons in the medial preoptic nucleus act as a thermostat. These structures are targets of histaminergic innervation and modulation. Activation of H1Rs in the anterior hypothalamus/preoptic area lower the set point of the hypothalamic thermostat, whereas H2Rs in the posterior hypothalamus are involved in the loss of body heat [351–353]. Body temperature and brain histaminergic activity exhibit circadian [340,354] and seasonal rhythms.

Histamine levels and turnover are elevated in hibernating ground squirrels in contrast to other transmitter systems [355]. Hibernating animals display a higher density of histaminergic fibers than euthermic animals in the hippocampus and SCN [356], in which wake-up signals may increase transcription of genes required for establishing circadian rhythms. Thus, histaminergic transmission during hibernation may be required to preserve not only metabolic and behavioral state but also neural circuit plasticity and function, suggesting an evolutionary conserved role of brain histamine in linking homeostatic and higher brain functions according to biological rhythms.

Learning and Memory

Histaminergic modulation of learning and memory is evident from lesions and pharmacological interventions in the tuberomamillary region [294,357–362] and from studies in histamine- and histamine receptor-deficient mice [212,363–365]. Seemingly conflicting evidences on the role of histamine in memory may be resolved by the notion that histamine effects on learning and memory strongly depend on not only task-inherent reinforcement contingencies, particularly novelty, but also rewarding (pleasure) and aversive (punishment) contexts [294,362,364,365]. Histamine promotes arousal and vigilance, particularly in novel environments [60], and novelty-induced arousal has motivational effects that can reinforce behavior. Thus, in keeping with its role in maintaining states of arousal and vigilance, histamine seems to be particularly important for the stabilization of memory traces formed by novel (arousing) experiences, both in pleasurable and in aversive contexts [296,360,364–366]. In other words, histamine may be specifically required to learn the new but not necessarily anew [296]. Although learning the new just as arousal implicates concerted actions of various transmitters including histamine and other biogenic amines, learning anew seems to depend mainly on noradrenergic and endocannabinoid influences [296]. Likewise, although the attentive recording (acquisition) of novel experiences requires a heightened state of arousal and vigilance, the transfer of recorded traces into long-term memory (consolidation) by replay and reverberation occurs during sleep, at times when histamine neurons are silent. Thus, histamine surges during novelty acquisition, for example, in the context of feeding rhythms [346], may act as a reinforcing signal for imprinting context (e.g., nutritional-metabolic)-dependent timing information on neural circuits implicated in consolidation of synaptic plasticity [175,317,319,367] and memory traces, for example, through the replay during subsequent sleep [306,368].

HDC-KO mice lack the ability to remain awake in a novel environment, concurrent with impairments in hippocampal theta and sustained cortical arousal [60]. They also show deficient episodic object memory (discrimination based on temporal relationships) but an increased negatively reinforced water-maze performance [365]. Likewise, HDC-KO mice show improved learning and memory retention of contextual fear conditioning along with enhanced hippocampal CA1 LTP before and decreased LTP after training [363]. Injection of histamine (icv) immediately after training normalized conditioned contextual fear responses in HDC-KO mice, whereas microinjection of histamine into the ventral hippocampus, amygdala, or nucleus acccumbens of rats impaired novel object-motivated exploratory behavior through H1R [369] or H2R activation [293,370–372]. In contrast, acute histamine infusion into the CA1 region of rats immediately after training, but not later, enhances consolidation of inhibitory avoidance memory through an H2R-dependent mechanism without altering locomotor activity, exploratory behavior, anxiety state, or retrieval of the avoidance response [360]. Notably, the effect of a loss of HDC function on object recognition, water-maze, and rotorod performance seem to be sex-dependent, emphasizing the importance of gender in the interpretation of the role of histaminergic neurotransmission in brain function [373].

H3Rs expressed by many neurons modulate the release of many transmitters and exhibit a high degree of heterogeneity and constitutive activity. Their contribution to both neuronal (axonal) plasticity and memory functions is thus very likely and is a major topic for the renewed interest in brain histamine as a drug target for disorders of memory including Alzheimer's disease [165]. Thioperamide (an H3R inverse agonist) enhances memory retention when administered after acquisition [374]. In the amygdala, H3R activation enhances consolidation of fear memory [375], and H3 antagonists impair fear memory [295] but may also exert facilitatory effects [376] through protean agonism. Interestingly, decreased histamine levels and reduced H3R-dependent histamine release specifically in the amygdala contribute to increased anxiety in mice deficient in apolipoprotein E [377], a lipoprotein implicated in neurite outgrowth and neurodegenerative diseases such as Alzheimer's. Systemic administration of R-α-methylhistamine, an H3 agonist, improves spatial memory in rats [378]. The results are consistent with the concept that the brain histamine system participates in limbic mechanisms of learning and memory, especially through the H3R.

HISTAMINE PATHOPHYSIOLOGY AND DISEASE

Levels of histidine (and some other amino acids) are significantly elevated in the brains of patients with hepatic encephalopathy [379] and in animals with a portacaval anastomosis, as a result of high ammonia levels [380]. Increased load of histidine leads to a higher synthesis but not turnover of brain histamine, with paradoxical effects on behavioral state control: hepatic encephalopathy patients suffer from sleepiness and have disturbed circadian rhythms. Likewise, portocaval-shunted rats display defects in histamine-induced plasticity [288] and circadian behavioral activity rhythms prototypic for hepatic encephalopathy [381]. Histamine receptors are deregulated in many brain disorders and neuropathologies, upregulated in hepatic encephalopathy [379], but downregulated in ageing, depression, Alzheimer's disease, and schizophrenia, as shown in functional PET imaging studies [192]. Histamine turnover is increased, and H1R binding is low in the frontal cortex of schizophrenic patients, although H2R antagonists can reduce negative symptoms in schizophrenia [217]. In contrast to low levels of histamine, higher levels inactivate NMDA receptors—in keeping with cognitive deficits. Histamine receptor expression is altered also in rats with an inbred preference for ethanol [382], emphasizing histamine's contribution to brain reward and memory functions [365]. Within the hypothalamus, only TMN neurons are affected [383] with tangle formation and degeneration in Alzheimer's disease [384] and Down syndrome [385]. In keeping with histamine's role in brain plasticity and repair, histaminergic endings take over the empty places left by degenerated dopaminergic axon varicosities in Parkinson's disease [386], whereas in Huntington's, not Parkinson's disease, there is a specific loss of H2R particularly in the putamen and globus pallidus [387]. Histaminergic activity has antiepileptic properties [307], H1 antihistamines can cause seizures, and H3R antagonists are anticonvulsive. Last but not least, histamine specifically controls itch [388,389] and modulates pain processing [390–392]. Histamine also plays a key role in autoimmunity and neuroinflammation [232,393], which is relevant, for example, in multiple sclerosis or primary headaches [394,395].

Central H1Rs play a major role in behavioral state control [195], but dysfunction also impact neuroendocrine functions associated with metabolic syndromes and obesity [346], major public health issues. H1Rs also mediate the adverse effects of atypical neuroleptics on body weight [178]. Finally, the H3R is the most promising target for treatment of brain disorders as its expression is confined to cells of the nervous system and tightly associated with the regulation of brain histamine function, both in health and in disease [165].

CONCLUSION

The brain histaminergic system is our major waking center that is deeply involved in many basic functions. It keeps the central nervous system alert and ready to react; it is the doorkeeper of consciousness. H1R and H2R mediate excitation and (long-term) potentiation of excitation, whereas the H3 autoreceptors provide a feedback control of synthesis, release, and electrical activity. As heteroreceptors they also control the varicosities of most of the other transmitter systems, making them a prime target for pharmaceutical research and development.

REFERENCES

1. Dale, H.H., Laidlaw, P.P. 1910. The physiological action of imidiazolethylamine. *J. Physiol.* (41):318.
2. Popielski, L. 1920. Beta-imidazolyläthylamin als mächtiger Erreger der Magendrüsen. *Pflugers Arch.* (178):214–236.
3. Feldberg, W. 1941. Histamine and anaphylaxis. *Annu. Rev. Physiol.* 3(1):671–694.
4. Kwiatkowski, H. 1941. Observations on the relation of histamine to reactive hyperaemia. *J. Physiol.* 100(2):147–158.
5. White, T. 1959. Formation and catabolism of histamine in brain tissue in vitro. *J. Physiol.* 149:34–42.
6. Bovet, D., Staub, A. 1937. Action protectrice des éthers phenoliques au cours de l'intoxication histaminique. *C. R. Seances Soc. Biol. Fil.* (124):547.
7. Monnier, M., Fallert, M., Battacharya, I.C. 1967. The waking action of histamine. *Experientia* 23(1):21–22.
8. Schwartz, J.C., Lampart, C., Rose, C., Rehault, M.C., Bischoff, S., Pollard, H. 1970. Development of hystaminergic systems in the newborn rat brain. *J. Physiol.* 62(Suppl 3):447.
9. Garbarg, M., Barbin, G., Feger, J., Schwartz, J.C. 1974. Histaminergic pathway in rat brain evidenced by lesions of the medial forebrain bundle. *Science* 186(4166):833–835.
10. Green, J.P. 1970. Histamine. In *Handbook of Neurochemistry*, ed. A. Lajtha, Vol. 10, pp. 221–250. New York, London: Plenum.
11. Black, J.W., Duncan, W.A., Durant, C.J., Ganellin, C.R., Parsons, E.M. 1972. Definition and antagonism of histamine H 2-receptors. *Nature* 236(5347):385–390.
12. Haas, H.L., Bucher, U.M. 1975. Histamine H2-receptors on single central neurones. *Nature* 255(5510):634–635.
13. Watanabe, T., Taguchi, Y., Shiosaka, S., Tanaka, J., Kubota, H. et al. 1984. Distribution of the histaminergic neuron system in the central nervous system of rats; a fluorescent immunohistochemical analysis with histidine decarboxylase as a marker. *Brain Res.* 295(1):13–25.
14. Panula, P., Yang, H.Y., Costa, E. 1984. Histamine-containing neurons in the rat hypothalamus. *Proc. Natl Acad. Sci. U.S.A.* 81(8):2572–2576.
15. Arrang, J.M., Garbarg, M., Schwartz, J.C. 1983. Auto-inhibition of brain histamine release mediated by a novel class (H3) of histamine receptor. *Nature* 302(5911):832–837.
16. Haas, H.L., Panula, P. 2003. The role of histamine and the tuberomamillary nucleus in the nervous system. *Nat. Rev. Neurosci.* 4(2):121–130.
17. Parsons, M.E., Ganellin, C.R. 2006. Histamine and its receptors. *Br. J. Pharmacol.* 147(Suppl 1):S127–S135.
18. Fleming, J.V., Fajardo, I., langlois, M.R., Sanchez-Jimenez, F., Wang, T.C. 2004. The C-terminus of rat L-histidine decarboxylase specifically inhibits enzymic activity and disrupts pyridoxal phosphate-dependent interactions with L-histidine substrate analogues. *Biochem. J.* 381(Pt 3):769–778.

19. Reite, O.B. 1972. Comparative physiology of histamine. *Physiol. Rev.* 52(3):778–819.
20. Moya-Garcia, A.A., Medina, M.A., Sanchez-Jimenez, F. 2005. Mammalian histidine decarboxylase: from structure to function. *Bioessays* 27(1):57–63.
21. Kuramasu, A., Saito, H., Suzuki, S., Watanabe, T., Ohtsu, H. 1998. Mast cell-/basophil-specific transcriptional regulation of human L-histidine decarboxylase gene by CpG methylation in the promoter region. *J. Biol. Chem.* 273(47):31607–31614.
22. Kollonitsch, J., Perkins, L.M., Patchett, A.A., Doldouras, G.A., Marburg, S. et al. 1978. Selective inhibitors of biosynthesis of aminergic neurotransmitters. *Nature* 274(5674):906–908.
23. Wouterlood, F.G., Sauren, Y.M., Steinbusch, H.W. 1986. Histaminergic neurons in the rat brain: correlative immunocytochemistry, Golgi impregnation, and electron microscopy. *J. Comp. Neurol.* 252(2):227–244.
24. Baudry, M., Martres, M.P., Schwartz, J.C. 1973. The subcellular localization of histidine decarboxylase in various regions of rat brain. *J. Neurochem.* 21(5):1301–1309.
25. Diewald, L., Heimrich, B., Busselberg, D., Watanabe, T., Haas, H.L. 1997. Histaminergic system in co-cultures of hippocampus and posterior hypothalamus: a morphological and electrophysiological study in the rat. *Eur. J. Neurosci.* 9(11):2406–2413.
26. Merickel, A., Edwards, R.H. 1995. Transport of histamine by vesicular monoamine transporter-2. *Neuropharmacology* 34(11):1543–1547.
27. Dismukes, K., Snyder, S.H. 1974. Histamine turnover in rat brain. *Brain Res.* 78(3):467–481.
28. Pollard, H., Bischoff, S., Schwartz, J.C. 1974. Turnover of histamine in rat brain and its decrease under barbiturate anesthesia. *J. Pharmacol. Exp. Ther.* 190(1):88–99.
29. Mochizuki, T., Yamatodani, A., Okakura, K., Takemura, M., Inagaki, N., Wada, H. 1991. In vivo release of neuronal histamine in the hypothalamus of rats measured by microdialysis. *Naunyn Schmiedebergs Arch. Pharmacol.* 343(2):190–195.
30. Strecker, R.E., Nalwalk, J., Dauphin, L.J., Thakkar, M.M., Chen, Y. et al. 2002. Extracellular histamine levels in the feline preoptic/anterior hypothalamic area during natural sleep-wakefulness and prolonged wakefulness: an in vivo microdialysis study. *Neuroscience* 113(3):663–670.
31. Philippu, A., Prast, H. 2001. Importance of histamine in modulatory processes, locomotion and memory. *Behav. Brain Res.* 124(2):151–159.
32. Itoh, Y., Oishi, R., Nishibori, M., Saeki, K. 1991. Characterization of histamine release from the rat hypothalamus as measured by in vivo microdialysis. *J. Neurochem.* 56(3):769–774.
33. Prast, H., Prast, M., Philippu, A. 1994. H3 autoreceptors and muscarinic acetylcholine receptors modulate histamine release in the anterior hypothalamus of freely moving rats. *Agents Actions* 41 Spec No:C64–C65.
34. Arrang, J.M., Gulat-Marnay, C., Defontaine, N., Schwartz, J.C. 1991. Regulation of histamine release in rat hypothalamus and hippocampus by presynaptic galanin receptors. *Peptides* 12(5):1113–1117.
35. Gulat-Marnay, C., Lafitte, A., Arrang, J.M., Schwartz, J.C. 1990. Modulation of histamine release in the rat brain by kappa-opioid receptors. *J. Neurochem.* 55(1):47–53.
36. Itoh, E., Fujimiya, M., Inui, A. 1999. Thioperamide, a histamine H3 receptor antagonist, powerfully suppresses peptide YY-induced food intake in rats. *Biol. Psychiatry* 45(4):475–481.
37. Barnes, W.G., Hough, L.B. 2002. Membrane-bound histamine N-methyltransferase in mouse brain: possible role in the synaptic inactivation of neuronal histamine. *J. Neurochem.* 82(5):1262–1271.
38. Prell, G.D., Green, J.P. 1986. Histamine as a neuroregulator. *Annu. Rev. Neurosci.* 9:209–254.

39. Schwartz, J.C., Arrang, J.M., Garbarg, M., Pollard, H., Ruat, M. 1991. Histaminergic transmission in the mammalian brain. *Physiol. Rev.* 71(1):1–51.
40. Nishibori, M., Tahara, A., Sawada, K., Sakiyama, J., Nakaya, N., Saeki, K. 2000. Neuronal and vascular localization of histamine N-methyltransferase in the bovine central nervous system. *Eur. J. Neurosci.* 12(2):415–424.
41. Prell, G.D., Khandelwal, J.K., Burns, R.S., Green, J.P. 1988. Histamine metabolites in cerebrospinal fluid of the rhesus monkey (Macaca mulatta): cisternal-lumbar concentration gradients. *J. Neurochem.* 50(4):1194–1199.
42. Prell, G.D., Morrishow, A.M., Duoyon, E., Lee, W.S. 1997. Inhibitors of histamine methylation in brain promote formation of imidazoleacetic acid, which interacts with GABA receptors. *J. Neurochem.* 68(1):142–151.
43. Hosli, L., Haas, H.L. 1971. Effects of histamine, histidine and imidazole acetic acid on neurones of the medulla oblongata of the cat. *Experientia* 27(11):1311–1312.
44. Pollard, H., Bischoff, S., Llorens-Cortes, C., Schwartz, J.C. 1976. Histidine decarboxylase and histamine in discrete nuclei of rat hypothalamus and the evidence for mast-cells in the median eminence. *Brain Res.* 118(3):509–513.
45. Hough, L.B., Khandelwal, J.K., Green, J.P. 1984. Histamine turnover in regions of rat brain. *Brain Res.* 291(1):103–109.
46. Silverman, A.J., Sutherland, A.K., Wilhelm, M., Silver, R. 2000. Mast cells migrate from blood to brain. *J. Neurosci.* 20(1):401–408.
47. Auvinen, S., Panula, P. 1988. Development of histamine-immunoreactive neurons in the rat brain. *J. Comp. Neurol.* 276(2):289–303.
48. Reiner, P.B., Semba, K., Fibiger, H.C., McGeer, E.G. 1988. Ontogeny of histidine-decarboxylase-immunoreactive neurons in the tuberomammillary nucleus of the rat hypothalamus: time of origin and development of transmitter phenotype. *J. Comp. Neurol.* 276(2):304–311.
49. Kinnunen, A., Panula, P. 1991. Histamine and tyrosine hydroxylase in developing rat brain. *Agents Actions* 33(1–2):108–111.
50. Eriksson, K.S., Peitsaro, N., Karlstedt, K., Kaslin, J., Panula, P. 1998. Development of the histaminergic neurons and expression of histidine decarboxylase mRNA in the zebrafish brain in the absence of all peripheral histaminergic systems. *Eur. J. Neurosci.* 10(12):3799–3812.
51. Renier, C., Faraco, J.H., Bourgin, P., Motley, T., Bonaventure, P. et al. 2007. Genomic and functional conservation of sedative-hypnotic targets in the zebrafish. *Pharmacogenet. Genomics* 17(4):237–253.
52. Peitsaro, N., Sundvik, M., Anichtchik, O.V., Kaslin, J., Panula, P. 2007. Identification of zebrafish histamine H(1), H(2) and H(3) receptors and effects of histaminergic ligands on behavior. *Biochem. Pharmacol.* 73(8):1205–1214.
53. Parmentier, R., Lin, J.S., Lyon, A. (Unpublished).
54. Ericson, H., Watanabe, T., Kohler, C. 1987. Morphological analysis of the tuberomammillary nucleus in the rat brain: delineation of subgroups with antibody against L-histidine decarboxylase as a marker. *J. Comp. Neurol.* 263(1):1–24.
55. Inagaki, N., Toda, K., Taniuchi, I., Panula, P., Yamatodani, A. et al. 1990. An analysis of histaminergic efferents of the tuberomammillary nucleus to the medial preoptic area and inferior colliculus of the rat. *Exp. Brain Res.* 80(2):374–380.
56. Wada, H., Inagaki, N., Yamatodani, A., Watanabe, T. 1991. Is the histaminergic neuron system a regulatory center for whole-brain activity? *Trends Neurosci.* 14(9):415–418.
57. Miklos, I.H., Kovacs, K.J. 2003. Functional heterogeneity of the responses of histaminergic neuron subpopulations to various stress challenges. *Eur. J. Neurosci.* 18(11):3069–3079.
58. Cenni, G., Blandina, P., Mackie, K., Nosi, D., Formigli, L. et al. 2006. Differential effect of cannabinoid agonists and endocannabinoids on histamine release from distinct regions of the rat brain. *Eur. J. Neurosci.* 24(6):1633–1644.

59. Sergeeva, O.A., Eriksson, K.S., Sharonova, I.N., Vorobjev, V.S., Haas, H.L. 2002. GABA(A) receptor heterogeneity in histaminergic neurons. *Eur. J. Neurosci.* 16(8): 1472–1482.

60. Parmentier, R., Ohtsu, H., Djebbara-Hannas, Z., Valatx, J.L., Watanabe, T., Lin, J.S. 2002. Anatomical, physiological, and pharmacological characteristics of histidine decarboxylase knock-out mice: evidence for the role of brain histamine in behavioral and sleep–wake control. *J. Neurosci.* 22(17):7695–7711.

61. Airaksinen, M.S., Panula, P. 1988. The histaminergic system in the guinea pig central nervous system: an immunocytochemical mapping study using an antiserum against histamine. *J. Comp. Neurol.* 273(2):163–186.

62. Smits, R.P., Steinbusch, H.W., Mulder, A.H. 1990. The localization of histidine decarboxylase-immunoreactive cell bodies in the guinea-pig brain. *J. Chem. Neuroanat.* 3(2):85–100.

63. Airaksinen, M.S., Flugge, G., Fuchs, E., Panula, P. 1989. Histaminergic system in the tree shrew brain. *J. Comp. Neurol.* 286(3):289–310.

64. Lin, J.S., Luppi, P.H., Salvert, D., Sakai, K., Jouvet, M. 1986. Histamine-immunoreactive neurons in the hypothalamus of cats. *C. R. Acad. Sci. III* 303(9):371–376.

65. Lin, J.S., Sakai, K., Jouvet, M. 1986. Role of hypothalamic histaminergic systems in the regulation of vigilance states in cats. *C. R. Acad. Sci. III* 303(11):469–474.

66. Panula, P., Airaksinen, M.S., Pirvola, U., Kotilainen, E. 1990. A histamine-containing neuronal system in human brain. *Neuroscience* 34(1):127–132.

67. Airaksinen, M.S., Paetau, A., Paljarvi, L., Reinikainen, K., Riekkinen, P. et al. 1991. Histamine neurons in human hypothalamus: anatomy in normal and Alzheimer diseased brains. *Neuroscience* 44(2):465–481.

68. Staines, W.A., Daddona, P.E., Nagy, J.I. 1987. The organization and hypothalamic projections of the tuberomammillary nucleus in the rat: an immunohistochemical study of adenosine deaminase-positive neurons and fibers. *Neuroscience* 23(2):571–596.

69. Ericson, H., Kohler, C., Blomqvist, A. 1991. GABA-like immunoreactivity in the tuberomammillary nucleus: an electron microscopic study in the rat. *J. Comp. Neurol.* 305(3):462–469.

70. Kukko-Lukjanov, T.K., Panula, P. 2003. Subcellular distribution of histamine, GABA and galanin in tuberomamillary neurons in vitro. *J. Chem. Neuroanat.* 25(4):279–292.

71. Reiner, P.B., McGeer, E.G. 1987. Electrophysiological properties of cortically projecting histamine neurons of the rat hypothalamus. *Neurosci. Lett.* 73(1):43–47.

72. Haas, H.L., Reiner, P.B. 1988. Membrane properties of histaminergic tuberomammillary neurones of the rat hypothalamus in vitro. *J. Physiol.* 399:633–646.

73. Uteshev, V., Stevens, D.R., Haas, H.L. 1995. A persistent sodium current in acutely isolated histaminergic neurons from rat hypothalamus. *Neuroscience* 66(1):143–149.

74. Takahashi, K., Lin, J.S., Sakai, K. 2006. Neuronal activity of histaminergic tuberomammillary neurons during wake-sleep states in the mouse. *J. Neurosci.* 26(40):10292–10298.

75. Lin, J.S., Hou, Y., Sakai, K., Jouvet, M. 1996. Histaminergic descending inputs to the mesopontine tegmentum and their role in the control of cortical activation and wakefulness in the cat. *J. Neurosci.* 16(4):1523–1537.

76. John, J., Wu, M.F., Boehmer, L.N., Siegel, J.M. 2004. Cataplexy-active neurons in the hypothalamus: implications for the role of histamine in sleep and waking behavior. *Neuron* 42(4):619–634.

77. Lin, J.S. 2000. Brain structures and mechanisms involved in the control of cortical activation and wakefulness, with emphasis on the posterior hypothalamus and histaminergic neurons. *Sleep Med. Rev.* 4(5):471–503.

78. Pape, H.C. 1996. Queer current and pacemaker: the hyperpolarization-activated cation current in neurons. *Annu. Rev. Physiol.* 58:299–327.

79. Kamondi, A., Reiner, P.B. 1991. Hyperpolarization-activated inward current in histaminergic tuberomammillary neurons of the rat hypothalamus. *J. Neurophysiol.* 66(6):1902–1911.

80. Stevens, D.R., Haas, H.L. 1996. Calcium-dependent prepotentials contribute to spontaneous activity in rat tuberomammillary neurons. *J. Physiol.* 493(Pt 3):747–754.

81. Stevens, D.R., Eriksson, K.S., Brown, R.E., Haas, H.L. 2001. The mechanism of spontaneous firing in histamine neurons. *Behav. Brain Res.* 124(2):105–112.

82. Greene, R.W., Haas, H.L., Reiner, P.B. 1990. Two transient outward currents in histamine neurones of the rat hypothalamus in vitro. *J. Physiol.* 420:149–163.

83. Jackson, A.C., Bean, B.P. 2007. State-dependent enhancement of subthreshold A-type potassium current by 4-aminopyridine in tuberomammillary nucleus neurons. *J. Neurosci.* 27(40):10785–10796.

84. Llinas, R.R., Alonso, A. 1992. Electrophysiology of the mammillary complex in vitro. I. Tuberomammillary and lateral mammillary neurons. *J. Neurophysiol.* 68(4):1307–1320.

85. Taddese, A., Bean, B.P. 2002. Subthreshold sodium current from rapidly inactivating sodium channels drives spontaneous firing of tuberomammillary neurons. *Neuron* 33(4):587–600.

86. Takeshita, Y., Watanabe, T., Sakata, T., Munakata, M., Ishibashi, H., Akaike, N. 1998. Histamine modulates high-voltage-activated calcium channels in neurons dissociated from the rat tuberomammillary nucleus. *Neuroscience* 87(4):797–805.

87. Uteshev, V.V., Knot, H.J. 2005. Somatic Ca(2+) dynamics in response to choline-mediated excitation in histaminergic tuberomammillary neurons. *Neuroscience* 134(1):133–143.

88. Wouterlood, F.G., Tuinhof, R. 1992. Subicular efferents to histaminergic neurons in the posterior hypothalamic region of the rat studied with PHA-L tracing combined with histidine decarboxylase immunocytochemistry. *J. Hirnforsch.* 33(4–5):451–465.

89. Ericson, H., Blomqvist, A., Kohler, C. 1991. Origin of neuronal inputs to the region of the tuberomammillary nucleus of the rat brain. *J. Comp. Neurol.* 311(1):45–64.

90. Yang, Q.Z., Hatton, G.I. 1997. Electrophysiology of excitatory and inhibitory afferents to rat histaminergic tuberomammillary nucleus neurons from hypothalamic and forebrain sites. *Brain Res.* 773(1–2):162–172.

91. Sakai, K., Yoshimoto, Y., Luppi, P.H., Fort, P., el Mansari, M. et al. 1990. Lower brainstem afferents to the cat posterior hypothalamus: a double-labeling study. *Brain Res. Bull.* 24(3):437–455.

92. Eriksson, K.S., Sergeeva, O.A., Selbach, O., Haas, H.L. 2004. Orexin (hypocretin)/dynorphin neurons control GABAergic inputs to tuberomammillary neurons. *Eur. J. Neurosci.* 19(5):1278–1284.

93. Stevens, D.R., Kuramasu, A., Eriksson, K.S., Selbach, O., Haas, H.L. 2004. Alpha 2-adrenergic receptor-mediated presynaptic inhibition of GABAergic IPSPs in rat histaminergic neurons. *Neuropharmacology* 46(7):1018–1022.

94. Sergeeva, O.A., Amberger, B.T., Eriksson, K.S., Scherer, A., Haas, H.L. 2003. Co-ordinated expression of 5-HT2C receptors with the NCX1 Na^+/Ca^{2+} exchanger in histaminergic neurones. *J. Neurochem.* 87(3):657–664.

95. Eriksson, K.S., Sergeeva, O., Brown, R.E., Haas, H.L. 2001. Orexin/hypocretin excites the histaminergic neurons of the tuberomammillary nucleus. *J. Neurosci.* 21(23):9273–9279.

96. Eriksson, K.S., Stevens, D.R., Haas, H.L. 2001. Serotonin excites tuberomammillary neurons by activation of $Na^{(+)}/Ca^{(2+)}$-exchange. *Neuropharmacology* 40(3):345–351.

97. Eriksson, K.S., Stevens, D.R., Haas, H.L. 2000. Opposite modulation of histaminergic neurons by nociceptin and morphine. *Neuropharmacology* 39(12):2492–2498.

98. Sergeeva, O.A., Amberger, B.T., Vorobjev, V.S., Eriksson, K.S., Haas, H.L. 2004. AMPA receptor properties and coexpression with sodium-calcium exchangers in rat hypothalamic neurons. *Eur. J. Neurosci.* 19(4):957–965.

99. Sergeeva, O.A., Amberger, B.T., Haas, H.L. 2007. Editing of AMPA and serotonin 2C receptors in individual central neurons, controlling wakefulness. *Cell Mol. Neurobiol.* 27(5):669–680.

100. Sergeeva, O.A., Eriksson, K.S., Haas, H.L. 2001. Glycine receptor mediated responses in rat histaminergic neurons. *Neurosci. Lett.* 300(1):5–8.

101. Steininger, T.L., Gong, H., McGinty, D., Szymusiak, R. 2001. Subregional organization of preoptic area/anterior hypothalamic projections to arousal-related monoaminergic cell groups. *J. Comp. Neurol.* 429(4):638–653.

102. Sherin, J.E., Elmquist, J.K., Torrealba, F., Saper, C.B. 1998. Innervation of histaminergic tuberomammillary neurons by GABAergic and galaninergic neurons in the ventrolateral preoptic nucleus of the rat. *J. Neurosci.* 18(12):4705–4721.

103. Saper, C.B., Cano, G., Scammell, T.E. 2005. Homeostatic, circadian, and emotional regulation of sleep. *J. Comp. Neurol.* 493(1):92–98.

104. Nelson, L.E., Guo, T.Z., Lu, J., Saper, C.B., Franks, N.P., Maze, M. 2002. The sedative component of anesthesia is mediated by GABA(A) receptors in an endogenous sleep pathway. *Nat. Neurosci.* 5(10):979–984.

105. Sergeeva, O.A., Andreeva, N., Garret, M., Scherer, A., Haas, H.L. 2005. Pharmacological properties of GABAA receptors in rat hypothalamic neurons expressing the epsilon-subunit. *J. Neurosci.* 25(1):88–95.

106. Stevens, D.R., Kuramasu, A., Haas, H.L. 1999. GABAB-receptor-mediated control of GABAergic inhibition in rat histaminergic neurons in vitro. *Eur. J. Neurosci.* 11(4):1148–1154.

107. Uteshev, V.V., Meyer, E.M., Papke, R.L. 2002. Activation and inhibition of native neuronal alpha-bungarotoxin-sensitive nicotinic ACh receptors. *Brain Res.* 948(1–2):33–46.

108. Uteshev, V.V., Stevens, D.R., Haas, H.L. 1996. Alpha-bungarotoxin-sensitive nicotinic responses in rat tuberomammillary neurons. *Pflugers Arch.* 432(4):607–613.

109. Uteshev, V.V., Meyer, E.M., Papke, R.L. 2003. Regulation of neuronal function by choline and 4OH-GTS-21 through alpha 7 nicotinic receptors. *J. Neurophysiol.* 89(4):1797–1806.

110. Sergeeva, O.A., Klyuch, B.P., Vandael, D., Haas, H.L. 2007. Dopaminergic excitation of histaminergic tuberomamillary neurons. *Acta Physiol.* (Oxf) 189:S653.

111. Sergeeva, O.A., Korotkova, T.M., Scherer, A., Brown, R.E., Haas, H.L. 2003. Co-expression of non-selective cation channels of the transient receptor potential canonical family in central aminergic neurones. *J. Neurochem.* 85(6):1547–1552.

112. Schmauss, C. 2003. Serotonin 2C receptors: suicide, serotonin, and runaway RNA editing. *Neuroscientist* 9(4):237–242.

113. Furukawa, K., Ishibashi, H., Akaike, N. 1994. ATP-induced inward current in neurons freshly dissociated from the tuberomammillary nucleus. *J. Neurophysiol.* 71(3):868–873.

114. Vorobjev, V.S., Sharonova, I.N., Haas, H.L., Sergeeva, O.A. 2003. Expression and function of P2X purinoceptors in rat histaminergic neurons. *Br. J. Pharmacol.* 138(5):1013–1019.

115. Vorobjev, V.S., Sharonova, I.N., Sergeeva, O.A., Haas, H.L. 2003. Modulation of ATP-induced currents by zinc in acutely isolated hypothalamic neurons of the rat. *Br. J. Pharmacol.* 139(5):919–926.

116. Sergeeva, O.A., Klyuch, B.P., Fleischer, W., Eriksson, K.S., Korotkova, T.M. et al. 2006. P2Y receptor-mediated excitation in the posterior hypothalamus. *Eur. J. Neurosci.* 24(5):1413–1426.

117. Hong, Z.Y., Huang, Z.L., Qu, W.M., Eguchi, N., Urade, Y., Hayaishi, O. 2005. An adenosine A receptor agonist induces sleep by increasing GABA release in the tuberomammillary nucleus to inhibit histaminergic systems in rats. *J. Neurochem.* 92(6):1542–1549.

118. Scammell, T.E., Gerashchenko, D.Y., Mochizuki, T., McCarthy, M.T., Estabrooke, I.V. et al. 2001. An adenosine A2a agonist increases sleep and induces fos in ventrolateral preoptic neurons. *Neuroscience* 107(4):653–663.

119. Alam, M.N., Kumar, S., Bashir, T., Suntsova, N., Methippara, M.M. et al. 2005. GABA-mediated control of hypocretin- but not melanin-concentrating hormone-immunoreactive neurones during sleep in rats. *J. Physiol.* 563(Pt 2):569–582.

120. Methippara, M.M., Alam, M.N., Szymusiak, R., McGinty, D. 2003. Preoptic area warming inhibits wake-active neurons in the perifornical lateral hypothalamus. *Brain Res.* 960(1–2):165–173.

121. Radulovacki, M., Virus, R.M., Djuricic-Nedelson, M., Green, R.D. 1984. Adenosine analogs and sleep in rats. *J Pharmacol. Exp. Ther.* 228(2):268–274.

122. Huston, J.P., Haas, H.L., Boix, F., Pfister, M., Decking, U. et al. 1996. Extracellular adenosine levels in neostriatum and hippocampus during rest and activity periods of rats. *Neuroscience* 73(1):99–107.

123. Porkka-Heiskanen, T., Strecker, R.E., Thakkar, M., Bjorkum, A.A., Greene, R.W., McCarley, R.W. 1997. Adenosine: a mediator of the sleep-inducing effects of prolonged wakefulness. *Science* 276(5316):1265–1268.

124. Haas, H.L., Selbach, O. 2000. Functions of neuronal adenosine receptors. *Naunyn Schmiedebergs Arch. Pharmacol.* 362(4–5):375–381.

125. Kohler, C., Ericson, H., Watanabe, T., Polak, J., Palay, S.L. et al. 1986. Galanin immunoreactivity in hypothalamic neurons: further evidence for multiple chemical messengers in the tuberomammillary nucleus. *J. Comp. Neurol.* 250(1):58–64.

126. Airaksinen, M.S., Alanen, S., Szabat, E., Visser, T.J., Panula, P. 1992. Multiple neurotransmitters in the tuberomammillary nucleus: comparison of rat, mouse, and guinea pig. *J. Comp. Neurol.* 323(1):103–116.

127. Trottier, S., Chotard, C., Traiffort, E., Unmehopa, U., Fisser, B. et al. 2002. Co-localization of histamine with GABA but not with galanin in the human tuberomamillary nucleus. *Brain Res.* 939(1–2):52–64.

128. Schonrock, B., Busselberg, D., Haas, H.L. 1991. Properties of tuberomammillary histamine neurones and their response to galanin. *Agents Actions* 33(1–2):135–137.

129. Zeitzer, J.M., Nishino, S., Mignot, E. 2006. The neurobiology of hypocretins (orexins), narcolepsy and related therapeutic interventions. *Trends Pharmacol. Sci.* 27(7):368–374.

130. Siegel, J.M., Boehmer, L.N. 2006. Narcolepsy and the hypocretin system—where motion meets emotion. *Nat. Clin. Pract. Neurol.* 2(10):548–556.

131. Saper, C.B., Chou, T.C., Scammell, T.E. 2001. The sleep switch: hypothalamic control of sleep and wakefulness. *Trends Neurosci.* 24(12):726–731.

132. Huang, Z.L., Qu, W.M., Li, W.D., Mochizuki, T., Eguchi, N. et al. 2001. Arousal effect of orexin A depends on activation of the histaminergic system. *Proc. Natl Acad. Sci. U.S.A.* 98(17):9965–9970.

133. Jorgensen, E.A., Knigge, U., Watanabe, T., Warberg, J., Kjaer, A. 2005. Histaminergic neurons are involved in the orexigenic effect of orexin-A. *Neuroendocrinology* 82(2):70–77.

134. Lin, L., Wisor, J., Shiba, T., Taheri, S., Yanai, K. et al. 2002. Measurement of hypocretin/orexin content in the mouse brain using an enzyme immunoassay: the effect of circadian time, age and genetic background. *Peptides* 23(12):2203–2211.

135. Gotoh, K., Fukagawa, K., Fukagawa, T., Noguchi, H., Kakuma, T. et al. 2005. Glucagon-like peptide-1, corticotropin-releasing hormone, and hypothalamic neuronal histamine interact in the leptin-signaling pathway to regulate feeding behavior. *FASEB J.* 19(9):1131–1133.

136. Gotoh, K., Fukagawa, K., Fukagawa, T., Noguchi, H., Kakuma, T. et al. 2007. Hypothalamic neuronal histamine mediates the thyrotropin-releasing hormone-induced suppression of food intake. *J. Neurochem.* 103(3):1102–1110.

137. Toftegaard, C.L., Knigge, U., Kjaer, A., Warberg, J. 2003. The role of hypothalamic histamine in leptin-induced suppression of short-term food intake in fasted rats. *Regul. Pept.* 111(1–3):83–90.

138. Tamiya, R., Hanada, M., Narita, N., Kawai, Y., Tohyama, M., Takagi, H. 1989. Neuropeptide Y afferents have synaptic interactions with histaminergic (histidine decarboxylase-immunoreactive) neurons in the rat brain. *Neurosci. Lett.* 99(3):241–245.

139. Ishizuka, T., Nomura, S., Hosoda, H., Kangawa, K., Watanabe, T., Yamatodani, A. 2006. A role of the histaminergic system for the control of feeding by orexigenic peptides. *Physiol. Behav.* 89(3):295–300.

140. Bajic, D., Hoang, Q.V., Nakajima, S., Nakajima, Y. 2004. Dissociated histaminergic neuron cultures from the tuberomammillary nucleus of rats: culture methods and ghrelin effects. *J. Neurosci. Methods* 132(2):177–184.

141. Riehl, J., Honda, K., Kwan, M., Hong, J., Mignot, E., Nishino, S. 2000. Chronic oral administration of CG-3703, a thyrotropin releasing hormone analog, increases wake and decreases cataplexy in canine narcolepsy. *Neuropsychopharmacology* 23(1):34–45.

142. Sergeeva, O.A., Parmentier, R., Vandael, D., Klyuch, B.P., Haas, H.L. 2007. Excitation of histaminergic neurons by thyrotropin-releasing hormone. *Soc. Neurosci. Abstr.*:199.2.

143. Chou, T.C., Scammell, T.E., Gooley, J.J., Gaus, S.E., Saper, C.B., Lu, J. 2003. Critical role of dorsomedial hypothalamic nucleus in a wide range of behavioral circadian rhythms. *J. Neurosci.* 23(33):10691–10702.

144. Tamiya, R., Hanada, M., Narita, N., Inagaki, S., Tohyama, M., Takagi, H. 1990. Histaminergic neurons receive substance P-ergic inputs in the posterior hypothalamus of the rat. *Exp. Brain Res.* 79(2):261–265.

145. Ishunina, T.A., van Heerikhuize, J.J., Ravid, R., Swaab, D.F. 2003. Estrogen receptors and metabolic activity in the human tuberomamillary nucleus: changes in relation to sex, aging and Alzheimer's disease. *Brain Res.* 988(1–2):84–96.

146. Huang, Z.L., Sato, Y., Mochizuki, T., Okada, T., Qu, W.M. et al. 2003. Prostaglandin E2 activates the histaminergic system via the EP4 receptor to induce wakefulness in rats. *J. Neurosci.* 23(14):5975–5983.

147. Ohshima, Y., Iwase, M., Izumizaki, M., Ishiguro, T., Kanamaru, M. et al. 2007. Hypoxic ventilatory response during light and dark periods and the involvement of histamine H1 receptor in mice. *Am. J. Physiol. Regul. Integr. Comp. Physiol.* 293(3):R1350–R1356.

148. Johnson, P.L., Moratalla, R., Lightman, S.L., Lowry, C.A. 2005. Are tuberomammillary histaminergic neurons involved in CO2-mediated arousal? *Exp. Neurol.* 193(1):228–233.

149. Williams, R.H., Jensen, L.T., Verkhratsky, A., Fugger, L., Burdakov, D. 2007. Control of hypothalamic orexin neurons by acid and CO2. *Proc. Natl Acad. Sci. U.S.A.* 104(25):10685–10690.

150. Kohler, C., Swanson, L.W., Haglund, L., Wu, J.Y. 1985. The cytoarchitecture, histochemistry and projections of the tuberomammillary nucleus in the rat. *Neuroscience* 16(1):85–110.

151. Panula, P., Pirvola, U., Auvinen, S., Airaksinen, M.S. 1989. Histamine-immunoreactive nerve fibers in the rat brain. *Neuroscience* 28(3):585–610.

152. Takeda, N., Inagaki, S., Taguchi, Y., Tohyama, M., Watanabe, T., Wada, H. 1984. Origins of histamine-containing fibers in the cerebral cortex of rats studied by immunohistochemistry with histidine decarboxylase as a marker and transection. *Brain Res.* 323(1):55–63.

153. Panula, P., Flugge, G., Fuchs, E., Pirvola, U., Auvinen, S., Airaksinen, M.S. 1989. Histamine-immunoreactive nerve fibers in the mammalian spinal cord. *Brain Res.* 484(1–2):234–239.

154. Lee, K.H., Broberger, C., Kim, U., McCormick, D.A. 2004. Histamine modulates thalamocortical activity by activating a chloride conductance in ferret perigeniculate neurons. *Proc. Natl Acad. Sci. U.S.A.* 101(17):6716–6721.

155. Hatton, G.I., Yang, Q.Z. 2001. Ionotropic histamine receptors and H2 receptors modulate supraoptic oxytocin neuronal excitability and dye coupling. *J. Neurosci.* 21(9):2974–2982.

156. Gengs, C., Leung, H.T., Skingsley, D.R., Iovchev, M.I., Yin, Z. et al. 2002. The target of Drosophila photoreceptor synaptic transmission is a histamine-gated chloride channel encoded by ort (hclA). *J. Biol. Chem.* 277(44):42113–42120.

157. Bekkers, J.M. 1993. Enhancement by histamine of NMDA-mediated synaptic transmission in the hippocampus. *Science* 261(5117):104–106.

158. Vorobjev, V.S., Sharonova, I.N., Walsh, I.B., Haas, H.L. 1993. Histamine potentiates N-methyl-D-aspartate responses in acutely isolated hippocampal neurons. *Neuron* 11(5):837–844.

159. Yanovsky, Y., Reymann, K., Haas, H.L. 1995. pH-dependent facilitation of synaptic transmission by histamine in the CA1 region of mouse hippocampus. *Eur. J. Neurosci.* 7(10):2017–2020.

160. Saybasili, H., Stevens, D.R., Haas, H.L. 1995. pH-dependent modulation of N-methyl-D-aspartate receptor-mediated synaptic currents by histamine in rat hippocampus in vitro. *Neurosci. Lett.* 199(3):225–227.

161. Williams, K. 1994. Subunit-specific potentiation of recombinant N-methyl-D-aspartate receptors by histamine. *Mol. Pharmacol.* 46(3):531–541.

162. Payne, G.W., Neuman, R.S. 1997. Effects of hypomagnesia on histamine H1 receptor-mediated facilitation of NMDA responses. *Br. J. Pharmacol.* 121(2):199–204.

163. de Esch, I.J., Thurmond, R.L., Jongejan, A., Leurs, R. 2005. The histamine H4 receptor as a new therapeutic target for inflammation. *Trends Pharmacol. Sci.* 26(9):462–469.

164. Hill, S.J., Ganellin, C.R., Timmerman, H., Schwartz, J.C., Shankley, N.P. et al. 1997. International Union of Pharmacology. XIII. Classification of histamine receptors. *Pharmacol. Rev.* 49(3):253–278.

165. Leurs, R., Bakker, R.A., Timmerman, H., de Esch, I.J. 2005. The histamine H3 receptor: from gene cloning to H3 receptor drugs. *Nat. Rev. Drug Discov.* 4(2):107–120.

166. Jongejan, A., Bruysters, M., Ballesteros, J.A., Haaksma, E., Bakker, R.A. et al. 2005. Linking agonist binding to histamine H1 receptor activation. *Nat. Chem. Biol.* 1(2):98–103.

167. Bakker, R.A., Nicholas, M.W., Smith, T.T., Burstein, E.S., Hacksell, U. et al. 2007. In vitro pharmacology of clinically used central nervous system-active drugs as inverse h1 receptor agonists. *J. Pharmacol. Exp. Ther.* 322(1):172–179.

168. Morisset, S., Rouleau, A., Ligneau, X., Gbahou, F., Tardivel-Lacombe, J. et al. 2000. High constitutive activity of native H3 receptors regulates histamine neurons in brain. *Nature* 408(6814):860–864.

169. Leurs, R., Hoffmann, M., Alewijnse, A.E., Smit, M.J., Timmerman, H. 2002. Methods to determine the constitutive activity of histamine H2 receptors. *Methods Enzymol.* 343:405–416.

170. Kuramasu, A., Sukegawa, J., Yanagisawa, T., Yanai, K. 2006. Recent advances in molecular pharmacology of the histamine systems: roles of C-terminal tails of histamine receptors. *J. Pharmacol. Sci.* 101(1):7–11.

171. Le Coniat, M., Traiffort, E., Ruat, M., Arrang, J.M., Berger, R. 1994. Chromosomal localization of the human histamine H1-receptor gene. *Hum. Genet.* 94(2):186–188.

172. Leurs, R., Church, M.K., Taglialatela, M. 2002. H1-antihistamines: inverse agonism, anti-inflammatory actions and cardiac effects. *Clin. Exp. Allergy* 32(4):489–498.
173. Wieland, K., Laak, A.M., Smit, M.J., Kuhne, R., Timmerman, H., Leurs, R. 1999. Mutational analysis of the antagonist-binding site of the histamine H(1) receptor. *J. Biol. Chem.* 274(42):29994–30000.
174. Leurs, R., Traiffort, E., Arrang, J.M., Tardivel-Lacombe, J., Ruat, M., Schwartz, J.C. 1994. Guinea pig histamine H1 receptor. II. Stable expression in Chinese hamster ovary cells reveals the interaction with three major signal transduction pathways. *J. Neurochem.* 62(2):519–527.
175. Selbach, O., Brown, R.E., Haas, H.L. 1997. Long-term increase of hippocampal excitability by histamine and cyclic AMP. *Neuropharmacology* 36(11–12):1539–1548.
176. Bakker, R.A., Casarosa, P., Timmerman, H., Smit, M.J., Leurs, R. 2004. Constitutively active Gq/11-coupled receptors enable signaling by co-expressed G(i/o)-coupled receptors. *J. Biol. Chem.* 279(7):5152–5161.
177. Brown, R.E., Sergeeva, O.A., Eriksson, K.S., Haas, H.L. 2002. Convergent excitation of dorsal raphe serotonin neurons by multiple arousal systems (orexin/hypocretin, histamine and noradrenaline). *J. Neurosci.* 22(20):8850–8859.
178. Kim, S.F., Huang, A.S., Snowman, A.M., Teuscher, C., Snyder, S.H. 2007. Antipsychotic drug-induced weight gain mediated by histamine H1 receptor-linked activation of hypothalamic AMP-kinase. *Proc. Natl Acad. Sci. U.S.A.* 104(9):3456–3459.
179. Bakker, R.A., Schoonus, S.B., Smit, M.J., Timmerman, H., Leurs, R. 2001. Histamine H(1)-receptor activation of nuclear factor-kappa B: roles for G beta gamma- and G alpha(q/11)-subunits in constitutive and agonist-mediated signaling. *Mol. Pharmacol.* 60(5):1133–1142.
180. Korotkova, T.M., Sergeeva, O.A., Ponomarenko, A.A., Haas, H.L. 2005. Histamine excites noradrenergic neurons in locus coeruleus in rats. *Neuropharmacology* 49(1):129–134.
181. McCormick, D.A., Williamson, A. 1991. Modulation of neuronal firing mode in cat and guinea pig LGNd by histamine: possible cellular mechanisms of histaminergic control of arousal. *J. Neurosci.* 11(10):3188–3199.
182. Zhou, F.W., Xu, J.J., Zhao, Y., LeDoux, M.S., Zhou, F.M. 2006. Opposite functions of histamine H1 and H2 receptors and H3 receptor in substantia nigra pars reticulata. *J. Neurophysiol.* 96(3):1581–1591.
183. Jin, C.L., Yang, L.X., Wu. X.H., Li, Q., Ding, M.P. et al. 2005. Effects of carnosine on amygdaloid-kindled seizures in sprague-dawley rats. *Neuroscience* 135(3):939–947.
184. Gorelova, N., Reiner, P.B. 1996. Histamine depolarizes cholinergic septal neurons. *J. Neurophysiol.* 75(2):707–714.
185. Xu, C., Michelsen, K.A., Wu, M., Morozova, E., Panula, P., Alreja, M. 2004. Histamine innervation and activation of septohippocampal GABAergic neurones: involvement of local ACh release. *J. Physiol.* 561(Pt 3):657–670.
186. Manahan-Vaughan, D., Reymann, K.G., Brown, R.E. 1998. In vivo electrophysiological investigations into the role of histamine in the dentate gyrus of the rat. *Neuroscience* 84(3):783–790.
187. Jahn, K., Haas, H.L., Hatt, H. 1995. Patch clamp study of histamine activated potassium currents on rabbit olfactory bulb neurons. *Naunyn Schmiedebergs Arch. Pharmacol.* 352(4):386–393.
188. Reiner, P.B., Kamondi, A. 1994. Mechanisms of antihistamine-induced sedation in the human brain: H1 receptor activation reduces a background leakage potassium current. *Neuroscience* 59(3):579–588.
189. Weiger, T., Stevens, D.R., Wunder, L., Haas, H.L. 1997. Histamine H1 receptors in C6 glial cells are coupled to calcium-dependent potassium channels via release of calcium from internal stores. *Naunyn Schmiedebergs Arch. Pharmacol.* 355(5):559–565.

190. Martinez-Mir, M.I., Pollard, H., Moreau, J., Arrang, J.M., Ruat, M. et al. 1990. Three histamine receptors (H1, H2 and H3) visualized in the brain of human and non-human primates. *Brain Res.* 526(2):322–327.

191. Yanai, K., Watanabe, T., Yokoyama, H., Hatazawa, J., Iwata, R. et al. 1992. Mapping of histamine H1 receptors in the human brain using [11C]pyrilamine and positron emission tomography. *J. Neurochem.* 59(1):128–136.

192. Yanai, K., Tashiro, M. 2007. The physiological and pathophysiological roles of neuronal histamine: an insight from human positron emission tomography studies. *Pharmacol. Ther.* 113(1):1–15.

193. Yanai, K., Watanabe, T., Meguro, K., Yokoyama, H., Sato, I. et al. 1992. Age-dependent decrease in histamine H1 receptor in human brains revealed by PET. *Neuroreport* 3(5):433–436.

194. Ma, R.Z., Gao, J., Meeker, N.D., Fillmore, P.D., Tung, K.S. et al. 2002. Identification of Bphs, an autoimmune disease locus, as histamine receptor H1. *Science* 297(5581):620–623.

195. Huang, Z.L., Mochizuki, T., Qu, W.M., Hong, Z.Y., Watanabe, T. et al. 2006. Altered sleep-wake characteristics and lack of arousal response to H3 receptor antagonist in histamine H1 receptor knockout mice. *Proc. Natl. Acad. Sci. U.S.A.* 103(12): 4687–4692.

196. Simons, F.E. 2004. Advances in H1-antihistamines. *N. Engl. J. Med.* 351(21): 2203–2217.

197. Bovet, D. 1950. Introduction to antihistamine agents and antergan derivative. *Ann. N. Y. Acad. Sci.* 50(9):1089–1126.

198. Richelson, E. 1978. Tricyclic antidepressants block histamine H1 receptors of mouse neuroblastoma cells. *Nature* 274(5667):176–177.

199. Traiffort, E., Vizuete, M.L., Tardivel-Lacombe, J., Souil, E., Schwartz, J.C., Ruat, M. 1995. The guinea pig histamine H2 receptor: gene cloning, tissue expression and chromosomal localization of its human counterpart. *Biochem. Biophys. Res. Commun.* 211(2):570–577.

200. Kobayashi, T., Inoue, I., Jenkins, N.A., Gilbert, D.J., Copeland, N.G., Watanabe, T. 1996. Cloning, RNA expression, and chromosomal location of a mouse histamine H2 receptor gene. *Genomics* 37(3):390–394.

201. Smit, M.J., Leurs, R., Alewijnse, A.E., Blauw, J., Nieuw Amerongen, G.P. et al. 1996. Inverse agonism of histamine H2 antagonist accounts for upregulation of spontaneously active histamine H2 receptors. *Proc. Natl Acad. Sci. U.S.A.* 93(13):6802–6807.

202. Fitzsimons, C.P., Lazar-Molnar, E., Tomoskozi, Z., Buzas, E., Rivera, E.S., Falus, A. 2001. Histamine deficiency induces tissue-specific down-regulation of histamine H2 receptor expression in histidine decarboxylase knockout mice. *FEBS Lett.* 508(2):245–248.

203. Ruat, M., Traiffort, E., Bouthenet, M.L., Schwartz, J.C., Hirschfeld, J. et al. 1990. Reversible and irreversible labeling and autoradiographic localization of the cerebral histamine H2 receptor using [125I]iodinated probes. *Proc. Natl Acad. Sci. U.S.A.* 87(5):1658–1662.

204. Vizuete, M.L., Traiffort, E., Bouthenet, M.L., Ruat, M., Souil, E. et al. 1997. Detailed mapping of the histamine H2 receptor and its gene transcripts in guinea-pig brain. *Neuroscience* 80(2):321–343.

205. Baudry, M., Martres, M.P., Schwartz, J.C. 1975. H1 and H2 receptors in the histamine-induced accumulation of cyclic AMP in guinea pig brain slices. *Nature* 253(5490):362–364.

206. Garbarg, M., Schwartz, J.C. 1988. Synergism between histamine H1- and H2-receptors in the cAMP response in guinea pig brain slices: effects of phorbol esters and calcium. *Mol. Pharmacol.* 33(1):38–43.

207. Traiffort, E., Ruat, M., Arrang, J.M., Leurs, R., Piomelli, D., Schwartz, J.C. 1992. Expression of a cloned rat histamine H2 receptor mediating inhibition of arachidonate release and activation of cAMP accumulation. *Proc. Natl Acad. Sci. U.S.A.* 89(7):2649–2653.

208. Pedarzani, P., Storm, J.F. 1995. Protein kinase A-independent modulation of ion channels in the brain by cyclic AMP. *Proc. Natl Acad. Sci. U.S.A.* 92(25): 11716–11720.

209. Haas, H.L., Konnerth, A. 1983. Histamine and noradrenaline decrease calcium-activated potassium conductance in hippocampal pyramidal cells. *Nature* 302(5907):432–434.

210. Pedarzani, P., Storm, J.F. 1993. PKA mediates the effects of monoamine transmitters on the K^+ current underlying the slow spike frequency adaptation in hippocampal neurons. *Neuron* 11(6):1023–1035.

211. Atzori, M., Lau, D., Tansey, E.P., Chow, A., Ozaita, A. et al. 2000. H2 histamine receptor-phosphorylation of Kv3.2 modulates interneuron fast spiking. *Nat. Neurosci.* 3(8):791–798.

212. Dai, H., Kaneko, K., Kato, H., Fujii, S., Jing, Y. et al. 2007. Selective cognitive dysfunction in mice lacking histamine H1 and H2 receptors. *Neurosci. Res.* 57(2):306–313.

213. Mobarakeh, J.I., Takahashi, K., Sakurada, S., Kuramasu, A., Yanai, K. 2006. Enhanced antinociceptive effects of morphine in histamine H2 receptor gene knockout mice. *Neuropharmacology* 51(3):612–622.

214. Teuscher, C., Poynter, M.E., Offner, H., Zamora, A., Watanabe, T. et al. 2004. Attenuation of Th1 effector cell responses and susceptibility to experimental allergic encephalomyelitis in histamine H2 receptor knockout mice is due to dysregulation of cytokine production by antigen-presenting cells. *Am. J. Pathol.* 164(3):883–892.

215. Lefranc, F., Yeaton, P., Brotchi, J., Kiss, R. 2006. Cimetidine, an unexpected antitumor agent, and its potential for the treatment of glioblastoma (review). *Int. J. Oncol.* 28(5):1021–1030.

216. Green, J.P., Maayani, S. 1977. Tricyclic antidepressant drugs block histamine H2 receptor in brain. *Nature* 269(5624):163–165.

217. Kaminsky, R., Moriarty, T.M., Bodine, J., Wolf, D.E., Davidson, M. 1990. Effect of famotidine on deficit symptoms of schizophrenia. *Lancet* 335(8701):1351–1352.

218. Lovenberg, T.W., Roland, B.L., Wilson, S.J., Jiang, X., Pyati, J. et al. 1999. Cloning and functional expression of the human histamine H3 receptor. *Mol. Pharmacol.* 55(6):1101–1107.

219. Arrang, J.M., Morisset, S., Gbahou, F. 2007. Constitutive activity of the histamine H(3) receptor. *Trends Pharmacol. Sci.* 28(7):350–357.

220. Gbahou, F., Rouleau, A., Morisset, S., Parmentier, R., Crochet, S. et al. 2003. Protean agonism at histamine H3 receptors in vitro and in vivo. *Proc. Natl Acad. Sci. U.S.A.* 100(19):11086–11091.

221. Bongers, G., Sallmen, T., Passani, M.B., Mariottini, C., Wendelin, D. et al. 2007. The Akt/GSK-3beta axis as a new signaling pathway of the histamine H(3) receptor. *J. Neurochem.* 103(1):248–258.

222. Arrang, J.M., Garbarg, M., Schwartz, J.C. 1987. Autoinhibition of histamine synthesis mediated by presynaptic H3-receptors. *Neuroscience* 23(1):149–157.

223. Arrang, J.M., Garbarg, M., Schwartz, J.C. 1985. Autoregulation of histamine release in brain by presynaptic H3-receptors. *Neuroscience* 15(2):553–562.

224. Schlicker, E., Werthwein, S., Zentner, J. 1999. Histamine H3 receptor-mediated inhibition of noradrenaline release in the human brain. *Fundam. Clin. Pharmacol.* 13(1):120–122.

225. Arrang, J.M., Drutel, G., Schwartz, J.C. 1995. Characterization of histamine H3 receptors regulating acetylcholine release in rat entorhinal cortex. *Br. J. Pharmacol.* 114(7):1518–1522.

226. Blandina, P., Giorgetti, M., Bartolini, L., Cecchi, M., Timmerman, H. et al. 1996. Inhibition of cortical acetylcholine release and cognitive performance by histamine H3 receptor activation in rats. *Br. J. Pharmacol.* 119(8):1656–1664.

227. Doreulee, N., Yanovsky, Y., Flagmeyer, I., Stevens, D.R., Haas, H.L., Brown, R.E. 2001. Histamine H(3) receptors depress synaptic transmission in the corticostriatal pathway. *Neuropharmacology* 40(1):106–113.

228. Brown, R.E., Reymann, K.G. 1996. Histamine H3 receptor-mediated depression of synaptic transmission in the dentate gyrus of the rat in vitro. *J. Physiol.* 496(Pt 1): 175–184.

229. Jang, I.S., Rhee, J.S., Watanabe, T., Akaike, N., Akaike, N. 2001. Histaminergic modulation of GABAergic transmission in rat ventromedial hypothalamic neurones. *J. Physiol.* 534(Pt 3):791–803.

230. Pillot, C., Heron, A., Schwartz, J.C., Arrang, J.M. 2003. Ciproxifan, a histamine H3-receptor antagonist/inverse agonist, modulates the effects of methamphetamine on neuropeptide mRNA expression in rat striatum. *Eur. J. Neurosci.* 17(2):307–314.

231. Tokita, S., Takahashi, K., Kotani, H. 2006. Recent advances in molecular pharmacology of the histamine systems: physiology and pharmacology of histamine H3 receptor: roles in feeding regulation and therapeutic potential for metabolic disorders. *J. Pharmacol. Sci.* 101(1):12–18.

232. Teuscher, C., Subramanian, M., Noubade, R., Gao, J.F., Offner, H. et al. 2007. Central histamine H3 receptor signaling negatively regulates susceptibility to autoimmune inflammatory disease of the CNS. *Proc. Natl Acad. Sci. U.S.A.* 104(24):10146–10151.

233. Gbahou, F., Vincent, L., Humbert-Claude, M., Tardivel-Lacombe, J., Chabret, C., Arrang, J.M. 2006. Compared pharmacology of human histamine H3 and H4 receptors: structure–activity relationships of histamine derivatives. *Br. J. Pharmacol.* 147(7):744–754.

234. Phillis, J.W., Tebecis, A.K., York, D.H. 1968. Depression of spinal motoneurones by noradrenaline, 5-hydroxytryptamine and histamine. *Eur. J. Pharmacol.* 4(4): 471–475.

235. Haas, H.L., Anderson, E.G., Hosli, L. 1973. Histamine and metabolites: their effects and interactions with convulsants on brain stem neurones. *Brain Res.* 51:269–278.

236. Whyment, A.D., Blanks, A.M., Lee, K., Renaud, L.P., Spanswick, D. 2006. Histamine excites neonatal rat sympathetic preganglionic neurons in vitro via activation of H1 receptors. *J. Neurophysiol.* 95(4):2492–2500.

237. Carpenter, D.O., Briggs, D.B., Strominger, N. 1983. Responses of neurons of canine area postrema to neurotransmitters and peptides. *Cell Mol. Neurobiol.* 3(2):113–126.

238. Khateb, A., Fort, P., Pegna, A., Jones, B.E., Muhlethaler, M. 1995. Cholinergic nucleus basalis neurons are excited by histamine in vitro. *Neuroscience* 69(2):495–506.

239. Cecchi, M., Passani, M.B., Bacciottini, L., Mannaioni, P.F., Blandina, P. 2001. Cortical acetylcholine release elicited by stimulation of histamine H1 receptors in the nucleus basalis magnocellularis: a dual-probe microdialysis study in the freely moving rat. *Eur. J. Neurosci.* 13(1):68–78.

240. Prast, H., Fischer, H., Philippu, A. 1994. Release of acetylcholine in the ventral striatum is influenced by histamine receptors. *Agents Actions* 41 Spec No:C85–C86.

241. McCormick, D.A., Williamson, A. 1989. Convergence and divergence of neurotransmitter action in human cerebral cortex. *Proc. Natl Acad. Sci. U.S.A.* 86(20):8098–8102.

242. Lakoski, J.M., Gallager, D.W., Aghajanian, G.K. 1984. Histamine-induced depression of serotoninergic dorsal raphe neurons: antagonism by cimetidine, a reevaluation. *Eur. J. Pharmacol.* 103(1–2):153–156.

243. Threlfell, S., Cragg, S.J., Kallo, I., Turi, G.F., Coen, C.W., Greenfield, S.A. 2004. Histamine H3 receptors inhibit serotonin release in substantia nigra pars reticulata. *J. Neurosci.* 24(40):8704–8710.

244. Schlicker, E., Fink, K., Detzner, M., Gothert, M. 1993. Histamine inhibits dopamine release in the mouse striatum via presynaptic H3 receptors. *J. Neural Transm. Gen. Sect.* 93(1):1–10.

245. Korotkova, T.M., Haas, H.L., Brown, R.E. 2002. Histamine excites GABAergic cells in the rat substantia nigra and ventral tegmental area in vitro. *Neurosci. Lett.* 320(3):133–136.

246. Lazarov, N.E., Gratzl, M. 2006. Selective expression of histamine receptors in rat mesencephalic trigeminal neurons. *Neurosci. Lett.* 404(1–2):67–71.

247. Sakata, T., Yoshimatsu, H., Masaki, T., Tsuda, K. 2003. Anti-obesity actions of mastication driven by histamine neurons in rats. *Exp. Biol. Med. (Maywood)* 228(10):1106–1110.

248. Inagaki, N., Yamatodani, A., Shinoda, K., Shiotani, Y., Tohyama, M. et al. 1987. The histaminergic innervation of the mesencephalic nucleus of the trigeminal nerve in rat brain: a light and electron microscopical study. *Brain Res.* 418(2):388–391.

249. Hutcheon, B., Puil, E., Spigelman, I. 1993. Histamine actions and comparison with substance P effects in trigeminal neurons. *Neuroscience* 55(2):521–529.

250. Ebersberger, A., Ringkamp, M., Reeh, P.W., Handwerker, H.O. 1997. Recordings from brain stem neurons responding to chemical stimulation of the subarachnoid space. *J. Neurophysiol.* 77(6):3122–3133.

251. Theoharides, T.C., Donelan, J., Kandere-Grzybowska, K., Konstantinidou, A. 2005. The role of mast cells in migraine pathophysiology. *Brain Res.: Brain Res. Rev.* 49(1):65–76.

252. Satayavivad, J., Kirsten, E.B. 1977. Iontophoretic studies of histamine and histamine antagonists in the feline vestibular nuclei. *Eur. J. Pharmacol.* 41(1):17–26.

253. Darlington, C.L., Gallagher, J.P., Smith, P.F. 1995. In vitro electrophysiological studies of the vestibular nucleus complex. *Prog. Neurobiol.* 45(4):335–346.

254. Takeda, N., Morita, M., Horii, A., Nishiike, S., Kitahara, T., Uno, A. 2001. Neural mechanisms of motion sickness. *J. Med. Invest.* 48(1–2):44–59.

255. Azuma, H., Sawada, S., Takeuchi, S., Higashiyama, K., Kakigi, A., Takeda, T. 2003. Expression of mRNA encoding the H1, H2, and H3 histamine receptors in the rat cochlea. *Neuroreport* 14(3):423–425.

256. Shen, B., Li, H.Z., Wang, J.J. 2002. Excitatory effects of histamine on cerebellar interpositus nuclear cells of rats through H(2) receptors in vitro. *Brain Res.* 948(1–2):64–71.

257. Lomax, P., Green, M.D. 1981. Histaminergic neurons in the hypothalamic thermoregulatory pathways. *Fed. Proc.* 40(13):2741–2745.

258. Szymusiak, R., Gvilia, I., McGinty, D. 2007. Hypothalamic control of sleep. *Sleep Med.* 8(4):291–301.

259. Cote, N.K., Harrington, M.E. 1993. Histamine phase shifts the circadian clock in a manner similar to light. *Brain Res.* 613(1):149–151.

260. Stehle, J. 1991. Effects of histamine on spontaneous electrical activity of neurons in rat suprachiasmatic nucleus. *Neurosci. Lett.* 130(2):217–220.

261. Karlstedt, K., Senkas, A., Ahman, M., Panula, P. 2001. Regional expression of the histamine H(2) receptor in adult and developing rat brain. *Neuroscience* 102(1):201–208.

262. Michelsen, K.A., Lozada, A., Kaslin, J., Karlstedt, K., Kukko-Lukjanov, T.K. et al. 2005. Histamine-immunoreactive neurons in the mouse and rat suprachiasmatic nucleus. *Eur. J. Neurosci.* 22(8):1997–2004.

263. Kjaer, A., Larsen, P.J., Knigge, U., Moller, M., Warberg, J. 1994. Histamine stimulates c-fos expression in hypothalamic vasopressin-, oxytocin-, and corticotropin-releasing hormone-containing neurons. *Endocrinology* 134(1):482–491.

264. Vizuete, M.L., Dimitriadou, V., Traiffort, E., Griffon, N., Heron, A., Schwartz, J.C. 1995. Endogenous histamine induces c-fos expression within paraventricular and supraoptic nuclei. *Neuroreport* 6(7):1041–1044.

265. Bennett, C.T., Pert, A. 1974. Antidiuresis produced by injections of histamine into the cat supraoptic nucleus. *Brain Res.* 78(1):151–156.
266. Tuomisto, L. 1986. Delayed ontogenesis of histamine in the hypothalamus of the homozygous Brattleboro rat. *Agents Actions* 18(1–2):219–221.
267. Haas, H.L., Wolf, P., Nussbaumer, J.C. 1975. Histamine: action on supraoptic and other hypothalamic neurones of the cat. *Brain Res.* 88(1):166–170.
268. Haas, H.L., Wolf, P. 1977. Central actions of histamine: microelectrophoretic studies. *Brain Res.* 122(2):269–279.
269. Li, Z., Miyata, S., Hatton, G.I. 1999. Inositol 1,4,5-trisphosphate-sensitive Ca^{2+} stores in rat supraoptic neurons: involvement in histamine-induced enhancement of depolarizing afterpotentials. *Neuroscience* 93(2):667–674.
270. Smith, B.N., Armstrong, W.E. 1996. The ionic dependence of the histamine-induced depolarization of vasopressin neurones in the rat supraoptic nucleus. *J. Physiol.* 495(Pt 2): 465–478.
271. Armstrong, W.E., Sladek, C.D. 1985. Evidence for excitatory actions of histamine on supraoptic neurons in vitro: mediation by an H1-type receptor. *Neuroscience* 16(2):307–322.
272. Hatton, G.I., Li, Z.H. 1998. Neurophysiology of magnocellular neuroendocrine cells: recent advances. *Prog. Brain Res.* 119:77–99.
273. Hatton, G.I., Yang, Q.Z. 1996. Synaptically released histamine increases dye coupling among vasopressinergic neurons of the supraoptic nucleus: mediation by H1 receptors and cyclic nucleotides. *J. Neurosci.* 16(1):123–129.
274. Yang, Q.Z., Hatton, G.I. 1994. Histamine mediates fast synaptic inhibition of rat supraoptic oxytocin neurons via chloride conductance activation. *Neuroscience* 61(4): 955–964.
275. Bealer, S.L., Crowley, W.R. 2001. Histaminergic control of oxytocin release in the paraventricular nucleus during lactation in rats. *Exp. Neurol.* 171(2):317–322.
276. Luckman, S.M., Larsen, P.J. 1997. Evidence for the involvement of histaminergic neurones in the regulation of the rat oxytocinergic system during pregnancy and parturition. *J. Physiol.* 501(Pt 3):649–655.
277. Knigge, U., Warberg, J. 1991. Neuroendocrine functions of histamine. *Agents Actions Suppl.* 33:29–53.
278. Bugajski, J., Gadek, A. 1983. Central H1- and H2-histaminergic stimulation of pituitary–adrenocortical response under stress in rats. *Neuroendocrinology* 36(6):424–430.
279. Netti, C., Guidobono, F., Olgiati, V.R., Sibilia, V., Pagani, F., Pecile, A. 1982. Influence of brain histaminergic system on episodic growth hormone secretion in the rat. *Neuroendocrinology* 35(1):43–47.
280. Haas, H.L. 1974. Histamine: action on single hypothalamic neurones. *Brain Res.* 76(2):363–366.
281. Renaud, L.P. 1976. Histamine microiontophoresis on identified hypothalamic neurons: 3 patterns of response in the ventromedial nucleus of the rat. *Brain Res.* 115(2):339–344.
282. Jorgenson, K.L., Kow, L.M., Pfaff, D.W. 1989. Histamine excites arcuate neurons in vitro through H1 receptors. *Brain Res.* 502(1):171–179.
283. Li, Y., Gao, X.B., Sakurai, T., van den Pol, A.N. 2002. Hypocretin/Orexin excites hypocretin neurons via a local glutamate neuron-A potential mechanism for orchestrating the hypothalamic arousal system. *Neuron* 36(6):1169–1181.
284. Pape, H.C., McCormick, D.A. 1995. Electrophysiological and pharmacological properties of interneurons in the cat dorsal lateral geniculate nucleus. *Neuroscience* 68(4):1105–1125.
285. Pillot, C., Heron, A., Cochois, V., Tardivel-Lacombe, J., Ligneau, X. et al. 2002. A detailed mapping of the histamine H(3) receptor and its gene transcripts in rat brain. *Neuroscience* 114(1):173–193.

286. Cumming, P., Damsma, G., Fibiger, H.C., Vincent, S.R. 1991. Characterization of extracellular histamine in the striatum and bed nucleus of the stria terminalis of the rat: an in vivo microdialysis study. *J. Neurochem.* 56(5):1797–1803.

287. Sittig, N., Davidowa, H. 2001. Histamine reduces firing and bursting of anterior and intralaminar thalamic neurons and activates striatal cells in anesthetized rats. *Behav. Brain Res.* 124(2):137–143.

288. Sergeeva, O.A., Schulz, D., Doreulee, N., Ponomarenko, A.A., Selbach, O. et al. 2005. Deficits in cortico-striatal synaptic plasticity and behavioral habituation in rats with portacaval anastomosis. *Neuroscience* 134(4):1091–1098.

289. Munakata, M., Akaike, N. 1994. Regulation of K^+ conductance by histamine H1 and H2 receptors in neurones dissociated from rat neostriatum. *J. Physiol.* 480(Pt 2): 233–245.

290. Bell, M.I., Richardson, P.J., Lee, K. 2000. Histamine depolarizes cholinergic interneurones in the rat striatum via a H(1)-receptor mediated action. *Br. J. Pharmacol.* 131(6):1135–1142.

291. Prast, H., Tran, M.H., Lamberti, C., Fischer, H., Kraus, M. et al. 1999. Histaminergic neurons modulate acetylcholine release in the ventral striatum: role of H1 and H2 histamine receptors. *Naunyn Schmiedebergs Arch. Pharmacol.* 360(5):552–557.

292. Bristow, L.J., Bennett, G.W. 1989. Effect of chronic intra-accumbens administration of the TRH analogue CG3509 on histamine-induced behaviour in the rat. *Br. J. Pharmacol.* 97(3):745–752.

293. Alvarez, E.O., Ruarte, M.B. 2004. Glutamic acid and histamine-sensitive neurons in the ventral hippocampus and the basolateral amygdala of the rat: functional interaction on memory and learning processes. *Behav. Brain Res.* 152(2):209–219.

294. Blandina, P., Efoudebe, M., Cenni, G., Mannaioni, P., Passani, M.B. 2004. Acetylcholine, histamine, and cognition: two sides of the same coin. *Learn. Mem.* 11(1):1–8.

295. Passani, M.B., Cangioli, I., Baldi, E., Bucherelli, C., Mannaioni, P.F., Blandina, P. 2001. Histamine H3 receptor-mediated impairment of contextual fear conditioning and in-vivo inhibition of cholinergic transmission in the rat basolateral amygdala. *Eur. J. Neurosci.* 14(9):1522–1532.

296. Bucherelli, C., Baldi, E., Mariottini, C., Passani, M.B., Blandina, P. 2006. Aversive memory reactivation engages in the amygdala only some neurotransmitters involved in consolidation. *Learn. Mem.* 13(4):426–430.

297. Kamei, C. 2001. Involvement of central histamine in amygdaloid kindled seizures in rats. *Behav. Brain Res.* 124(2):243–250.

298. Toyota, H., Ito, C., Yanai, K., Sato, M., Watanabe, T. 1999. Histamine H1 receptor binding capacities in the amygdalas of the amygdaloid kindled rat. *J. Neurochem.* 72(5):2177–2180.

299. Jiang, X., Chen, A., Li, H. 2005. Histaminergic modulation of excitatory synaptic transmission in the rat basolateral amygdala. *Neuroscience* 131(3):691–703.

300. Brown, R.E., Haas, H.L. 1999. On the mechanism of histaminergic inhibition of glutamate release in the rat dentate gyrus. *J. Physiol.* 515(Pt 3):777–786.

301. Weiler, H.T., Hasenohrl, R.U., van Landeghem, A.A., van Landeghem, M., Brankack, J. et al. 1998. Differential modulation of hippocampal signal transfer by tuberomammillary nucleus stimulation in freely moving rats dependent on behavioral state. *Synapse* 28(4):294–301.

302. Greene, R.W., Haas, H.L. 1990. Effects of histamine on dentate granule cells in vitro. *Neuroscience* 34(2):299–303.

303. Gerber, U., Gahwiler, B.H. 1994. GABAB and adenosine receptors mediate enhancement of the K^+ current, IAHP, by reducing adenylyl cyclase activity in rat CA3 hippocampal neurons. *J. Neurophysiol.* 72(5):2360–2367.

304. Kostopoulos, G., Psarropoulou, C., Haas, H.L. 1988. Membrane properties, response to amines and to tetanic stimulation of hippocampal neurons in the genetically epileptic mutant mouse tottering. *Exp. Brain Res.* 72(1):45–50.

305. Yanovsky, Y., Haas, H.L. 1998. Histamine increases the bursting activity of pyramidal cells in the CA3 region of mouse hippocampus. *Neurosci. Lett.* 240(2):110–112.

306. Buzsaki, G., Draguhn, A. 2004. Neuronal oscillations in cortical networks. *Science* 304(5679):1926–1929.

307. Yokoyama, H. 2001. The role of central histaminergic neuron system as an anticonvulsive mechanism in developing brain. *Brain Dev.* 23(7):542–547.

308. Haas, H.L., Greene, R.W. 1986. Effects of histamine on hippocampal pyramidal cells of the rat in vitro. *Exp. Brain Res.* 62(1):123–130.

309. Knoche, A., Yokoyama, H., Ponomarenko, A., Frisch, C., Huston, J., Haas, H.L. 2003. High-frequency oscillation in the hippocampus of the behaving rat and its modulation by the histaminergic system. *Hippocampus* 13(2):273–280.

310. Ponomarenko, A.A., Knoche, A., Korotkova, T.M., Haas, H.L. 2003. Aminergic control of high-frequency (approximately 200 Hz) network oscillations in the hippocampus of the behaving rat. *Neurosci. Lett.* 348(2):101–104.

311. Phillis, J.W., Tebecis, A.K., York, D.H. 1968. Histamine and some antihistamines: their actions on cerebral cortical neurones. *Br. J. Pharmacol. Chemother.* 33(3): 426–440.

312. Haas, H.L., Wolf, P., Palacios, J.M., Garbarg, M., Barbin, G., Schwartz, J.C. 1978. Hypersensitivity to histamine in the guinea-pig brain: microiontophoretic and biochemical studies. *Brain Res.* 156(2):275–291.

313. Lledo, P.M., Alonso. M., Grubb. M.S. 2006. Adult neurogenesis and functional plasticity in neuronal circuits. *Nat. Rev. Neurosci.* 7(3):179–193.

314. Brown, R.E., Stevens, D.R., Haas, H.L. 2001. The physiology of brain histamine. *Prog. Neurobiol.* 63(6):637–672.

315. Yanovsky, Y., Brankack, J., Haas, H.L. 1995. Differences of CA3 bursting in DBA/1 and DBA/2 inbred mouse strains with divergent shuttle box performance. *Neuroscience* 64(2):319–325.

316. Buzsaki, G., Haas, H.L., Anderson, E.G. 1987. Long-term potentiation induced by physiologically relevant stimulus patterns. *Brain Res.* 435(1–2):331–333.

317. Selbach, O., Doreulee, N., Bohla, C., Eriksson, K.S., Sergeeva, O.A. et al. 2004. Orexins/hypocretins cause sharp wave- and theta-related synaptic plasticity in the hippocampus via glutamatergic, gabaergic, noradrenergic, and cholinergic signaling. *Neuroscience* 127(2):519–528.

318. Reymann, K.G., Frey, J.U. 2007. The late maintenance of hippocampal LTP: requirements, phases, 'synaptic tagging', 'late-associativity' and implications. *Neuropharmacology* 52(1):24–40.

319. Selbach, O., Stehle, J., Haas, H.L. 2007. Hippocampal long-term synaptic plasticity is controlled by histamine, hypocretins (orexins) and clock genes. *Soc. Neurosci. Abstr.*: 928.13.

320. Inagaki, N., Fukui, H., Ito, S., Yamatodani, A., Wada, H. 1991. Single type-2 astrocytes show multiple independent sites of Ca^{2+} signaling in response to histamine. *Proc. Natl Acad. Sci. U.S.A.* 88(10):4215–4219.

321. Jung, S., Pfeiffer, F., Deitmer, J.W. 2000. Histamine-induced calcium entry in rat cerebellar astrocytes: evidence for capacitative and non-capacitative mechanisms. *J. Physiol.* 527(Pt 3):549–561.

322. Shelton, M.K., McCarthy, K.D. 2000. Hippocampal astrocytes exhibit Ca^{2+}-elevating muscarinic cholinergic and histaminergic receptors in situ. *J. Neurochem.* 74(2):555–563.

323. Juric, D.M., Miklic, S., Carman-Krzan, M. 2006. Monoaminergic neuronal activity up-regulates BDNF synthesis in cultured neonatal rat astrocytes. *Brain Res.* 1108(1):54–62.
324. Abbott, N.J. 2000. Inflammatory mediators and modulation of blood–brain barrier permeability. *Cell Mol. Neurobiol.* 20(2):131–147.
325. Karlstedt, K., Nissinen, M., Michelsen, K.A., Panula, P. 2001. Multiple sites of L-histidine decarboxylase expression in mouse suggest novel developmental functions for histamine. *Dev. Dyn.* 221(1):81–91.
326. Palkovits, M., Deli, M.A., Gallatz, K., Toth, Z.E., Buzas, E., Falus, A. 2007. Highly activated c-fos expression in specific brain regions (ependyma, circumventricular organs, choroid plexus) of histidine decarboxylase deficient mice in response to formalin-induced acute pain. *Neuropharmacology* 53(1):101–112.
327. Von Economo, C. 1926. Die Pathologie des Schlafes. In *Handbuch des Normalen und Pathologischen Physiologie*, eds. A. Von Bethe, G. Von Bergmann, G. Embden, A. Ellinger, pp. 591–610. Berlin: Springer.
328. Lin, J.S., Sakai, K., Jouvet, M. 1988. Evidence for histaminergic arousal mechanisms in the hypothalamus of cat. *Neuropharmacology* 27(2):111–122.
329. Wu, M.F., Gulyani, S.A., Yau, E., Mignot, E., Phan, B., Siegel, J.M. 1999. Locus coeruleus neurons: cessation of activity during cataplexy. *Neuroscience* 91(4):1389–1399.
330. Ligneau, X., Lin, J., Vanni-Mercier, G., Jouvet, M., Muir, J.L. et al. 1998. Neurochemical and behavioral effects of ciproxifan, a potent histamine H3-receptor antagonist. *J. Pharmacol. Exp. Ther.* 287(2):658–666.
331. Monti, J.M., Jantos, H., Boussard, M., Altier, H., Orellana, C., Olivera, S. 1991. Effects of selective activation or blockade of the histamine H3 receptor on sleep and wakefulness. *Eur. J. Pharmacol.* 205(3):283–287.
332. Monti, J.M., Jantos, H., Ponzoni, A., Monti, D. 1996. Sleep and waking during acute histamine H3 agonist BP 2.94 or H3 antagonist carboperamide (MR 16155) administration in rats. *Neuropsychopharmacology* 15(1):31–35.
333. Monti, J.M., Pellejero, T., Jantos, H. 1986. Effects of H1- and H2-histamine receptor agonists and antagonists on sleep and wakefulness in the rat. *J. Neural Transm.* 66(1):1–11.
334. Parmentier, R., Anaclet, C., Guhennec, C., Brousseau, E., Bricout, D. et al. 2007. The brain H(3)-receptor as a novel therapeutic target for vigilance and sleep–wake disorders. *Biochem. Pharmacol.* 73(8):1157–1171.
335. Lin, J.S., Sakai, K., Jouvet, M. 1994. Hypothalamo-preoptic histaminergic projections in sleep–wake control in the cat. *Eur. J. Neurosci.* 6(4):618–625.
336. Vanni-Mercier, G., Gigout, S., Debilly, G., Lin, J.S. 2003. Waking selective neurons in the posterior hypothalamus and their response to histamine H3-receptor ligands: an electrophysiological study in freely moving cats. *Behav. Brain Res.* 144(1–2):227–241.
337. Nelson, L.E., Lu, J., Guo, T., Saper, C.B., Franks, N.P., Maze, M. 2003. The alpha2-adrenoceptor agonist dexmedetomidine converges on an endogenous sleep-promoting pathway to exert its sedative effects. *Anesthesiology* 98(2):428–436.
338. Scammell, T.E., Estabrooke, I.V., McCarthy, M.T., Chemelli, R.M., Yanagisawa, M. et al. 2000. Hypothalamic arousal regions are activated during modafinil-induced wakefulness. *J. Neurosci.* 20(22):8620–8628.
339. Orr, E., Quay, W.B. 1975. Hypothalamic 24-hour rhythms in histamine, histidine, decarboxylase and histamine-N-methyltransferase. *Endocrinology* 96(4):941–945.
340. Mochizuki, T., Yamatodani, A., Okakura, K., Horii, A., Inagaki, N., Wada, H. 1992. Circadian rhythm of histamine release from the hypothalamus of freely moving rats. *Physiol. Behav.* 51(2):391–394.
341. Onoe, H., Watanabe, Y., Ono, K., Koyama, Y., Hayaishi, O. 1992. Prostaglandin E2 exerts an awaking effect in the posterior hypothalamus at a site distinct from that mediating its febrile action in the anterior hypothalamus. *J. Neurosci.* 12(7):2715–2725.

342. Siegel, J.M. 2004. Hypocretin (orexin): role in normal behavior and neuropathology. *Annu. Rev. Psychol.* 55:125–148.
343. Steininger, T.L., Alam, M.N., Gong, H., Szymusiak, R., McGinty, D. 1999. Sleep–waking discharge of neurons in the posterior lateral hypothalamus of the albino rat. *Brain Res.* 840(1–2):138–147.
344. Siegel, J.M., Nienhuis, R., Fahringer, H.M., Paul, R., Shiromani, P. et al. 1991. Neuronal activity in narcolepsy: identification of cataplexy-related cells in the medial medulla. *Science* 252(5010):1315–1318.
345. Lu, J., Bjorkum, A.A., Xu, M., Gaus, S.E., Shiromani, P.J., Saper, C.B. 2002. Selective activation of the extended ventrolateral preoptic nucleus during rapid eye movement sleep. *J. Neurosci.* 22(11):4568–4576.
346. Masaki, T., Yoshimatsu, H. 2006. The hypothalamic H1 receptor: a novel therapeutic target for disrupting diurnal feeding rhythm and obesity. *Trends Pharmacol. Sci.* 27(5):279–284.
347. Jorgensen, E.A., Knigge, U., Warberg, J., Kjaer, A. 2007. Histamine and the regulation of body weight. *Neuroendocrinology* 86(3):210–214.
348. Ookuma, K., Sakata, T., Fukagawa, K., Yoshimatsu, H., Kurokawa, M. et al. 1993. Neuronal histamine in the hypothalamus suppresses food intake in rats. *Brain Res.* 628(1–2):235–242.
349. Masaki, T., Yoshimatsu, H., Chiba, S., Watanabe, T., Sakata, T. 2001. Central infusion of histamine reduces fat accumulation and upregulates UCP family in leptin-resistant obese mice. *Diabetes* 50(2):376–384.
350. Fujise, T., Yoshimatsu, H., Kurokawa, M., Oohara, A., Kang, M. et al. 1998. Satiation and masticatory function modulated by brain histamine in rats. *Proc. Soc. Exp. Biol. Med.* 217(2):228–234.
351. Green, M.D., Cox, B., Lomax, P. 1976. Sites and mechanisms of action of histamine in the central thermoregulatory pathways of the rat. *Neuropharmacology* 15(5): 321–324.
352. Clark, W.G., Cumby, H.R. 1976. Biphasic changes in body temperature produced by intracerebroventricular injections of histamine in the cat. *J. Physiol.* 261(1):235–253.
353. Tsai, C.L., Matsumura, K., Nakayama, T., Itowi, N., Yamatodani, A., Wada, H. 1989. Effects of histamine on thermosensitive neurons in rat preoptic slice preparations. *Neurosci. Lett.* 102(2–3):297–302.
354. McGinty, D., Szymusiak, R. 1990. Keeping cool: a hypothesis about the mechanisms and functions of slow-wave sleep. *Trends Neurosci.* 13(12):480–487.
355. Sallmen, T., Beckman, A.L., Stanton, T.L., Eriksson, K.S., Tarhanen, J. et al. 1999. Major changes in the brain histamine system of the ground squirrel citellus lateralis during hibernation. *J. Neurosci.* 19(5):1824–1835.
356. Sallmen, T., Lozada, A.F., Anichtchik, O.V., Beckman, A.L., Leurs, R., Panula, P. 2003. Changes in hippocampal histamine receptors across the hibernation cycle in ground squirrels. *Hippocampus* 13(6):745–754.
357. Klapdor, K., Hasenohrl, R.U., Huston, J.P. 1994. Facilitation of learning in adult and aged rats following bilateral lesions of the tuberomammillary nucleus region. *Behav. Brain Res.* 61(1):113–116.
358. Onodera, K., Yamatodani, A., Watanabe, T., Wada, H. 1994. Neuropharmacology of the histaminergic neuron system in the brain and its relationship with behavioral disorders. *Prog. Neurobiol.* 42(6):685–702.
359. de Almeida, M.A., Izquierdo, I. 1986. Memory facilitation by histamine. *Arch. Int. Pharmacodyn. Ther.* 283(2):193–198.
360. da Silva, W.C., Bonini, J.S., Bevilaqua, L.R., Izquierdo, I., Cammarota, M. 2006. Histamine enhances inhibitory avoidance memory consolidation through a H2 receptor-dependent mechanism. *Neurobiol. Learn. Mem.* 86(1):100–106.

361. Netto, C.A., Izquierdo, I. 1985. Posterior hypothalamic deafferentation abolishes the amnestic effect of electroconvulsive shock in rats. *Psychoneuroendocrinology* 10(2):159–163.

362. Passani, M.B., Giannoni, P., Bucherelli, C., Baldi, E., Blandina, P. 2007. Histamine in the brain: beyond sleep and memory. *Biochem. Pharmacol.* 73(8):1113–1122.

363. Liu, L., Zhang, S., Zhu, Y., Fu, Q., Zhu, Y. et al. 2007. Improved learning and memory of contextual fear conditioning and hippocampal CA1 long-term potentiation in histidine decarboxylase knock-out mice. *Hippocampus* 17(8):634–641.

364. Dere, E., Souza-Silva, M.A., Spieler, R.E., Lin, J.S., Ohtsu, H. et al. 2004. Changes in motoric, exploratory and emotional behaviours and neuronal acetylcholine content and 5-HT turnover in histidine decarboxylase-KO mice. *Eur. J. Neurosci.* 20(4):1051–1058.

365. Dere, E., Souza-Silva, M.A., Topic, B., Spieler, R.E., Haas, H.L., Huston, J.P. 2003. Histidine-decarboxylase knockout mice show deficient nonreinforced episodic object memory, improved negatively reinforced water-maze performance, and increased neo- and ventro-striatal dopamine turnover. *Learn. Mem.* 10(6):510–519.

366. Giovannini, M.G., Efoudebe, M., Passani, M.B., Baldi, E., Bucherelli, C. et al. 2003. Improvement in fear memory by histamine-elicited ERK2 activation in hippocampal CA3 cells. *J. Neurosci.* 23(27):9016–9023.

367. Brown, R.E., Fedorov, N.B., Haas, H.L., Reymann, K.G. 1995. Histaminergic modulation of synaptic plasticity in area CA1 of rat hippocampal slices. *Neuropharmacology* 34(2):181–190.

368. Selbach, O., Haas, H.L. 2006. Hypocretins: the timing of sleep and waking. *Chronobiol. Int.* 23(1–2):63–70.

369. Alvarez, E.O., Alvarez, P.A. 2007. Motivated exploratory behaviour in the rat: the role of hippocampus and the histaminergic neurotransmission. *Behav. Brain Res.* 186(1):118–125.

370. Alvarez, E.O., Ruarte, M.B. 2002. Histaminergic neurons of the ventral hippocampus and the baso-lateral amygdala of the rat: functional interaction on memory and learning mechanisms. *Behav. Brain Res.* 128(1):81–90.

371. Alvarez, E.O., Banzan, A.M. 2001. Functional regional distribution of histamine receptors in the rat hippocampus: modulation of learning of an active avoidance response. *J. Neural Transm.* 108(11):1249–1261.

372. Alvarez, E.O., Ruarte, M.B., Banzan, A.M. 2001. Histaminergic systems of the limbic complex on learning and motivation. *Behav. Brain Res.* 124(2):195–202.

373. Acevedo, S.F., Pfankuch, T., Ohtsu, H., Raber, J. 2006. Anxiety and cognition in female histidine decarboxylase knockout (Hdc(−/−)) mice. *Behav. Brain Res.* 168(1):92–99.

374. Orsetti, M., Ferretti, C., Gamalero, R., Ghi, P. 2002. Histamine H3-receptor blockade in the rat nucleus basalis magnocellularis improves place recognition memory. *Psychopharmacology* (Berl) 159(2):133–137.

375. Cangioli, I., Baldi, E., Mannaioni, P.F., Bucherelli, C., Blandina, P., Passani, M.B. 2002. Activation of histaminergic H3 receptors in the rat basolateral amygdala improves expression of fear memory and enhances acetylcholine release. *Eur. J. Neurosci.* 16(3):521–528.

376. Baldi, E., Bucherelli, C., Schunack, W., Cenni, G., Blandina, P., Passani, M.B. 2005. The H3 receptor protean agonist proxyfan enhances the expression of fear memory in the rat. *Neuropharmacology* 48(2):246–251.

377. Van Meer, P., Pfankuch, T., Raber, J. 2007. Reduced histamine levels and H(3) receptor antagonist-induced histamine release in the amygdala of Apoe−/− mice. *J. Neurochem.* 103(1):124–130.

378. Rubio, S., Begega, A., Santin, L.J., Arias, J.L. 2002. Improvement of spatial memory by (R)-alpha-methylhistamine, a histamine H(3)-receptor agonist, on the Morris water-maze in rat. *Behav. Brain Res.* 129(1–2):77–82.

379. Lozeva, V., Tuomisto, L., Sola, D., Plumed, C., Hippelainen, M., Butterworth, R. 2001. Increased density of brain histamine H(1) receptors in rats with portacaval anastomosis and in cirrhotic patients with chronic hepatic encephalopathy. *Hepatology* 33(6):1370–1376.

380. Fogel, W.A., Andrzejewski, W., Maslinski, C. 1991. Brain histamine in rats with hepatic encephalopathy. *J. Neurochem.* 56(1):38–43.

381. Lozeva, V., Valjakka, A., Anttila, E., MacDonald, E., Hippelainen, M., Tuomisto, L. 1999. Brain histamine levels and neocortical slow-wave activity in rats with portacaval anastomosis. *Hepatology* 29(2):340–346.

382. Lintunen, M., Hyytia, P., Sallmen, T., Karlstedt, K., Tuomisto, L. et al. 2001. Increased brain histamine in an alcohol-preferring rat line and modulation of ethanol consumption by H(3) receptor mechanisms. *FASEB J.* 15(6):1074–1076.

383. Nakamura, S., Takemura, M., Ohnishi, K., Suenaga, T., Nishimura, M. et al. 1993. Loss of large neurons and occurrence of neurofibrillary tangles in the tuberomammillary nucleus of patients with Alzheimer's disease. *Neurosci. Lett.* 151(2):196–199.

384. Panula, P., Rinne, J., Kuokkanen, K., Eriksson, K.S., Sallmen, T. et al. 1998. Neuronal histamine deficit in Alzheimer's disease. *Neuroscience* 82(4):993–997.

385. Schneider, C., Risser, D., Kirchner, L., Kitzmuller, E., Cairns, N. et al. 1997. Similar deficits of central histaminergic system in patients with Down syndrome and Alzheimer disease. *Neurosci. Lett.* 222(3):183–186.

386. Anichtchik, O.V., Peitsaro, N., Rinne, J.O., Kalimo, H., Panula, P. 2001. Distribution and modulation of histamine H(3) receptors in basal ganglia and frontal cortex of healthy controls and patients with Parkinson's disease. *Neurobiol. Dis.* 8(4):707–716.

387. Martinez-Mir, M.I., Pollard, H., Moreau, J., Traiffort, E., Ruat, M. et al. 1993. Loss of striatal histamine H2 receptors in Huntington's chorea but not in Parkinson's disease: comparison with animal models. *Synapse* 15(3):209–220.

388. Ikoma, A., Steinhoff, M., Stander, S., Yosipovitch, G., Schmelz, M. 2006. The neurobiology of itch. *Nat. Rev. Neurosci.* 7(7):535–547.

389. Andrew, D., Craig, A.D. 2001. Spinothalamic lamina I neurons selectively sensitive to histamine: a central neural pathway for itch. *Nat. Neurosci.* 4(1):72–77.

390. Cannon, K.E., Chazot, P.L., Hann, V., Shenton, F., Hough, L.B., Rice, F.L. 2007. Immunohistochemical localization of histamine H3 receptors in rodent skin, dorsal root ganglia, superior cervical ganglia, and spinal cord: potential antinociceptive targets. *Pain* 129(1–2):76–92.

391. Hough, L.B., Nalwalk, J.W., Barnes, W.G., Leurs, R., Menge, W.M. et al. 2000. A third life for burimamide. Discovery and characterization of a novel class of non-opioid analgesics derived from histamine antagonists. *Ann. N. Y. Acad. Sci.* 909:25–40.

392. Mobarakeh, J.I., Takahashi, K., Sakurada, S., Nishino, S., Watanabe, H. et al. 2005. Enhanced antinociception by intracerebroventricularly administered orexin A in histamine H1 or H2 receptor gene knockout mice. *Pain* 118(1–2):254–262.

393. Musio, S., Gallo, B., Scabeni, S., Lapilla, M., Poliani, P.L. et al. 2006. A key regulatory role for histamine in experimental autoimmune encephalomyelitis: disease exacerbation in histidine decarboxylase-deficient mice. *J. Immunol.* 176(1):17–26.

394. Guerrero, R.O., Cardenas, M.A., Ocampo, A.A., Pacheco, M.F. 1999. Histamine as a therapeutic alternative in migraine prophylaxis: a randomized, placebo-controlled, double-blind study. *Headache* 39(8):576–580.

395. Togha, M., Ashrafian, H., Tajik, P. 2006. Open-label trial of cinnarizine in migraine prophylaxis. *Headache* 46(3):498–502.

Section B

The Third Histamine Receptor

4 Phylogeny, Gene Structure, Expression, and Signaling

Pertti Panula, CongYu Jin,
Kaj Karlstedt, and Remko A. Bakker

CONTENTS

Identification of the Histamine H$_3$ Receptor 83
Histamine H3R Signal Transduction 84
Gene Structure and Isoforms 84
Expression in Vertebrate Tissues 87
Developmental Expression 88
Expression in Human Brain 89
    General Expression Patterns 89
    Prefrontal Cortex 89
    Temporal Cortex 89
    Thalamus 89
    Hippocampal Formation and Entorhinal Cortex 91
    Basal Ganglia 92
Regulation of H3R Expression in Physiological
    and Pathophysiological Conditions 92
    General Considerations 92
    Hibernation 93
    Ischemia, Epilepsy, and Brain Trauma 94
    Addiction and Alcohol-Related Behavior 95
    Vestibular Compensation 96
Acknowledgments 96
References 97

IDENTIFICATION OF THE HISTAMINE H$_3$ RECEPTOR

The histamine H$_3$ receptor (H3R), which mediates a negative feedback on the release of histamine from rat brain slices, was identified in 1983 [1]. The receptor received significant interest ever since this first pharmacological description as shown in several authoritative reviews on various aspects of its biology. The cloning of the human H3R cDNA in 1999 [2] has subsequently led to a rapid expansion in the knowledge on the molecular mechanisms of the H3R actions. Currently, the H3R has shown promise as a potential therapeutic target in the central nervous system (CNS) for the treatment of various diseases, including obesity and cognitive disorders (for detailed reviews see Refs 3–8). The first isolated hH3R cDNA encodes a 445 amino acid protein (hH3R$_{445}$), and initial suggestions of the G-protein-coupled receptor (GPCR) nature of the H3R based on H3R agonist-induced [^{35}S]GTPγS binding [9,10], GTP- and pertussis toxin (PTX) sensitivity of H3R radioligand binding, and responses [9,11] were confirmed. The identification of the H3R at the molecular level subsequently allowed a great boost in H3R research. Not only this resulted in a great increase in the understanding of the H3R at the molecular level, including the identification of numerous H3R splice variants, but also numerous pharmaceutical companies have programs to identify selective and potent H3R antagonists. The progress that has been made in the development of H3R ligands has been elaborately reviewed elsewhere [3,4,12].

HISTAMINE H3R SIGNAL TRANSDUCTION

The cloning of the H3R cDNA allowed detailed studies of its function and molecular mechanisms following its activation. Those studies have indicated the ability of the H3R to modulate several intracellular signal transduction pathways. These include the Gα$_{i/o}$-dependent inhibition of adenylyl cyclase (AC), activation of phospholipase A$_2$ (PLA$_2$), the phosphorylation of Akt, and the mitogen-activated kinases (MAPK), and the inhibition of the Na$^+$/H$^+$ exchanger [13,14] and K$^+$-induced Ca^{2+} mobilization [15,16]. Of these, the activation of Gα$_{i/o}$ proteins, the inhibition of AC, and the activation of PLA$_2$ and MAPK are the best studied. The heterologous expression of the human H3R confirmed initial suggestions on the Gα$_{i/o}$-coupled nature of the H3R as the activation of the receptor led to the PTX-sensitive inhibition of forskolin-induced cAMP formation [13,17–20]. Besides assays that measure the intracellular levels of cAMP, to measure the activation of Gα$_{i/o}$ proteins directly, [^{35}S]GTPγS-binding assays are also commonly performed for assaying H3R activity. Activity of the H3R on either AC or [^{35}S]GTPγS binding independently from agonists, that is, spontaneous or constitutive activity, can be readily detected. Various H3R antagonists including thioperamide, clobenpropit, and ciproxyfan have been shown to inhibit this constitutive H3R activity and hence are inverse H3R agonists [13,17]. The H3R-mediated activation of Gα$_{i/o}$ proteins may also result in the activation of PLA$_2$ as well as in a G$_{βγ}$-mediated activation of MAPK [21,22] and the phospho-inositol-3-kinase (PI3K)/protein kinase B (PKB, also known as Akt)/GSK-3β pathway (Figure 4.1). As discussed later in this chapter, plastic changes in H3R mRNA expression occur in several pathophysiological conditions, which make the MAPK and Akt signaling of H3R functionally important in brain trauma, ischemia, and excitotoxicity.

GENE STRUCTURE AND ISOFORMS

Molecular identification of the first human H3R in 1999 [2] also allowed studies on this receptor in other species. Since then the H3R has been characterized at least in guinea pig [23], rat [22,24,25], mouse [26,27], dog (GenBank accession # AY 231165;

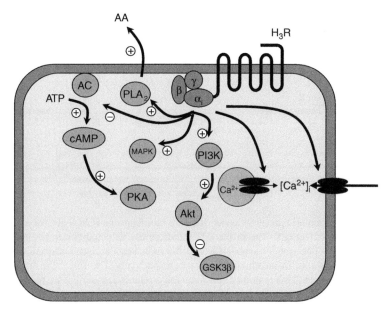

FIGURE 4.1 H3R-mediated signal transduction. The H3R can modulate several signal transduction pathways, including the inhibition of AC, the activation of MAPK and PLA_2, as well as the modulation of intracellular calcium levels through Ca^{2+} channels and the Akt/GSK-3b axis.

AY231166), hamster [28], monkey [29], rabbit (GenBank accession # DQ826506), and zebrafish [30]. The H3R was found to have several different variants (isoforms) with differential coupling to second messenger systems, and isoforms were detected not only in man [31] and rat [17,22], but also in guinea pig [23] and mouse [27]. Heterogeneity had been observed in binding properties of H3R ligands to membranes, suggesting the existence of receptor subtypes [32,33]. Alternative splicing event during gene transcription is probably the main cause for the occurrence of these receptor modifications. Many GPCRs are transcribed from intronless genes but, for example, the human H3R gene is suggested to consist of either three exons and two introns [31,34] or four exons and three introns [19,35], facilitating the rearrangements of the cDNA sequences and ultimately the receptor proteins. H3R variability is further increased by several polymorphisms, resulting in single amino acid alteration in the coding sequence [5,36].

In rat, the H3R gene is located on chromosome 20, and it contains three or four introns. Three different functional isoforms (H3A, H3B, and H3C) and one nonfunctional truncated isoform (H3T) were identified [22]. Using polymerase chain reaction (PCR), the full-length isoform appears to predominate in most rat brain regions [17]. With a set of oligonucleotide probes and *in situ* hybridization, the expression patterns of the functional isoforms were determined. The strategy for probe design is described in Figure 4.2. The hybridization signal given by the probe detecting the H3C transcript was strong in striatum, olfactory tubercle, cortical layers V and VIb, pyramidal layers of hippocampal fields CA1 and CA2, dorsal thalamic nuclei,

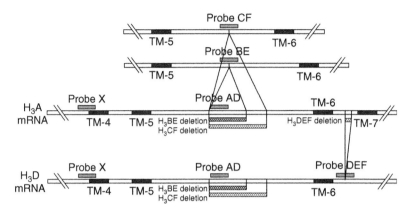

FIGURE 4.2 A schematic presentation of different rat histamine H3R isoforms and probes used in *in situ* hybridizations. The probe AD indicates the detected site in the full-length intracellular loop 3. The site for probes CF and BE indicates the region used to detect the long and short deletion in intracellular loop three, respectively. The splice site between the putative transmembrane (TM) regions 6 and 7 and the produced transcripts are recognized by the probe marked DEF. All indicated isoforms are detected by the upstream oligonucleotide probe marked as probe X.

ventromedial hypothalamic nucleus, locus coeruleus, tuberomammillary nucleus, trapezoid body, and cerebellar Purkinje cells. Moderate H3C expression was seen in layer II of the cerebral cortex and low in medial septum, diagonal band, and substantia inominata [22]. The H3A isoform expression was most prominent in the dorsal part of dentate gyrus, and the expression levels in pyramidal layer of hippocampal field CA1 was strongest in ventral hippocampus [22]. The overall expression of H3B was very weak, with the highest levels seen in ventral and ventrolateral tuberomammillary nuclei [22]. A representative set of images showing the mid-thalamic-level expression of the three indicated H3 isoforms can be seen in Figure 4.3. The total H3R expression can be estimated from a section hybridized with a probe that detects all isoforms (see Figure 4.2 for probe design).

In the rat H3 gene, there is a putative intron between the predicted transmembrane (TM) regions 6 and 7. It has recently been seen that splicing events at this site create a frameshift deletion that eliminates the main stop codon replacing the last 53 amino acids with a new set of 105 amino acids, thus altering and extending the carboxyterminal part of the receptor. This splicing also eliminates the TM7 region, creating a receptor that is predicted to have only six TM regions (6TM-rH3 isoforms) with the carboxyterminal tail flipped to an extracellular position [37]. Combination of the splicing of this fourth intron and alternative splicing of the third intron results in three additional isoforms defined as histamine receptors H3D, H3E, and H3F, respectively (see Figure 4.1 for a schematic presentation). Although these 6TM receptors are unable to bind histamine and other known and tested histamine receptor ligands, they seem to have a crucial effect on signaling acting as dominant-negative isoforms [37]. Their expression pattern, at least in the rat brain, overlaps substantially with the expression pattern of the classical 7TM-histamine H3 receptors (7TM-rH3Rs). Expression studies conducted with 6TM-rH3-specific

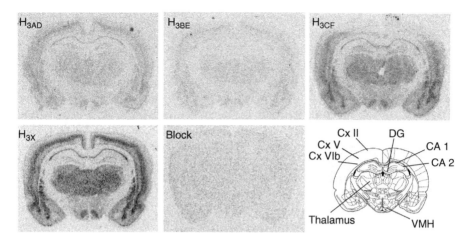

FIGURE 4.3 Midthalamic level sections from rat brain after *in situ* hybridization with specific oligonucleotides for H3AD, H3BE, and H3CF isoforms. The section hybridized with the H3X probe indicates the overall expression of all H3 isoforms, and the *block* section is from a control experiment where excess application (100-fold) of cold probe is shown to block the specific signal. Note the strong expression in the cortical laminae, dorsal thalamus, verntromedial hypothalamic nucleus, amygdale, and the pyramidal layer of CA1 subfield of the hippocampus. (Cx VIb, cerebral cortex layer VIb; Cx V, cerebral cortex layer V; Cx II, cerebral cortex layer II; DG, dentate gyrus; CA1 pyramidal layers of hippocampal fields CA1; CA2, pyramidal layers of hippocampal fields CA2; and VMH, ventromedial thalamic nuclei.)

oligonucleotides show that these isoforms could be coupled to a novel physiological mechanism controlling the overall activity of the histaminergic system, as will be discussed in more detail later in this chapter.

The H3R gene structure is well preserved in vertebrate evolution. The zebrafish receptor has also three exons, and the protein sequence shows 42–50% similarity to mouse, rat, dog, and human receptors [30].

EXPRESSION IN VERTEBRATE TISSUES

H3R is best known as a CNS receptor, although its expression has also been demonstrated in peripheral organs such as the gut, heart, and skin. The identification of H4R as a major peripheral histamine receptor has rendered pharmacological evidence somewhat difficult to interpret, as these two closely related receptors share many ligands. Many studies provide evidence for only mRNA or protein expression rather than both, or pharmacological effects, which are difficult to interpret. Until all these methods have yielded parallel results, care should be taken in the interpretation of results for peripheral H3R. In the brain, the results are more clear-cut, as H3R expression in several regions is abundant, and consistent evidence with several methods has been easy to collect.

In the rat brain, H3R is widely expressed in all parts of the brain (telencephalon, diencephalon, mesencephalon, myelencephalon, cerebellum, and spinal cord)

[22,38]. In agreement with the autoreceptor nature of H3R, the histaminergic tubero-mamillary neurons express high levels of mRNA, as do the serotonergic raphe neurons. In telencephalon, for example, the olfactory tubercle, cerebral cortex (laminae V and VIb), striatum, hippocampus (pyramidal layers of CA1 and CA2), and amygdala express H3R. In diencephalon, the ventromedial nucleus expresses H3R in addition to the TMN neurons. In the cerebellum, the highest expression is in Purkinje cells. In the mouse brain, H3R expression resembles that of the rat brain: abundant expression in the cerebral cortex, striatum, TMN neurons, and dorsal thalamus [27]. Rouleau et al. [27] also point out some significant differences to the rat expression: low expression was found in the mouse stria terminalis, and the expression in the thalamic nuclei was more uneven than in the rat. In the hippocampus, CA1 area in the mouse showed low expression in contrast to the rat. These results fit rather well with the localization of H3R protein in CA3 and dentate gyrus of the hippocampus, lamina V of the cerebral cortex, the olfactory tubercle, Purkinje cell layer of the cerebellum, substantia nigra, globus pallidus, thalamus, and striatum [39].

In zebrafish, H3R mRNA is detected by PCR in the brain and also in the heart and spleen [30]. It is interesting that the H4R has not yet been identified in the zebrafish genome, and it remains possible that H3R serves corresponding functions in fish. However, histamine is certainly made only in the brain of the zebrafish [40], and more detailed studies on the expression of histidine decarboxylase should be carried out using high-resolution *in situ* hybridization. *In situ* hybridization of H3R has not been carried out, but H3R radioligand binding is high in the optic tectum and dorsal zone of periventricular hypothalamus, and lower binding can be found in other parts of the hypothalamus, torus semicircularis, and dorsal tegmental area [41].

DEVELOPMENTAL EXPRESSION

In agreement with the multiple functions in the body, both histidine decarboxylase (HDC) and H3R are expressed widely during development. In addition to the nervous system, embryonal rat kidney, heart, liver, thymus, epithelial cells in skin, and gastrointestinal tract have been reported to express H3R mRNA using PCR and *in situ* hybridization methods [42]. Several isoforms of H3R were amplified from embryonal rat adipose tissue and liver [42]. Using oligonucleotide probes, Karlstedt et al. [40] reported a distinct but limited expression of H3R mRNA in the developing brown adipose tissue and CNS. The high expression of H3R mRNA in the brown adipose tissue during fetal development suggests that at this age, histamine through H3R may be an important direct regulator of metabolism. Soon after birth, the expression became nondetectable for *in situ* hybridization, which suggests rapid downregulation in brown adipose tissue. In the rat CNS, H3R expression is detectable on day E14 [42], and it is high already on day E16 in the thalamus, hypothalamus, and midbrain [40]. Many areas, which show modest expression in adults, such as spinal cord, display significant expression during fetal life [40,42]. One study also reports H3R mRNA expression in spinal ganglia [42], whereas another detected distinct peripheral H3R mRNA only in the brown adipose tissue [40]. The difference in these two studies may be in part due to differences in sensitivity of the methods, because one used RNA probes [42] whereas the other applied synthetic oligonucleotide probes [40]. Using antibodies against synthetic peptides conjugated to carrier proteins, H3R-like immunoreactivity has been localized to medium-sized to large dorsal root gangli neurons in the rat and mouse, and in a subset of principal sympathetic ganglion cells [43]. So far, no evidence about the presence of H3R mRNA in sympathetic ganglion cells has been published.

EXPRESSION IN HUMAN BRAIN

GENERAL EXPRESSION PATTERNS

So far, the expression pattern of H3Rs has been studied in several crucial human fore-brain regions including the cortex, thalamus, and basal ganglia. Receptor expression in some midbrain areas such as substantia nigra has also been reported [44]. Both *in situ* hybridization and receptor-binding autoradiography have been applied to reveal the mRNA expression sites and receptor localization.

PREFRONTAL CORTEX

In the prefrontal cortex, three histamine receptors (H1R, H2R, and H3R) show lami-nar preference in their mRNA expression patterns (Figures 4.4A through 4.4C and 4.5). The mRNA expression of H3R is detected in the gray matter with the highest expression level in the cortical layer 5 and the lowest expression level in layer 1. This laminar distribution pattern is similar throughout the eulaminate, dysgranular, and agranular prefrontal cortical areas in the human brain [45].

Compared to the mRNA expression pattern, the distribution pattern of H3R binding detected by $[^3H]N^\alpha$-methylhistamine is fairly even in the gray matter of the human prefrontal cortex and a thin layer of white matter is adjacent to the gray matter (Figures 4.4D and 4.5). Slightly higher density of $[^3H]N^\alpha$-methylhistamine-binding sites is seen in the middle cortical layers (deep lamina III and lamina IV) where the densest thalamic inputs are found, whereas the lowest binding density is seen in the superficial layer 1 and deep layer 6 [45].

TEMPORAL CORTEX

In the temporal cortex, H3R-binding sites detected by $[^3H]N^\alpha$-methylhistamine are also mainly seen in the gray matter (Figure 4.4E). Similar to that of the prefrontal cortex, the highest density of $[^3H]N^\alpha$-methylhistamine-binding sites is seen in the middle cortical layers (layers 3 and 4), whereas the lowest density is seen in the deep layer 6 (Jin and Panula, in preparation). However, one previous study reported a slightly different binding pattern using $[^3H](R)\alpha$-methylhistamine as a ligand [46]; the external cortical layers showed higher binding densities in both prefrontal and temporal cortices.

THALAMUS

H3R mRNA is expressed at a high intensity in the human dorsal thalamus [47] (Figures 4.4F and 4.5), the only part of thalamus that projects to the cortex. In general, high to moderate expression level is seen in most of the principal relay nuclei (anterior, lateral, and medial nuclei; lateral geniculate nucleus), midline and internal

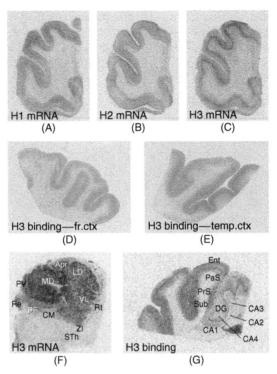

FIGURE 4.4 mRNA expression patterns of histamine receptors and H3R radioligand ($[^3H]N^\alpha$-methylhistamine)-binding patterns in the human brain. (A) H1R mRNA expression pattern in the human prefrontal cortex. The expression level is highest in layers 1, 5, and 6. (B) H2R mRNA expression pattern in the human prefrontal cortex. The expression level is highest in layer 2. (C) H3R mRNA expression pattern in the human prefrontal cortex. The expression level is highest in layer 5. (D) $[^3H]N^\alpha$-methylhistamine binding pattern in the human dorsal lateral prefrontal cortex. (E) $[^3H]N^\alpha$-methylhistamine binding pattern in the human superior temporal cortex. (F) H3R mRNA expression pattern in the human thalamus. (G) $[^3H]N^\alpha$-methylhistamine binding pattern in the human anterior hippocampal formation and entorhinal cortex. (APr, anteroprinciple thalamic nucleus; CM, centromedian nucleus; DG, dentate gyrus; Ent, entorhinal cortex; PaS, parasubiculum; PrS, presubiculum; LD, laterodorsal nucleus; MD, mediodorsal nucleus; PF, parafascicular nucleus; PV, paraventricular thalamic nucleus; Re, reuniens; Rt, reticular nucleus; Sub, subthalamic nucleus; VL, ventrolateral nucleus; and ZI, zona incerta.)

medullary laminar nuclei, whereas the expression level is low in the medial geniculate nucleus, posterior thalamic region (pulvinar), and the ventral thalamus (reticular nucleus and zona incerta). The expression is particularly abundant in the associate relays that project to the prefrontal cortex, such as the mediodorsal thalamic nucleus.

H3R-binding sites are detectable using $[^3H]N^\alpha$-methylhistamine [47] or $[^3H](R)$ α-methylhistamine as ligands. The highest density of binding sites was seen in the midline nuclei (reuniens, paraventricular, and subhabenula), mediodorsal nucleus, some of the internal medullary laminar nuclei (parafascicular, paratenial, and

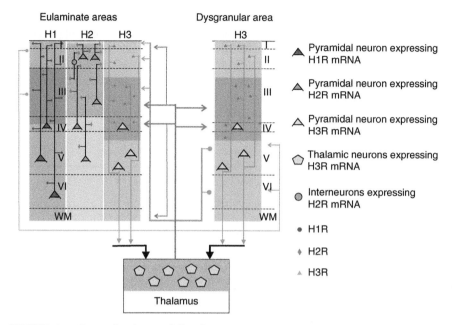

FIGURE 4.5 (See color insert following page 148.) Summary of the mRNA expression and receptor ligand-binding patterns of three histamine receptors (H1, H2, and H3) in the human prefrontal cortex (using eulaminate areas as an example), and the possible connections between the cortical areas and within the thalamocortical system. The presence of mRNA in the cell bodies and distribution of the receptor protein within the axons and dendrites underlies the discrepancy between the mRNA expression and receptor ligand-binding patterns. Most of the neurons expressing H1 and H3R mRNA are located in the deep cortical layers of the eulaminate areas. Most neurons expressing H2R mRNA are located in the superficial cortical layers. H1R and H2R expressed by the pyramidal neurons might locate on their ascending apical dendrites and contribute to the detected receptor ligand-binding sites in the upper cortical layers. H3R expressed by the pyramidal neurons in the deep layers might be located on their axonal terminals in the upper layers. The pyramidal neurons in the deep layers of the dysgranular areas also send axonal projections to the upper layers of the eulaminate areas; therefore, part of the H3R expressed by the pyramidal neurons in the dysgranular areas might be located on the axonal terminals in the upper layers of the eulaminate areas and contribute to the detectable receptor ligand-binding sites there. In addition, pyramidal neurons in lamina V project to the dorsal thalamus, and neurons in dorsal thalamus project to the cortex, mostly targeting the middle layers (laminae III, IV). Thus, some of the detected H3R ligand-binding sites in the middle cortical layers are located on the terminals of the dorsal thalamic inputs, and vice versa. It cannot be overlooked that part of the H2R-expressing neurons in the upper layers are interneurons.

fasciculosus), and parts of the pulvinar (medial, inferior, and diffuse). The binding level is generally low in other parts of the thalamus.

HIPPOCAMPAL FORMATION AND ENTORHINAL CORTEX

H3R radioligand [^{3}H]N$^\alpha$-methylhistamine binding is detected through all parts of the hippocampal formation and entorhinal cortex (Jin and Panula, unpublished;

Figure 4.4G). The binding is most prominent in the dentate gyrus, high in the subicular complex and entorhinal cortex, and moderate to low in the hippocampal CA1–4 regions. In the hippocampus, H3R binding is prominent in CA1 and distributes in a decreasing order in CA3, CA4, and CA2. Similar to the other cortical areas, a layer preference is observed also in the subicular complex and entorhinal cortex. In the subicular complex, the binding density is high in the deep layer of subiculum and the superficial layers of presubiculum and parasubiculum. In the entorhinal cortex, the binding density is higher in the superficial and deep layers than the middle layers.

BASAL GANGLIA

H3R is abundant in the basal ganglia, where several key circuits are regulated by this receptor [38,48,49]. Using neurotoxins, Cumming et al. [49] found that the abundant striatal H3R ligand binding in the rat originates largely, if not exclusively, from local striatal neurons rather than nigrostiratal projection neurons. In agreement with this, H3R mRNA expression is abundant in the caudate nucleus and putamen, low in the globus pallidus, very low or absent in the substantia nigra [44,50]. On the contrary, the level of H3R radioligand ([^{3}H]N$^\alpha$-methylhistamine or [^{3}H](R)α-methylhistamine) binding is very high in the substantia nigra and globus pallidus, but moderate in the putamen and caudate nucleus [44]. Measured from the autoradiography films, binding density order in normal human postmortem brain is substantia nigra ≥ putamen ≥ globus pallidus externum ≥ globus pallidus internum ≥ frontal cortex [44]. Moreover, in the subthalamic nucleus, there is a low level of both H3R mRNA expression and [^{3}H]N$^\alpha$-methylhistamine binding detected [47], but no visible [^{3}H](R)α-methylhistamine-binding sites [51]. In addition, H3R radioligand [^{3}H](R)α-methylhistamine-binding level is high in the nucleus accumbens [51].

In a postmortem study, the H3R radioligand binding was significantly higher in the substantia nigra of Parkinson's disease (PD) patients than in normal age-matched controls [44]. No significant difference was found among binding levels in putamen, pallidum externum, and pallidum internum. However, expression of H3R mRNA in pallidum externum was higher among Parkinsonian than control brains.

REGULATION OF H3R EXPRESSION IN PHYSIOLOGICAL AND PATHOPHYSIOLOGICAL CONDITIONS

GENERAL CONSIDERATIONS

The role of H3R as an auto- and heteroreceptor expressed widely in the CNS is in line with the suggested role of histamine as a general regulator of neuronal activation and involvement in several complex functions such as sleep and hibernation [52]. Accurate localization of the receptor within different domains of the cell can be obtained with antibodies against H3R, which have been available recently [39,40,53]. Immunohistochemistry has the great advantage of high resolution, but it suffers from a difficulty to exclude the possibility of cross-reacting proteins. Although preadsorption controls improve the specificity, the possibility of unknown endogenous proteins, which are not available for testing, renders it difficult to use immunohistochemistry alone for specific localization studies. *In situ* hybridization with long RNA probes or oligo-DNA probes gives additional support for the existence of specific gene products in tissues and cells. Provided that radioactive probes are used, quantification with automated imaging systems and standards gives a possibility to selectively identify differences in gene expression in distinct types of neurons and glial cells in the brain. Receptor-binding autoradiography is very useful for analysis of active, ligand-binding receptors in areas of the brain. Although *in situ* hybridization detects mRNA even in the absence of protein synthesis, and immunocytochemistry reveals protein distribution of both active and inactive receptor, ligand-binding autoradiography can reliably quantify active ligand-binding receptors. Active receptors can also be localized with [^{35}S]GTP-γ-S-binding method, which indicates ligand-induced activation of intracellular G-protein binding [10]. For best results, all these methods are used in combination. The mRNA signal in *in situ* hybridization samples is usually in the cell bodies and proximal dendrites rather than in terminal areas, where active receptors reside. Immunocytochemistry reveals the receptor protein in terminal areas as well, but is blind to the activity state. Use of tagged receptors in live cells is a powerful method, which allows detailed analysis of receptor trafficking both in cultured cells and in brain.

Anatomical methods are complemented with quantitative PCR, which can identify the receptor isoforms and their abundance. Western blotting can be used to identify the isoforms and quantify receptor protein. However, these methods do not allow analysis of networks where the receptor is active.

HIBERNATION

Hibernating animals undergo periodic changes between the hibernating and the euthermic states. During hibernation bouts, the metabolic rate of the golden-mantled ground squirrel falls to 1/20 of that during the euthermic state, and the body temperature drops close to 0°C or even lower. The histamine levels and turnover are, contrary to most other transmitters, higher during hibernation than during euthermic state [54], which renders it likely that histamine is involved in regulation or either maintenance of the hibernation bout or its termination. Despite the significant changes in histamine throughout the hibernation cycle, the general organization of the brain histaminergic system in golden-mantled ground squirrel is similar to that of other mammals, although more extensive (denser fiber networks) than that of the rat or mouse. Because the hippocampus displays clear electroencephalic activity throughout the hibernation bout, this area is of particular interest. Indeed, histamine infused in the hippocampus with osmotic minipumps just before the time of expected arousal from the bout significantly extends the expected bout length [55], suggesting that histamine may actively maintain the bout and control its length. It is not completely understood as to which of the histamine receptors is most important in this process, because all three (H1–H3) are present in ground squirrel hippocampus. The H1R and H2R ligand binding increase in hippocampus during hibernation, whereas the mRNA expression, receptor ligand binding, and [^{35}S]GTP-γ-S binding decrease for H3R during the hibernation bout [56]. H3R mRNA expression and receptor ligand binding in the caudate and putamen are higher during hibernation than arousal, suggesting that histamine may actively regulate basal ganglia throughout the hibernation cycle [57]. High H3R ligand binding was seen in the globus pallidus and zona reticulate of the substantia nigra. Using the [^{35}S]GTP-γ-S method, it was evident that histamine H3R can be activated throughout the hibernation cycle [57]. It is thus possible that histaminergic regulation through H3R is responsible for the reduction of the dopaminergic transmission during hibernation [56]. It is possible that the brain stem systems known to regulate hibernation regulate hypothalamus (e.g., TMN), which in turn controls the septum and hippocampus, which are also crucial in this circuitry. Whether the ascending peripheral input needed for the regulation is mediated entirely through the brain stem or also through hypothalamus is not currently known.

ISCHEMIA, EPILEPSY, AND BRAIN TRAUMA

In a four-vessel occlusion model of ischemia and reperfusion, rats show an increase in H3R mRNA expression in the caudate-putamen, and a decrease in the globus pallidus and entire thalamus. These changes are associated with increased H3R ligand binding in cortex, caudate-putamen, globus pallidus, and hippocampus [58]. These changes may be associated with the observed increase in striatal histamine release following middle cerebral artery occlusion [59]. Increased histamine might protect target neurons from damage through the activation of H1R.

Kainic acid-induced seizures in rat are a widely used model of temporal lobe epilepsy. Systemic kainic acid induces a cascade of behavioral and structural changes, which allow studies on the symptoms and findings of temporal lobe epilepsy, for example, convulsions, neuronal degeneration and plasticity, synaptic reorganization, and reactive glial pathology. In kainic acid-induced epilepsy, the changes are first seen in dendrites of neurons and astrocyte cells. Widespread neuronal degeneration then follows. The sites affected include the hippocampus, amygdala, piriform cortex, septum, and thalamus [60–62]. Kainic acid-induced seizures are probably generated in the hippocampal field CA3, followed by the activation of CA1 neurons. The activation then spreads to other limbic structures, including piriform cortex and amygdala.

Activation of the central histamine system seems to alleviate the symptoms in various forms of convulsions, and inhibition of the histaminergic system increases convulsions [63–65].

H3R antagonists have been reported to protect against seizures by increasing histamine release [66–69], although conflicting results have also been reported [63]. Hypothalamic histaminergic TMN neurons protect hippocampal neurons *in vitro* against kainic acid-induced damage, and the effect is specific for histamine in this system [70]. Because H3R activation is connected to regulation of Ca^{2+} channels and signaling cascades are related to plasticity, such as the MAPK and Akt systems, histamine through H3R is potentially important in either protection of neurons against damage or cell death signaling. To understand these mechanisms, it is useful to see how H3R is regulated in seizures. Potentially, these experiments might also suggest functional differences between the isoforms, the significance of which is unclear.

Systemic kainic acid induces a short and transient increase in histamine levels in the striatum, hippocampus, piriform cortex, and amygdala. This increase occurs between 6 and 24 h after kainic acid administration, and the peak is already declining 3 days after kainic acid. In addition to high-performance liquid chromatography (HPLC) measurements and identification of the amine, the density of histamine-immunoreactive nerve fibers in these areas increases [71]. This period is too short for sprouting of nerve fibers originating from the TMN, and other HDC-expressing cells have not been found in kainic acid-treated rats. Thus, it is possible that kainic acid alters the kinetics of histamine synthesis, perhaps by increasing uptake of L-histidine to be metabolized to histamine by HDC. Availability of L-histidine seems to be a major regulatory factor in histamine synthesis, because systemic injections of L-histidine [72,73] or portocaval anastomosis [74,75], associated with a significant increase in neutral amino acids, are associated with significant elevations of brain histamine. The full-length H3RA form mRNA undergoes interesting, rapid, and transient upregulation in the hippocampal field CA3, followed by CA1 region, amygdale, and piriform cortex. The deletion isoforms H3RB and H3RC do not show similar changes [76]. The relative overexpression of the H3RA isoform, which is efficiently coupled to MAPK- and Akt-signaling pathways, may thus have significant roles in plasticity associated with kainic acid-induced neurodegeneration or subsequent recovery. There is already evidence of the significance of MAPK-signaling route in H3R-mediated formation of fear memory [77], and the Akt pathway is important in the protection against apoptosis.

Pentylenetetrazole induces generalized tonic-clonic seizures in rat. In this model, expression of the full-length H3RA isoform mRNA also increases in cerebral cortex, caudate putamen, and piriform cortex, but the increase becomes evident as late as 48 h after treatment [37]. Interestingly, this increase is associated with a concomitant decrease in H3R isoforms with the alternative, putatively extracellular C-terminus in some areas [37]. In cell lines, the isoforms with the alternative C-terminus act as dominant-negative isoforms, which inhibit normal trafficking of the active, ligand-binding isoforms. It is possible that the differential regulation of the isoforms in experimental epilepsy is controlled to modify histaminergic signaling in these pathological conditions. However, the mechanisms of the regulation are currently poorly understood.

Brain trauma models, including the fluid percussion model [78,79], can yield useful information of impacts of mechanical trauma on brain structures and neurotransmitter functions. When fluid percussion trauma is directed to the left parietotemporal cortical area of the rat, a bilateral decrease in H3R binding in cortical areas is seen, whereas the thalamic H3R binding is increased bilaterally. Surprisingly, the H3R mRNA expression is decreased in ipsilateral thalamus but not in ipsilateral cortex [79]. This result suggests that the thalamus is vulnerable to traumatic damage and the afferent thalamic inputs are a site for H3R upregulation.

ADDICTION AND ALCOHOL-RELATED BEHAVIOR

Rat strains that differ in their alcohol-related behavior (alcohol preference and alcohol-induced motor impairment) differ significantly in their brain histamine content [71,80] and H3R ligand brain regional binding. Alcohol-preferring AA rats have significantly higher histamine levels in frontal cortex, septum, hypothalamus, hippocampus, and midbrain than alcohol-avoiding ANA rats. Also *tele*-methylhistamine levels are higher in many brain areas, suggesting higher histamine turnover rate in

AA rats [71]. H3R ligand binding is 13–35% lower in primary motor and insular cortex, nucleus accumbens, and hippocampus of alcohol-preferring AA than alcohol-avoiding ANA rats [71]. Two H3R inverse agonists, thioperamide and clobenpropit, dose-dependently suppress alcohol self-administration of AA rats, and an agonist R-α-methylhistamine increases it. Ethanol preference and intake thus seem to be causally linked to brain histamine release and H3R mechanisms. However, which circuitries and transmitters are most important in this regulation is not known. For example, dopamine and GABA release may be affected in several brain regions.

Alcohol causes motor incoordination in rats. This can be quantified with tilting plain, accelerated rotarod, or horizontal wire test (see Ref. 80). Alcohol-sensitive rats have been produced by selective outbreeding for high and low alcohol sensitivity after moderate alcohol administration [80]. The alcohol-sensitive ANT rats have lower histamine levels in several brain areas (frontal cortex, septum, hypothalamus, hippocampus, and thalamus) than the alcohol-tolerant AT rats [80], and higher H3R ligand binding and G-protein activation than alcohol-tolerant rats [80]. Lowering the brain histamine levels with α-fluoromethylhistidine increases the sensitivity of the alcohol-tolerant rats to alcohol [80], suggesting that histaminergic mechanisms are important for motor control. Currently, it is not known whether this effect is due to a cerebellar mechanism or regulation of muscle tone.

VESTIBULAR COMPENSATION

Unilateral labyrinthectomy in the rat results in ocular and motor postural syndrome characterized by spontaneous nystagmus, barrel rotation, and circling behavior. These symptoms diminish during the following week resulting in a condition called vestibular compensation. Betahistine, a drug with partial H1R agonistic and H3R antagonistic properties, facilitates the recovery, suggesting involvement of a histaminergic mechanism in the process. In the rat, unilateral labyrinthectomy is associated with bilateral increase in H3R mRNA expression during the first 24 h, followed by a decline that reaches control levels during the first week [81]. H3R ligand binding increases ipsilaterally at 48 h postlesion. The H3R may be localized on GABAergic medial vestibular interneurons, or terminals of glutamatergic second-order medial vestibular neurons. These neurons may contribute to commissural disinhibition, which contributes to vestibular compensation.

In the cat, unilateral labyrinthectomy increases HDC expression in the TMN and decreases ipsilateral H3R binding in the medial vestibular nucleus [82]. Both betahistine and thioperamide increase the expression of HDC mRNA in the TMN and decrease the H3R ligand binding in the vestibular nuclei and TMN after unilateral labyrinthectomy [83]. A bilateral decline in density of histaminergic fibers also follows unilateral vestibular lesions, suggesting that the system undergoes plastic changes [84] during the time of recovery.

ACKNOWLEDGMENTS

Original research has been supported by the Academy of Finland, the Finnish Parkinson Foundation, Sigrid Juselius Foundation, and Magnus Ehrnrooth Foundation.

REFERENCES

1. Arrang, J.M., Garbarg, M. and Schwartz, J.C. 1983. Auto-inhibition of brain histamine release mediated by a novel class (H3) of histamine receptor. *Nature* 302: 832–837.
2. Lovenberg, T.W., Roland, B.L., Wilson, S.J., Jiang, X., Pyati, J., Huvar, A., Jackson, M.R. and Erlander, M.G. 1999. Cloning and functional expression of the human histamine H3 receptor. *Mol Pharmacol* 55: 1101–1107.
3. Celanire, S., Wijtmans, M., Talaga, P., Leurs, R. and de Esch, I.J. 2005. Keynote review: Histamine H(3) receptor antagonists reach out for the clinic. *Drug Discov Today* 10: 1613–1627.
4. Esbenshade, T.A., Fox, G.B. and Cowart, M.D. 2006. Histamine H3 receptor antagonists: preclinical promise for treating obesity and cognitive disorders. *Mol Interv* 6: 77–88, 59.
5. Leurs, R., Bakker, R.A., Timmerman, H. and de Esch, I.J. 2005. The histamine H3 receptor: from gene cloning to H3 receptor drugs. *Nat Rev Drug Discov* 4: 107–120.
6. Bongers, G., Bakker, R.A. and Leurs, R. 2007. Molecular aspects of the histamine H3 receptor. *Biochem Pharmacol* 73: 1195–1204.
7. Hancock, A.A., Diehl, M.S., Fey, T.A., Bush, E.N., Faghih, R., Miller, T.R., Krueger, K.M., Pratt, J.K., Cowart, M.D., Dickinson, R.W., Shapiro, R., Knourek-Segel, V.E., Droz, B.A., McDowell, C.A., Krishna, G., Brune, M.E., Esbenshade, T.A. and Jacobson, P.B. 2005. Antiobesity evaluation of histamine H3 receptor (H3R) antagonist analogs of A-331440 with improved safety and efficacy. *Inflamm Res* 54 (Suppl 1): S27–S29.
8. Hancock, A.A., Bennani, Y.L., Bush, E.N., Esbenshade, T.A., Faghih, R., Fox, G.B., Jacobson, P., Knourek-Segel, V., Krueger, K.M., Nuss, M.E., Pan, J.B., Shapiro, R., Witte, D.G. and Yao, B.B. 2004. Antiobesity effects of A-331440, a novel non-imidazole histamine H3 receptor antagonist. *Eur J Pharmacol* 487: 183–197.
9. Clark, E.A. and Hill, S.J. 1996. Sensitivity of histamine H3 receptor agonist-stimulated [35S]GTP gamma[S] binding to pertussis toxin. *Eur J Pharmacol* 296: 223–225.
10. Laitinen, J.T. and Jokinen, M. 1998. Guanosine 5'-(gamma-[35S]thio)triphosphate auto-radiography allows selective detection of histamine H3 receptor-dependent G protein activation in rat brain tissue sections. *J Neurochem* 71: 808–816.
11. Jansen, F.P., Wu, T.S., Voss, H.P., Steinbusch, H.W., Vollinga, R.C., Rademaker, B., Bast, A. and Timmerman, H. 1994. Characterization of the binding of the first selective radiolabelled histamine H_3 receptor antagonist, [125I]-iodophenpropit, to rat brain. *Br J Pharmacol* 113: 355–362.
12. Stark, H., Kathmann, M., Schlicker, E., Schunack, W., Schlegel, B. and Sippl, W. 2004. Medicinal chemical and pharmacological aspects of imidazole-containing histamine H3 receptor antagonists. *Mini Rev Med Chem* 4: 965–977.
13. Wieland, K., Bongers, G., Yamamoto, Y., Hashimoto, T., Yamatodani, A., Menge, W.M., Timmerman, H., Lovenberg, T.W. and Leurs, R. 2001. Constitutive activity of histamine H(3) receptors stably expressed in SK-N-MC cells: display of agonism and inverse agonism by H(3) antagonists. *J Pharmacol Exp Ther* 299: 908–914.
14. Silver, R.B., Mackins, C.J., Smith, N.C., Koritchneva, I.L., Lefkowitz, K., Lovenberg, T.W. and Levi, R. 2001. Coupling of histamine H3 receptors to neuronal Na^+/H^+ exchange: a novel protective mechanism in myocardial ischemia. *Proc Natl Acad Sci USA* 98: 2855–2859.
15. Silver, R.B., Poonwasi, K.S., Seyedi, N., Wilson, S.J., Lovenberg, T.W. and Levi, R. 2002. Decreased intracellular calcium mediates the histamine H_3 receptor-induced attenuation of norepinephrine exocytosis from cardiac sympathetic nerve endings. *Proc Natl Acad Sci USA* 99: 501–506.
16. Seyedi, N., Mackins, C.J., Machida, T., Reid, A.C., Silver, R.B. and Levi, R. 2005. Histamine H_3 receptor-induced attenuation of norepinephrine exocytosis: a decreased protein kinase A activity mediates a reduction in intracellular calcium. *J Pharmacol Exp Ther* 312: 272–280.

17. Morisset, S., Rouleau, A., Ligneau, X., Gbahou, F., Tardivel-Lacombe, J., Stark, H., Schunack, W., Ganellin, C.R., Schwartz, J.C. and Arrang, J.M. 2000. High constitutive activity of native H3 receptors regulates histamine neurons in brain. *Nature* 408: 860–864.

18. Gomez-Ramirez, J., Ortiz, J. and Blanco, I. 2002. Presynaptic H-3 autoreceptors modulate histamine synthesis through cAMP pathway. *Mol Pharmacol* 61: 239–245.

19. Coge, F., Guenin, S.P., Audinot, V., Renouard-Try, A., Beauverger, P., Macia, C., Ouvry, C., Nagel, N., Rique, H., Boutin, J.A. and Galizzi, J.P. 2001. Genomic organization and characterization of splice variants of the human histamine H3 receptor. *Biochem J* 355: 279–288.

20. Uveges, A.J., Kowal, D., Zhang, Y., Spangler, T.B., Dunlop, J., Semus, S. and Jones, P.G. 2002. The role of transmembrane helix 5 in agonist binding to the human H3 receptor. *J Pharmacol Exp Ther* 301: 451–458.

21. Levi, R., Seyedi, N., Schaefer, U., Estephan, R., Mackins, C.J., Tyler, E. and Silver, R.B. 2007. Histamine H_3 receptor signaling in cardiac sympathetic nerves: Identification of a novel MAPK-PLA2-COX-PGE2-EP3R pathway. *Biochem Pharmacol* 73: 1146–1156.

22. Drutel, G., Peitsaro, N., Karlstedt, K., Wieland, K., Smit, M.J., Timmerman, H., Panula, P. and Leurs. R. 2001. Identification of rat H3 receptor isoforms with different brain expression and signaling properties. *Mol Pharmacol* 59: 1–8.

23. Tardivel-Lacombe, J., Rouleau, A., Heron, A., Morisset, S., Pillot, C., Cochois, V., Schwartz, J.C. and Arrang, J.M. 2000. Cloning and cerebral expression of the guinea pig histamine H3 receptor: evidence for two isoforms. *Neuroreport* 11: 755–759.

24. Lovenberg, T.W., Pyati, J., Chang, H., Wilson, S.J. and Erlander, M.G. 2000. Cloning of rat histamine H(3) receptor reveals distinct species pharmacological profiles. *J Pharmacol Exp Ther* 293: 771–778.

25. Morisset, S., Sasse, A., Gbahou, F., Heron, A., Ligneau, X., Tardivel-Lacombe, J., Schwartz, J.C. and Arrang, J.M. 2001. The rat H3 receptor: gene organization and multiple isoforms. *Biochem Biophys Res Commun* 280: 75–80.

26. Chen, J., Liu, C. and Lovenberg, T.W. 2003. Molecular and pharmacological characterization of the mouse histamine H3 receptor. *Eur J Pharmacol* 467: 57–65.

27. Rouleau, A., Heron, A., Cochois, V., Pillot, C., Schwartz, J.C. and Arrang, J.M. 2004. Cloning and expression of the mouse histamine H3 receptor: evidence for multiple isoforms. *J Neurochem* 90: 1331–1338.

28. Barrett, P., Ross, A.W., Balik, A., Littlewood, P.A., Mercer, J.G., Moar, K.M., Sallmen, T., Kaslin, J., Panula, P., Schuhler, S., Ebling, F.J., Ubeaud, C. and Morgan, P.J. 2005. Photoperiodic regulation of histamine H3 receptor and VGF messenger ribonucleic acid in the arcuate nucleus of the Siberian hamster. *Endocrinology* 146: 1930–1939.

29. Yao, B.B., Sharma, R., Cassar, S., Esbenshade, T.A. and Hancock, A.A. 2003. Cloning and pharmacological characterization of the monkey histamine H3 receptor. *Eur J Pharmacol* 482: 49–60.

30. Peitsaro, N., Sundvik, M., Anichtchik, O.V., Kaslin, J. and Panula, P. 2007. Identification of zebrafish histamine H1, H2 and H3 receptors and effects of histaminergic ligands on behavior. *Biochem Pharmacol* 73: 1205–1214.

31. Tardivel-Lacombe, J., Morisset, S., Gbahou, F., Schwartz, J.C. and Arrang, J.M. 2001. Chromosomal mapping and organization of the human histamine H3 receptor gene. *Neuroreport* 12: 321–324.

32. West, R.E., Jr., Zweig, A., Granzow, R.T., Siegel, M.I. and Egan, R.W. 1990. Biexponential kinetics of (R)-alpha-[3H]methylhistamine binding to the rat brain H3 histamine receptor. *J Neurochem* 55: 1612–1616.

33. Harper, E.A., Shankley, N.P. and Black, J.W. 1999. Evidence that histamine homologues discriminate between H_3 receptors in guinea-pig cerebral cortex and ileum longitudinal muscle myenteric plexus. *Br J Pharmacol* 128: 751–759.

34. Wiedemann, P., Bonisch, H., Oerters, F. and Bruss, M. 2002. Structure of the human histamine H3 receptor gene (HRH3) and identification of naturally occurring variations. *J Neural Transm* 109: 443–453.
35. Wellendorph, P., Goodman, M.W., Burstein, E.S., Nash, N.R., Brann, M.R. and Weiner, D.M. 2002. Molecular cloning and pharmacology of functionally distinct isoforms of the human histamine H(3) receptor. *Neuropharmacology* 42: 929–940.
36. Hancock, A.A., Esbenshade, T.A., Krueger, K.M. and Yao, B.B. 2003. Genetic and pharmacological aspects of histamine H3 receptor heterogeneity. *Life Sci* 73: 3043–3072.
37. Bakker, R.A., Lozada, A.F., van Marle, A., Shenton, F.C., Drutel, G., Karlstedt, K., Hoffmann, M., Lintunen, M., Yamamoto, Y., van Rijn, R.M., Chazot, P.L., Panula, P. and Leurs, R. 2006. Discovery of naturally occurring splice variants of the rat histamine H3 receptor that act as dominant-negative isoforms. *Mol Pharmacol* 69: 1194–1206.
38. Pillot, C., Heron, A., Cochois, V., Tardivel-Lacombe, J., Ligneau, X., Schwartz, J.C. and Arrang, J.M. 2002. A detailed mapping of the histamine H(3) receptor and its gene transcripts in rat brain. *Neuroscience* 114: 173–193.
39. Chazot, P.L., Hann, V., Wilson, C., Lees, G. and Thompson, C.L. 2001. Immunological identification of the mammalian H3 histamine receptor in the mouse brain. *Neuroreport* 12: 259–262.
40. Karlstedt, K., Ahman, M.J., Anichtchik, O.V., Soinila, S. and Panula, P. 2003. Expression of the H3 receptor in the developing CNS and brown fat suggests novel roles for histamine. *Mol Cell Neurosci* 24: 614–622.
41. Peitsaro, N., Anichtchik, O.V. and Panula, P. 2000. Identification of a histamine H(3)-like receptor in the zebrafish (Danio rerio) brain. *J Neurochem* 75: 718–724.
42. Heron, A., Rouleau, A., Cochois, V., Pillot, C., Schwartz, J.C. and Arrang, J.M. 2001. Expression analysis of the histamine H-3 receptor in developing rat tissues. *Mech Develop* 105: 167–173.
43. Cannon, K.E., Chazot, P.L., Hann, V., Shenton, F., Hough, L.B. and Rice, F.L. 2007. Immunohistochemical localization of histamine H3 receptors in rodent skin, dorsal root ganglia, superior cervical ganglia, and spinal cord: potential antinociceptive targets. *Pain* 129: 76–92.
44. Anichtchik, O.V., Peitsaro, N., Rinne, J.O., Kalimo, H. and Panula, P. 2001. Distribution and modulation of histamine H(3) receptors in basal ganglia and frontal cortex of healthy controls and patients with Parkinson's disease. *Neurobiol Dis* 8: 707–716.
45. Jin, C.Y. and Panula, P. 2005. The laminar histamine receptor system in human prefrontal cortex suggests multiple levels of histaminergic regulation. *Neuroscience* 132: 137–149.
46. Martinez-Mir, M.I., Pollard, H., Moreau, J., Arrang, J.M., Ruat, M., Traiffort, E., Schwartz, J.C. and Palacios, J.M. 1990. Three histamine receptors (H1, H2 and H3) visualized in the brain of human and non-human primates. *Brain Res* 526: 322–327.
47. Jin, C.Y., Kalimo, H. and Panula, P. 2002. The histaminergic system in human thalamus: correlation of innervation to receptor expression. *Eur J Neurosci* 15:1125–1138.
48. Pollard, H., Moreau, J., Arrang, J.M. and Schwartz, J.C. 1993. A detailed autoradiographic mapping of histamine H3 receptors in rat brain areas. *Neuroscience* 52: 169–189.
49. Cumming, P., Shaw, C. and Vincent, S.R. 1991. High affinity histamine binding site is the H3 receptor: characterization and autoradiographic localization in rat brain. *Synapse* 8: 144–151.
50. Anichtchik, O.V., Huotari, M., Peitsaro, N., Haycock, J.W., Mannisto, P.T. and Panula, P. 2000. Modulation of histamine H3 receptors in the brain of 6-hydroxydopamine-lesioned rats. *Eur J Neurosci* 12: 3823–3832.
51. Goodchild, R.E., Court, J.A., Hobson, I., Piggott, M.A., Perry, R.H., Ince, P., Jaros, E. and Perry, E.K. 1999. Distribution of histamine H_3 receptor binding in the normal human basal

ganglia: comparison with Huntington's and Parkinson's disease cases. *Eur J Neurosci* 11: 449–456.

52. Haas, H. and Panula, P. 2003. The role of histamine and the tuberomamillary nucleus in the nervous system. *Nature Rev Neurosci* 4: 121–130.
53. Karlstedt, K., Senkas, A., Ahman, M. and Panula, P. 2001. Regional expression of the histamine H(2) receptor in adult and developing rat brain. *Neuroscience* 102: 201–208.
54. Sallmen, T., Beckman, A.L., Stanton, T.L., Eriksson, K.S., Tarhanen, J., Tuomisto, L. and Panula, P. 1999. Major changes in the brain histamine system of the ground squirrel Citellus lateralis during hibernation. *J Neurosci* 19: 1824–1835.
55. Sallmen, T., Lozada, A.F., Beckman, A.L. and Panula, P. 2003. Intrahippocampal histamine delays arousal from hibernation. *Brain Res* 966: 317–320.
56. Sallmen, T., Lozada, A.F., Anichtchik, O.V., Beckman, A.L., Leurs, R. and Panula, P. 2003. Changes in hippocampal histamine receptors across the hibernation cycle in ground squirrels. *Hippocampus* 13: 745–754.
57. Sallmen, T., Lozada, A.F., Anichtchik, O.V., Beckman, A.L. and Panula, P. 2003. Increased brain histamine H3 receptor expression during hibernation in golden-mantled ground squirrels. *BMC Neurosci* 4: 24.
58. Lozada, A., Munyao, N., Sallmen, T., Lintunen, M., Leurs, R., Lindsberg, P.J. and Panula, P. 2005. Postischemic regulation of central histamine receptors. *Neuroscience* 136: 371–379.
59. Adachi, N., Itoh, Y., Oishi, R. and Saeki, K. 1992. Direct evidence for increased continuous histamine release in the striatum of conscious freely moving rats produced by middle cerebral artery occlusion. *J Cereb Blood Flow Metab* 12: 477–483.
60. Sperk, G. 1994. Kainic acid seizures in the rat. *Prog Neurobiol* 42: 1–32.
61. Schwob, J.E., Fuller, T., Price, J.L. and Olney, J.W. 1980. Widespread patterns of neuronal damage following systemic or intracerebral injections of kainic acid: a histological study. *Neuroscience* 5: 991–1014.
62. Ben Ari, Y. 1985. Limbic seizure and brain damage produced by kainic acid: mechanisms and relevance to human temporal lobe epilepsy. *Neuroscience* 14: 375–403.
63. Scherkl, R., Hashem, A. and Frey, H.H. 1991. Histamine in brain—its role in regulation of seizure susceptibility. *Epilepsy Res* 10: 111–118.
64. Tuomisto, L. and Tacke, U. 1986. Is histamine an anticonvulsive inhibitory transmitter? *Neuropharmacology* 25: 955–958.
65. Tuomisto, L., Tacke, U. and Willman, A. 1987. Inhibition of sound-induced convulsions by metoprine in the audiogenic seizure susceptible rat. *Agents Actions* 20: 252–254.
66. Yokoyama, H., Onodera, K., Iinuma, K. and Watanabe, T. 1993. Effect of thioperamide, a histamine H3 receptor antagonist, on electrically induced convulsions in mice. *Eur J Pharmacol* 234: 129–133.
67. Yokoyama, H., Onodera, K., Maeyama, K., Sakurai, E., Iinuma, K., Leurs, R., Timmerman, H. and Watanabe, T. 1994. Clobenpropit (VUF-9153), a new histamine H3 receptor antagonist, inhibits electrically induced convulsions in mice. *Eur J Pharmacol* 260: 23–28.
68. Vohora, D., Pal, S.N. and Pillai, K.K. 2000. Thioperamide, a selective histamine H3 receptor antagonist, protects against PTZ-induced seizures in mice. *Life Sci* 66: L297–L301.
69. Vohora, D., Pal, S.N. and Pillai, K.K. 2001. Histamine and selective H_3 receptor ligands: a possible role in the mechanism and management of epilepsy. *Pharmacol Biochem Behav* 68: 735–741.
70. Kukko-Lukjanov, T.K., Soini, S., Taira, T., Michelsen, K.A., Panula, P. and Holopainen, I.E. 2006. Histaminergic neurons protect the developing hippocampus from kainic acid-induced neuronal damage in an organotypic coculture system. *J Neurosci* 26: 1088–1097.

71. Lintunen, M., Hyytia, P., Sallmen, T., Karlstedt, K., Tuomisto, L., Leurs, R., Kiianmaa, K., Korpi, E.R. and Panula, P. 2001. Increased brain histamine in an alcohol-preferring rat line and modulation of ethanol consumption by H(3) receptor mechanisms. *FASEB J* 15: 1074–1076.

72. Schwartz, J.C., Lampart, C. and Rose, C. 1972. Histamine formation in rat brain in vivo: effects of histidine loads. *J Neurochem* 19: 801–810.

73. Green, H. and Erickson, R.W. 1967. Effect of some drugs upon the histamine concentration of guinea pig brain. *Arch Int Pharmacodyn Ther* 166: 121–126.

74. Fogel, W.A., Andrzejewski, W. and Maslinski, C. 1991. Brain histamine in rats with hepatic encephalopathy. *J Neurochem* 56: 38–43.

75. Fogel, W.A., Michelsen, K.A., Panula, P., Sasiak, K. and Andrzejewski, W. 2001. Cerebral and gastric histamine system is altered after portocaval shunt. *J Physiol Pharmacol* 52: 657–670.

76. Lintunen, M., Sallmen, T., Karlstedt, K. and Panula, P. 2005. Transient changes in the limbic histaminergic system after systemic kainic acid-induced seizures. *Neurobiol Dis* 20: 155–169.

77. Giovannini, M.G., Efoudebe, M., Passani, M.B., Baldi, E., Bucherelli, C., Giachi, F., Corradetti, R. and Blandina, P. 2003. Improvement in fear memory by histamine-elicited ERK2 activation in hippocampal CA3 cells. *J Neurosci* 23: 9016–9023.

78. Pierce, J.E., Smith, D.H., Trojanowski, J.Q. and McIntosh, T.K. 1998. Enduring cognitive, neurobehavioral and histopathological changes persist for up to one year following severe experimental brain injury in rats. *Neuroscience* 87: 359–369.

79. Lozada, A., Maegele, M., Stark, H., Neugebauer, E.M. and Panula, P. 2005. Traumatic brain injury results in mast cell increase and changes in regulation of central histamine receptors. *Neuropathol Appl Neurobiol* 31: 150–162.

80. Lintunen, M., Raatesalmi, K., Sallmen, T., Anichtchik, O., Karlstedt, K., Kaslin, J., Kiianmaa, K., Korpi, E.R. and Panula, P. 2002. Low brain histamine content affects ethanol-induced motor impairment. *Neurobiol Dis* 9: 94–105.

81. Lozada, A.F., Aarnisalo, A.A., Karlstedt, K., Stark, H. and Panula, P. 2004. Plasticity of histamine H-3 receptor expression and binding in the vestibular nuclei after labyrinthectomy in rat. *BMC Neurosci* 5.

82. Tighilet, B., Trottier, S., Mourre, C. and Lacour, M. 2006. Changes in the histaminergic system during vestibular compensation in the cat. *J Physiol* 573: 723–739.

83. Tighilet, B., Mourre, C., Trottier, S. and Lacour, M. 2007. Histaminergic ligands improve vestibular compensation in the cat: behavioural, neurochemical and molecular evidence. *Eur J Pharmacol* 568: 149–163.

84. Lacour, M. and Tighilet, B. 2000. Vestibular compensation in the cat: the role of the histaminergic system. *Acta Otolaryngol Suppl* 544: 15–18.

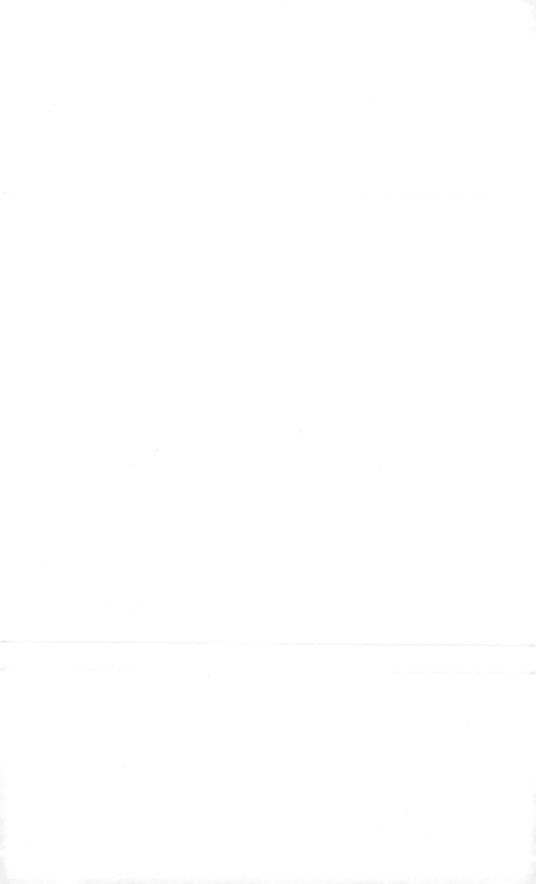

5 Drug Discovery: From Hits to Clinical Candidates

Sylvain Celanire, Florence Lebon, and Holger Stark

CONTENTS

Introduction.. 103
The H₃ Receptor: A Highly Competitive Target 104
Natural Products as Potent H₃ Receptor Ligands.. 105
Imidazole-Based H₃ Receptor Modulators.. 108
    Agonists and Agonistic Compounds 108
    Antagonists.. 109
    Issues within Imidazole Chemical Class... 110
Drug Discovery Research of Nonimidazole-Based
    H₃ Receptor Antagonists.. 111
    Academic Pioneers in the Nonimidazole H₃ Chemical Class........... 111
    Pharmaceutical Companies' Drug Discovery Programs:
    From Hits to Clinical Leads 112
Recent Advance in H₃ Receptor Ligand Computer-Aided
    Drug Design... 133
    Introduction 133
    Histamine H₃ Receptor Antagonists *In Silico* Models...................... 135
    Conclusion 143
Radiolabeled and Fluorescent H₃ Receptor Ligands.................................... 143
Multitarget-Oriented H₃ Receptor Drug Design 146
    Drug Combinations 146
    Hybrid Compounds 146
Preclinical and Clinical Studies of H₃ Receptor Drug Candidates............... 149
Conclusion and Future Perspectives 151
References.. 152

INTRODUCTION

In recent years, numerous highly recommendable review articles have been published, demonstrating the high interest in histamine H_3 receptor (H_3R) ligands and the broad spectrum of different lead structures [1–7]. This publication should add some new and most recent findings from a structural and chemical point of view and have a somewhat different focus on important issues in this scientific field. The section, "The H_3 Receptor: A Highly Competitive Target," refers to the competitive aspect of the H_3R field and the involvement of worldwide pharmaceutical companies. Then, the medicinal chemistry of H_3R ligands (agonists, antagonists, and inverse agonists), disclosed by both academic groups and pharmaceutical companies, is thoroughly reviewed, with a particular focus on druglike properties and developability profile (in the sections, "Natural Products as Potent H_3 Receptor Ligands," "Imidazole-Based H_3 Receptor Modulators," and "Drug Discovery Research of Nonimidazole-Based H_3 Receptor Antagonists"). A computer-aided drug design description in the section, "Recent Advance in H_3R Ligand Computer-Aided Drug Design," guides to the molecular biology of the H_3R and the different *in silico* approaches. New pharmacological radiolabeled and fluorescent tools to study *in vitro* and *in vivo* biological responses are detailed in the section, "Radiolabeled and Fluorescent H_3 Receptor Ligands". The section, "Multitarget-Oriented H_3 Receptor Drug Design," is distinctly dedicated to novel opportunities in the multitarget H_3R drug design. Finally, the section, "Preclinical and Clinical Studies of H_3 Receptor Drug Candidates," refers to the preclinical and clinical studies involving new H_3R chemical entities identified as drug candidates.

THE H_3 RECEPTOR: A HIGHLY COMPETITIVE TARGET

Since the first generation of imidazole-based H_3 antagonists, this chemical class of compounds has been the center of drug discovery programs across academic groups and pharmaceutical companies, with around 50 patent applications being published between 1995 and 2006 [8,9]. The limited therapeutic use of imidazole-based compounds, together with the discovery of the constitutive activity of the histamine H_3R by several groups and the successful cloning of the human H_3R by the group of Lovenberg [10] at Johnson & Johnson (J&J) Process Research and Development (PRD) have clearly influenced the whole field of drug discovery research. The discontinuation of Gliatech's clinical lead GT2331 (*vide infra*) in clinical trials and the identification of functional activity discrepancies across species (e.g., neutral antagonism in rodent H_3 and full agonism activity in human H_3) reoriented medicinal chemistry programs worldwide toward nonimidazole chemical series. As shown in Figure 5.1, the number of patent applications filed within this distinct chemical class has continued to rise since 1999, with nearly 50 published patent applications for the year 2006 alone [8,9,11]. Interestingly enough, the number of patents filed up to June 2007 raised the total number filed for the year 2005 alone, which maintain a high degree of chemical space within the nonimidazole class of H_3 antagonists.

Furthermore, the number of patent applications filed and published per company since 1999 and up to June 2007 is represented in Figure 5.2 [8,9]. We could reasonably rank the top 10 pharmaceutical companies, led by J&J PRD and GlaxoSmithKline (GSK), followed by Abbott Laboratories, Pfizer, Hoffmann-La Roche, Banyu Pharm., Eli Lilly & Co, Novo-Nordisk, Schering Corp., and Bioprojet (in collaboration with Ferrer International and several academic universities). It is worth mentioning that both Pfizer and Hoffman-La Roche, lately involved in the H_3 field, are pursuing intensive H_3 drug discovery programs, securing their chemical series with patent applications filing. Companies such as AstraZeneca, Sanofi-Aventis,

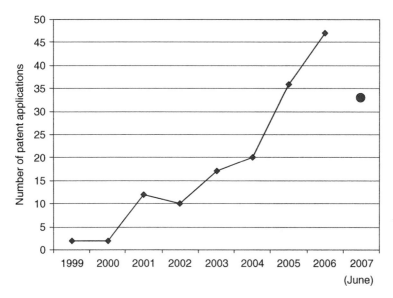

FIGURE 5.1 Number of patent applications in the nonimidazole series: evolution from 1999 to June 2007.

Athersys, Laboratoires Servier, UCB Pharma, Neurogen, and Arena Pharmaceuticals have also recently reported novel H_3 modulators, whereas J&J PRD, Merck, Lundbeck, and Kyowa H.K. Ltd. have claimed combination of H_3R ligands and other drugs (see section Multitarget-Oriented H_3 Receptor Drug Design) or new therapeutic uses of selected H_3 ligands (e.g., stroke and depression).

NATURAL PRODUCTS AS POTENT H_3 RECEPTOR LIGANDS

Despite the early finding of histamine as an important mediator of different physiological and pathophysiological functions [12], only a very few number of compounds have been identified as natural products displaying histamine H_3R affinity [13]. The imidazole-containing compounds verongamine (**1**) and carcinine (**2**) (β-alanylhistamine; Figure 5.3) belong to an early claimed general construction pattern for histamine H_3R antagonists, in which an N-containing heterocycle as basic moiety is linked through a spacer to a polar functionality, which may also be then connected through another spacer or directly to a lipophilic moiety. With modifications and extensions, this blue print is more or less still true for most of the antagonist compounds. Verongamine and related tyrosine-derived products have been isolated from marine sponge *Verongula gigantea* of the order Verongida [304] and also prepared in total synthesis [14]. Verongamine is a histamine H_3R antagonist of low potency (pIC_{50} 5.6). The same is true for carcinine (**2**) (pK_i 6.5) [13,15]. Interestingly, the related dipeptidyl precursor carnosine (**3**) (β-alanyl-L-histidine) displayed different histaminelike effects of which some could be antagonized by the histamine H_3R antagonist thioperamide [16–18]. Both histamine derivatives **2** and **3** have been detected in different human tissues and showed antioxidant properties [19].

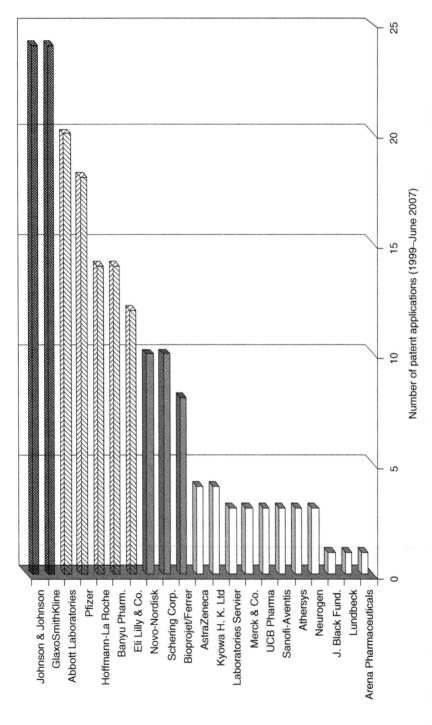

FIGURE 5.2   Number of patent applications per company within the nonimidazole H_3 chemical series, from 1999 to June 2007.

Verongamine (1)

R = H Carcinine (2)
R = COOH Carnosine (3)

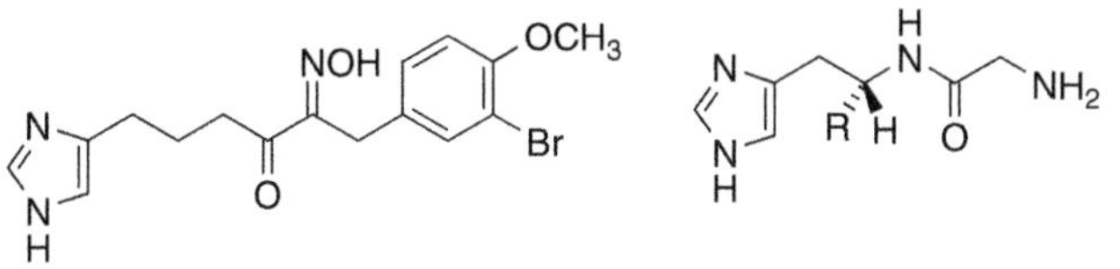

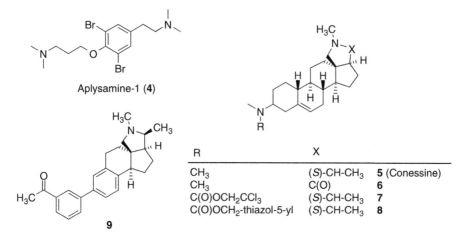

FIGURE 5.3 Imidazole-base natural product with histamine H_3 affinity.

Aplysamine-1 (4)

9

R	X	
CH_3	(*S*)-CH-CH_3	5 (Conessine)
CH_3	C(O)	6
C(O)OCH_2CCl_3	(*S*)-CH-CH_3	7
C(O)OCH_2-thiazol-5-yl	(*S*)-CH-CH_3	8

FIGURE 5.4 Nonimidazole natural products with histamine H_3 affinity.

Also from a marine sponge of Verongidae family, *Aplysina* sp., aplysamine-1 (**4**) has been detected as a moderate potent antagonist and one of the first nonimidazole compounds (Figure 5.4) [20]. Later investigations on structure–activity relationships (SAR) demonstrate that the related debromo tyramine-based derivative is about five times more potent than **4** (pK_i 8.2 versus 7.5, respectively) [21]. One of the most interesting findings in natural products is the detection of the azacyclosteroid conessine (**5**) as potent (pK_i 8.3), and brain-penetrating histamine H_3R antagonist by high-throughput screening (HTS) from Abbott Labs [22–24]. This alkaloid does not possess any aromatic moiety and demonstrates a strict geometry of functionalities. Therefore, it is an excellent tool for computational models. The importance of both basic centers was investigated by amide (ring E, **6**, pK_i 6.3) or carbamate formation (exocyclic N-containing functionality, **7**, pK_i 7.7). Different carbamate, amide, amine, alcohol, ester, ether, ketone, and alkene derivatives are described related to the variation on compound **8**. Further derivative (**9**) containing aromatic A and B rings were also allowed, maintaining H_3R affinity (pK_i 9.9–6.1). Synthetic approaches to such compounds are described by Kopach et al. [25] and Jiang and Xu [26]. The reason for broad variations of the amino functionality was based on the poor pharmacokinetic properties of conessine (**5**). Although it showed a high brain/blood concentration ratio, its extremely low central nervous system (CNS) clearance, low selectivity versus α_2-adrenoceptors (pK_i 8.0), and potential to induce phospholipidosis (probably due to its cationic amphiphilic feature) were the most important drawbacks [27,28]. Recently, conessine has also been isolated from the stem bark of African *Funtumia elastica*, Apocynaceae, and showed moderate anti-plasmodial activity [29]. The utility of natural products as sources of novel structures is well known although they will not necessarily be the final drug entity [30].

IMIDAZOLE-BASED H_3 RECEPTOR MODULATORS

Since the discovery of the histamine H_3R in 1983 [31], the development of potent and selective agonists and antagonists has been mainly based on modifications of the endogeneous ligand. As most imidazole variations led to a dramatic loss of affinity, further optimization was focused on side-chain modifications.

Agonists and Agonistic Compounds

In 1987, the existence of the H_3R was confirmed by the use of the selective agonist R-α-methylhistamine (**10**) (Figure 5.5). The orientation of the methyl group is the same as that of the carboxy group in L-histidine. Simple methylation of the side chain led to potent and selective compounds as also shown with N^α-methylhistamine (**11**), whereas 4-methylated imidazole derivative showed H_4R preference [32,33]. The basic amino functionality could be exchanged by an isothiourea (imetit, **12**) or isourea moiety. Steric restrictions by incorporation of a pyrrolidine moiety (SCH 50971, **13**) (VUF 4864) [34], by a tetrahydrofuran spacer (imifuramine) [35] or by different cyclopropyl groups (AEIC) [36] in specific stereochemical orientations may maintain H_3R affinity. Surprisingly, the tertiary amine in methimepip (**14**) [36–38] and the aromatic pyridine nitrogen in immethridine (**15**) might replace the primary amino group of histamine [39]. Compound **15** is a potent H_3R agonist (pK_i 9.1, pEC_{50} 9.1 [α = 0.8] [histamine; α = 1]). In receptor screening, it showed a low H_4R partial agonism activity and low affinities at α_{2A} receptor subtype, together with good physicochemical and *in vitro* Absorption, Distribution, Metabolism, Excretion (ADME) properties [40]. Recently, N^α,N^α-dimethylimbutamine has been reported as a selective histamine H_3R agonist, which can be seen as a less restricted methimepip analog [41]. To overcome poor bioavailability, high first-pass effects or other unwanted

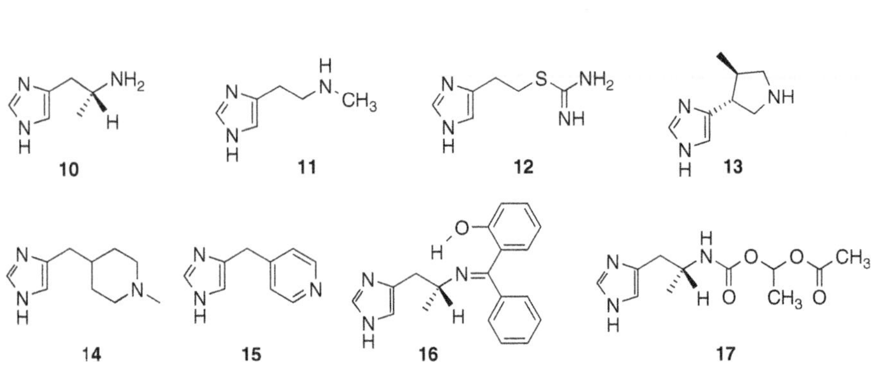

FIGURE 5.5 Imidazole H_3 agonists, including methimepip (**14**), immethridine (**15**), and clinical BP-2.94 (**16**).

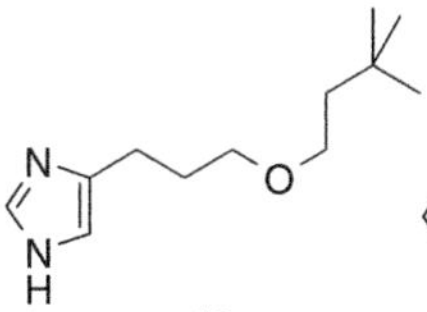

FIGURE 5.6   Imidazole H_3 ligands with *protean agonism* properties, including GT2331 (**20**).

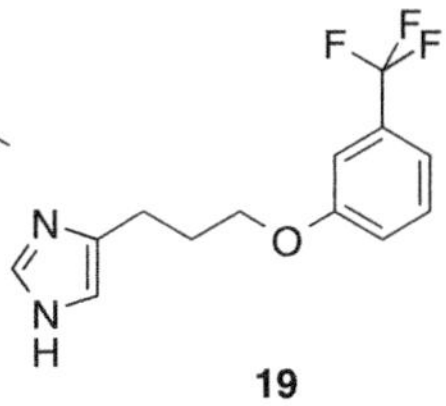

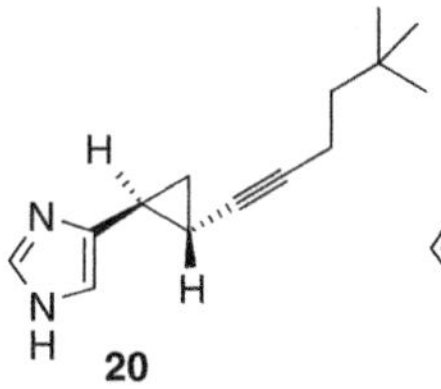

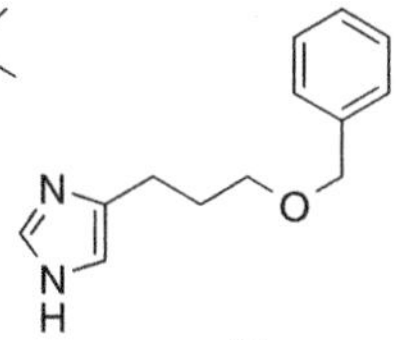

pharmacokinetic problems observed for most of the aminergic H_3 agonists, prodrugs such as the azomethine BP2.94 (**16**) [42,43] or the acyloxyalkylcarbamate (**17**) [44] have been prepared, showing great improvement in their pharmacodynamic and distribution properties. Compound **16** is in clinical phase II, although development seems to be halted as no reports have occurred for a while.

Under physiological conditions, the protonated amino functionality had been assumed an essential moiety for agonist activity. Therefore, it was surprising that compounds, which belong to the general construction pattern of antagonists, showed partial to full agonist properties depending on the test system. For compounds **18** (Freie Universitate Berlin [FUB] 407) and **19** (University College of London [UCL] 1470) (Figure 5.6), it was shown that a restricted binding mode on a lipophilic pocket seems to be necessary for agonist properties, whereas slight modifications increased antagonist properties [45–47]. The same statement seems to be true for compound **20** (GT-2331) and related compounds [48–50], as this compound was previously claimed as antagonist in rodents showing in later stages of testing full agonism profile in human. The situation is getting even more complex with proxyfan (**21**) and related structures as they displayed the full spectra of pharmacological properties from inverse agonists to full agonists depending on the test system and the conditions [51,52]. Therefore, this class of compounds belongs to protean agonists based on theoretical models on modulations of G-protein-coupled receptors [53]. Agonist properties have so far been reported for imidazole-derived compounds only. The aforementioned nonbasic compounds also displayed some antagonist properties. Slight variations could easily lead to inverse agonists or neutral antagonists without any remaining agonist properties but with high H_3R affinity.

Antagonists

There is great structural overlap between the classes of partial agonists, nonbasic agonists or protean ligands and antagonists/inverse agonists because they share the aforementioned structural blueprint. These features are also shared by the reference antagonists in this area, which are the thiourea derivative thioperamide (**22**) as the first potent ligand, clobenpropit (**23**) as an analog of the isothiourea compound imetit, and ciproxifan (**24**) as a selective compound with high *in vitro* and *in vivo* potency (Figure 5.7) [54]. Regardless of the current focus on nonimidazole leads, these structures are useful pharmacological tools for the sake of comparison because plenty of pharmacological data have been obtained. However, one should keep in mind that they share some moderate H_4R affinities (pK_i 7.3–7.6, **22**; 7.9, **23**; 5.7, **24**)

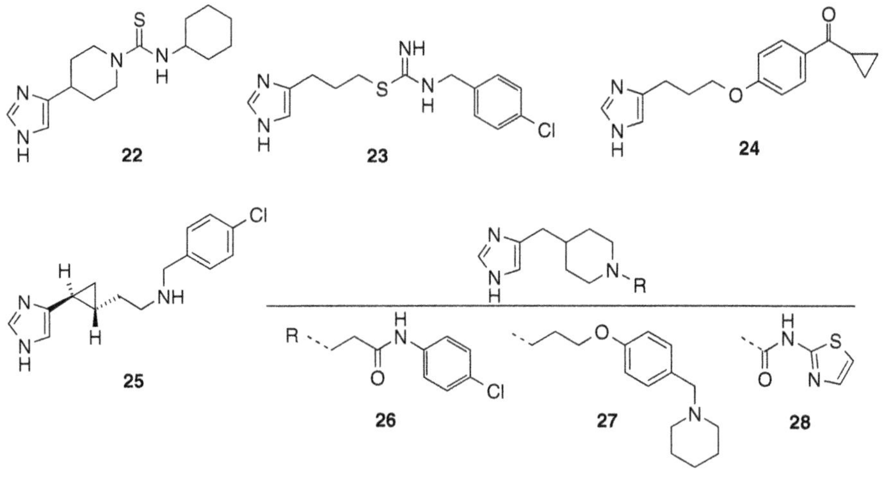

FIGURE 5.7 Imidazole H_3 antagonists, including thioperamide (**22**), clobenpropit (**23**), and ciproxifan (**24**).

[55] and clobenpropit is acting as H_4R agonist. As imidazole-containing compounds possess a high potential for interaction with cytochrome P450 isoenzymes [56], investigation on these reference structures showed interactions in the low micromolar concentration range for all of them [57].

The fluent structural transition from agonists to antagonists is well presented with agonist derivatives [58–60]. Indeed, the cyclopropyl derivative **25** displayed antagonism potency (pIC_{50} 8.1) and is comparable to less restricted compounds from the Leurs group [38]. The immepip derivatives **26**, **27**, and **28** showed pK_i values of 9.4, 8.5, and 8.4, respectively. Although compound **26** showed a pIC_{50} value of 7.4 on CYP2D6 (CYP3A4 pIC_{50} 4.7), compounds **27** and **28** displayed a better profile with pIC_{50} values of 4.9 and 5.7, respectively. Unfortunately, compound **27** showed extremely poor absorption and distribution in different species. A prodrug approach related to the one described for the agonists has also been recently reported for antagonists based on imidazole derivatization [61]. Many imidazole-containing compounds of recent series use this moiety as polar group instead of the histamine-like pharmacophore (*vide infra*).

Issues within Imidazole Chemical Class

The therapeutic use of imidazole-based H_3 ligands, and particularly H_3 antagonists, has suffered from many liabilities. As already mentioned, the imidazole ring is known for its potential to bind the iron atom in the heme of cytochrome P450 isoenzymes (CYP450). Therefore, many imidazole-based H_3 blockers have displayed high inhibition of the main CYP450 enzymes such as CYP2D6 and CYP3A4. Imidazole-containing compounds may thus compromise the metabolism of coadministered drugs, resulting in undesired drug–drug interactions [62] and extrapyramidal symptoms [13,56,63]. Furthermore, evidence of low oral bioavailability (e.g., thioperamide) and low brain penetration led a number of research groups in both academia and pharmaceutical companies to turn to the development of nonimidazole-containing compounds with more favorable druglike properties.

These few examples already make clear that the focus on the development of histamine H_3R antagonists has dramatically changed. Although 10 years ago, affinity and selectivity were mostly addressed, functional activities and *in vitro/in vivo* DMPK issues are recurrent for most current imidazole-based leads. The affinity at the so-called nontargets and pharmacokinetic problems rises dramatically with further pharmacological and clinical development. Cytochrome P450 (CYP_{450}) interactions, cardiac ion channels, and blood/brain ratios are now the topics to deal with.

DRUG DISCOVERY RESEARCH OF NONIMIDAZOLE-BASED H_3 RECEPTOR ANTAGONISTS

Academic Pioneers in the Nonimidazole H_3 Chemical Class

One of the first patents on potent histamine H_3R antagonists without an imidazole moiety came from the James Black group describing different types of guanidines [64]. Almost simultaneously, the consortium of Bioprojet and different academic groups filed a broad patent application on alkylamine-based compounds [65–70], leading to the discovery of BF-2.649 (former FUB649 (**29**); Figure 5.8) [71,72]. Indeed, BF-2.649 showed an ED_{50} value of 1.6 mg/kg and a maximal effect elicited at 10 mg/kg (p.o.) and 3–5 mg/kg (i.p.) in an *ex vivo* binding assay. Good oral absorption in mice with fast distribution (C_{max} of 30 min) and good brain penetration ($C_{max\ brain}/C_{max\ plasma}$ ratio of 23.5) are clear attributes to druglike behavior. Related compounds with an alternative substitution pattern showed reduced affinities at CYP_{450} isoenzymes, for example, pIC_{50} values at CYP2D6 7.2 µM (**29**), 4.7 (**30**), and <4 (**31**). BF-2.649 already showed promising preclinical data concerning affinity, selectivity, absorption, distribution, and pharmacological activities at sleep–wake state, cognitive impairment, epilepsy, and different models of psychiatric diseases. Compounds displaying variations of the ether functionality or nonaromatic analogs were also potent, but did not reach the profile of the parent compound [73,74]. Owing to some structural limitations of imidazole-based antagonists, maintenance of H_3R affinity within different piperidine-based compounds and analogs is clearly shown in Figure 5.8, with compounds **32** (pK_i 7.4; ED_{50} 2.4 mg/kg p.o.) and **33** (pK_i 8.6) [75–77].

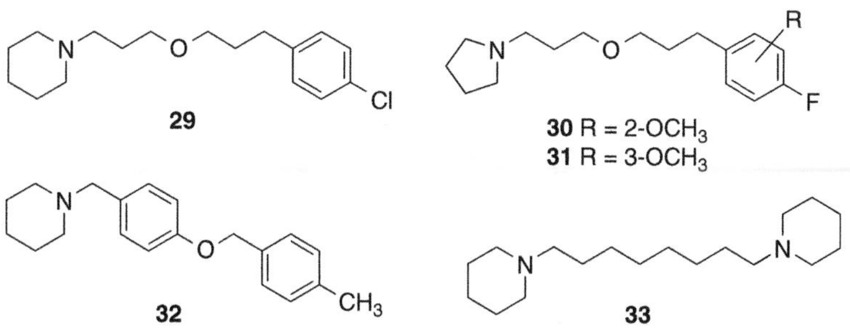

FIGURE 5.8 Identification of BF-2.649 (tiprolisant; **29**) and derivatives from Bioprojet. Novel ligands (**32** and **33**) from academic groups.

Earlier, academic groups from the Netherlands, Italy, Finland, United Kingdom, France, and Germany described their lead structures, whereas later on, the part was taken over by pharmaceutical companies.

Pharmaceutical Companies' Drug Discovery Programs: From Hits to Clinical Leads

Johnson & Johnson PRD: Targeting Provigilant Drugs

As shown by the number of patent applications filed within the past 7 years, J&J PRD (including both Ortho McNeil and Janssen Pharmaceutica) is considered as one of the main player in H_3R drug discovery research. Since their successful efforts to clone the human H_3R in 1999, J&J PRD recently entered clinical phase with their proprietary H_3R compound JNJ-17216498 (structure not yet disclosed), currently in phase II trials for the treatment of sleep/wake disorders and narcolepsy [8,9,78]. Frequently disclosed, their medicinal chemistry programs were mainly focused on improving pharmacokinetic properties (e.g., brain resident half-life), brain receptor occupancy, and distribution to identify the adequate profile to target such disease (e.g., increase daytime wakefulness without impacting night sleep).

An initial HTS campaign, using recombinant hH_3R, resulted in the discovery of RWJ-20085 (**34**, JNJ-280566; Figure 5.9) [79], originally developed in a calcium channel blocker program (pIC_{50} 6.2; [^{3}H]nitrendipine binding) [80]. Interestingly, JNJ-280566 displayed weak affinity at the hH_3R (pK_i 5.6) [81] and was therefore subjected to systematic modifications. First, shifting to lower alkylamino groups successfully boosted the potency, with a maximum obtained with the cyclic piperidino analog (**35**, hH_3R pK_i 8.5), whereas its less basic morpholino analog showed a 1.4-log unit decreased affinity (structure not shown). The piperidino-propoxy-, propylamino-, butyl-, and ethylethynyl-linkage conferred optimal activity, whatever the position of the methyl group onto the imidazopyridine moiety (e.g., hH_3R: **36**, pK_i 8.7; **37**, pK_i 8.2). Particularly, compound **36** (JNJ-6379490) exhibited good antagonism potency (pA_2 8.7) and selectivity over other histamine receptor subtypes and a panel of 50 targets (ca. 3-log-unit). Despite adequate pharmacokinetic profile (see Table 5.1) and CNS penetration properties in an *ex vivo* binding assay (ED_{50} of

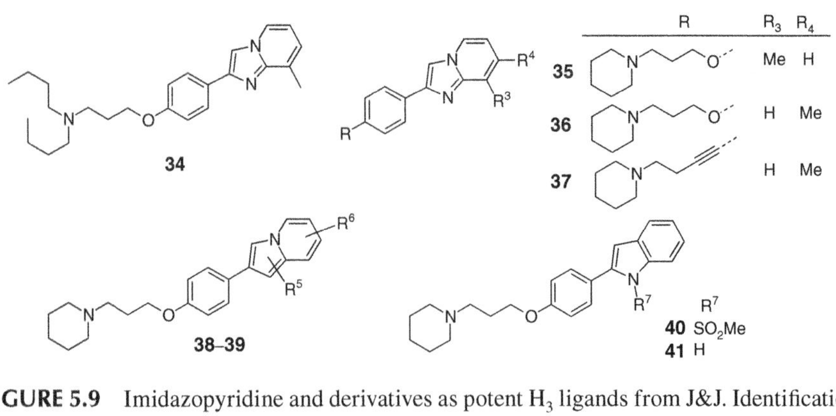

FIGURE 5.9 Imidazopyridine and derivatives as potent H_3 ligands from J&J. Identification of JNJ-280566 (**34**) and JNJ-6379490 (**36**).

TABLE 5.1

Summary of Pharmacokinetics Properties for Selected H$_3$ Antagonists

Compound	Name	Oral F (%)[a]	Vdss (L/kg)[a]	CL (L/h kg)[a]	$t_{1/2}$ (h)[a]
29	BF2.649	84	nr	nr	~2
36	JNJ-6379490	57	nr	nr	5.2
44	JNJ-5207852	>85	>100	nr	>13
51	Unknown	nr	3.55	12.8[b]	3.2
52	Unknown	nr	1.72	21.6[b]	0.92
56	A-304121	86	17.8	2.7	4.4
58	A-317920	35	2.3	2.3	0.7
65	A-349821	>100	6.3	3.2	1.3
		33[c]	2.3[c]	0.6[c]	2.6[c]
68	ABT-239	53	9.3	3.2	5.3
		74[c]	2.3[c]	0.8[c]	8.3[c]
72	A-424835	38	7.5	1.2	4.3
73	A-431404	57	12.2	1.8	4.8
74	A-698418	14	9.3	2.8	2.3
76	A-687136	17	12.2	2.7	2.6
77	A-688057	26	15.9	3.4	2.9
		30[c]	3.2[c]	1.3[c]	1.7[c]
84	Unknown	55	6.0	0.6	6.9
89	Unknown	70	7.4	0.53	8.3
90	Unknown	90	6.3	0.84	5.3
98	GSK189254	83	4.3	2.4	1.6
99	GSK207040	88	5.4	1.7	2.9
113	GSK334429	91	3.1	1.4	2.1
116	Unknown	80	nr	1.4	2.0
		90[c]	nr	0.6[c]	5.0[c]
126	NNC-0038-1202	85	nr	3.1	~3
137	Unknown	59	nr	nr	>10
210f	Unknown	21	9.6	1.1	9.3

Note: F%, oral bioavailability; Vdss, volume of distribution; CL, blood clearance; $t_{1/2}$, half-life.

[a] Values for rat species.

[b] CL expressed in milliliter per minute per kilogram after intravenous administration.

[c] Values for dog species.

0.2 mg/kg; i.p., rat), JNJ-6379490 has showed toxicity in dogs, which preclude its use from further development [79].

Efforts were then pursued around the imidazopyridine scaffold, with alternative heterocyclic ring systems [82]. Indolizidine-analog of JNJ-6379490 showed 1.5-fold decrease affinity (R^5 = H; R^6 = Me; **38** hH$_3$ pK_i 7.4), whereas the methyl group was better tolerated when located on the five-membered ring. Unsubstituted indolizidine (R^5 = R^6 = H; **39**) and N-methylsulfonyl indole gave similar affinity (e.g., **40** pK_i 7.9), whereas NH-free indole compound **41** showed weaker hH$_3$ affinity. Compound **39** was further profiled, showing good antagonism potency (pA_2 8.5), good permeability

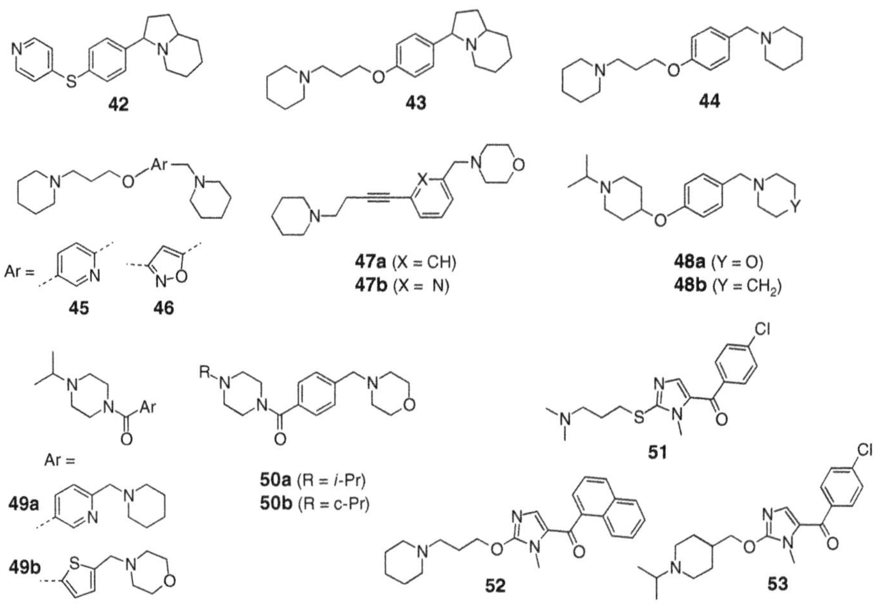

FIGURE 5.10 H$_3$ ligands developed by J&J. Identification of JNJ-10266386 (**42**), JNJ-5207852 (**44**), JNJ-10181457 (**47a**), JNJ-7737782 (**48a**), and JNJ-132600 (**51**).

properties in a Caco-2 assay (Papps $= 14.1 \times 10^{-6}$ cm/s) and favorable pharmacokinetic profile. The rapid metabolic clearance in human liver microsomes ($t_{1/2} \sim 10$ min) has limited the therapeutic scope of this imidazopyridine series. Efforts were therefore pursued toward the replacement of this heterocyclic ring system, while keeping a basic feature required for high affinity (Figure 5.10). One of the strategies was based on an initial HTS hit, bearing a similar saturated indolizidine (**42**, JNJ-10266386) [79] displaying weak hH$_3$R affinity (pK_i 6.5). Applying the aforementioned piperidinopropoxy moiety led to high hH$_3$R affinity compound **43** (pK_i 9.5) [83]. Interestingly, this dibasic feature is supposed to similarly operate on the natural product aplysamine **4** (Figure 5.4). This led J&J researchers to study SAR around aplysamine-based derivatives [21]. Shortening the right-hand-side ethyl chain did not influence the hH$_3$R affinity, but removing bromine atoms led to a fivefold increase compared with aplysamine affinity (pK_i 7.5). Combining both the actions and replacing the dimethylamino group by a piperidine at both the terminal sites provided a subnanomolar affinity H$_3$ ligand (**44**, hH$_3$ pK_i 9.4; rH$_3$ pK_i 9.0), identified as JNJ-5207852 [79,84]. This model further led to the design of derivatives around 4-(aminoalkoxy)benzylamines to study the SAR [85,86]. Most acyclic and cyclic amines, bearing polar groups or lipophilic residues, are tolerated at both the terminal sites, affinity ranging from pK_i 7.9 to pK_i 9.3. Replacing the nitrogen atom by a CH group has dramatically reduced the hH$_3$-binding affinity by 2- to 3-log unit. Therefore, one of the most active compounds in the series remains the *bis*-piperidine JNJ-5207852, with nanomolar to subnanomolar affinity (rH$_3$ pK_i 8.9; rat cortex H$_3$ (rctxH$_3$) pK_i 9.3), subnanomolar antagonism potency (pA_2 9.8), and 3-log unit selectivity versus histamine receptor subtypes and 50 off-targets (CEREP). JNJ-5207852 has also demonstrated excellent brain penetration and full H_3R occupancy at 1 mg/kg, with an ED_{50} of 0.12 mg/kg (s.c., rat). However, despite excellent oral bioavailability in rat ($F > 85\%$), JNJ-5207852 displayed unfavorable long half-life and high volume of distribution (see Table 5.1). Indeed, a rat biodistribution study revealed high concentration in kidney, lung, and liver; much higher than uptake in different brain regions such as cerebral cortex, hippocampus, and striatum [87]. More importantly, JNJ-5207852 induced phospholipidosis in rats [79], a known potential toxicity issue often observed in the case of cationic amphiphilic molecules bearing more than one basic center.

In the second round of optimization, while keeping piperidinomethyl group at the right-hand side of the structure, the phenyl central core could be successfully replaced by a six-membered heteroaromatic ring (e.g., pyridyl 45 hH_3 pK_i 9.1), the five-membered ring pyrazolyl surrogate showing 1-log unit decrease in hH_3R affinity (46) [88]. As mentioned earlier, the propoxy linker could also be switched to butyl-1-ynyl spacer, resulting in high-potent H_3 ligands, as exemplified in Figure 5.10 by compounds 47a (hH_3 pK_i 8.9) and its pyridyl meta-analog 47b (hH_3 pK_i 8.1) [89]. The less basic morpholino derivatives 47a (JNJ-10181457) showed slightly reduced H_3-binding affinity at hH_3 and rH_3 (rH_3 pK_i 8.1) but displayed high antagonism potency at hH_3 (pA_2 9.2). Interestingly, JNJ-10181457 had a more favorable pharmacokinetic profile compared with JNJ-5207852, with a maximal H_3 occupancy of 85% after 1 h in a rat *ex vivo* binding experiment (10 mg/kg, p.o.), whereas a parallel PK/PD study revealed a shorter brain residency ($<10\%$ H_3 occupancy after 24 h) ($\sim100\%$ after 48 h for JNJ-5207852).

To improve brain receptor occupancy, scientists at J&J PRD have pursued their search of novel H_3 antagonists belonging to their established dibasic pharmacophore and investigated linker rigidification (see also section Recent Advance in H_3 Receptor Ligand Computer-Aided Drug Design). Indeed, SAR around the conformational restricted *iso*-propyl piperidin-4-oxyphenyl framework provided highly potent H_3 antagonists, as exemplified by compounds 48a (hH_3 pK_i 8.7; pA_2 9.3) and 48b (hH_3 pK_i 9.2; pA_2 9.9) [90,91]. On the basis of previous investigations, the profile of morpholino derivative 48a (JNJ-7737782) was more detailed, with high selectivity on a panel of 50 targets (CEREP, $<18\%$ inhibition at 1 µM) but with a lower binding affinity for the rH_3R (pK_i 7.8). JNJ-7737782 has demonstrated *in vivo* efficacy in a rat Electroencephalogram (EEG) EEG model of wakefulness, supporting the therapeutic use of H_3 antagonists in sleep/wake disorders and narcolepsy.

More SAR investigations were disclosed by Carruthers and coworkers at the last European Histamine Research Society (EHRS) meeting in 2006, with the concomitant replacement of both phenyl central core and aminopropoxy spacer by a heteroaryl piperazinylcarboxamide framework [92,93]. Indeed, a large variety of heterocycles were introduced and screened against hH_3R, as exemplified by compounds 49a (hH_3 pK_i 9.0) and 49b (hH_3 pK_i 7.5). Compound 49a was further profiled, showing nanomolar affinity for the rH_3R, high antagonism properties (pA_2 9.2), and high selectivity in a CEREP screen. With good solubility and Caco-2 permeability, compound 49a has showed acceptable brain penetration with an ED_{50} of 6 mg/kg (*ex vivo* binding), oral bioavailability ($F = 50$–70%), and good *in vitro* ADME profile.

Interestingly enough, the phenyl analog **50a** has been recently highlighted in two patent applications together with its *N*-cyclopropyl piperazine analog **50b** [94]. A comparison study has been disclosed in which both compounds displayed nanomolar antagonism potency (**50a**, pA_2 8.4; **50b**, pA_2 9.0) and adequate pharmacokinetic profile in rat (see Table 5.1). It is worth mentioning that the introduction of the cyclopropyl group proved to lower the basic properties of compound **50b** (pK_a measured = 6.5; 5.3) compared with compound **50a** (pK_a measured = 7.6; 6.2), which may offer a greater permeability and volume of distribution profile.

Finally, other five-membered heterocycles have been investigated by J&J PRD: starting from the initial HTS hit JNJ-132600 (**51**, hH$_3$ pK_i 8.2, rH$_3$ pK_i 8.0; pA_2 8.7) [79], *N*-methylimidazole derivatives have been claimed in patent applications (e.g., **52**) [95] or compound **53** (hH$_3$ pK_i 8.4), for which a scale-up synthesis has also been reported [96].

Abbott Laboratories: Drug Design of Novel Cognitive Enhancers
Among the first players in the drug design of H$_3$R antagonist/inverse agonists, Abbott Laboratories—Neurosciences has been extremely active in terms of patent applications filling and medicinal chemistry program public disclosure. With two potential clinical candidates, namely, ABT-834 and ABT-239, Art Hancock and his team had to overcome many challenges to keep their chemical series alive from genotoxicity, phospholipidosis, and even cardiac proarrhythmia potential [97,98]. Their drug discovery program from HTS to candidate delivery is emphasized hereafter through the identification of chemically diverse H$_3$ antagonists/inverse agonists (Figure 5.11) [97,99].

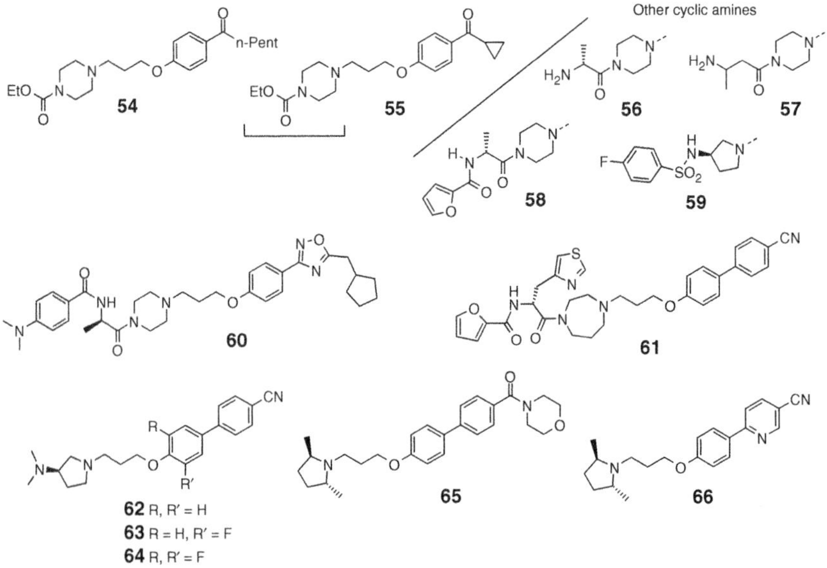

FIGURE 5.11 Selected H$_3$ ligands from Abbott Laboratories: identification of A-923 (**54**), A-304121 (**56**), A-308830 (**57**), A-317920 (**58**), A-320436 (**61**), A-331440 (**62**), A-417022 (**63**), A-423579 (**64**), A-349821 (**65**), and A-389985 (**66**).

Indeed, HTS hit A-923 (**54**), belonging to the earlier-defined pharmacophore, showed high affinity on rH_3R (pK_i 8.6), but suffered from poor bioavailability and selectivity versus histamine H_1R and H_2R subtypes. A hit-to-lead phase led to the design of new potent H_3 ligands around the piperazino-propoxyphenyl cyclopropyl-ketone scaffold, bearing a D-amino acid motif. This work directly led to the analog **55** (rH_3 pK_i 8.3) and discovery of the highly selective and orally bioavailable A-304121 (**56**, tartrate salt; rH_3 pK_i 8.9) and analog A-308830 (**57**, rH_3 pK_i 9.3) [100,101]. However, A-304121 is 3-log unit less potent at the hH_3R (pK_i 6.1), showing weak functional antagonism activity (pA_2 6.8) and more dramatically inducing multiorgan phospholipidosis and skeletal muscle waste in a 2-week rat toxicity study [97,102,103]. Suppressing the basicity of this cationic amphiphilic druglike scaffold by key substitution on the nitrogen atom of the piperazine moiety led to the identification of A-317920 (**58**), with no phospholipidosis potential [102,103]. Despite this improvement, A-317920 still demonstrated low affinity for the hH_3R (pK_i 7.0) compared with the rH_3R (pK_i 9.1) and moderate oral bioavailability (see Table 5.1), precluding its use as a development candidate. Further pharmacomodulation on both right- and left-hand-side parts of the propoxyphenyl motif successfully led to compound **59** with nanomolar affinity at both hH_3R and rH_3R (pK_i 8.8) [104,105]. Alternatively, the replacement of the cyclopropyl ketone by diverse substituted heteroaryl (e.g., cyclopentylmethyl oxadiazole) and aryl groups (e.g., *para*-cyanophenyl) provides high H_3 affinity piperazine-based compound **60** (hH_3 pK_i 7.8; rH_3 pK_i 8.6) [106,107] and homopiperazine analog **61** (identified as A-320436; hH_3 pK_i 8.8; rH_3 pK_i 9.3) [108,109]. Despite high selectivity versus several biogenic amines and transporters, A-320436 showed poor brain penetration and low oral bioavailability in rat ($F = 3.5\%$). Further screening of basic fragments onto this biphenyl scaffold provided new high-affinity ligands such as compound **62** (A-331440), which became the lead candidate in the antiobesity program of Abbott Laboratory (Figure 5.11) [110–114]. Indeed, A-331440 displayed nanomolar affinity at both hH_3 (pK_i 8.7) and rH_3R (pK_i 8.2) and moderate oral bioavailability in rat. However, a positive result in an *in vitro* micronucleus assay for potential genotoxicity forced Abbott to discontinue this proof-of-concept antiobesity candidate. Optimization around A-331440 lead compound successfully provided genotoxicity-free H_3R ligands, namely, A-417022 (**63**, hH_3 pK_i 8.4; rH_3 pK_i 8.2) and A-423579 (**64**, hH_3 pK_i 8.7; rH_3 pK_i 8.3) [115,116]. No development has been reported so far. Switching from (*R*)-3-dimethylaminopyrrolidine to 2,5-dimethylpyrrolidine (structure not shown, hH_3 pK_i 9.2; rH_3 pK_i 8.2) provides further improvement toward subnanomolar hH_3 ligands. The combination of both right-hand-side aryl modifications and the enantiopure (*2R,5R*)-dimethylpyrrolidine led finally to the identification of promising H_3 antagonists/inverse agonists in these series, such as A-349821 (**65**) and A-389985 (**66**) [117,118]. Both compounds showed high H_3 affinity (**65**, hH_3 pK_i 9.3, rH_3 pK_i 8.8 and **66**, hH_3 pK_i 9.2; rH_3 pK_i 8.6). More interestingly, A-349821 displayed competitive antagonism (pK_b 9.3) and inverse agonism ($pEC_{50} = 9.1$) properties in the $[^{35}S]$-GTPγS-binding assay, together with a high selectivity versus a large panel of receptors. In addition, A-349821 showed excellent pharmacokinetic properties in several species (see Table 5.1), neither with P-glycoprotein substrate liabilities nor with toxicity in a 2-week rat study [97–99,119]. Despite efficacy in cognitive models, A-349821 suffers from low CNS penetration (brain/plasma ratio = 0.6), and more dramatically, cardiovascular side effects, that is, prolonged cardiac action potential (QT interval duration), in the anesthetized dog model. By considering effective blood levels, these adverse cardiovascular effects subsequently provided a low safety margin, precluding its consideration as a development candidate [97,99].

To alleviate the cardiac toxicity of the former lead A-349821, its prototypical aminopropoxyphenyl framework was rigidified, a concept that has been often used to design druglike compounds by decreasing the number of rotatable bonds and linearity. Therefore, the 2-aminoethyl-benzofuran motif was modified to the more conformational restricted derivative that could enhance CNS penetration, and potentially improve the cardiac safety margin. Efficient chemical synthesis toward polyfunctionalized benzofuran derivatives successfully provided novel, highly potent, and selective H$_3$ antagonists (Figure 5.12). Indeed, compound **67** (A-360175), bearing the simplified (2R)-methylpyrrolidine as a basic part, provided the first fingerprint of a new generation of highly potent H$_3$ antagonists [120–122]. It displayed a 10-fold improvement on hH$_3$R (pK$_i$ 9.4) and rH$_3$R (pK$_i$ 9.0) affinity, together with competitive antagonism (pK$_b$ 9.3) and inverse agonism (pEC$_{50}$ 8.9) properties in the [^{35}S]-GTPγS-binding assay [122,123]. The *para*-cyanophenyl switch did not influence the binding affinity on either hH$_3$R or rH$_3$R and led to the identification of A-358239 (**68**), known as ABT-239 (hH$_3$ pK$_i$ 9.4; rH$_3$ pK$_i$ 8.9; pEC$_{50 \text{ inv.}}$ 8.9; pK$_b$ 9.0) [124,125]. Extensive preclinical studies have been performed on ABT-239 [126,127]. Displaying high selectivity versus a large panel of receptors, including other histamine receptor subtypes (150-fold to >10,000-fold), ABT-239 showed low *in vitro* metabolism on multispecies hepatocytes, excellent pharmacokinetic profile (see Table 5.1), and rather high plasma protein binding (PPB = 94% [rat]; 97% [human]) [107,128]. Interestingly enough, its (S)-enantiomer (A-631972, structure not shown) revealed similar binding affinity (hH$_3$ pK$_i$ 9.2; rH$_3$ pK$_i$ 8.6) but less selectivity versus α$_{2C}$ adrenergic receptor (α$_{2C}$AR pK$_i$ 7.2) [129]. Novel lead candidate ABT-239 (**68**) has showed high CNS penetration (brain/plasma ratio >20), and demonstrated broad efficacy in several behavioral tests, with high therapeutic index after acute, 2-week and 4-week chronic toxicity studies [99,127]. On the basis of the previous discontinuation of A-349821 for low cardiac safety margin, ABT-239 was further evaluated in dog and monkey cardiovascular safety studies. Although no cardiovascular side effects were observed in the canine model at more than 180-fold effective blood exposure level [130], a monkey telemetry study at effective concentration demonstrated QT prolongation, and thereby a low safety margin (around 30-fold) precluding its use for further development [97,131]. A solution to detect cardiotoxicity potential of new

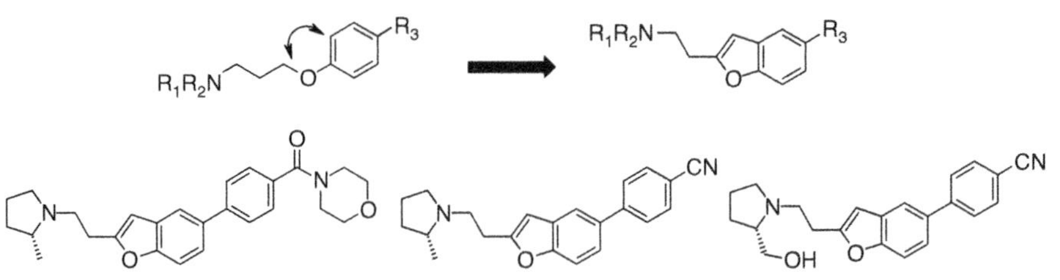

FIGURE 5.12 Rigidification strategy developed by Abbott Laboratories: identification of A-360175 (**67**), ABT-239 (**68**), and A-354396 (**69**).

chemical entities earlier in the drug discovery process has been the medium to HTS of compounds in the hERG potassium ion channel (either on radiolabeled ligand displacement binding assay or on patch-clamp technology), known to be involved in some cardiac proarrhythmia effects. Indeed, the recent disclosure of hERG binding affinity of ABT-239 (pK_i 6.7), displaying ~2.5-log unit selectivity versus the hH_3R affinity, is first in the search of hERG-free H_3 antagonists [132].

Pursuing therefore their search to deliver H_3 inverse agonists with optimal druglike properties, scientists at Abbott Laboratories explored the SAR around the benzofuran scaffold. More than 50 amines were introduced at the left-hand-side chain but did not improve the overall pharmacological properties observed with the (R)-2-methyl pyrrolidine. It is worth mentioning that the introduction of a hydroxyl function near the basic center did not dramatically influence the binding mode of compound 69 (A-354396; Figure 5.12), displaying nanomolar affinity on hH_3R and rH_3R, as well as good antagonism properties [123,131]. As shown in Figure 5.13, the right-hand-side chemical modulation has provided a large number of ABT-239-like derivatives, in which diverse electron-withdrawing/donating functional groups were introduced, not only onto the benzofuran central core but also on the aryl and heteroaryl group linked to it [107]. Particularly, compounds 70, 71 (A-424835), and 72 (A-431404) displayed high affinity, with highly potent hH_3R inverse agonism and competitive

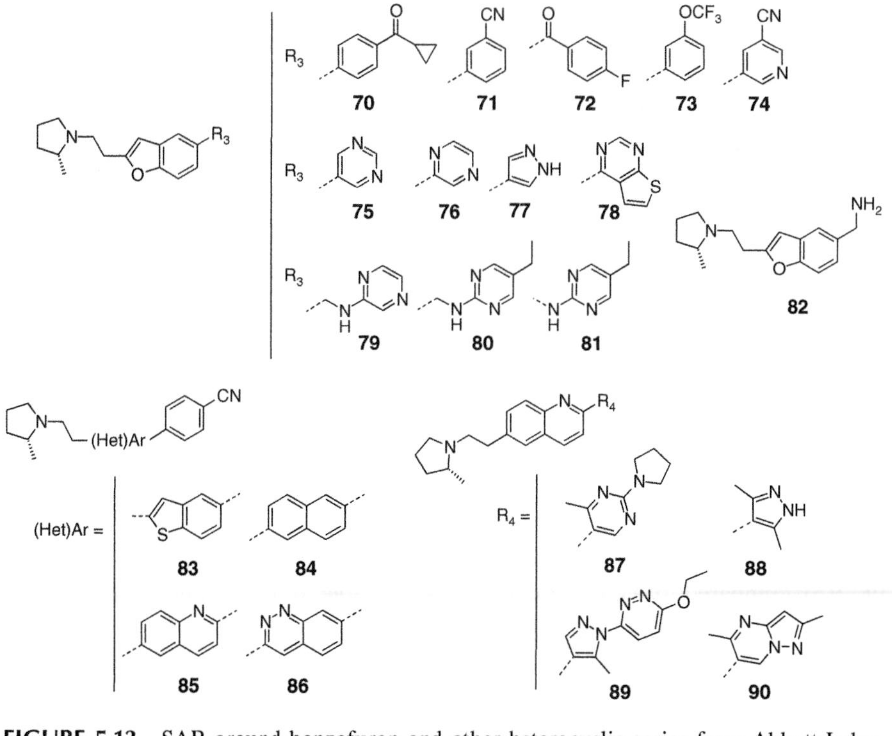

FIGURE 5.13 SAR around benzofuran and other heterocyclic series from Abbott Laboratories: identification of A-424835 (71), A-431404 (72), A-698418 (74), A-687136 (76), A-688057 (77), and A-748835 (88).

antagonism properties (**70**, pK_i 9.5; **71**, pK_i 9.5, pEC_{50} 8.7, pK_b 9.1; and **72**, pK_i 8.0, pEC_{50} 9.0, pK_b 9.2) in an hH_3 [^{35}S]GTPγS-binding assay. With good pharmacokinetics properties and high brain–plasma ratio (21x–61x) (see Table 5.1), selected compounds, 71 and 72, proved to be active in several models of cognitive and attention disorders. Although replacement of cyano group by trifluoromethoxy group led to a dramatically drop of binding affinity (**73**, hH_3 pK_i 8.0; rH_3 pK_i 6.9), switching to the cyano-pyridine led to a successful improvement in terms of *in vitro* biology profile (**74**, identified as A-698418; $hH_3\,pK_i$ 10.1, $rH_3\,pK_i$ 9.6) with 3-log unit selectivity versus α_{2C} and α_{1A} adrenergic receptors as well as dopamine transporter (DAT) [132]. A-698418 showed subnanomolar inverse agonism properties (pEC_{50} 9.5) but suffered from CNS adverse effects at low doses. Its adequate half-life ($t_{1/2}$ = 2.4 h) (see Table 5.1) still allowed the profiling of A-698418 in rodent models of cognition, showing efficacy at 0.03 mg/kg (i.p.). Shifting to pyrimidine 75 and pyridazine 76 led to similar hH_3R affinity and inverse agonism properties (pK_i 10.1 and 9.8, respectively; pEC_{50} 9.1 for both) [132–134]. Binding affinities for the rH_3R were lower for both compounds, more pronounced for 75 (A-687136) with a 1-log unit decrease and improved selectivity versus DAT. Despite a 10-fold improvement in observed CNS side effects, appearing at a dose >28 μmol/kg, A-687136 demonstrated poor pharmacokinetic properties in rat (see Table 5.1). The five-membered ring pyrazole 77 (A-688057) showed slightly reduced *in vitro* hH_3/rH_3R-binding affinity, selectivity, and inverse agonism potency (hH_3 pEC_{50} 8.8), and potent competitive antagonism properties in an electric field stimulation experiment in guinea pig (gpH_3 pA_2 8.1). Pharmacokinetic profile of A-688057 proved to be superior to A-698418 and A-687136, but did not match ABT-239 profile. Moderate PPB across five species was reported (64–87%) and its *in vitro* ADME profile revealed low CYPs inhibition at 2 μM except for the CYP2D6 isoform (IC_{50} 0.87 μM). On the basis of aforementioned cardiotoxicity issues, preclinical tests were performed for A-688057. Unlike ABT-239, A-688057 and its congeners A-698418 and A-687136 displayed a better selectivity profile on hERG-binding affinity (e.g., A-688057, pK_i <5.0) [97,132]. In addition, genotoxicity (micronucleus assay), mutagenicity (AMES test), and phospholipidosis (*in vitro* assay) were not induced by A-688057. The first CNS adverse effects (i.p., mice), such as tremor and ataxia, were noticed above 84 μmol/kg, with lethality from 280 μmol/kg, making A-688057 the cleanest of this set of compounds. A-688057 has been profiled for *in vivo* activity, showing efficacy in rodent model of cognition, attention, and impulsivity. The exact status of A-688057 in Abbott pipeline remains undisclosed.

Further derivatization toward heteroaryl or aminodiazine as a replacement of the initial *para*-cyanophenyl group led to the discovery of novel, potent H_3R antagonists (**78–81**) with comparable superior affinity (e.g., **78** hH_3 pK_i 10.2; rH_3 pK_i 9.8), compared to ABT-239 [135]. However, none of the compounds prepared, including these selected ones, proved superior in terms of pharmacokinetic properties (rat species), displaying low-to-moderate oral bioavailability, high plasma clearance, and reduced half-life, which might explain a moderate efficacy in models of cognition. It is also worth mentioning that the aminomethyl pyrimidine **80** showed a markedly reduced phospholipidosis index compared with its dibasic pyrimidine-free analog **82** [132].

Because the initial benzofuran ring affords optimal druglike properties combined to the (R)-2-methylpyrrolidine basic part, further SAR exploration around aromatic and heteroaromatic surrogates has followed and successfully provided high-affinity antagonists such as benzothiophenes (**83**, hH_3 pK_i 9.5), naphthalenes (**84**, hH_3 pK_i 9.7; rH_3 pK_i 8.6), and quinolines (**85**, hH_3 pK_i 9.2; rH_3 pK_i 8.3) [136–138]. Interestingly, cinnoline (**86**) showed a reduced binding on hH_3 (hH_3 pK_i 8.5; rH_3 pK_i 8.2) [139]. Early 2007, Black et al. [140] reported SAR around compound **84** and the influence of various secondary amines on the hH_3 and rH_3 affinity. Shifting from the 2-methyl to the linear or branched ethyl, *iso*-propyl and *iso*-butyl pyrrolidine dramatically reduced both hH_3 and rH_3 affinity (up to 3-log unit decrease, structures not shown). Despite an improved pharmacokinetic profile (see Table 5.1), recent *in vitro* cardiotoxicology studies on compound **84** showed similar hERG channel affinity to ABT-239 [141]. Fine-tuning chemical optimization to get rid of hERG activity has proven to be successful, as exemplified by A-688057 (**77**) but remains challenging in terms of pharmacokinetic and brain penetration profile.

Further SARs have also been explored, particularly the replacement of the *para*-cyanophenyl moiety by nearly 50 mono- (**87**, **88**), bi- (**89**, **90**), and tricyclic heteroaryls [139]. In this context, selected compounds described in Figure 5.13 have shown high affinity (hH_3 pK_i 9.0–9.7; rH_3 pK_i 8.6–9.4) and potency (hH_3 GTPγS, inverse agonism pEC_{50} = 9.1 [**87**], 9.2 [**89**], 9.0 [**90**]), and for some, excellent pharmacokinetic properties compared to ABT-239 (see Table 5.1) [142]. Adequate brain penetration and associated lower to moderate PPB across species (64–89%) were also demonstrated. Compounds **87**, **90**, and more recently **88** (A-748835) showed good efficacy in models of cognition and attention disorders. In a particular aspect, compound **90** did not show significant CYP450s inhibition issues, phospholipidosis, mutagenic, or clastogenic liabilities. In another recent disclosed study, the acute and daily dosing (5 days, 0.1 mg/kg, i.p.) of A-748835 did not alter rat brain H_3R-binding site expression, neither the efficacy nor the potency in an (R)-alphamethyl histam (RAMH)-induced drinking model [143]. No affinity on hERG K^+ channel has been reported to date.

Such intensive efforts, performed by Abbott Laboratory scientists, to combine *in vitro* potency, *in vivo* efficacy, adequate pharmacokinetic profile reinforced by the lack of any cardiotoxicity issues would certainly lead to promising clinical candidates in the near future.

GlaxoSmithKline: Drug Discovery Strategies in Central Nervous System and Non-Central Nervous System Areas

Drugs Targeting Dementia, Pain, and Narcolepsy Disorders

With more than 20 patent applications within 2 years and two drug candidates in clinical trials, GSK is another key leader in the histamine H_3 field. Since the first disclosure of their H_3 medicinal chemistry program in 2004 [144], the tremendous efforts around the discovery of their first clinical candidate GSK189254 have been unveiled [145,146].

HTS of the in-house GSK compound collection has resulted in the identification of compound **91** (Figure 5.14) [147]. Initially designed during a lead optimization phase of novel human urotensin-II (hUT) receptor antagonists, such as SB-436811 (**92**; hUT pK_i 6.7) [148], compound **91** (hUT pK_i 5.6) displayed potent H_3 antagonism activity (hH_3 fpK_b 8.6) despite an acyclic dimethylamino group, a basic part

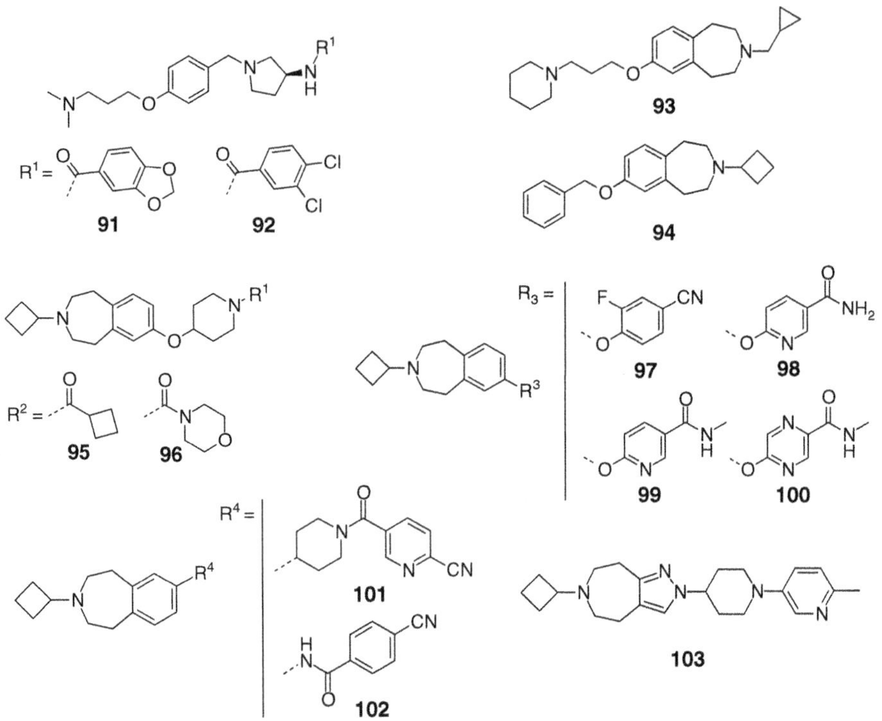

FIGURE 5.14 From HTS hits to the identification of H_3 drug candidates GSK189254 (**99**) and GSK207040 (**100**) from GSK.

known for weak affinity within the early discovered aminopropoxyphenyl-based H_3 antagonists. Poor pharmacokinetic properties led researchers to seek new scaffolds with better druglike properties. A conformational restricted template of initial hit **91** at the right-hand side provided bicyclic compound **93**, the first entry into the benzazepane ring system [149]. This dibasic compound effectively showed high antagonism activity (hH_3 pK_b 9.3). The initial replacement of the aminopropoxy side chain by a benzyloxy group (structure not shown) slightly influenced the affinity but, more importantly, highlighted the fact that compound **93** may act in a reverse mode at the hH_3R (see Recent Advance in H_3R Ligand Computer-Aided Drug Design). Therefore, this novel H_3 chemotype was further derivatized to study the scope of alkyl groups compatible with H_3 affinity. Among diverse sterically hindered acyclic and cyclic alkyl groups linked to the basic nitrogen atom of the core structure, the N-cyclobutyl group (**94**) provided the best-balanced properties between hH_3 potency (fpK_i 9.6) and *in vitro* PK profile (i.e., low CYP450s inhibition). However, owing to high metabolic clearance on human and rat liver microsomes (e.g., Cl_{int} >50 min/mL/g protein), a second round of optimization was performed. Novel rigidified N-acylpiperidyloxy group showed reduced hH_3 potency (**95**; fpK_i 8.9) but markedly improved ADME properties, weak CYP2D6 inhibition, and lower intrinsic clearance on both human and rat microsomes (Cl_{int} <3.9 min/mL/g protein). The more polar morpholinourea **96** maintained the potency (fpK_i 9.1) and demonstrated improved intrinsic clearance (Cl_{int} <1.4 min/mL/g protein) but only showed a moderate oral H_3R occupancy in the rat brain. This problem was tackled by switching to diversely substituted, planar (hetero)aromatic rings [150]. As examples, although lipophilic 2-fluoro-*para*-cyanophenyl group (**97**; hH_3 fpK_i 8.8) did not afford an appropriate affinity/ADME balance, nicotinamide **98** greatly afford improved potency (hH_3 fpK_i 9.3) and rat brain H_3 occupancy (81% at 3 mg/kg, p.o.) together with a low human intrinsic clearance (Cl_{int} = 0.7 min/mL/g protein). Its potential to inhibit CYP2D6 isoform led to the start of a fine-tuned SAR around the amide substitution. Increasing the bulk size of acyclic or cyclic alkylamine maintains the potency at hH_3 (fpK_i >9.5) and low intrinsic clearance across species. More interestingly, the *N*-methyl analog (**99**) showed the best *in vitro* ADME profile among the whole range of amines introduced (e.g., ethyl, *iso*-propyl, and pyrrolidinyl) (structures not shown). Indeed, compound **99** (GSK189254) had subnanomolar to nanomolar affinity (hH_3R recombinant/cortex pK_i 9.9/9.6; rat hH_3R recombinant/rcortex pK_i 9.2/8.6) together with an excellent selectivity profile over a large panel of targets (CEREP) [151,152]. GSK189254 displayed potent competitive antagonism (pA_2 9.1) and inverse agonism activity (pEC_{50} 8.2), with good physicochemical properties (log D_{oct} = 0.9; solubility >5 mg/mL, at pH 7.4). Oral administration in rat brain cortex of GSK189254 revealed high H_3 occupancy (ED_{50} = 0.17 mg/kg in *ex vivo* binding assay), predicting a good brain penetration. Together with an excellent pharmacokinetic profile (see Table 5.1), a good brain–plasma ratio of 1.2:1 at steady state (PPB = 61%), GSK189254 demonstrated efficacy in several rodent preclinical models of dementia and sleep/wake disorders [153]. *In vivo* microdialysis studies recently completed its pharmacological profile, showing a clear modulation of key neurotransmitters (e.g., HA and ACh) in different brain regions involved in arousal, learning, and memory processes [154].

The replacement of the pyridine nucleus by a pyridazine ring (**100**, GSK207040) did not alter any of the primary screening parameters, that is, subnanomolar affinity (hH_3R pK_i 9.7) and excellent brain penetration properties from *ex vivo* binding studies (oral ED_{50} = 0.03 mg/kg) [155]. GSK207040 displayed subnanomolar affinity at native H_3R expressed in human-, rat-, and pig brain cortex (pK_i = 9.7 [hctx]; 9.1 [rctx]; 9.5 [pctx]), whereas having lower nanomolar affinity at mouse- and dog cortex H_3 (pK_i < 9.0). High selectivity at the other histamine receptor subtypes (>1000-fold) and over a panel of around 50 targets has been demonstrated, together with good functional antagonism (pA_2 9.23). With high brain penetration and excellent pharmacokinetic profile (see Table 5.1), GSK207040 demonstrated *in vivo* activity in rodent models of scopolamine-induced amnesia and capsaicin-induced secondary allodynia.

Since the identification of GSK189254 as an excellent development candidate, scientists further explored the initial benzoazepane central core as a privilege drug-like scaffold. Some examples of other analogous structures (**101**, **102**) and more recently pyrrazolo-azepane **103**, have also been claimed as potent H_3 antagonists (Figure 5.14) [156–158].

Alternative spacers were also investigated, leading to piperidinyloxy chemical series as represented in Figure 5.15. The introduction of *N*-(hetero)aryl piperidine group provided potent H_3 antagonists in the nanomolar to subnanomolar affinity range, as exemplified by selected compounds (**104**, **105**, and **106**) (hH_3 pK_b 8.9–10.2) [159]. Interestingly, introduction of polar substituents led to an improved intrinsic

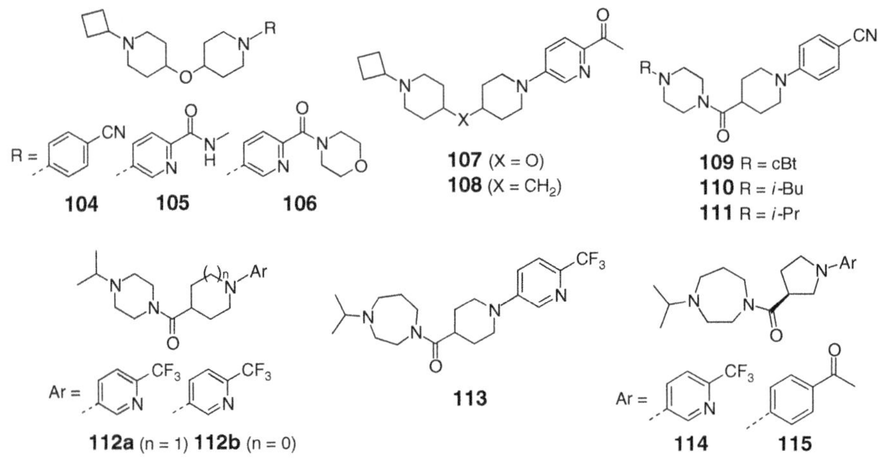

FIGURE 5.15 Selected H_3 ligands reported by GSK: identification of GSK357868 (**105**), GSK334429 (**113**), and GSK678103 (**115**) as potent H_3R antagonists.

clearance (Cl_{int} human <1.8 mL/min/g protein), more pronounced on the rat species (Cl_{rat} ranging from 6.1 mL/min/g (**104**) to <0.5 mL/min/g (**106**)). Compound **105** (GSK357868) showed more favorable profile among the disclosed compounds, displaying an oral ED_{50} value of 0.08 mg/kg in the *ex vivo* binding assay and a good brain–blood ratio of 2:1, predicting an adequate CNS penetration. The influence of the ether linker was further initiated with a selected panel of aryl and heteroaryl series. Indeed, the replacement of the bridged oxygen atom by a methylene linker within the 2-acetyl-5-yl derivatives (**107** and **108**) resulted in higher potency (hH_3R pK_b 10.5 and 9.9, respectively) [160]. Moreover, the introduction of the cyclobutyl group resulted in improved potency and affinity at both hH_3R and rH_3R, when compared to methyl, *iso*-propyl, and cyclopropylmethyl groups (data not shown). Particularly, compound **108** showed oral efficacy in the *ex vivo* binding assay (84% H_3R occupancy at 3 mg/kg, p.o., 3 h postdose) and low to moderate intrinsic clearance on rat and human liver microsomes (Cl_{int} <6 mL/min/g protein).

Scientists at GSK have also investigated the replacement of the 1-subtituted-piperidin-4-yloxy by a 1-subtituted-piperazin-4-ylcarbonyl group while varying the aryl/heteroaryl on the right-hand-side part [161]. Compared to previous *para*-cyanophenyl derivative **104**, cyclobutyl, *iso*-butyl, and *iso*-propyl groups provide less potent compounds (i.e., **109**, **110**, and **111**, respectively, pK_b ranging from 8.8 to 9.2). The *iso*-propyl piperazine derivative **111** has, however, showed the best *in vitro* clearance profile (Cl_{int} = 0.3 [human] and 1.1 [rat] mL/min/g protein) together with a good oral brain penetration (ED_{50} = 1.3 mg/kg, *ex vivo* binding) and adequate brain/blood ratio (1.2:1). Further derivatization onto the piperidinyl right-hand-side substituents provided 2-trifluoromethyl-pyridin-5-yl **112a** analogs with an overall improved potency (hH_3R pK_b >9.6), on human metabolic clearance (Cl_{int} <0.8 mL/min/g) and on brain penetration properties, with an oral ED_{50} <0.57 mg/kg. Lower N-pyridinyl pyrrolidinyl (**112b**) analogs have resulted in reduced potency, and more importantly, in lower brain penetration properties [162]. Shifting from trifluoromethyl-pyridin-5-yl piperazine to its homopiperazine analog led to the identification of the highly potent antagonist GSK334429 (**113**, hH$_3$ pK_b 9.7), showing a 10-fold improvement in binding affinity at rat recombinant H$_3$R (pK_i 9.0). Indeed, it displayed subnanomolar affinity at native H$_3$R expressed in human-, rat-, mouse-, and pig brain cortex (pK_i 9.1–9.6), although having nanomolar affinity at dog cortex H$_3$R [155]. Sharing similar *in vitro* profile (selectivity and potency) as GSK189254, GSK334429 displayed good oral efficacy in the *ex vivo* binding assay (*ED*$_{50}$ = 0.35 mg/kg; brain/blood ratio of 0.8:1), adequate *in vitro* clearance (e.g., *Cl*$_{int}$ hum <0.5 mL/min/g protein) and moderate PPB (PPB = 66%). Together with good to excellent pharmacokinetic profile (see Table 5.1), GSK334429 has demonstrated *in vivo* efficacy in rodent models of scopolamine-induced amnesia and capsaicin-induced secondary allodynia.

On the basis of these excellent pharmacological and pharmacodynamic properties, GSK scientists applied the homopiperazine feature to the lower *N*-trifluoromethylpyridinyl and *N*-phenyl pyrrolidine analogs, namely, compounds **114** and **115**, exemplified in Figure 5.15 as their enantiopure (*R*)-form [162]. In contrast to compound **114**, showing a 10-fold decrease in antagonism potency, higher *in vitro* clearance and low oral H$_3$ occupancy in rat, its *N*-cyclobutyl analog (structure not shown), however, restored subnanomolar potency (pK_b >10) and good oral brain penetration (H$_3$R occupancy of 94% at 3 mg/kg, 3 h postdose). Within the *N-iso*-propyl homopiperazine series, 4-phenylacetyl **115** (GSK678103) showed improved potency (~1-log unit), good *in vitro* clearance for both human and rat species (*Cl*$_{int}$ <0.6 mL/min/kg), and oral brain penetration (H$_3$ occupancy of 89% at 3 mg/kg, p.o., 3 h postdose), with an ED$_{50}$ of 0.37 mg/kg, similar to that of GSK334429. Furthermore, GSK678103, in further studies, has demonstrated nanomolar affinity at rH$_3$ (pK_i 9.0), low CYP450s inhibition (*IC*$_{50}$ >100 µM) and a good brain/blood ratio of 2.6:1. Since the public report of this medicinal chemistry program, GSK recently disclosed a novel phase I clinical candidate GSK239512 (structure not disclosed) for the treatment of dementia [145].

Drugs Targeting Inflammation and Allergic Rhinitis
On the basis of the intensive medicinal chemistry program developed at GSK for the discovery of CNS drug candidates, some chemical opportunities have recently emerged in the non-CNS area. Indeed, the identification of compounds **116** [163] and recently **117** [164] within the aforementioned piperidyloxy-based series has been specifically claimed for the treatment of inflammatory and allergic disorders field (Figure 5.16). Particularly, compound **116** showed subnanomolar functional antagonism (pK_b 9.5) and good pharmacokinetic properties in rat and dog species (see Table 5.1). Its low brain-penetrating properties with increased plasma level make these compounds attractive for H$_3$-mediated peripheral disorders.

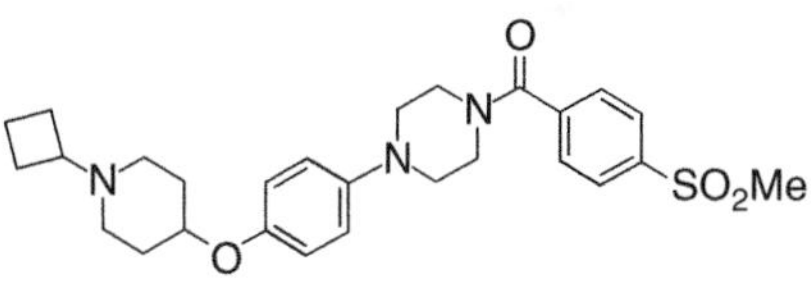

116 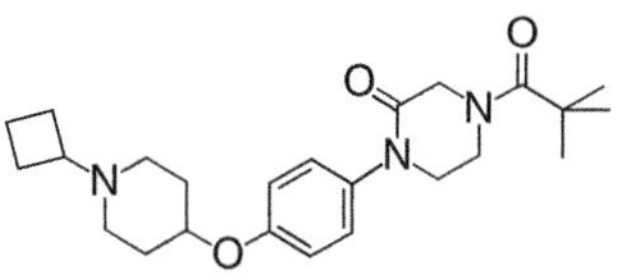   **117**

FIGURE 5.16 H$_3$R antagonists claimed by GSK for treatment of inflammatory disorders.

Novo-Nordisk: Medicinal Chemistry Program Targeting Antiobesity Agents
After having been earlier involved in the development of imidazole-based H_3 antagonists, scientists from Novo-Nordisk focused their research from 2003 onward around nonimidazole derivatives. Preliminary investigation around monoacyldiamine-based synthesis, either by solid-support or by solution-based methodologies, led to the screening of around 700 compounds using H_3-binding assay. Focused libraries were further prepared in the monoacyl piperazine chemical series with potent H_3 antagonism properties using a GTPγS functional assay [165]. Selected branched and cyclic alkyl-piperazines showed subnanomolar antagonism potency, as exemplified by compounds **118**, **119**, **120**, and **121** (e.g., 119 hH_3 pK_i 9.1) (Figure 5.17), whereas increasing the bulkiness of the alkyl group has resulted in less-potent compounds (e.g., **121**, hH_3 pK_i 6.3). Cyclopentyl-piperazine **120** (NNC 0038-1049) displayed nanomolar antagonism potency and has been used as an excellent pharmacological tool in rodent models of obesity. Further SAR exploration around 3-pentyl-piperazine **119** with various linker types and substituted aryl groups was initiated. Indeed, the replacement of the keto function by an oxygen atom maintains nanomolar potency (**122**). The linker pattern and dibasic feature had showed a strong influence on potency, as exemplified by ethyloxyphenyl **123** (hH_3 pK_i 7.0) and 4-dimethylaminophenyl-acetamide **124** (hH_3 pK_i 9.0). Switching the piperazine basic part to a new 2-([pyrrolidin-1-yl]methyl)pyrrolidine chemotype led to a dramatic decrease of potency into the micromolar range (**125**, hH_3 pK_i 5.7) [166]. On the basis of the previous investigation performed around the linker topography, the butan-1,4-dione was converted into a

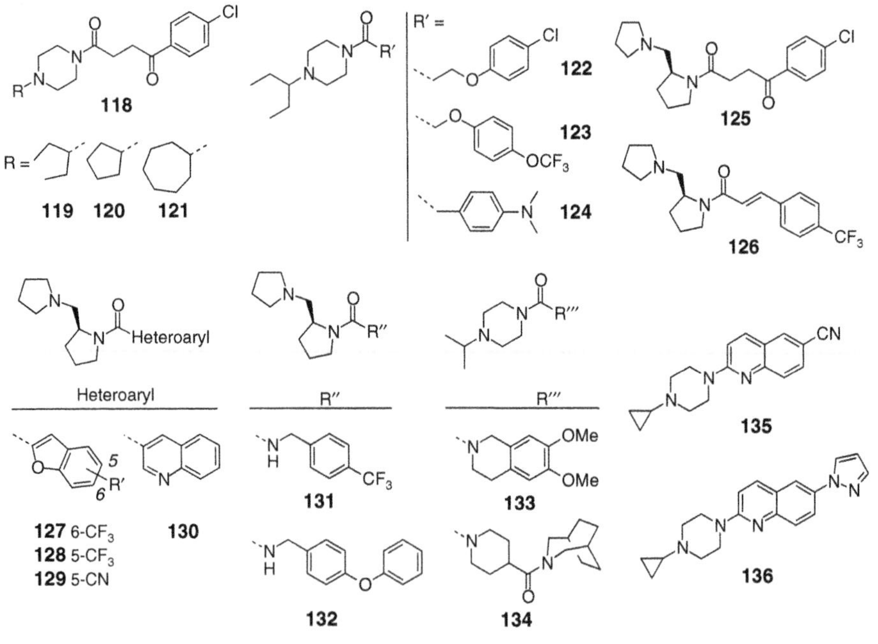

FIGURE 5.17 Selected H_3 ligands investigated by Novo-Nordisk and identification of NNC-0038-1049 (**120**), NNC-0038-1202 (**126**), and NNC-0038-2238 (**134**).

cinnamic rigidified linker, which successfully restored the initial nanomolar potency observed in the piperazine series for some dihydro analogs (**126**, NNC 0038-1202, hH$_3$ pK_i 8.3). NNC 0038-1202 was further characterized, displaying weak affinity at the rH$_3$ (pK_i 7.1) but good selectivity against a panel of 75 receptors (CEREP). *In vitro* ADME profiling revealed low CYP$_{450}$ inhibition at the 2D6 and 3A4 enzyme isoforms (*IC*$_{50}$ > 65 μM) and low micromolar activity at the CYP1A2 isoforms. Moreover, NNC 0038-1202 showed an adequate pharmacokinetic profile (see Table 5.1). The replacement of trifluoromethyl group by polar substituents such as nitrile, sulfonylmethyl, methoxy, or ketone slightly influences the antagonism potency (pK_i 7.9–8.6). Rigidification of the cinnamic linker with the phenyl moiety into a benzofuran ring system provided novel potent H$_3$ antagonists **127** (hH$_3$ pK_i 7.8), with a more pronounced nanomolar hH$_3$R activity for the 5-substituted derivatives, as exemplified by compounds **128** (pK_i 8.4) and **129** (pK_i 8.3) [167]. It is worth mentioning that the bicyclic quinoline analog **130** resulted in weaker potency (pK_i <6.8). Cross-screened on CYP450 isoforms, namely, CYP1A2, 2D6, and 3A4 subtypes, compound **130** showed low to moderate inhibition of all three isoforms than for lead NNC-0038-1202 and trifluoromethoxy analog (30 and 31% at 10 μM, respectively), whereas its cyano derivative (hH$_3$ pK_i 8.2, structure not shown) has shown a better profile on main CYP450 isoforms (<10% at 10 μM). More importantly, early assessment of the cardiac proarrhythmia potential of lead compound NNC-0038-1202 has revealed high hERG-channel inhibition in the astemizole-binding assay (73% at 10 μM). In a search to identify hERG-free H$_3$ antagonists, scientists at Novo-Nordisk pursued their investigation toward a lead-hopping strategy [168]. Applied to the cinnamic derivatives, the more polar trifluoromethyl benzylurea analogs **131** revealed not only weaker antagonism potency (hH$_3$ pK_i 6.8), but a markedly reduced hERG inhibition (20% at 10 μM) also. A large chemical diversity was explored (more than 300 ureas obtained) in which the substituted benzyl ureas were found to be the most potent compounds from the series. As exemplified by compound **132**, the introduction of lipophilic residues provided encouraging improvement in hH$_3$ potency (hH$_3$ pK_i 7.6) and simultaneously gave higher hERG inhibition (62%). Several conformationally constrained features are also known to reduce hERG-binding potential. A parallel synthesis of alkylpiperazine-based compounds was therefore investigated, including a wide diversity of polar, lipophilic, or bulky groups. Gratifyingly, improved H$_3$ antagonism potency was noticed (around 20 molecules reported, hH$_3$ pK_i 7.3–8.2) together with low hERG inhibition, as exemplified by selected compounds **133** and **134** (hERG-inh. <10% at 10 μM). NNC-0038-2238 (**134**; hH$_3$ pK_i 7.9, hERG-inh. 8% at 10 μM) has shown a low propensity to interact with CYP1A2, CYP2D6, and CYP3A4 (*IC*$_{50}$ > 25 μM). On the basis of the knowledge acquired within the alkylpiperazine series, the same group investigated novel compounds displaying lower molecular weight and polar surface area as well as fewer rotatable bonds, as a strategy to improving brain penetration to centrally bind to H$_3$R [169]. First, the *N*-alkylpiperanylquinoline was investigated, showing a more pronounced potency for cyclopropylpiperazinyl-quinolines. As exemplified by compounds **135** (hH$_3$ pK_i 8.3) and **136** (hH$_3$ pK_i 9.0), the introduction of small polar substituents or even heterocycles led to the most potent H$_3$ antagonist in this series. Therefore, combining both binding data and *in vitro* ADME-Tox-(ADMET) properties proved to be a successful strategy at Novo-Nordisk in their H$_3$R drug discovery program.

Eli Lilly & Co, Laboratoires Servier, Hoffman-La Roche, and Pfizer:
Drug Design Efforts toward Novel H₃ Receptor Antagonists

Since 2003, researchers from Eli Lilly & Co have focused their medicinal chemistry program on novel *N*-benzoyl 2-(pyrrolidin-1-ylmethyl) pyrrolidine derivatives. Indeed, early claimed compound **137** displayed nanomolar potency (hH₃ pK_i 9.0) with adequate pharmacokinetic properties in rat (oral F = 59%) (Figure 5.18) [170,171]. Interestingly, Lilly scientists further claimed novel potent H₃ antagonists in which part of the spacer is modified and fused to the phenyl-core (**138**) [172] and for some others, the aminopropoxy linker is removed, as shown in claimed compound **139** [173]. In this case, a dramatic decrease in hH₃R-binding affinity is noticed (pK_i 7.1), but this modification proved that the *N*-benzoyl 2-(pyrrolidin-1-ylmethyl) pyrrolidine fragment could serve as a potent surrogate of the classic aminopropoxyphenyl framework. Further investigation from Lilly scientists led to novel potent H₃ antagonists, as exemplified by claimed compound **140a–e** (hH₃ pK_i 7.3–8.5) [174–177].

From the same group, another class of compound within the aminopropoxyquinoline series has been recently reported [178]. Starting from tetrahydroisoquinoline (THiQ) scaffold **141**, identified following medium-throughput screening campaign, and displaying nanomolar antagonism potency (hH₃ pK_i 8.6), a selected diversity of lipophilic (e.g., ethyl and cyclohexylmethyl) or polar (e.g., thiophenoyl and phenylsulfonyl) residues onto the nitrogen atom were investigated around the THiQ and the tetrahydroquinoline (THQ) analogs (Figure 5.19). The 6- and 7-substituted THiQs (**142** and **143**, respectively) were generally more potent than their 5- and 8-substituted THQ regioisomers, with a more pronounced subnanomolar affinity for the di-basic one (e.g., **142a**, hH₃ pK_i 9.3; **143a**, hH₃ pK_i 9.3). With the exception of THiQ **143b** (hH₃ pK_i 9.5), the introduction of a phenylsulfonyl group onto all nitrogen-regioisomers led to 10-fold less potent compounds. Further derivatization of the central core was explored, and particularly, the access to the benzoazepane ring system, as exemplified by selected compound **144a,b**, displaying high potency (e.g., **144b**, hH₃ pK_i 9.7; rH₃ pK_i 8.9) [179]. The introduction of polar groups (acyl, methylsulfonyl) led to monobasic compounds with weaker affinity (~1-log unit decrease) at the rH₃R than at the hH₃R. Compounds **143a** and **144b** were further profiled, displaying nanomolar hH₃R inverse agonism potency in a GTPγS-binding assay (**143a** pIC_{50} 9.0;

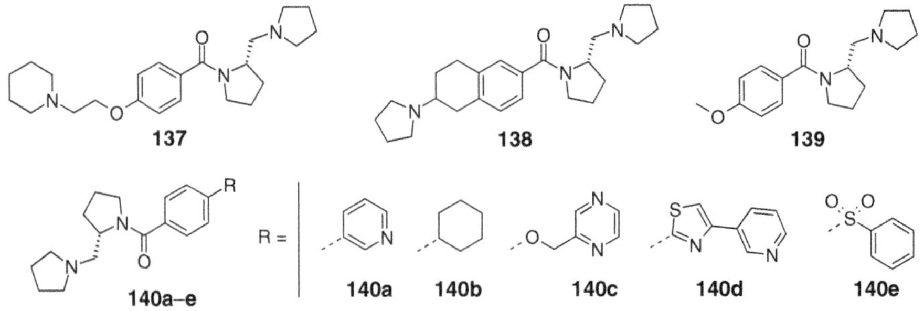

FIGURE 5.18 Pyrrolidinomethylpyrrolidine carbamoyls as potent H₃R antagonists claimed by Eli Lilly & Co.

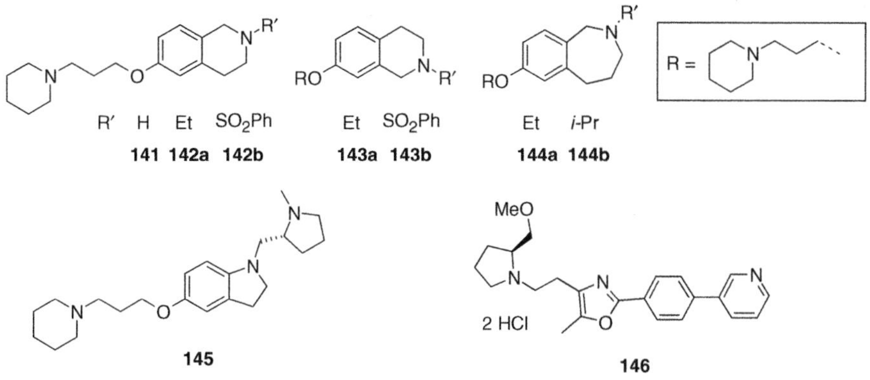

FIGURE 5.19 Tetrahydroisoquinoline, benzazepine, indoline, and tricyclic derivatives as potent H₃R antagonists described and claimed by Eli Lilly & Co.

144b pIC_{50} 8.8) as well as more than 1500-fold selectivity versus the other histamine receptor subtypes. Both compounds had good oral brain penetration as observed in a rat *ex vivo* binding assay, with an IC_{50} of 1.1 and 5.3 mg/kg for compounds **143a** and **144b**, respectively. Moreover, both compounds showed adequate pharmacokinetic properties in rat (>69% oral bioavailability). In a patent application, indoline **145** was also claimed as a potent H₃ antagonist (pK_i 9.3) [180], demonstrating that the benzo-fused cyclic amine represented an attractive scaffold that both Lilly and GSK have successfully explored. Another distinct chemical class has also been claimed by the same group around the aminoalkyloxazolyl phenyl derivatives, as exemplified by compound **146** with potent H₃ antagonism properties (hH₃ pK_i 7.8).

Scientists at Laboratoires Servier recently disclosed their medicinal chemistry program [181]. On the basis of a database-mining approach, they first developed an *in silico* tool from an initial set of 15,000 compounds and applied molecular descriptors and druglike property filters, to generate a final database set for screening against the H₃R. Chemically diverse hits were found (Figure 5.20), as exemplified by compound **147** (S750-1), **148** (S01743-1), and **149** (S08676-1), displaying weak to moderate antagonism properties (e.g., **147**, hH₃ pK_i 7.3). Particularly, S750-1 showed 1-log-unit less affinity for the rH₃, moderate metabolic clearance, and moderately increased endogenous cerebral concentration of N^τ-methyl histamine by 48% (30 mg/kg in mice, p.o.), a marker of H₃ antagonism activity *in vivo*. It is worth mentioning that the resolution of S750-1 gave the pure enantiomer S36639-1 (hH₃ pK_i 7.4), approximately five times more potent than its isomer S36640-1. Moreover, as S750-1 was negative in an *in vitro* toxicity AMES (II) test, this provided confidence to pursue this novel octahydro-2H-pyrrido[1,2-a]pyrazine chemical series in a hit-to-lead phase [182]. Focused on increasing potency while keeping a good pharmacokinetic profile, structural modifications such as linker size, central polar group, and right-hand-side phenyl substitution have resulted in the identification of compounds **150** (S36662-1) and **151** (S36620-1) with similar affinity (hH₃ pK_i ~7.3). Both showed good antagonism potency (pK_b ~7.5) in a GTPγS-binding assay. Interestingly, the replacement of the trimethoxyphenyl by a *para*-cyano phenyl group resulted in

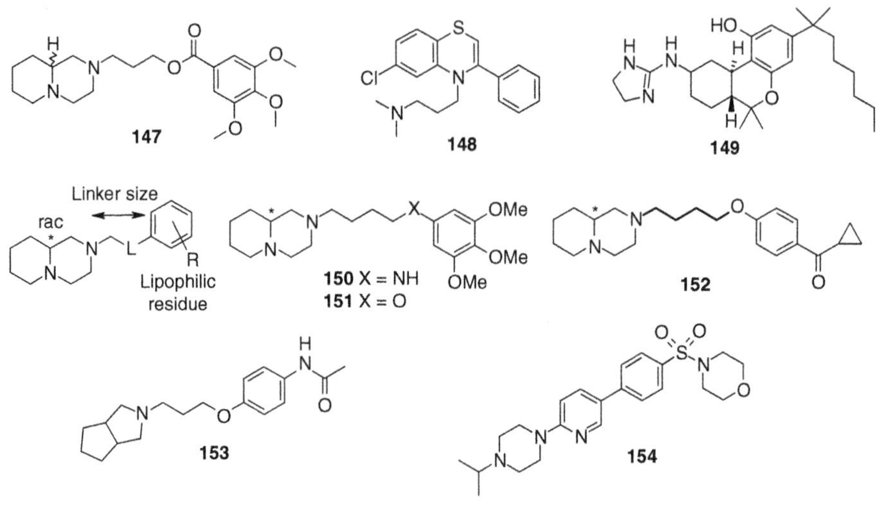

FIGURE 5.20 Selected H_3R antagonists described and claimed by Laboratoires Servier: identification of S36662-1 (**150**), S36620-1 (**151**), and S38761-1 (**152**).

a 1-log-unit improvement on the hH_3 affinity in the case of butoxy (structure not shown, hH_3 pK_i 7.0–7.6), compared to its propoxy analogs. Further exploration of phenyl substitution led to the identification of S38761-1 (**152**); displaying nanomolar affinity (hH_3 pK_i 8.1; rH_3 pK_i 7.6); high increase of central N^τ-methyl histamine; and good metabolic stability on human, rat, and monkey liver microsomes. The same group has also claimed similar azabicyclic-alkylphenoxy-based compounds as well as novel heterocycles as potent H_3 ligands in patent applications, as exemplified by selected compounds **153** and **154** , respectively [183,184].

Newly entered in the H_3 field, scientists from Hoffman-La Roche presented, at the Annual EHRS Meeting in 2006, a short SAR study about H_3 inverse agonists for the treatment of obesity, a therapeutic field mainly dominated by Novo-Nordisk and Abbott Laboratories [185]. On the basis of the well-known pharmacophore model (*vide infra*), they have explored the naphthalene and quinoline chemical series linked to the common aminopropoxy linker (Figure 5.21) [186]. This led to a first compound **155a** displaying good affinity and inverse agonism properties (hH_3 pK_i 7.6; pEC_{50} 7.6, GTPγS assay) as well as a 3-log-unit higher selectivity at the other histamine receptor subtypes. Shifting the 4-methoxypiperidine onto the carboxamide moiety not only led to a lower affinity compound (**155b**, hH_3 pK_i 7.0) but also successfully improved metabolic stability on rat liver microsomes (Cl_{int} = 8 μL/min/mg protein) compared to **155a** (Cl_{int} = 67 μL/min/mg protein). Similar bicyclic carboxamide derivatives have been claimed in several patent applications, displaying good hH_3 affinity, as exemplified by quinoline **156** (hH_3 pK_i 7.1) [187] or indole derivatives **157** [188]. Interestingly, Roche medicinal chemists recently reported fused pyrazino-indole in which the amide is linked to the indole nitrogen (**158** hH_3 pK_i 8.2) [189]. This scaffold is closely related to their antiobesity $5HT_{2C}$ receptor agonist program targeting antiobesity agents, in which the classic aminopropoxy spacer is missing, such as in compound **159** ($h5HT_{2C}$ pK_i 8.4) [190]. Any specific affinity data on serotonin

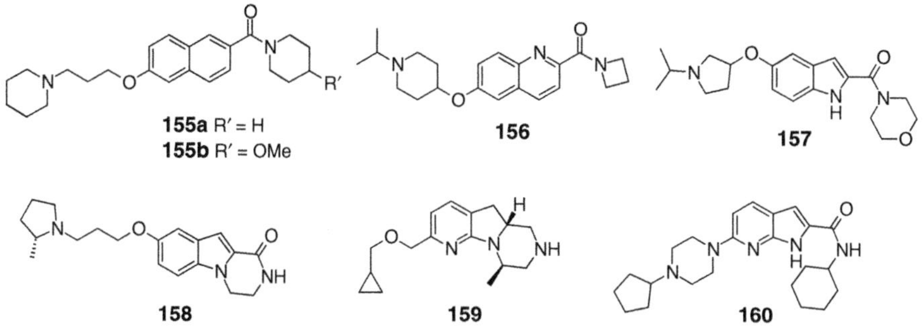

FIGURE 5.21 Selected H$_3$R ligands (**155–159**) described and claimed by Hoffman-La Roche.

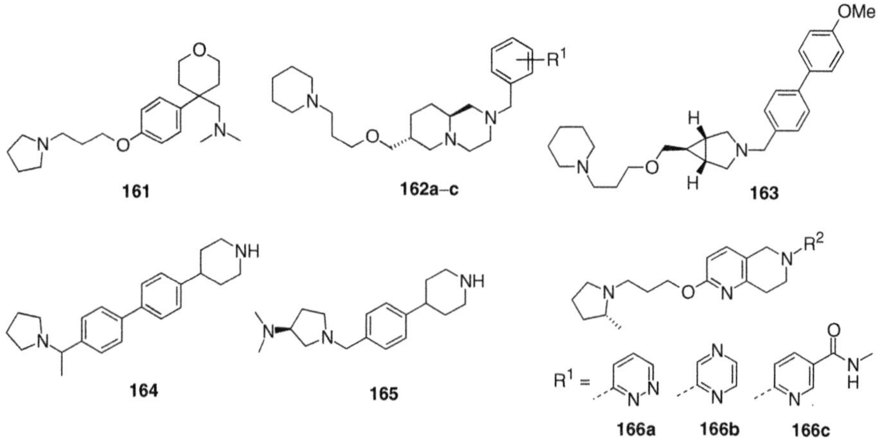

FIGURE 5.22 Selected H$_3$ ligands claimed by Pfizer.

receptors are disclosed in their H$_3$-related patent applications, but the low potential for phospholipidosis and hERG potassium channel of compound **158** is undoubtedly a good starting point for new derivatives in their H$_3$R program. Such chemical framework has therefore been intelligently used for the drug design of H$_3$R ligands, with cyclopentyl piperazinyl moiety as a surrogate of the classical spacer, as exemplified by compound **160** (hH$_3$ pK_i 7.4) [191].

New structural classes have appeared in several patent applications from Pfizer since 2005, sharing the known aminopropoxyphenyl feature (*vide infra*), such as compound **161** with subnanomolar affinity at hH$_3$ (pK_i 9.4), potentially due to its dibasic feature (Figure 5.22) [192]. However, novel aza and diazabicyclic structures revealed submicromolar to nanomolar affinity at native H$_3$R expressed in rat cortex, as exemplified by selected claimed compounds **162a** (R = H, rH$_3$ pK_i 6.9), **162b** (R = 4-SO$_2$Me, rH$_3$ pK_i 7.4), **162c** (R = 3-F, rH$_3$ pK_i 8.0), and **163** (rH$_3$ pK_i 7.5) [193–195]. Some substituted benzylamine derivatives have also been claimed in several patent applications, as exemplified by dibasic compounds **164** (rH$_3$R pK_i 8.0) and **165** (rH$_3$ pK_i 7.5) [196,197]. More interestingly, recently claimed tetrahydronaphthyridine derivatives have been screened on H_3 (functional cAMP assay) and hERG potassium ion channel (competition binding on [^{3}H]-dofetilide radioligand) [198]. Selected compounds **166a–c**, sharing the common aminopropoxy spacer, displayed similar hH_3 potency (pK_i ~8.0) and 1,000- to 10,000-fold selectivity versus hERG K^+ channel (**166a**, pK_i 4.3; **166b**, pK_i 4.9, and **166c**, pK_i 4.0).

Banyu Pharmaceutical, Athersys, AstraZeneca, Sanofi-Aventis, Neurogen, Schering-Plough, UCB Pharma, and Arena Pharmaceuticals: New Chemical Entities as H_3 Receptor Modulators

Researchers at Banyu Pharmaceutical have reported new chemical series in several patent applications including novel oxo-pyridine-, oxo-quinazoline-, and fused tricyclic-based structures displaying nanomolar activity at hH_3 (e.g., **167**, hH_3 pIC_{50} 9.5; **168**, hH_3 pEC_{50} 9.6, GTPγS) (Figure 5.23) [199,200]. In efforts designed to replace the aminopropoxyphenyl spacer, carbamoyl spirocyclohexyl derivatives were identified as highly potent H_3 antagonists (e.g., **169**, hH_3 pIC_{50} 10.1) [201]. Indeed, the Athersys group has claimed novel indolizidinol alkynylaryl-based derivatives such as **170** (hH_3 pIC_{50} 8.0) [202]. Researchers at AstraZeneca have claimed phenyl carboxamide (**171**) and benzyl-urea (**172**) derivatives [203,204]. Sanofi-Aventis group is also active in the H_3R field, claiming novel nonimidazole-containing antagonists in patent applications, including compounds **173** (no specific activity described) and **174** (hH_3 pK_i 10.2) together with *in vivo* activity in a rat antiobesity model [205,206].

In 2006, Neurogen entered the H_3 arena with newly claimed chemical entities such as compounds **175** and **176** as representatives (no specific data) [207,208]. Since their long-term involvement in the histamine H_1/H_3 field, scientists at Schering Corp. have identified novel nonimidazole H_3 antagonists that do not belong to the classical aminopropoxyphenyl framework. Indeed, piperidinomethyl-aminopyridines (**177a,b**), and more recently amino-alkoxyphenyl-benzimidazole-based compounds

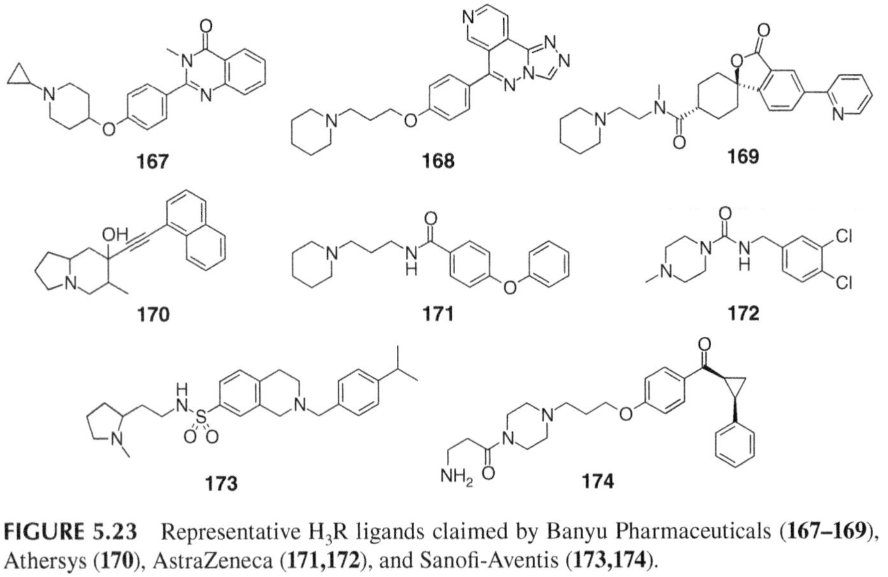

FIGURE 5.23 Representative H_3R ligands claimed by Banyu Pharmaceuticals (**167–169**), Athersys (**170**), AstraZeneca (**171,172**), and Sanofi-Aventis (**173,174**).

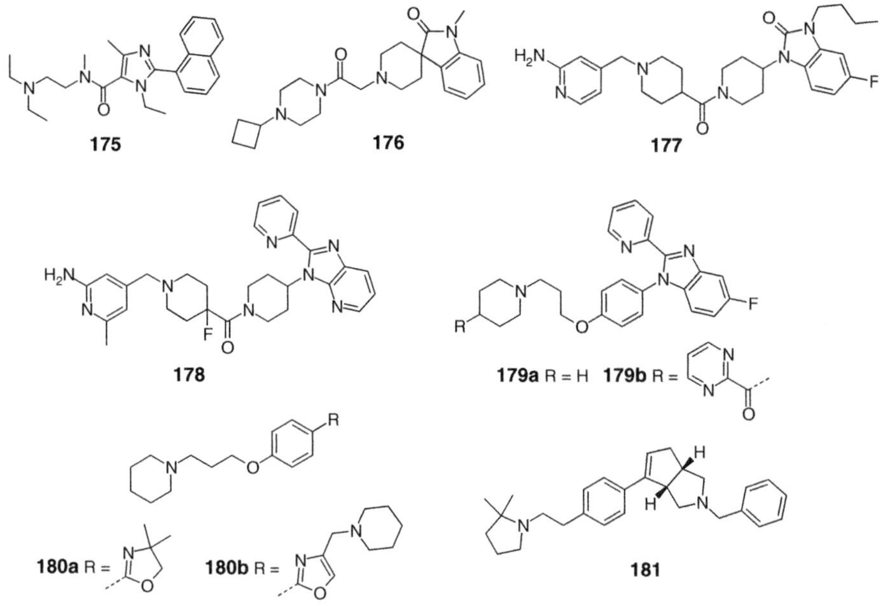

FIGURE 5.24 Representative H$_3$R ligands claimed by Neurogen (**175a–b**), Schering Corp. (**176–179a,b**), UCB Pharma (**180a,b**), and Arena Pharmaceuticals (**181**).

(e.g., **178a** hH$_3$ pK_i 9.0; **178b**), have been claimed in a number of patent applications by this group (Figure 5.24) [209–212]. Involved in the histamine H$_1$R field earlier, with the antihistaminic blockbuster drug Zyrtec® (cetirizine) for the treatment of allergic rhinitis, scientists at biopharmaceutical company UCB Pharma pursued their efforts toward the discovery of novel histamine H$_3$ ligands. In two patent applications, novel oxazoline and oxazole-based structures have been reported, with compounds **179** and **180** as selected examples (no specific data described) [213,214].

Finally, in 2007 Arena Pharmaceuticals entered the H$_3$ field with aza-bicyclic derivatives as H$_3$ modulators (e.g., **181**, hH$_3$ pK_i 9.2). Analogs have also been claimed with therapeutic potential in sleep wake disorders [215]. No patent applications have been reported so far.

RECENT ADVANCE IN H$_3$ RECEPTOR LIGAND COMPUTER-AIDED DRUG DESIGN

Introduction

Molecular modeling studies published within the histamine H$_3$ field have remained limited compared to the vast variety of H$_3$ ligands that have been disclosed over the past few years [6]. Besides the obvious Intellectual Property (IP) reasons that will limit publication of three dimensional (3-D) knowledge, several studies suggest that different classes of histamine H$_3$R antagonists may interact with different sets of receptor site points. Since a very low number of mutational studies have been published for the H$_3$R, the absence of validating mutagenesis data has to a certain extent hampered the interpretation of SAR in terms of receptor binding. Still, the existence of a large dataset of experimentally tested H_3 antagonists as well as mutation studies in the H_1R–H_4R has guided the generation and validation of *in silico* models. In the absence of crystallographic structural data of the H_3R, the reported modeling studies (Table 5.2) have relied on ligand-based modeling techniques such as pharmacophore mapping and 3-D-QSAR models and 3-D receptor homology modeling—two approaches that have proven particularly successful for investigating GPCR/antagonist binding. These models, which will be discussed hereafter, provide a greater understanding of the bioactive conformation and binding mode of both imidazole- and nonimidazole-containing antagonists compared to the 2-D prototypical representation of H_3R antagonist-binding features as shown in Figure 5.25 [6]. This knowledge can then serve as a basis for the design of highly potent H_3R binders or for virtual screening purposes.

TABLE 5.2
In Silico 3-D Models for H_3R Antagonists Reported within the Histamine H_3 Field

Model	Compounds Studied	Hypothesis	References
Pharmacophore model	Imidazole-containing antagonists	IBS	216
Pharmacophore models	Antagonists	Interaction with D114 and E206	236
3-D-QSAR	Nonimidazole antagonists		238
rH_3R model bovine rhodopsin	Imidazole-containing antagonists	IBS	220
	Extended to nonimidazole compound		227
rH_3R and hH_3R model bovine rhodopsin	Imidazole-containing antagonists		228
rH_3R and hH_3R endothelinR model	Agonists and antagonists	Interaction with D114	230
hH_3R bovine rhodopsin	Nonimidazole antagonists	Interaction with D114 and E206	235
hH_3R bovine rhodopsin	Antagonists		236

Note: IBS, imidazole-binding site.

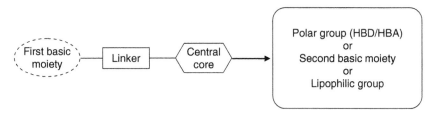

FIGURE 5.25 (See color insert following page 148.) Prototypical pharmacophore for histamine H_3R antagonists: a basic moiety is connected through a linker (often propyloxy chain) to an aromatic central core, which can be further substituted by lipophilic groups, basic moieties, or H-bond donors or acceptors.

Histamine H₃ Receptor Antagonists *In Silico* Models

A pharmacophore model for imidazole-containing antagonists was proposed by De Esch et al. [216], which reveals four hydrogen-bonding site points and two distinct lipophilic pockets available for antagonist binding. The model that is exemplified in Figure 5.26A [216] is based on the hypothesis that all imidazole-containing ligands bind to the same receptor site. This essential role of the imidazole ring derives from studies where substituting or replacing the imidazole moiety by other functional groups leads to a dramatically reduced or a total loss of H_3R activity. Besides the imidazole group, most of the antagonists considered in their study contain an additional NH moiety, which can interact with a hydrogen-bonding acceptor site. A previous study conducted by the same group on imidazole-containing ligands, whether agonists or antagonists, suggested interaction for this NH moiety with the highly conserved aspartic acid D114 [217]. Since the linker group connecting both moieties in antagonists is significantly longer than in agonists, the model suggested an alternate conformation of the highly conserved aspartic acid D114, according to whether it is binding to agonists or antagonists. Such a molecular *switch* between agonistic versus antagonistic activity was similarly proposed for the histamine H_1R [218].

Revealing the existence of lipophilic pockets 1 and 2 for antagonists binding explained the observed differences in the SAR of histamine H_3R antagonists [216]. Antagonists, such as clobenpropit (**23**), occupy pocket 1, whereas the lipophilic tail of thioperamide (**22**) interacts with hydrophobic pocket 2. Information about the shape of pocket 2 was obtained by the incorporation of a Quantum Structure-Activity Relationship study conducted on 15 thioperamide derivatives, which showed a correlation ($r = .93$) between the pA_2 and the dihedral angle φ between the thiourea and

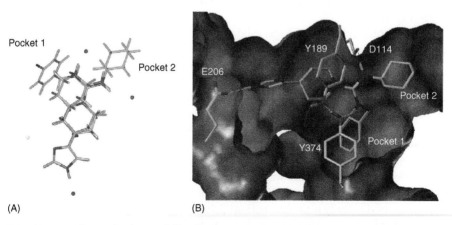

(A)   (B)

FIGURE 5.26 (See color insert following page 148.)   (A) The binding site for histamine H_3 receptor antagonists proposed by De Esch et al., can be described by four hydrogen-bonding site points and two lipophilic pockets. (B) Compound **183** bound to Lorenzi et al., [220] 3-D rH_3R model showing an interaction pattern involving residues E206, D114, Y189, Y374 as well as lipophilic pockets 1 and 2. (Reprinted from De Esch, I.J.P., Mills, J.E.J., Perkins, T.D.J. et al., *J. Med. Chem.*, 44, 1666–1674, 2001; Lorenzi, S., Mor, M., Bordi, F. et al., *Bioorg. Med. Chem.*, 13, 5647–5657, 2005. With permission from Elsevier.)

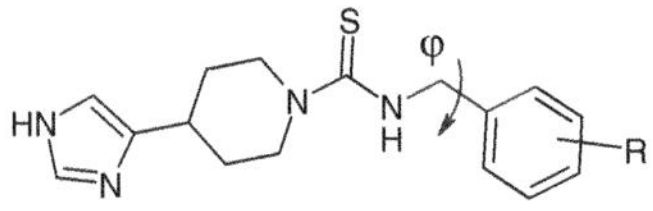

FIGURE 5.27 Thioperamide derivatives. Correlation between the pA_2 and the dihedral angle φ between the thiourea and the benzyl moiety and the calculated electron density δ on the substituted carbon atom, following the equation $pA_2 = -0.02(\pm 0.003)$ φ $- 0.93(\pm 0.16)$ δ $+ 4.81(\pm 0.42)$.

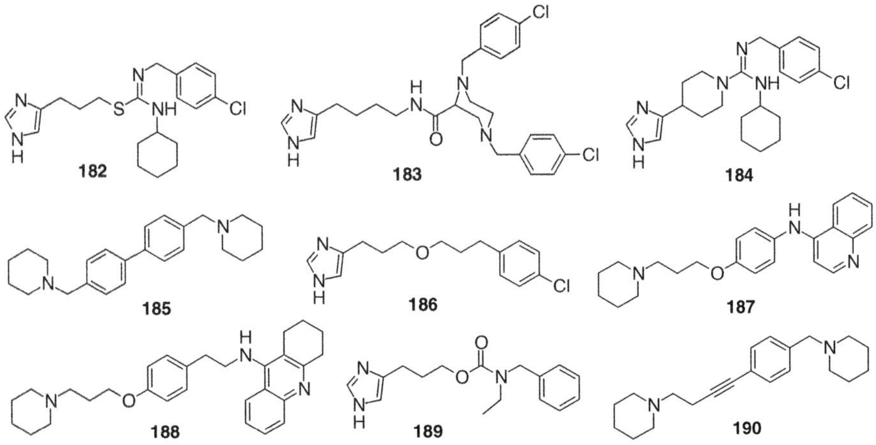

FIGURE 5.28 Selected H_3R ligands used in the computer-aided drug design studies.

the benzyl moiety and the calculated electron density δ on the substituted carbon atom (Figure 5.27) [219].

The pharmacophore model was validated through the synthesis of a novel series of clobenpropit-based antagonists with high H_3R affinity, designed to interact with all four hydrogen-bonding sites and the two hydrophobic pockets as exemplified by VUF5228 (**182**) (Figure 5.28). Branched compounds (e.g., **183**), published from the Schering research group, further supported this pharmacophore model (Figure 5.25) [220].

The existence of two lipophilic pockets was further suggested by docking imidazole-containing antagonists into a 3-D model of the rat histamine H_3R, built by comparative modeling from the crystallographic coordinates of bovine rhodopsin [220]. As in the previous study, the existence of an imidazole-binding site for imidazole-containing ligands was postulated. On the basis of mutational studies reported on the histamine H_1–H_4R regarding histamine binding, the underlying hypothesis of this study is the interaction of the imidazole ring with amino acid E206 [221–225]. The resulting model, in good agreement with the previously mentioned pharmacophore model, reveals a cavity allowing accommodation of antagonists such as clobenpropit or thioperamide through interaction with residues E206 (TM5), D114 (TM3) as well as two tyrosine residues, Y189 belonging to the extracellular loop 2 and Y374 in TM6 (Figure 5.26B [220]). The latter residue, which is conserved among the histamine receptors, could be critical for the antagonist behavior since it is spatially close to W371, suggested to be involved in receptor activation [226].

The two pockets identified are mainly lipophilic in nature. The bigger one, pocket 1, is deeply inserted between helices 3, 6, and 7 and is surrounded by L117, C370, W371, F367, W402, and N404, whereas pocket 2 is delimited by Y91, W110, H187, F398, W399, and W402. The model was able to accommodate compounds VUF5228 (**182**) and **184**, both of which contain two lipophilic groups, giving a pattern of interaction in the model similar to those of clobenpropit and thioperamide. The model was further shown to accommodate a series of rigidified nonimidazole compounds with a similar pattern of interaction [227]. The results related to this series will be discussed later and compared to other reported binding modes for nonimidazole H_3 ligands.

A similar region of interaction for H_3 imidazole-containing ligands was proposed by Stark et al. [228] in an effort to rationalize binding differences looked for some antagonists between the rat histamine H_3 (rH_3) and the human histamine H_3R (hH_3). Although the rat and the human receptor have above 90% overall homology, they differ by only five amino acids at the level of the transmembrane domain, two of which, residues V_r122A_h and A_r119T_h, are described to account for the observed species dependent binding properties [229,230]. Two 3-D homology models were constructed for the histamine rH_3R and hH_3R on the basis of the crystallographic coordinates of bovine rhodopsin. Docking of ciproxifan, clobenpropit, thioperamide, and 11 iodoproxyfan derivatives into both models resulted in a pattern of interaction where the tautomerism of the imidazole ring allows the molecules to interact with two glutamate residues, E206 and E191 (Figure 5.29A [228]). The latter glutamate residue is located on the extracellular loop 2, which folds into the binding pocket, similar to the previous model where Y189 was highlighted. Y115 (TM3) further stabilizes the imidazole ring in this position. D114 makes no direct hydrogen bond

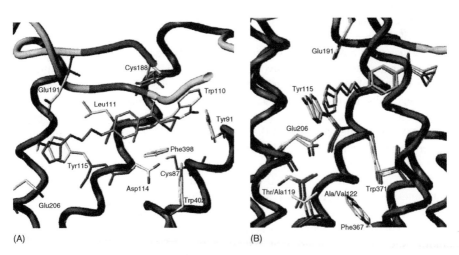

(A)   (B)

FIGURE 5.29 (See color insert following page 148.)   (A) Possible interaction sites proposed by Stark et al., between ciproxifan (violet) and the rH_3R are shown (helices in front of the ligand are not displayed for reasons of clarity). (B) Influence of amino acids A119T and V122A on the binding site and on the binding of ciproxifan (rH_3R residues are colored white and bound ciproxifan orange, hH_3R residues are colored green and bound ciproxifan green). (Reprinted from Stark, H., Sippl, W., Ligneau, X. et al., *Bioorg. Med. Chem. Lett.*, 11, 951–954, 2001. With permission from Elsevier.)

to any of the investigated ligands with the exception of clobenpropit, in which the carboxylate group of the aspartic residue interacts with the polar isothiourea group of the ligand. Although the global orientation of the antagonists was found to be very similar in both receptor models, A_r119T_h and V_r122A_h mutations were found to indirectly influence the geometry of the imidazole-binding pocket, as these two residues are located in proximity to E206 and Y115 (Figure 5.29B).

The existence of a specific imidazole-binding site for all imidazole-containing histamine H_3R ligands and the role of the interaction between the imidazole ring and E206 are challenged by mutagenesis experiments, indicating that E206A mutation does not significantly modify the K_D value of iodoproxyfan [221], which further suggests the possibility of alternative binding sites.

A second study, which analyzed how the amino acid changes between the human and the rat H_3R might be responsible for the pharmacological differences observed for some antagonists, considered both imidazole and nonimidazole H_3R ligands [230]. Molecular models in this case were developed by analogy with earlier work on the dopamine D_1 and endothelin receptors, leading to very different binding hypothesis. The assumption in this study is the interaction of the most basic moiety of the compounds with amino acid D114 on TM3. The compounds are further inserted into a cleft between TM2, 3, 6, and 7 parallel to the transmembrane helices (Figure 5.30A [230]). A similar binding region and an *upright* ligand orientation have also been described recently in a homology model of the dopamine D_2 receptor [231]. This region between TM3, 6, and 7 was able to accommodate the lipophilic group of clobenpropit in the model developed by Lorenzi et al. [220] (pocket 1) and previously discussed. However, in the present case, the compounds are inserted more deeply into the cavity than previously reported. In this orientation, agonists are suggested to have a second crucial interaction with D80 on TM2, a residue shown to be important for functional activity of different GPCRs [232], whereas antagonists would not interact with D80. In the structure of bovine rhodopsin, it has been suggested that this residue is present in its protonated state [233] and involved in a hydrogen-bond network with intramolecular water molecules [234]. Using the model, species selectivity is rationalized by a direct influence of residues 119 and 122, both in proximity to the site occupied by the ligands. In particular, the larger side chain of valine at position 122 in the rH_3R makes a smaller cavity than the alanine of the hH_3R would make, leading to tighter interaction with the lipophilic groups of thioperamide or A-304121 (**56**), the most species-selective H_3R inverse agonist (Figure 5.30B). This model, in which histamine spans from D114 to D80 without interacting with E206, is challenged by mutagenesis data, where E206A mutation was reported to significantly influence histamine binding [221].

A recent study considering a series of nonimidazole antagonists suggests a binding site for H_3R binders that extends between D114 and E206 in the hH_3R based on the analysis of mutagenesis data on the $H_1R–H_4R$ [235]. One of the compounds analyzed (JNJ-5207852) contains two piperidine groups separated by the traditional propyloxybenzyl scaffold. When docked manually into the hypothetical binding cleft, this compound interacts through the basic moieties with D114 and E206 (Figure 5.31A [235]). The aromatic ring interacts with the aromatic side chain of Y115 in a stacking mode and is further in close contact with the aromatic ring

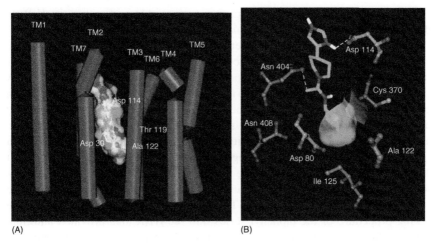

(A)   (B)

FIGURE 5.30 (See color insert following page 148.) (A) As proposed by Yao et al., the H_3 ligands are placed in the H_3 receptor TMs (red) between TM2, 3, 6, and 7. All ligands interact with D114 on TM3, and the agonists are able to interact with D80 on TM2 also. The residues suggested to be important for human and rat receptor specificity (at position **119** and **122**) of some ligands are on H_3R near the lower portion of the ligands. (B) Thioperamide is placed in the binding site of human (orange) receptor model. The protonated imidazole interacts with D114 on TM3. The thiocarbonyl interacts with Asn 404 on TM7. This places the cyclohexyl ring in the cavity between TM3 and TM6. (Reprinted from Yao, B.B., Hutchins, C.N., Carr, T.L. et al. *Neuropharmacol.*, 44, 773–786, 2003. With permission from Elsevier.)

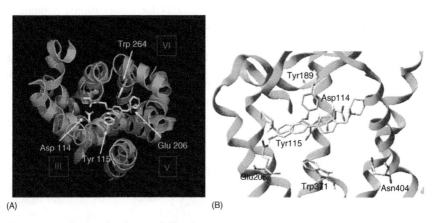

(A)   (B)

FIGURE 5.31 (See color insert following page 148.) (A) H_3 receptor model proposed by Axe et al., with compound y bound in the putative binding site, showing the interaction with several key amino acid residue side chains in the helical bundle. (B) Compound **185** (yellow carbons) within the H_3R model proposed by Morini et al. [227]. Only selected amino acids are represented, with gray carbons, and only polar hydrogens are depicted. The protein backbone is represented by a ribbon; for clarity, a portion of TM6 is not shown. (Reprinted from Axe, F.U., Bembenek, S.D., and Szalma, S., *J. Mol. Graph. Model,* 24, 456–464, 2006; Morini, G., Comini, M., Rivara, M. et al., *Bioorg. Med. Chem. Lett.*, 16, 4063–4067, 2006. With permission from Elsevier.)

of W371. In agreement with the interaction pattern observed within the H₃R, the authors developed a three-point pharmacophore model, with two basic centers and an aromatic ring. A series of rigidified nonimidazole compounds, which display high affinity for the H₃R, was reported to bind an rH₃R model in a similar manner (Figure 5.31B) [227]. The most potent compound of the series contains two piperidine basic moieties linked by a rigid biphenyl scaffold (**185**, Figure 5.28) and interacts with the rH₃R through residues D114 and E206 as well as Y189 and Y115. The proximity of D114 to Y115 allows this stacking interaction to take place at a precise distance between the basic nitrogen and the aromatic moiety, afforded in most antagonists by the propyloxy length. Apodaca et al. [85] indeed noted a 15- to 40-fold reduction in activity when the propylene linker was shortened to an ethylene linker. Similarly, increasing the length of the spacer in the biphenyl series led to a decrease in H₃R-binding affinity. The authors further noted that the automated docking procedure of the biphenyl series into the rH₃R also provided additional binding solutions similar to the ones proposed by Yao et al. [230] in which the piperidine nitrogen interacts with D114 although the compound is deeply inserted in a lipophilic cleft between TM3, 6, and 7.

A successful attempt to use a homology model of the hH₃R for virtual screening purposes was described recently [236,237]. To obtain a model suitable for subsequent ligand docking, ligand information was included in the model-building process to refine the placement of amino acids. In this *inverse docking* strategy, the ligand is used to retrieve the most suitable binding site from an ensemble of alternative binding sites. The resulting binding site was able to accommodate large hH₃R antagonists. In the model, the binding region spans between D114 and E206 as previously suggested by several groups and favors interaction with D114 for monocationic compounds. Accordingly, compound FUB181 (**186**, Figure 5.28) interacts with D114 rather than with E206, and the protonated moiety is further stabilized by the aromatic cluster consisting of W110, F291, and W292 (Figure 5.32A). The flexible or aromatic linker lies in a cleft restrained by L294, a site that is occupied by glycine residues in most other biogenic aminergic GPCRs. Two lipophilic pockets are present for

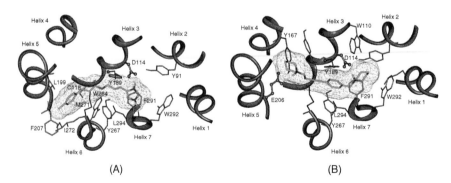

(A)   (B)

FIGURE 5.32 (See color insert following page 148.)   (A) FUB181 (**186**) in the hH₃R-binding site. (B) Ligand **190** in the hH₃R-binding site. (Reprinted from Schlegel, B. The human histamine H₃-receptor: A molecular modelling study of G-protein coupled receptor. Dissertation, Cuvillier Verlag, Göttingen, September 25, 2005. With permission.)

antagonists binding and are located between helices 3, 4, 5, and 6 (Figures 5.32A and 5.32B [236]). The existence of two binding pockets had been suggested by previous pharmacophore and receptor-binding modeling studies [216,220]. However, in these studies, a unique imidazole-binding site was postulated, which located the binding pockets between TM3, 6, and 7.

The resulting model was used for a docking study using the program GOLD and the scoring function GoldScore on a dataset comprising known hH_3R ligands and randomly selected Derwent World Drug Index (WDI) ligands. The model was able to discriminate hH_3R antagonists from non-hH_3R compounds, retrieving only 11.4% WDI ligands among the 80% top-ranked hH_3R antagonists.

The authors compared the docking strategy to a pharmacophore-based screening in which three different potent hH_3R antagonists—FUB836 (**187**), FUB833 (**188**), FUB209 (**189**), and linear phenylakyne **190** (Figure 5.28)—were used as templates for the generation of pharmacophore models. Each pharmacophore model contains binding features and volume constraints, based on the van der Waals volume of the compounds as well as exclusion spheres encompassing forbidden occupancy regions (Figure 5.33 [236]). By combining the three models, 93% of known H_3R antagonists were retrieved, whereas 2.5% potential H_3R antagonists were obtained from WDI and the MDB (Maybridge) showing a good discrimination between H_3-focused and random libraries. To further filter out inactive or moderately active compounds, a more stringent filter was applied (Figure 5.33C). Although the positive ionisable moiety/imidazole group and the spacer moiety were required in all models, of all

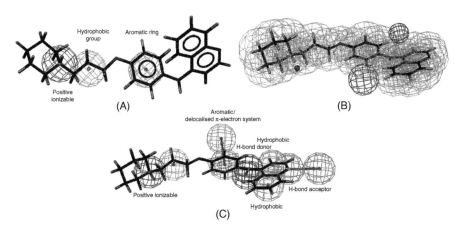

FIGURE 5.33 (See color insert following page 148.)   (A) Pharmacophoric features defined on the alleged bioactive conformation of FUB836. (B) The complete pharmacophore model additionally includes a shape query (blue spheres) and forbidden volumes (back spheres). (C) Features in FUB836 used for the definition of a leave-one out pharmacophore model. Although the positive ionisable moiety/imidazole group and the spacer moiety were required in all models, of all other features, each was allowed to be missed in a combinatorial way. (Reprinted from Schlegel, B. The human histamine H_3-receptor: A molecular modelling study of G-protein coupled receptor. Dissertation, Cuvillier Verlag, Göttingen, September 25, 2005. With permission.)

other features, each was allowed to be missed in a combinatorial way. Both the hH$_3$R model and the pharmacophore models were able to retrieve a significant portion of the known H$_3$R antagonists once again showing the great potential of those two common strategies of *in silico* screening.

Recently, a pharmacophore model was published for nonimidazole antagonists and used for further alignment in 3-D-QSAR studies using CoMFA and CoMSIA with a set of 106 histamine H$_3$R antagonists with activity range spanning five orders of magnitude [238]. Studied compounds came from J&J PRD and Bioprojet/FUB research program described earlier. The five-point pharmacophore features a positive basic nitrogen, three hydrophobic regions, and one acceptor site with a lone pair of vectors in agreement with previously reported models (Figures 5.34A and 5.34B; compound **48b** as an example). The authors point out that the protonated basic nitrogen reported in the western part of the prototypical pharmacophore is in their case replaced by a lipophilic moiety. However, an inverted orientation in which the western part contains the basic protonated moiety and the eastern part contains the lipophilic moiety is also plausible.

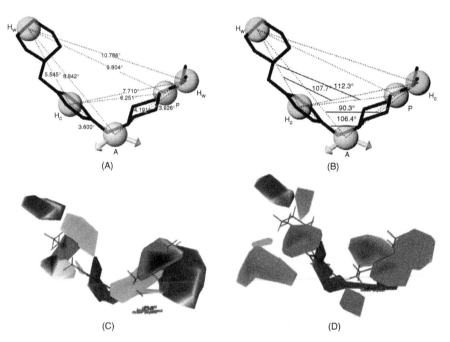

(A)   (B)

(C)   (D)

FIGURE 5.34 (See color insert following page 148.) (A) Pharmacophore features and distances mapped onto compound **49a**. (B) Pharmacophore features and angles mapped onto compound **49a**. Positive basic nitrogen feature is indicated by sphere P, hydrophobic spheres by Hw, Hc, He, acceptor as sphere A with a lone pair of vectors. (C) Contour maps for CoMSIA model (steric-favored region—pink, disfavored region—blue, electropositive-favored region—orange, yellow, and electronegative-favored region—cyan). (Reprinted from Narkhede, S.S. and Degani, M.S., *QSAR & Combi. Sci.*, 26, 744–753, 2007. With permission from Wiley-VCH.) (D) CoMSIA model (donor-favored region—red, acceptor-favored region—green, and hydrophobic-favored region—blue).

The pharmacophore-based 3-D-QSAR, CoMFA, and CoMSIA models developed show a good correlation between the predicted and the observed activities within the training and test sets with r_{cv}^2 of .53 and .46 and *predictive* r^2 value of .76 and .82 for CoMFA and CoMSIA models, respectively. The contour maps of molecular property fields, represented in Figures 5.34C and 5.34D, offer a visual representation of the antagonist's structural requisite for histamine H_3R binding. As mentioned, molecules with a bulky protonated site, which enter sterically unfavored regions (blue), result in lower activities. Small sterically disfavored region is highlighted for the spacer between the protonated site and the hydrophobic Hc region in agreement with previously discussed histamine hH_3R model, which showed that the flexible or aromatic spacer of H_3R antagonists lay in a cleft restrained by L294. Next to the hydrophobic region Hc, three different regions can be found: a donor-favored region (red), an acceptor-favored region (green), and a hydrophobic-favored region (blue) in agreement with the prototypical pharmacophore.

Conclusion

Over the past few years, *in silico* models within the histamine H_3 field have been developed based on SAR data, species selectivity, and mutagenesis data. These models provide important insights regarding the binding of antagonists to the histamine H_3R, and several groups within pharmaceutical companies have reported the successful use of such *in silico* models in their H_3 drug discovery programs [181,185]. However, this review also shows that different starting hypotheses can lead to very different binding models. In the absence of crystallographic structural data, multiple and compound-specific mutagenesis data would be required to discriminate between the various binding hypotheses formulated. As crystallographic techniques for transmembrane proteins are progressing, further insights into GPCR/antagonist binding could be down the road.

RADIOLABELED AND FLUORESCENT H_3 RECEPTOR LIGANDS

Along with the preclinical development of potent drug candidates, the need for radiolabeled H_3 ligands has been crucial to study the histamine H_3R–ligand interactions and therefore to run appropriate *in vitro* binding and functional screening assays. The pharmacology of imidazole-based radioligands has been reviewed by Timmerman, Leurs, and coworkers [239,240]; this section will focus on the H_3 radioligands found to date and some recent developments in fluorescent H_3 antagonists.

Indeed, Esbenshade et al. [241] and Yao et al. [242] from Abbott Laboratories have reported the first tritiated nonimidazole H_3 antagonist, namely [^{3}H]-A-317920 **191** (specific activity: 86 Ci/mmol) (Figure 5.35). *In vitro* binding studies of [^{3}H]-A-317920 revealed that desirable signal to noise ratios were obtained, with affinities at the rH_3 (pK_d 9.2) and hH_3 (pK_d 7.4), in compaison with binding affinities observed for unlabelled A-317920 (rH_3 pK_i 9.2; hH_3 pK_i 7.0), derived from [^{3}H]-NαMH competition binding assays. However, the relative low binding affinity of [^{3}H]-A-317920 for the hH_3R led Abbott scientists to search for a more balanced rat/human affinity H_3 antagonist. Successfully, preclinical candidate A-349821 had fulfilled

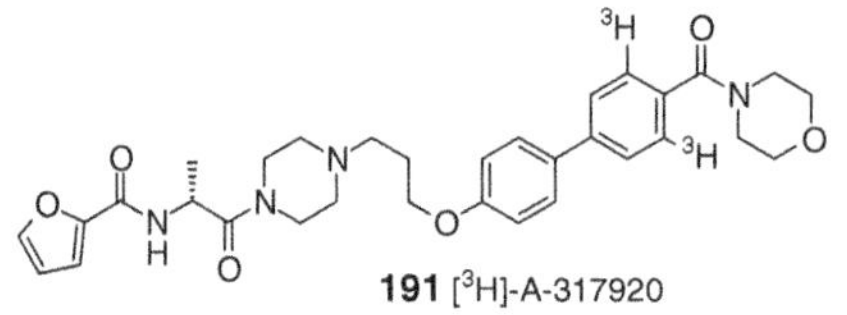

191 $[^3H]$-A-317920

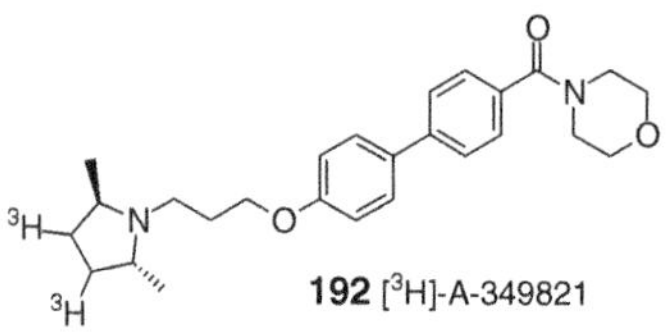

192 $[^3H]$-A-349821

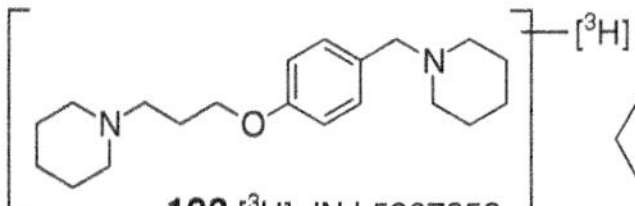

193 $[^3H]$-JNJ-5207852

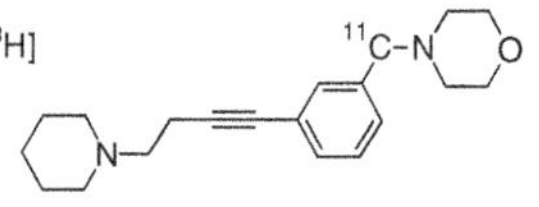

194 $[^{11}C]$-JNJ-10181457

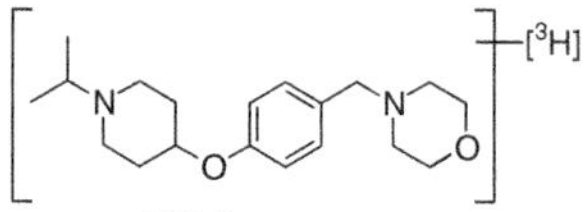

195 $[^3H]$-JNJ-773782

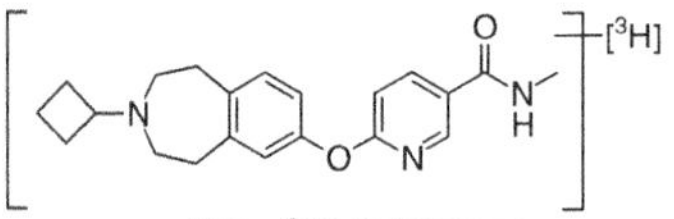

196a $[^3H]$-GSK189254

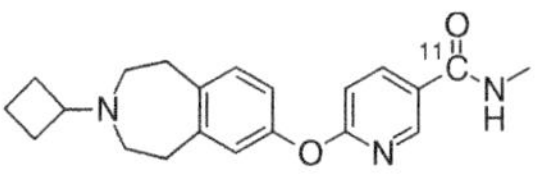

196b $[^{11}C]$-GSK189254

FIGURE 5.35 Radiolabeled nonimidazole H_3 antagonists of A-317920, A-349821, JNJ-10181457, JNJ-5207852, JNJ-7737782, and GSK289254.

this requirement, with nanomolar to subnanomolar affinity for rH_3R (pK_i 9.0) and hH_3R (pK_i 9.5). Its tritiated labeled equivalent, $[^3H]$-A-349821 **192**, showed similar high-affinity binding and specificity for hH_3 (pK_i 10.5), with at least 10-fold higher affinity than at the rH_3R (pK_i 9.7) and rcortexH_3R (pK_i 9.3) [243]. It has also been demonstrated that $[^3H]$-A-349821 displacement binding experiments of a series of Abbott compounds suggest recognition of a single H_3-binding site compared to H_3 agonists, thereby discriminating high and low H_3 affinity receptor sites.

In 2004, scientists at J&J reported the radiolabeling of their preclinical compound, JNJ-5207852 [244]. *In vitro* binding studies of tritiated $[^3H]$-JNJ-5207852 **193** revealed high affinity (rH_3 pK_d 8.7; hH_3 pK_d 8.8), close to the binding data obtained for the unlabelled JNJ-5207852 (rH_3 pK_i 8.9; hH_3 pK_i 9.2). CNS distribution in mouse brain, using autoradiography, demonstrated high receptor occupancy and extensive labeling in cortex, hypothalamus, and striatum, consistent with the reported H_3R site brain distribution. As previously described, JNJ-5207852 has showed unfavorable pharmacokinetics, leading to the identification of a follow-up compound, JNJ-10181457. Later in 2006, Airaksinen et al. [245] reported the radiosynthesis and biodistribution studies of $[^{11}C]$-JNJ-10181457 (**194**). Labeled $[^{11}C]$-JNJ-10181457 provided high-specific radioactivity (56 GBq/μmol) and showed high H_3R brain uptake in mice and rat at a dose of 10 mg/kg (i.p.), with a maximum at 30 min for the hippocampus and cerebral cortex region. Additional biodistribution studies, however, revealed high uptake in peripheral organ such as kidney, lung, and liver, superior to the brain regions of interest, which preclude further investigations as a PET ligand. From the same group, Dvorak and coworkers [85] have reported the tritiated JNJ-7737782 (**195**) in *in vitro* autoradiography studies, demonstrating extensive H_3 binding in known rich brain regions such as cortex striatum and substantia nigra.

Clinical drug candidate GSK189254, developed by GSK, has also been radiolabeled as [³H]-GSK189254 (**196a**, specific activity: 81 Ci/mmol) [146]. *In vitro* binding studies have revealed subnanomolar-binding affinity at rctxH$_3$ (pK_d 10.1) and hctxH$_3$ (pK_d 10.3), consistent with binding affinities of unlabeled GSK189354. It is worth mentioning that elegant syntheses of two [¹¹C]-GSK189254 derivatives have been recently published in a patent application (e.g., **196b**) [246]. In addition, *in vitro* autoradiography studies demonstrated high uptake not only in cortex, hippocampus, striatum, and hypothalamus brain regions in rat but also in human cortex and hippocampus. For the first time, GSK scientists revealed strong evidence of dense H$_3$ binding in nondisease human cortex and brain regions of early-to-late-stage Alzheimer's disease patients. Together with proof-of-concept in preclinical rodent models of cognitive disorders, these new results support the role of histamine H$_3$R antagonists, such as GSK189254, as novel therapeutic agents for the treatment of dementia of Alzheimer's type.

The development of new research tools for studying receptor–ligand interactions is therefore of great interest. In parallel to the identification of potent, brain penetrating, radiolabeled drug candidates for PET and SPECT monitoring, novel nonradioactive ligands such as fluorescent tagged molecules could provide alternative solution for labeling receptor, biodistribution in tissues, or binding assays. As part of their drug discovery program, Cowart et al. [247] from Abbott laboratories developed new probe ligands around the benzofuran chemical series to which ABT-239 belongs. As shown in Figure 5.36, known fluorescent-based fragments, such as nitrobenzodioxaolyl (**197**) and tetramethylrhodamine (**198**), were introduced at the terminal amino site of the previously described compound **82**. Despite their high molecular weight and less drug-likeness, both exemplified compounds displayed subnanomolar affinity at rH$_3$R and hH$_3$R, with fluorescent properties, which may be useful for *in vitro* binding studies [247].

Recently, Stark and coworkers reported novel, highly potent, fluorescent H$_3$ antagonists bearing the known piperidinopropoxyphenyl framework. From a focused SAR study (18 examples), compounds **199** and **200** have exhibited subnanomolar

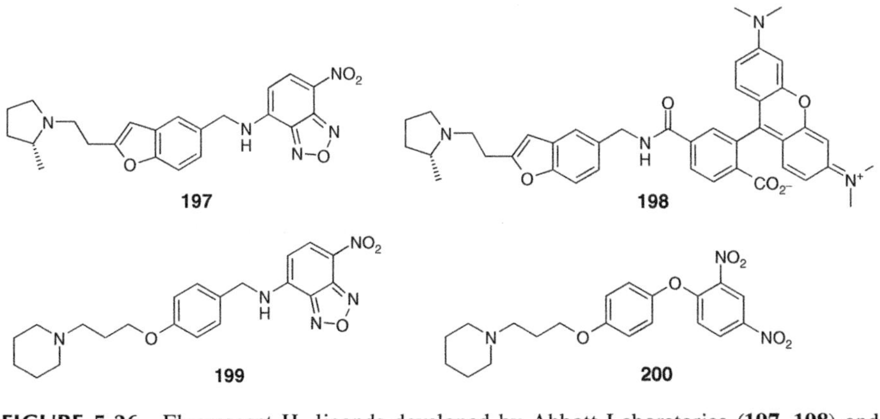

FIGURE 5.36 Fluorescent H$_3$ ligands developed by Abbott Laboratories (**197, 198**) and Bioprojet/JWG University of Frankfurt (**199, 200**).

hH_3 affinity. Interestingly, compound **199** has demonstrated *in vivo* efficacy in the modulation of brain N^τ-methyl histamine (oral ED_{50} of 0.39 mg/kg in mice) [248].

MULTITARGET-ORIENTED H_3 RECEPTOR DRUG DESIGN

In contrast to the classical concept "one disease—one target—one drug," the multiple targeting approaches by a single chemical entity or a combination of compounds are often realized with marketed drugs for complex diseases. In some cases, Paul Ehrlich's *magic bullet* to a *magic shotgun* way proved to be advantageous in some therapy when the whole is greater than the sum of the parts [249,250].

Drug Combinations

The combination of an H_3R ligand with another ligand of a different pharmacological profile has been the topic of numerous pharmacological studies. Depending on the targets, the models and the ligands additive, synergistical, adverse, or no effects have been observed. Peripheral disorders such as nasal allergic response or nasal congestion have been treated in models with H_3R ligands in combination with H_1R antagonists. Surprisingly, some studies suggested H_3R agonist [251], whereas others suggested antagonists for an effective therapy [252,253]. At the moment, it is not clear whether H_4-mediated or unspecific effects, complex regulations, different target tissues, or compounds immanent properties caused these differences [254]. Actually, the dual H_1/H_3 antagonist behavior is the most preferred line in this class of antagonists [255], and recent claiming has additionally introduced H_4R antagonism [256]. Combination of an H_3R antagonist with aminergic reuptake-inhibitors [257] or other antidepressant/antipsychotic compounds [258] has been the center of interest of some academic group and pharmaceutical companies (*vide infra*).

Hybrid Compounds

Hybrid compounds combine at least two different pharmacological properties in one molecule. There are different approaches to achieve these properties. In most cases, two pharmacophore fragments or scaffolds have to be designed as one compound. This can be achieved by the combination of two pharmacophores:

1. By a cleavable linker resulting *in vivo* into two separate compounds
2. By a stable linker
3. By addition of the two fragments
4. By an integrated approach having a structural overlap of both [259]

The difficulty for the realization is rising with the given numbering. Depending on the definition of the pharmacophore, some differences in the approaches may be claimed. The strategic orientation for such a directed compound design has to orientate on the complexity of the disease and the optimization of treatment. An integrated approach and an additional approach on imidazole-based dual H_1R/H_3R antagonists have been realized by **201** (pK_i 7.1 [H_1] and 7.1 [H_3]) [260] and **202** (pK_i 8.2 [hH_1] and 7.8 [hH_3]) [261,262], whereas a nonimidazole compound by a linker approach is represented with **203** (pK_i 7.3 [H_1] and 10.6 [H_3]) (Figure 5.37) [263].

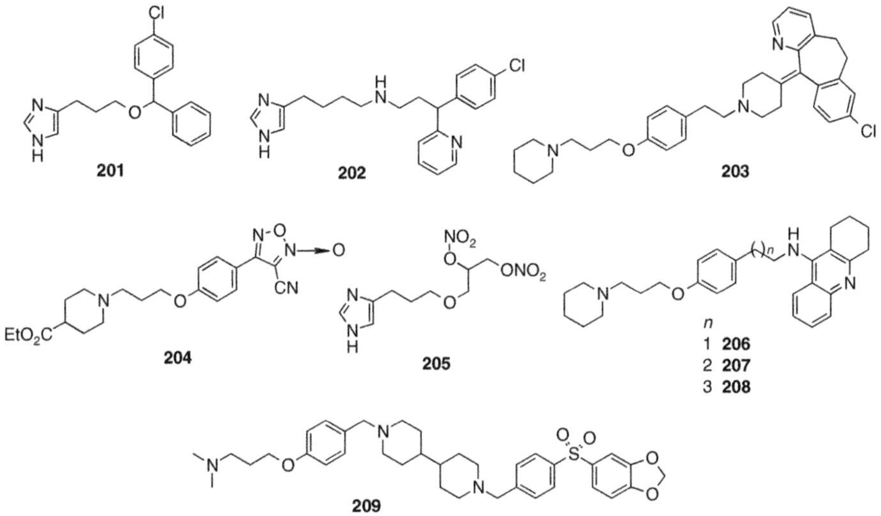

FIGURE 5.37 Hybrid H_3 compounds: dual H_3-H_1 ligands (**201–203**), dual H_3-NO synthase ligands (**204–205**), dual H_3-HMTase ligands (**206–208**), and dual H_3-M_2 ligands (**209**).

Typical fragments of H_1 antagonists can be found in all of these compounds (e.g., diphenhydramine, chlorpheniramine, and desloratidine). Although it is not clear whether these compounds are entering the blood brain barrier, it might be an advantage for an exclusive peripheral action if they possess a comparable pharmacokinetic profile to that of second generation of H_1 antagonists.

Concerning learning and memory, NO is another important neurotransmitter. The Torino group dealt with different *in vitro* NO-releasing principles in different classes of antagonists for potential synergy of both effects (pA_2 6.4 [H_3], NO release: 19% [**204**]; pA_2 6.03 [H_3], NO release: 20% [**205**]; pA_2 7.81 [H_3], 83% NO-dependent relaxation) [264–266]. In antiamnesic compounds, hybrid approaches have often been realized [267,268]. Inhibition of acetylcholinesterase (AChE) enzyme plays a significant role for these effects. As it was shown that tacrine markedly inhibits histamine *N*-methyltransferase (HMT) enzyme as well as AChE, such approach was a good starting point for hybrid structures. The tacrine-derived imidazole and especially nonimidazole compounds were highly affine H_3R ligands with HMT inhibitory potencies [269–272] and additional beneficial properties. Compounds **206**, **207**, and **208** showed pK_i values (H_3) of 9.5, 8.6, and 8.7; pIC_{50} values (HMT) of 7.3, 7.0, and 7.3; pIC_{50} values (AChE) of 8.6, 8.1, and 8.5; as well as pIC_{50} values for butyrylcholinesterase as a potentially compensating metabolic enzyme of 8.1, 8.0, and 8.0, respectively (Figure 5.37) [273]. This is an impressive example of a balanced potency at four targets simultaneously of clearly designed compounds without serendipity in finding. A structural basis of different drugs acting at HMT can be extracted from x-ray studies [274]. A combination of the H_3 antagonist thioperamide and tacrine was shown to improve performance on a spontaneous alternation task in mice synergistically [275]. From a structural point, these compounds are comparable to the fluorescence-tagged derivatives. Dual H_3/muscarinic M_2 receptor antagonists, which are optionally comedicated with an AChE inhibitor, are another logical approach to treat cognitive disorders as represented with different bipiperidines (**209**: pK_i 8.2 [H$_3$]; 10.3 [M$_2$]) [276].

As psychiatric diseases are a therapeutically unsatisfying field and an urgent need for enhanced medications exists [277], histamine H$_3$R antagonists have been hybridized with aminergic reuptake inhibitors, mostly selective serotonin reuptake inhibitors (SSRI) (Stark et al., unpublished results). On the basis of the structure of sertraline and *in-house* developments at J&J PRD, isoquinoline derivatives are found to be promising structural overlap for hybrid structures by an integrated approach. These 1,2,3,4-THiQs have been varied by optimization of the piperidino group of the H$_3$ pharmacophore [278], substitution pattern of the aromatic SSRI pharmacophore [279], heteroaromatic replacement, rigidification [280], and introduction of hetero-atoms [281]. Compounds **210a–g**, **211**, and **212a–d** showed remarkable affinities at H$_3$Rs and simultaneously at serotonin transporter (SERT) (Figure 5.38).

Stereochemistry for most compounds has been characterized as *cis*-configuration having for selected compounds determined the S-configuration at the dibenzylic position (position 4) as the most preferred one. Stereochemical aspects affect H$_3$ binding of a factor of about 3, whereas the eudismic ratio for SERT affinities is about 3-log units with the eutomer on the other stereoisomer. Interestingly, the 2,6-naphthyridines, such as 212a, showed a pronounced SERT stereoselectivity. Comparable 2,5-derivatives (nomenclature as 1,6-naphthyridines) were less active, whereas 2,8-derivatives (nomenclature as 1,7-naphthyridines) showed promising profiles. Racemic compound **212a** showed a modest oral bioavailability ($F = 16\%$) with slow brain penetration ($C_{max} = 1.28$ μM at 24 h) leading to a delayed but prolonged pharmacological response in mice ($t_{1/2} = 15.7$ h). Similar pharmacokinetic profile (see Table 5.1) was obtained for compound (+)–210f, which showed, however, an ED$_{50}$ of 0.1 mg/kg for SERT and of 0.05 mg/kg at H$_3$Rs measured by receptor occupancy with moderate affinities for norepinephrine and DATs. These multitarget approaches have faced the problems of the rightly balanced activities. Different tissue distribution, receptor densities, cross-talks, etc., make the already difficult situation much more complex with multitarget drugs. Nevertheless, most of the drugs used for psychiatric diseases can be classified as *dirty drugs* having

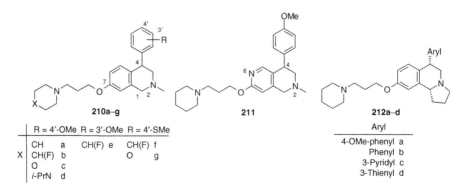

FIGURE 5.38   Dual H$_3$-SSRI ligands (**210–212**) from J&J PRD.

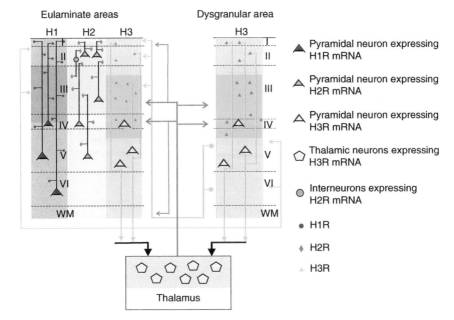

COLOR FIGURE 4.5 Summary of the mRNA expression and receptor ligand-binding patterns of three histamine receptors (H1, H2, and H3) in the human prefrontal cortex (using eulaminate areas as an example), and the possible connections between the cortical areas and within the thalamocortical system. The presence of mRNA in the cell bodies and distribution of the receptor protein within the axons and dendrites underlies the discrepancy between the mRNA expression and receptor ligand-binding patterns. Most of the neurons expressing H1 and H3R mRNA are located in the deep cortical layers of the eulaminate areas. Most neurons expressing H2R mRNA are located in the superficial cortical layers. H1R and H2R expressed by the pyramidal neurons might locate on their ascending apical dendrites and contribute to the detected receptor ligand-binding sites in the upper cortical layers. H3R expressed by the pyramidal neurons in the deep layers might be located on their axonal terminals in the upper layers. The pyramidal neurons in the deep layers of the dysgranular areas also send axonal projections to the upper layers of the eulaminate areas; therefore, part of the H3R expressed by the pyramidal neurons in the dysgranular areas might be located on the axonal terminals in the upper layers of the eulaminate areas and contribute to the detectable receptor ligand-binding sites there. In addition, pyramidal neurons in lamina V project to the dorsal thalamus, and neurons in dorsal thalamus project to the cortex, mostly targeting the middle layers (laminae III, IV). Thus, some of the detected H3R ligand-binding sites in the middle cortical layers are located on the terminals of the dorsal thalamic inputs, and vice versa. It cannot be overlooked that part of the H2R-expressing neurons in the upper layers are interneurons.

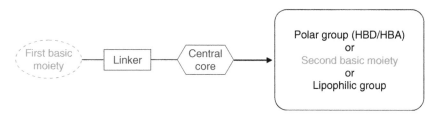

COLOR FIGURE 5.25 Prototypical pharmacophore for histamine H₃R antagonists: a basic moiety is connected through a linker (often propyloxy chain) to an aromatic central core, which can be further substituted by lipophilic groups, basic moieties, or H-bond donors or acceptors.

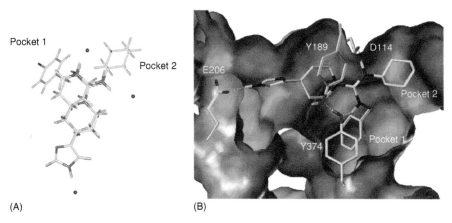

COLOR FIGURE 5.26 (A) The binding site for histamine H₃ receptor antagonists proposed by De Esch et al. [216] can be described by four hydrogen-bonding site points and two lipophilic pockets. (B) Compound **183** bound to Lorenzi et al. [220] 3-D rH₃R model showing an interaction pattern involving residues E206, D114, Y189, Y374 as well as lipophilic pockets 1 and 2. (Reprinted from De Esch, I.J.P., Mills, J.E.J., Perkins, T.D.J. et al. *J. Med. Chem.*, 44, 1666–1674, 2001; Lorenzi, S., Mor, M., Bordi, F. et al. *Bioorg. Med. Chem.*, 13, 5647–5657, 2005. With permission from Elsevier.)

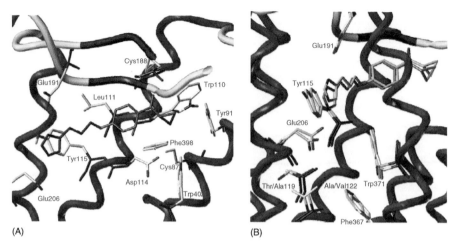

(A)   (B)

COLOR FIGURE 5.29 (A) Possible interaction sites proposed by Stark et al. [228] between ciproxifan (violet) and the rH$_3$R are shown (helices in front of the ligand are not displayed for reasons of clarity). (B) Influence of amino acids A119T and V122A on the binding site and on the binding of ciproxifan (rH$_3$R residues are colored white and bound ciproxifan orange, hH$_3$R residues are colored green and bound ciproxifan green). (Reprinted from Stark, H., Sippl, W., Ligneau, X. et al. *Bioorg. Med. Chem. Lett.*, 11, 951–952, 2001. With permission from Elsevier.)

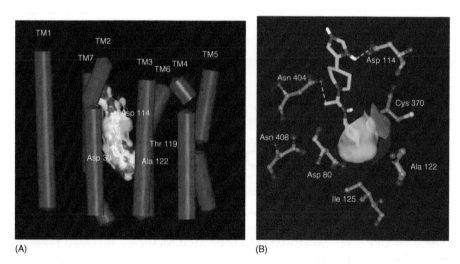

(A)   (B)

COLOR FIGURE 5.30 (A) As proposed by Yao et al. [230], the H$_3$ ligands are placed in the H$_3$ receptor TMs (red) between TM2, 3, 6, and 7. All ligands interact with D114 on TM3, and the agonists are able to interact with D80 on TM2 also. The residues suggested to be important for human and rat receptor specificity (at position **119** and **122**) of some ligands are on H$_3$R near the lower portion of the ligands. (B) Thioperamide is placed in the binding site of human (orange) receptor model. The protonated imidazole interacts with D114 on TM3. The thiocarbonyl interacts with Asn 404 on TM7. This places the cyclohexyl ring in the cavity between TM3 and TM6. (Reprinted from Yao, B.B., Hutchins, C.N., Carr, T.L. et al. *Neuropharmacol.*, 44, 773–786, 2003. With permission from Elsevier.)

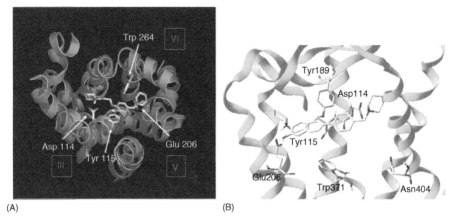

(A)   (B)

COLOR FIGURE 5.31 (A) H_3 receptor model proposed by Axe et al. [235] with compound y bound in the putative binding site, showing the interaction with several key amino acid residue side chains in the helical bundle. (B) Compound **185** (yellow carbons) within the H_3R model proposed by Morini et al. [227]. Only selected amino acids are represented, with gray carbons, and only polar hydrogens are depicted. The protein backbone is represented by a ribbon; for clarity, a portion of TM6 is not shown. (Reprinted from Axe, F.U., Bembenek, S.D., and Szalma, S., *J. Mol. Graph. Model,* 24, 456–464, 2006; Morini, G., Comini, M., Rivara, M. et al., *Bioorg. Med. Chem. Lett.*, 16, 4063–4067, 2006. With permission from Elsevier.)

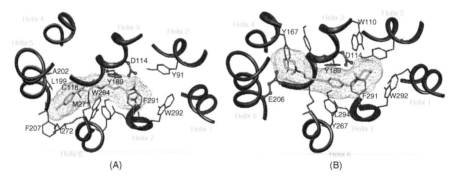

(A)   (B)

COLOR FIGURE 5.32 (A) FUB181 (**186**) in the hH_3R-binding site. (B) Ligand **190** in the hH_3R-binding site. (Reprinted from Schlegel, B. The human histamine H_3-receptor: A molecular modelling study of G-protein coupled receptor. Dissertation, Cuvillier Verlag, Göttingen, September 25, 2005. With permission.)

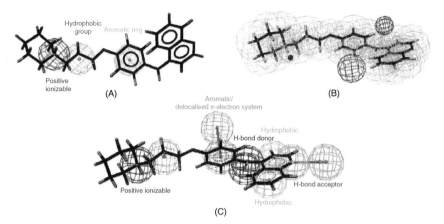

COLOR FIGURE 5.33 (A) Pharmacophoric features defined on the alleged bioactive conformation of FUB836. (B) The complete pharmacophore model additionally includes a shape query (blue spheres) and forbidden volumes (back spheres). (C) Features in FUB836 used for the definition of a leave-one out pharmacophore model. Although the positive ionisable moiety/imidazole group and the spacer moiety were required in all models, of all other features, each was allowed to be missed in a combinatorial way. (Reprinted from Schlegel, B. The human histamine H_3-receptor: A molecular modelling study of G-protein coupled receptor. Dissertation, Cuvillier Verlag, Göttingen, September 25, 2005. With permission.)

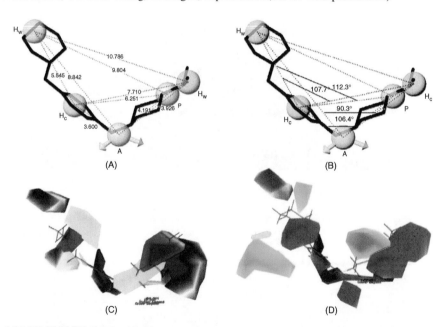

COLOR FIGURE 5.34 (A) Pharmacophore features and distances mapped onto compound **49a**. (B) Pharmacophore features and angles mapped onto compound **49a**. Positive basic nitrogen feature is indicated by sphere P, hydrophobic spheres by Hw, Hc, He, acceptor as sphere A with a lone pair of vectors. (C) Contour maps for CoMSIA model (steric-favored region—pink, disfavored region—blue, electropositive-favored region—orange, yellow, and electronegative-favored region—cyan). (Reprinted from Narkhede, S.S. and Degani, M.S., *QSAR & Combi. Sci.*, 26, 744–753, 2007. With permission from Wiley-VCH.) (D) CoMSIA model (donor-favored region—red, acceptor-favored region—green, and hydrophobic-favored region—blue).

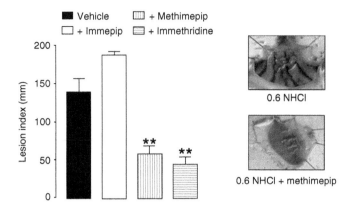

COLOR FIGURE 6.3 Effects of the dual H_3/H_4 receptor agonist immepip (30 mg/kg s.c.) and the selective H_3 receptor agonists methimepip (30 mg/kg s.c.), and immethridine (30 mg/kg s.c.) on the gastric damage induced by HCl 0.6 N i.g. (■) in the conscious rat. On the ordinate lesion index, values are mean ±SEM from 8–10 rats. **$p < .01$ versus vehicle (saline). (See Morini, G., Grandi, D., Krause, M., Schunack, W., *Inflamm. Res.* 46, S101–S102, 1997 for methodological details.)

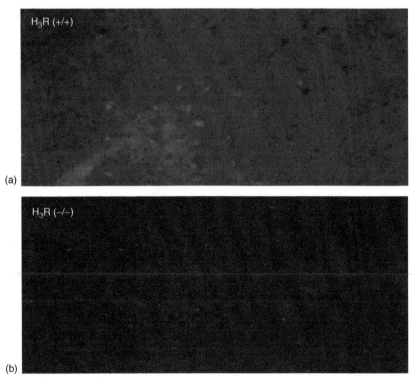

COLOR FIGURE 12.1 High expression of the histamine H_3R in the mammalian SN. Immunohistochemical labeling of the H_3 histamine receptor in the SN using a selective anti-H_3 349-358 histamine receptor antibody [6]. (a) Wild-type mouse; (b) $H_3(-/-)$ mouse. (Image produced by Dr. Keri Cannon in the laboratories of Dr. Frank Rice and Professor Lindsay Hough, Albany, NY.)

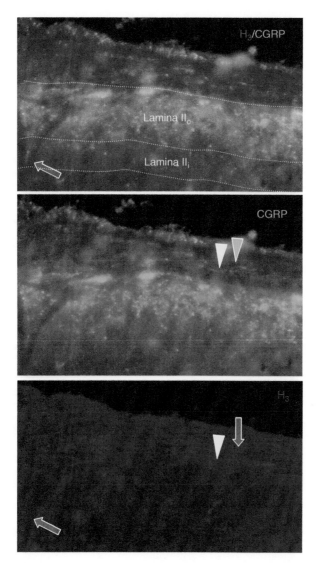

COLOR FIGURE 12.2 The histamine H_3R is expressed on a subpopulation of Aδ fibers in the spinal cord. Immunhistochemical double labeling of the H_3 histamine receptor (red) and CGRP (green) in the dorsal horn of the mouse spinal cord, showing CGRP-positive fibers with (yellow arrow) and without (red arrow) H_3R-LI ramified extensively in lamina II. These and other published data show that periarterial, peptidergic, and H_3R-containing Aδ fibers may be sources of high-threshold mechanical nociception [54]. (Image produced by Dr. Keri Cannon in the laboratories of Dr. Frank Rice and Professor Lindsay Hough, Albany, NY.)

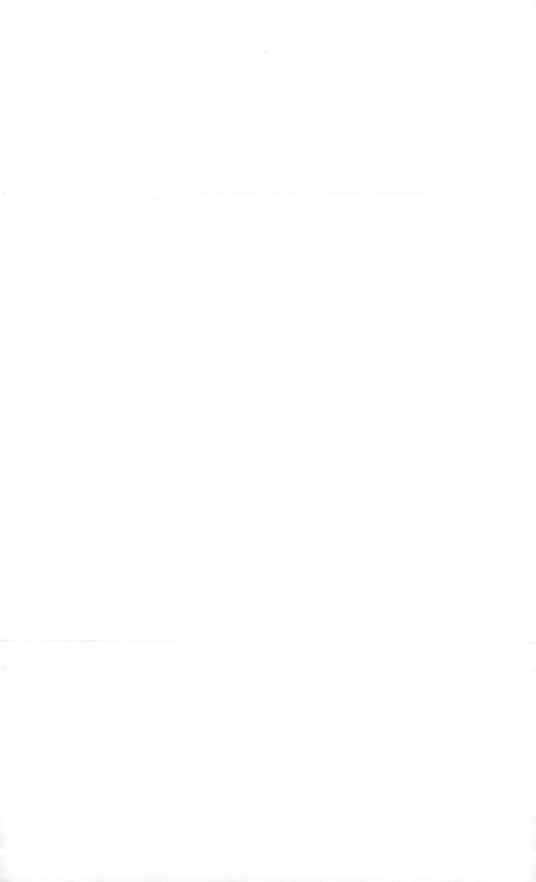

much more than one target with pharmacological profiling. The targeted promiscuity of these compounds may open new therapeutics with a so far unknown original therapeutic profile.

PRECLINICAL AND CLINICAL STUDIES OF H₃ RECEPTOR DRUG CANDIDATES

Since the pharmacological identification of the histamine H_3R in 1983, academic groups and pharmaceutical companies shared a highly competitive field with more than 150 patent applications published before 2007. Since the early clinical failure of the imidazole-based compound GT2331 (**20**) from the former Gliatech Company, no proof-of-concept in human in a defined therapeutic indication was revealed until 2006. Appreciating the narrowing chemical space over the years, pharmaceutical companies are accelerating preclinical studies of their own drug candidates to enter quickly into clinical trials and acquire knowledge on the therapeutic efficacy, tolerability, as well as the potential safety issues. Indeed, companies involved in the H_3 field have been faced with many challenges ranging from target selectivity, species differences, metabolic interactions, inadequate pharmacokinetics, or lack of efficacy in animal models, to toxicity issues, cardiovascular, or CNS adverse effects. Clinical status of previously identified H_3 antagonists is summarized in Figure 5.39 [282] and detailed in the following text.

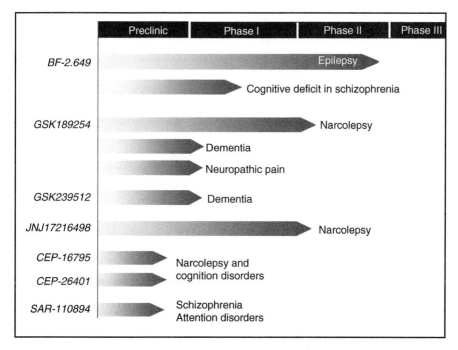

FIGURE 5.39 Preclinical and clinical status of new H_3 chemical entities (June 30, 2007). Lin, J.S., Dauvilliers, Y., Arnulf, I. et al. 2008. *Neurobiol. Dis.*, 30, 1, 2008. With permission.)

As an example, the drug discovery program of Abbott Laboratories has been faced with genotoxicity of their preclinical antiobesity agent A-331440 as well as cardiac QTc prolongation in nonrodent species induced by ABT-239, precluding its clinical development due to a low safety margin. Nevertheless, Abbott Laboratories are actively pursuing their efforts with new chemical series with better safety profile. No follow-up clinical candidate has emerged up to date.

In May 2005, a novel orally active H_3 antagonist, identified as JNJ17216498 from J&J PRD, has entered into phase I clinical trials (source: Prompt; IMS Research). Results demonstrate good tolerability and pharmacokinetic profile. In March 2007, J&J has initiated a phase II with JNJ-17216498 to study its safety and effectiveness (capsules containing 10 or 50 mg) compared to modafinil (400 mg) and placebo in patients with narcolepsy, with and without cataplexy [78]. Approximately 64 adult patients will be enrolled in this phase II randomized, double-blind, placebo, and comparator-controlled, parallel group, multicenter study. Modafinil, developed by Cephalon, is a drug currently approved to treat narcolepsy. Interestingly, Cephalon also entered the histamine H_3R field and reported to develop novel H_3 antagonists for the treatment of wake/cognition disorders. IND filings are expected in 2008 for the H_3 antagonists CEP-16795 [283] and CEP-26401 [284]. No chemical structures or patent applications have been reported to date.

As key active player in the worldwide H_3R drug discovery research, the first H_3 drug candidate from GSK, namely, GSK189254, is developed for the symptomatic treatment of Alzheimer's disease [285] with efficacy in several preclinical models of cognitive disorders, and entered phase I clinical trials for the treatment of dementia in March 2005 [145]. Interestingly, earlier, GSK189254 was reported to be part of GSK psychiatry pipeline for the treatment of schizophrenia [286] and is still involved, in 2006, in this area, targeting the cognitive dysfunction symptoms [287]. In August 2006, a phase II clinical trial has been initiated with GSK189254 for the treatment of narcolepsy (70 patients) [288]. Late 2006, a phase I clinical trial of GSK189254 (up to 100 μg once daily) in comparison with duloxetine (up to 60 mg daily) has started to determine the safety and efficacy of GSK189254 in the electrical hyperalgesia (EH) model in healthy volunteers (40 patients), for the treatment of neuropathic pain [289]. Indeed, GSK189254 has demonstrated efficacy in preclinical models of mechanical hyperalgesia and allodynia in the chronic constriction injury test. Recently, GSK announced, in its product pipeline, a novel phase I drug candidate, namely, GSK239512 (structure unknown), for the treatment of dementia [145]. Indeed, this 12-people enrollment study started in May 2007 defined the primary outcomes on human brain receptor occupancy using [^{11}C]-GSK-189254 PET ligand as well as the safety of the drug and plasma concentrations after oral administration as secondary outcomes [290]. Interestingly, another phase I/II clinical trial involving GSK's GW784568X drug candidate has been initiated in mid-2006 for the treatment of allergic rhinitis [291]. Structurally unknown, this development candidate has recently been reported to be linked to the single claimed compound **117** from GSK's H_3 medicinal chemistry program [292], due to its low CNS penetration. It remains to be confirmed, as this compound displayed low affinity for the H_1R, and more importantly, such concept has been developed by the group of Aslanian from Schering-Plough Corp., in which a coadministration of an H_1R antagonist is required for efficacy [293].

Early 2007, Bioprojet/Ferrer companies and the well-established international academic consortium from UCL (U.K.), INSERM (France), Johann Wolfgang Goethe University (JWGU), and FUB (Germany) have reported the preclinical pharmacological profile of their H_3 antagonist FUB-649, known as BF-2.649 (tiprolisant). Codeveloped by Bioprojet and Ferrer, BF-2.649 has indeed demonstrated efficacy in several preclinical models of cognition, sleep/wake disorders, and schizophrenia [71]. In October 2005, BF-2.649 entered phase Ib/II, double-blind, placebo-controlled, clinical trial for the treatment of cognitive disorders in 60 patients suffering from schizophrenia [8,9,294,295]. Interestingly, more than 10 exploratory phase II clinical trials have been initiated with BF-2.649 in France and Spain (source: Pharmaproject). Since the Gliatech GT2331 discontinuation, BF-2.649 is the first nonimidazole H_3 antagonist/inverse agonist to succeed in phase II clinical trials in 2006. Indeed, BF2.649 showed efficacy in the treatment of patients (10 males enrolled) suffering from obstructive sleep apnea with once a day dosing (40 mg) during 3–7 days [296]. It is also tolerated in volunteers receiving 5 mg of olanzapine simultaneously. The olanzapine-induced hunger sensation was reduced to placebo level with BF-2.649. In addition, BF-2.649 has demonstrated broad efficacy not only in preclinical rodent models of absence epilepsy, GAERS, and pharmacoresistant epilepsy but also in human clinical trial in photosensitive seizure and pharmacoresistant epilepsy tests [297]. Most impressively, 12 patients with photosensitive epilepsy have been treated with different dosages of BF2.649 (20, 40, and 60 mg) leading dose-dependent from partial to total suppression of photoparoxysmal response with or without comedications (e.g., as sodium valproate). BF-2.649 has proved to be well tolerated in *add-on* therapy with current antiepileptic drugs such as Keppra (UCB Pharma) or Depakine (Sanofi-Aventis) [298]. More recently, BF-2.649 has progressed to Phase 2 clinical trial showing efficacy in narcoleptic patients having excessive daytime sleepiness (EDS).

Finally, in February 2007, Sanofi-Aventis reported the identification of SAR-110894 as a novel H_3 antagonist (structure unknown), currently at the preclinical stage for the treatment of schizophrenia and attention-deficit disorders [299].

CONCLUSION AND FUTURE PERSPECTIVES

Since the discovery of the histamine H_3R in the 1980s and the cloning of human H_3R 7 years ago, the quest for innovative H_3 antagonist as potential clinical candidates for the treatment of unmet medical needs within the CNS and non-CNS therapeutic axes has never been so intense these past 2 years. The H_3 drug discovery process has been constantly refined from the original idea to the proof-of-concept in human.

The exponential patent application filings and public disclosures of widely diverse chemical series demonstrated the ability of medicinal chemists to identify key features for high-affinity ligands and transformed their creativity into innovative compounds. Such work has been gratefully supported by computer-aided drug design activities. The different *in silico* approaches described earlier highlighted the combined efforts of computational chemists and biologists to study the ligand–receptor interactions. Recent QSAR studies around Abbott's arylbenzofuran series [300] as well as refined 3-D pharmacophore ligand-based design strategies from Hoffman-La Roche [301] successfully afford a complementary approach in the early drug discovery phase. Large HTS campaign is the most common starting point for a medicinal chemical strategy. Interestingly, Acadia Pharmaceuticals recently developed a proprietary receptor selection and amplification technology (R-SAT) proliferation assay to measure antagonism and inverse agonism activities [302]. Screening over 250,000 small molecules led to the identification of 15 distinct nonimidazole chemical classes with nanomolar to subnanomolar potency compounds. One of their leads, namely AC-381, showed efficacy in a rat-feeding model.

Later, during the lead optimization phase, the known liabilities of many preclinical compounds targeting CNS disorders such as poor pharmacokinetics, phospholipidosis, low brain penetration, cardiovascular toxicity leading to lack of efficacy or low therapeutic index have been drastically tackled by pharmaceuticals companies. Indeed, the H_3 *first-in-class* drug on the CNS market is still eagerly awaited. To this end, companies such as Abbott Labs, GSK, and J&J PRD have successfully introduced these critical parameters within their own screening decision cascade, with focused SAR studies on hERG K^+ channel activity, *in vitro* metabolic clearance, brain H_3R occupancy, or brain/plasma ratio.

Finally, current clinical phases of drug candidates developed by GSK, J&J PRD, and Bioprojet would certainly inform about the potential and the clinical safety of such unique H_3 ligand to provide new therapeutic solutions for the treatment of severe CNS-related diseases. The combination/dual therapy of multitargeted H_3 ligands may also be a promising alternative strategy for the treatment of CNS disorders, where multiple neurotransmitters are involved [303].

The tremendous drug discovery efforts achieved by H_3 research scientists all over the world are therefore gratefully acknowledged, and in the coming years we might therefore expect novel histamine H_3R drugs since the histamine H_1 and H_2 blockbuster drug era.

REFERENCES

1. Aslanian, R. and Shih, N.Y. 2004. Recent progress in histamine H3 receptor chemistry. *Ann. Rep. Med. Chem.* 39:57–66.
2. Stark, H., Kathmann, M., Schlicker, E. et al. 2004. Medicinal chemical and pharmacological aspects of imidazole-containing histamine H3 receptor antagonists. *Mini-Rev. Med. Chem.* 4:965–977.
3. De Esch, I.J.P. and Belzar, K.J. 2004. Histamine H3 receptor agonists. *Mini-Rev. Med. Chem.* 4:955–963.
4. Cowart, M., Altenbach, R., Black, L. et al. 2004. Medicinal chemistry and biological properties of non-imidazole histamine H3 antagonists. *Mini-Rev. Med. Chem.* 4:979–992.
5. Leurs, R., Bakker, R.A., Timmerman, H. et al. 2005. The histamine H3 receptor: From gene cloning to H3 receptor drugs. *Nat. Rev. Drug Disc.* 4:107–120.
6. Celanire, S., Wijtmans, M., Talaga, P. et al. 2005. Keynote review: Histamine H3 receptor antagonists reach out for the clinic. *Drug Disc. Today* 10:1613–1627.
7. Letavic, M.A., Barbier, A.J., Dvorak, C.A. et al. 2006. Recent medicinal chemistry of the histamine H3 receptor. *Prog. Med. Chem.* 44:181–206.
8. IDdb3. 2007. *Investigational Drugs Database (IDdb)*. Thomson Current Drugs. Thomson Scientific. http://www. iddb3.com.
9. *Derwent Discovery World Drug Alert Plus* 2007. Thomson Scientific. https://www. derwent-discovery.com/.

10. Lovenberg, T.W., Pyati, J., Chang, H. et al. 2000. Cloning of rat histamine H3 receptor reveals distinct species pharmacological profiles. *J. Pharmacol. Exp. Ther.* 293:771–778.

11. Berlin, M. and Boyce, C.W. 2007. Recent advances in the development of histamine H3 antagonists. *Expert Opin. Ther. Pat.* 17:675–687.

12. Dale, H. and Laidlaw, P. 1910. The physiological action of beta-iminazolylethylamine. *J. Physiol.* 41:318–344.

13. De Luca, L. 2006. Naturally occurring and synthetic imidazoles: Their chemistry and their biological activities. *Curr. Med. Chem.* 13:1–23.

14. Boehlow, T.R., Harburn, J.J., and Spilling, C.D. 2001. Approaches to the synthesis of some tyrosine-derived marine sponge metabolites: Synthesis of verongamine and purealidin N. *J. Org. Chem.* 66:3111–3118.

15. Chen, Z., Sakurai, E., Hu, W. et al. 2004. Pharmacological effects of carcinine on histaminergic neurons in the brain. *Br. J. Pharmacol.* 143:573–580.

16. Tanida, M., Niijima, A., Fukuda, Y. et al. 2005. Dose-dependent effects of l-carnosine on the renal sympathetic nerve and blood pressure in urethane-anesthetized rats. *Am. J. Physiol.* 288:R447–R455.

17. Shen, Y., Hu, W.W., Fan, Y.Y. et al. 2007. Carnosine protects against NMDA-induced neurotoxicity in differentiated rat PC12 cells through carnosine-histidine-histamine pathway and H1/H3 receptors. *Biochem. Pharmacol.* 73:709–717.

18. Nagai, K., Niijima, A., Yamano, T. et al. 2003. Possible role of l-carnosine in the regulation of blood glucose through controlling autonomic nerves. *Exp. Biol. Med.* 228:1138–1145.

19. Babizhayev, M., Seguin, M., Gueyene, J. et al. 1994. l-Carnosine (β-alanyl-l-histidine) and carcinine (β-alanylhistamine) act as natural antioxidants with hydroxyl-radical-scavenging and lipid-peroxidase activities. *Biochemistry* 304:509–516.

20. Pompni, S.A. and Gullo, V.P. 1994. US5352707A.

21. Swanson, D.M., Wilson, S.J., Boggs, J.D. et al. 2006. Aplysamine-1 and related analogs as histamine H3 receptor antagonists. *Bioorg. Med. Chem. Lett.* 16:897–900.

22. Zhao, C., Bennani, Y.L., Gopalakrishnan, S. et al. 2005. Discovery of novel natural alkaloid conessine as potent histamine H3 receptor antagonist, *230th ACS National Meeting,* Washington, DC, August 28 to September 1, 2005. Abst. MEDI-104.

23. Zhao, C., Sun, M., Cowart, M.D. et al. 2005. WO2005100377A1.

24. Zhao, C., Sun, M., Cowart, M.D. et al. 2005. US2005227953A1.

25. Kopach, M.E., Fray, A.H., and Meyers, A.I. 1996. An asymmetric route to the conanine BCDE ring system. A formal total synthesis of (+)-conessine. *J. Am. Chem. Soc.* 118:9876–9883.

26. Jiang, B. and Xu, M. 2004. Highly enantioselective construction of fused pyrrolidine systems that contain a quarternary stereocenter: Concise formal synthesis of (+)-conessine. *Angew. Chem. Int. Ed.* 43:2543–2546.

27. Anderson, N. and Borlak, J. 2006. Drug-induced phospholipidosis. *FEBS Lett.* 580:5533–5540.

28. Reasor, M.J. and Kacew, S. 2001. Drug-induced phospholipidosis: Are there functional consequences. *Exp. Biol. Med.* 226:825–830.

29. Zirihi, G.N., Grellier, P., Guede-Guina, F. et al. 2005. Isolation, characterization and antiplasmodial activity of steroidal alkaloids from *Funtumia elastica* (Preuss) Stapf. *Bioorg. Med. Chem. Lett.* 15:2637–2640.

30. Newman, D.J., Cragg, C.G., and Snader, K.M. 2003. Natural products as source of new drugs over the period 1981–2002. *J. Nat. Prod.* 66:1022–1037.

31. Arrang, J.M., Garbarg, M., and Schwartz, J.C. 1983. Autoinhibition of brain histamine release mediated by a novel class (H3) of histamine receptor. *Nature* 302:832–837.

32. Lim, H.D., van Rijn, R.M., Ling, P. et al. 2005. Evaluation of histamine H1-, H2-, and H3-receptor ligands at the human histamine H4 receptor: Identification of 4-methylhistamine

as the first potent and selective H4 receptor agonist. *J. Pharmacol. Exp. Ther.* 314:1310–1321.

33. Gbahou, F., Vincent, L., Humbert-Claude, M. et al. 2006. Compared pharmacology of human histamine H3 and H4 receptors: Structure-activity relationships of histamine derivatives. *Br. J. Pharmacol.* 147:744–754.

34. Kitbunnadaj, R., Zuiderveld, O.P., De Esch, I.J.P. et al. 2003. Synthesis and structure–activity relationships of conformationally constrained histamine H3 receptor agonists. *J. Med. Chem.* 46:5445–5457.

35. Harusawa, S., Araki, L., Imazu, T. et al. 2003. Synthesis of (+-)-trans- or cis-(5-amino methyltetrahydrofuranyl)imidazole by Mitsunobu cyclization: Synthetic studies toward novel histamine H3 or H4-ligands. *Chem. Pharm. Bull.* 51:325–329.

36. Kitbunnadaj, R., Hashimoto, T., Poli, E. et al. 2005. N-Substituted piperidinyl alkyl imidazoles: Discovery of methimepip as a potent and selective histamine H3 receptor agonist. *J. Med. Chem.* 48:2100–2107.

37. Kitbunnadaj, R., Hoffmann, M., Fratantoni, S.A. et al. 2005. New high affinity H3 receptor agonists without a basic side chain. *Bioorg. Med. Chem.* 13:6309–6323.

38. Kazuta, Y., Hirano, K., Natsume, K. et al. 2003. Cyclopropane-based conformational restriction of histamine. (1S,2S)-2-(2-Aminoethyl)-1-(1H-imidazol-4-yl)cyclopropane, a highly selective agonist for the histamine H3 receptor, having a *cis*-cyclopropane structure. *J. Med. Chem.* 46:1980–1988.

39. Kitbunnadaj, R., Zuiderveld, O.P., Christophe, B. et al. 2004. Identification of 4-(1H-Imidazol-4(5)-ylmethyl)pyridine (immethridine) as a novel, potent, and highly selective histamine H3 receptor agonist. *J. Med. Chem.* 47:2414–2417.

40. Celanire, S., Gillard, M., Christophe, B. et al. 2007. Pharmacological characterization, *in vitro* and *in vivo* ADME properties of immethridine, a potent and highly selective histamine H3R agonist. *35th Eur. Histamine Res. Soc.* Delphi, Greece, Abst. P5.

41. Govoni, M., Lim, H.D., El Atmioui, D. et al. 2006. A chemical switch for the modulation of the functional activity of higher homologues of histamine on the human histamine H3 receptor: Effect of various substitutions at the primary amino function. *J. Med. Chem.* 49:2549–2557.

42. Krause, M., Stark, H., Schunack, W. 2001. Azomethine prodrugs of (R)-a-methylhistamine, a highly potent and selective histamine H3-receptor agonist. *Curr. Med. Chem.* 8:1329–1340.

43. Fozard, J.R. 2000. BP-294 (Ste Civile Bioprojet). *Curr. Opin. Investig. Drugs* 1:86–89.

44. Stark, H., Krause, M., Rouleau, A. et al. 2001. Enzyme-catalyzed prodrug approaches for the histamine H3-receptor agonist (R)-a-methylhistamine. *Bioorg. Med. Chem. Lett.* 9:191–198.

45. Sasse, A., Ligneau, X., Rouleau, A. et al. 2002. Influence of bulky substituents on histamine H3 receptor agonist/antagonist properties. *J. Med. Chem.* 45:4000–4010.

46. Pelloux-Leon, N., Fkyerat, A., Piripitsi, A. et al. 2004. Meta-substituted aryl(thio)ethers as potent partial agonists (or antagonists) for the histamine H3 receptor lacking a nitrogen atom in the side chain. *J. Med. Chem.* 47:3264–3274.

47. Meier, G., Krause, M., Huels, A. et al. 2004. 4-(w-(Alkyloxy)alkyl)-1H-imidazole derivatives as histamine H3 receptor antagonists/agonists. *J. Med. Chem.* 47:2678–2687.

48. Tedford, C.E., Hoffmann, M., Seyedi, N. et al. 1998. High antagonist potency of GT-2227 and GT-2331, new histamine H3 receptor antagonists, in two functional models. *Eur. J. Pharmacol.* 351:307–311.

49. Liu, H., Kerdesky, F.A., Black, L.A. et al. 2004. An efficient multigram synthesis of the potent histamine H3 antagonist GT-2331 and the reassessment of the absolute configuration. *J. Org. Chem.* 69:192–194.

50. Ito, S., Yoshimoto, R., Miyamoto, Y. et al. 2006. Detailed pharmacological characterization of GT-2331 for the rat histamine H3 receptor. *Eur. J. Pharmacol.* 529:40–46.

51. Morisset, S., Rouleau, A., Lineau, X. et al. 2000. High constitutive activity of native H3 receptors regulates histamine neurons in brain. *Nature* 408:860–864.

52. Gbahou, F., Rouleau, A., Morisset, S. et al. 2003. Protean agonism at histamine H3 receptors *in vitro* and *in vivo*. *Proc. Natl Acad. Sci. U.S.A.* 100:11086–11091.

53. Kenakin, T. 2001. Inverse, protean, and ligand-selective agonism: Matters of receptor conformation. *FASEB J.* 15:598–611.

54. Stark, H. 2004. Turning from monogamy to strategic promiscuity. *Drug Disc. Today* 9:736–737.

55. De Esch, I.J.P., Thurmond, R.L., Jongejan, A. et al. 2005. The histamine H4 receptor as a new therapeutic target for inflammation. *Trends Pharmacol. Sci.* 26:462–469.

56. Zhang, M., Ballard, M.E., Pan, L. et al. 2005. Lack of cataleptogenic potentiation with non-imidazole H3 receptor antagonists reveals potential drug–drug interactions between imidazole-based H3 receptor antagonists and antipsychotic drugs. *Brain Res.* 1045:142–149.

57. Yang, R., Hey, J.A., Aslanian, R. et al. 2002. Coordination of histamine H3 receptor antagonists with human adrenal cytochrome P450 enzymes. *Pharmacology* 66:128–135.

58. Watanabe, M., Kazuta, Y., Hayashi, H. et al. 2006. Stereochemical diversity-oriented conformational restriction strategy. Development of potent histamine H3 and/or H4 receptor antagonists with an imidazolylcyclopropane structure. *J. Med. Chem.* 49:5587–5596.

59. Vaccaro, W.D., Sher, R., Berlin, M. et al. 2006. Novel histamine H3 receptor antagonists based on the 4-[(1H-imidazol-4-yl)methyl]piperidine scaffold. *Bioorg. Med. Chem. Lett.* 16:395–399.

60. Berlin, M., Ting, P.C., Vaccaro, W.D. et al. 2006. Reduction of CYP450 inhibition in the 4-[(1H-imidazol-4-yl)methyl]piperidine series of histamine H3 receptor antagonists. *Bioorg. Med. Chem. Lett.* 16:989–994.

61. Rivara, M., Vacondio, F., Silva, C. et al. 2008. Synthesis and stability in biological of 1H-imidazole-1-carboxylates of RS203, an antagonist of the histamine H3 receptor. *Chem. Biodivers.* 5:140–152.

62. Lin, J.H. and Lu, A.Y. 1998. Inhibition and induction of cytochrome P450 and the clinical implications. *Clin. Pharmacokinet.* 35:361–390.

63. Pillot, C., Ortiz, J., Heron, A. et al. 2002. Ciproxifan, a histamine H3-receptor antagonist/inverse agonist, potentiates neurochemical and behavioral effects of haloperidol in the rat. *J. Neuroscience* 22:7272–7280.

64. Kalindjian, S.B., Buck, I.M., Linney, I.D. et al. 1999. WO9942458A1.

65. Schwartz, J-C., Arrang, J-M., Garbarg, M. et al. 2000. EP978512A1.

66. Schwartz, J. and Lecomte, J. 2006. WO2006103546A2.

67. Schwartz, J. and Lecomte, J. 2006. WO2006103537A2.

68. Bertrand, I., Capet, M., Lecomte, J-M. et al. 2006. WO2006117611A1.

69. Bertrand, I., Capet, M., Lecomte, J-M. et al. 2006. WO2006117609A2.

70. Meier, G., Apelt, J., Reichert, U. et al. 2001. Influence of imidazole replacement in different structural classes of histamine H3-receptor antagonists. *Eur. J. Pharm. Sci.* 13:249–259.

71. Ligneau, X., Landais, L., Perrin, D. et al. 2007. Brain histamine and schizophrenia: Potential therapeutic applications of H3-receptor inverse agonists studied with BF2.649. *Biochem. Pharmacol.* 73:1215–1224.

72. Ligneau, X., Perrin, D., Landais, L. et al. 2007. BF2.649 [1-{3-[3-(4-chlorophenyl)propoxy]propyl}piperidine, hydrochloride], a nonimidazole inverse agonist/antagonist at the human histamine H3 receptor: Preclinical pharmacology. *J. Pharmacol. Exp. Ther.* 320:365–375.

73. Lazewska, D., Kiec-Kononowicz, K., Elz, S. et al. 2005. Piperidine-containing histamine H3 receptor antagonists of the carbamate series: The alkyl derivatives. *Pharmazie* 60:403–410.

74. Lazewska, D., Ligneau, X., Schwartz, J.C. et al. 2006. Ether derivatives of 3-piperidino-propan-1-ol as non-imidazole histamine H3 receptor antagonists. *Bioorg. Med. Chem.* 14:3522–3529.
75. Miko, T., Ligneau, X., Pertz, H.H. et al. 2003. Novel nonimidazole histamine H3 receptor antagonists: 1-(4-(Phenoxymethyl)benzyl)piperidines and related compounds. *J. Med. Chem.* 46:1523–1530.
76. Miko, T., Ligneau, X., Pertz, H.H. et al. 2004. Structural variations of 1-(4-(phenoxymethyl)benzyl)piperidines as nonimidazole histamine H3 receptor antagonists. *Bioorg. Med. Chem.* 12:2727–2736.
77. Bertoni, S., Flammini, L., Manenti, V. et al. 2007. *In vitro* pharmacology at human histamine H3 receptors and brain access of non-imidazole alkylpiperidine derivatives. *Pharmacol. Res.* 55:111–116.
78. A safety and effectiveness study of a single dose of JNJ-17216498 in patients with narcolepsy, http://clinicaltrials.gov/show/NCT00424931.
79. Bonaventure, P., Letavic, M., Dugovic, C. et al. 2007. Histamine H3 receptor antagonists: From target identification to drug leads. *Biochem. Pharmacol.* 73:1084–1096.
80. Sanfilippo, P.J., Urbanski, M., Press, J.B. et al. 1988. Synthesis of (aryloxy)alkylamines. 2. Novel imidazo-fused heterocycles with calcium channel blocking and local anesthetic activity. *J. Med. Chem.* 31:2221–2227.
81. Shah, C., McAtee, L., Breitenbucher, J.G. et al. 2002. Novel human histamine H3 receptor antagonists. *Bioorg. Med. Chem. Lett.* 12:3309–3312.
82. Chai, W., Breitenbucher, J.G., Kwok, A. et al. 2003. Non-imidazole heterocyclic histamine H3 receptor antagonists. *Bioorg. Med. Chem. Lett.* 13:1767–1770.
83. Apodaca, R., Carruthers, N.I., Carson, J.R. et al. 2002. WO2002024695A2.
84. Apodaca, R., Carruthers, N.I., Dvorak, C.A. et al. 2002. WO200212214A2.
85. Apodaca, R., Dvorak, C.A., Xiao, W. et al. 2003. A new class of diamine-based human histamine H3 receptor antagonists: 4-(Aminoalkoxy)benzylamines. *J. Med. Chem.* 46:3938–3944.
86. Apodaca, R.L., Dvorak, C.A., Shah, C.R. et al. 2004. WO2004037257A1.
87. Airaksinen, A.J., Jablonowski, J.A., van der Mey, M. et al. 2006. Radiosynthesis and biodistribution of a histamine H3 receptor antagonist 4-[3-(4-piperidin-1-yl-but-1-ynyl)-[11C]benzyl]-morpholine: Evaluation of a potential PET ligand. *Nucl. Med. Biol.* 33:801–810.
88. Carruthers, N.I., Shah, C.R., Swanson, D.M. et al. 2005. US2005222151A1.
89. Apodaca, R., Xiao, W., Jablonoski, J.A. et al. 2003. WO2003050099A1.
90. Dvorak, C.A., Apodaca, R., Barbier, A.J. et al. 2005. 4-phenoxypiperidines: Potent, conformationally restricted, non-imidazole histamine H3 antagonists. *J. Med. Chem.* 48:2229–2238.
91. Apodaca, R., Carruthers, N.I., Dvorak, C.A. et al. 2002. WO200212190A2.
92. Apodaca, R.L., Jablonowski, J.A., Ly, K.S. et al. 2004. WO2004037801A1.
93. Carruthers, N.I., Shah, C.R., Swanson, D.M. et al. 2005. US2005222129A1.
94. Allison, B.D., Carruthers, N.I., Grice, C.A. et al. 2007. US2007066821A1.
95. Bogenstaetter, M., Carruthers, N.I. and Jablonowski, J.A. 2002. WO2002079168A1.
96. Mani, N.S., Jablonowski, J.A., and Jones, T.K. 2004. A scalable synthesis of a histamine H3 receptor antagonist. *J. Org. Chem.* 69:8115–8117.
97. Hancock, A.A. 2006. The challenge of drug discovery of a GPCR target: Analysis of preclinical pharmacology of histamine H3 antagonists/inverse agonists. *Biochem. Pharmacol.* 71:1103–1113.
98. Esbenshade, T.A., Fox, G.B., and Cowart, M.D. 2006. Histamine H3 receptor antagonists: Preclinical promise for treating obesity and cognitive disorders. *Mol. Interv.* 6:77–88, 59.

99. Bennani, Y. 2005. Selective tissue targeting as a strategy for CNS drugs: Application to H3 blockers. *Interplay of Chemistry and Biology in Integrative Drug Discovery* meeting, Miami, FL, March.
100. Faghih, R., Dwight, W., Gentles, R. et al. 2002. Structure–activity relationships of non-imidazole H(3) receptor ligands. Part 1. *Bioorg. Med. Chem. Lett.* 12:2031–2034.
101. Faghih, R., Dwight, W., Black, L. et al. 2002. Structure–activity relationships of non-imidazole H3 receptor ligands. Part 2: Binding preference for d-amino acids motifs. *Bioorg. Med. Chem. Lett.* 12:2035–2037.
102. Esbenshade, T.A., Krueger, K.M., Miller, T.R. et al. 2003. Two novel and selective non-imidazole histamine H3 receptor antagonists A-304121 and A-317920: I. In vitro pharmacological effects. *J. Pharmacol. Exp. Ther.* 305:887–896.
103. Fox, G.B., Pan, J.B., Radek, R.J. et al. 2003. Two novel and selective nonimidazole H3 receptor antagonists A-304121 and A-317920: II. In vivo behavioral and neurophysiological characterization. *J. Pharmacol. Exp. Ther.* 305:897–908.
104. Vasudevan, A., Conner, S.E., Gentles, R.G. et al. 2002. Synthesis and evaluation of potent pyrrolidine H3 antagonists. *Bioorg. Med. Chem. Lett.* 12:3055–3058.
105. Bennani, Y.L., Faghih, R., Dwight, W.J. et al. 2002. WO200206223A1.
106. Gfesser, G.A., Zhang, H., Dinges, J. et al. 2004. Structure–activity relationships of non-imidazole H3 receptor ligands. Part 3: 5-Substituted 3-phenyl-1,2,4-oxadiazoles as potent antagonists. *Bioorg. Med. Chem. Lett.* 14:673–676.
107. Gfesser, G.A., Faghih, R., Bennani, Y.L. et al. 2005. Structure–activity relationships of arylbenzofuran H3 receptor antagonists. *Bioorg. Med. Chem. Lett.* 15:2559–2563.
108. Curtis, M.P., Dwight, W., Pratt, J. et al. 2004. D-amino acid homopiperazine amides: Discovery of A-320436, a potent and selective non-imidazole histamine H(3)-receptor antagonist. *Arch. Pharm.* 337:219–229.
109. Bennani, Y.L., Black, L.A., Dwight, W.J. et al. 2001. US2001049367A1.
110. Hancock, A.A., Bush, E.N., Jacobson, P.B. et al. 2004. Histamine H3 antagonists in models of obesity. *Inflamm. Res.* 53:S47-S48.
111. Hancock, A.A., Bennani, Y.L., Bush, E.N. et al. 2004. Antiobesity effects of A-331440, a novel non-imidazole histamine H3 receptor antagonist. *Eur. J. Pharmacol.* 487:183–197.
112. Hancock, A.A., Diehl, M.S., Fey, T.A. et al. 2005. Antiobesity evaluation of histamine H3 receptor (H3R) antagonist analogs of A-331440 with improved safety and efficacy. *Inflamm. Res.* 54:S27-S29.
113. Hancock, A.A. and Brune, M.E. 2005. Assessment of pharmacology and potential anti-obesity properties of H3 receptor antagonists/inverse agonists. *Expert Opin. Invest. Drugs* 14:223–241.
114. Hancock, A.A., Bitner, R.S., Krueger, K.M. et al. 2006. Distinctions and contradistinctions between antiobesity histamine H3 receptor (H3R) antagonists compared to cognition-enhancing H3 receptor antagonists. *Inflamm. Res.* 55:S42–S44.
115. Hancock, A.A., Diehl, M.S., Faghih, R. et al. 2004. In vitro optimization of structure activity relationships of analogs of A-331440 combining radioligand receptor binding assays and micronucleus assays of potential antiobesity histamine H3 receptor antagonists. *Basic Clin. Pharmacol. Tox.* 95:144–152.
116. Fey, T.A., Bush, E.A., Dickinson, R.A. et al. 2004. Effects of A-423579, a novel histamine-3 receptor antagonist in rodent models of diet-induced obesity. *Experimental Biology,* Washington, DC, April 17–21. Abst. #394.5.
117. Bennani, Y.L. and Faghih, R. 2002. WO200240461A2.
118. Faghih, R., Dwight, W., Pan, J.B. et al. 2003. Synthesis and SAR of aminoalkoxy-biaryl-4-carboxamides: Novel and selective histamine H3 receptor antagonists. *Bioorg. Med. Chem. Lett.* 13:1325–1328.

119. Esbenshade, T.A., Fox, G.B., Krueger, K.M. et al. 2004. Pharmacological and behavioral properties of A-349821, a selective and potent human histamine H3 receptor antagonist. *Biochem. Pharmacol.* 68:933–945.

120. Cowart, M., Faghih, R., Gfesser, G. et al. 2004. The medicinal chemistry of novel H(3) antagonists. *Inflamm. Res.* 53(Suppl 1):S69–S70.

121. Cowart, M., Pratt, J.K., Stewart, A.O. et al. 2004. A new class of potent non-imidazole H3 antagonists: 2-Aminoethylbenzofurans. *Bioorg. Med. Chem. Lett.* 14:689–693.

122. Cowart, M., Faghih, R., Curtis, M.P. et al. 2005. 4-(2-[2-(2(R)-Methylpyrrolidin-1-yl)ethyl]benzofuran-5-yl)benzonitrile and related 2-aminoethylbenzofuran H3 receptor antagonists potently enhance cognition and attention. *J. Med. Chem.* 48:38–55.

123. Miller, T.R., Krueger, K.M., Baranowski, J.L. et al. 2004. Pharmacological properties of novel, non-imidazole benzofuran H3 receptor antagonists. *Experimental Biology*, Washington, DC, April 17–21. Abst. #396.3.

124. Pu, Y.M., Grieme, T., Gupta, A. et al. 2005. A facile and scaleable synthesis of ABT-239, a benzofuranoid H3 antagonist. *Org. Proc. Res. Dev.* 9:45–50.

125. Ku, Y.Y., Pu, Y.M., Grieme, T. et al. 2006. An efficient and convergent synthesis of the potent and selective H3 antagonist ABT-239. *Tetrahedron* 62:4584–4589.

126. Esbenshade, T.A., Fox, G.B., Krueger, K.M. et al. 2005. Pharmacological properties of ABT-239 [4-(2-{2-[(2R)-2-methylpyrrolidinyl]ethyl}-benzofuran-5-yl)benzonitrile]: I. Potent and selective histamine H3 receptor antagonist with drug-like properties. *J. Pharmacol. Exp. Ther.* 313:165–175.

127. Fox, G.B., Esbenshade, T.A., Pan, J.B. et al. 2005. Pharmacological properties of ABT-239 [4-(2-{2-[(2R)-2-methylpyrrolidinyl]ethyl}-benzofuran-5-yl)benzonitrile]: II. Neurophysiological characterization and broad preclinical efficacy in cognition and schizophrenia of a potent and selective histamine H3 receptor antagonist. *J. Pharmacol. Exp. Ther.* 313:176–190.

128. Esbenshade, T.A., Wetter, J., Marsh, K. et al. 2005. ABT-239, a potent human histamine H3 receptor antagonist with favorable drug-like properties. *Experimental Biol.*, San Diego, CA, March 31 to April 5. Abst. #321.7.

129. Milicic, I., Krueger, K., Miller, T. et al. 2005. Pharmacological properties of the S-enantiomer of the histamine H3 receptor antagonist ABT-239: An inverse agonist with no anti-obesity effects. *Experimental Biol.*, San Diego, CA, March 31 to April 5. Abst. #85.9.

130. Preusser, L.C., Fryer, R.M., Esbenshade, T.A. et al. 2005. ABT-239, a novel H3 receptor antagonist: Demonstration of a benign cardiovascular profile in the anesthetized canine. *Experimental Biol.*, San Diego, CA, March 31 to April 5. Abst. #87.14.

131. Esbenshade, T.A. 2006. Preclinical pursuit of enhanced safety of H3 antagonists/inverse agonists for neuropsychiatric disease. *The Histamine H3 Receptor: Clinical Applications of Antagonist/Inverse Agonists. 25th Biennial Congress of the Collegium Internationale Neuro-Psychopharmacologicum.* Chicago, IL, July 7–13.

132. Cowart, M., Gfesser, G.A., Browman, K.E. et al. 2007. Novel heterocyclic-substituted benzofuran histamine H3 receptor antagonists: In vitro properties, drug-likeness, and behavioral activity. *Biochem. Pharmacol.* 73:1243–1255.

133. Cowart, M., Faghih, R., Gfesser, G. et al. 2005. Achievement of behavioral efficacy and improved potency in new heterocyclic analogs of benzofuran H3 antagonists. *Inflamm. Res.* 54:S25–S26.

134. Sun, M., Zhao, C., Gfesser, G.A. et al. 2005. Synthesis and SAR of 5-amino- and 5-(Aminomethyl)benzofuran histamine H3 receptor antagonists with improved potency. *J. Med. Chem.* 48:6482–6490.

135. Cowart, M.D., Sun, M., Altenbach, R.A. et al. 2005. Bicyclic heteroaromatic histamine H3 antagonists: Synthesis, potency, and in vivo profiles of analogs optimized for drug-likeness. *XIII RSC-SCI Med. Chem. Symp.* September 22, Cambridge, U.K.

136. Altenbach, R.J., Black, L.A., Chang, S-J. et al. 2005. US2005256309A1.
137. Cowart, M.D., Ku, Y., Chang, S-J. et al. 2004. WO2004101559A1.
138. Altenbach, R.J., Black, L.A., Chang, S-J., et al. 2005. US2005256118A1.
139. Liu, H., Altenbach, R.J., Miller, T.R. et al. 2005. Design, synthesis, and structure-activity relationship of novel non-imidazole histamine H3 antagonists. *230th ACS National Meeting*, Washington, DC, August 28 to September 1. Abst. MEDI-103.
140. Black, L.A., Nersesian, D.L., Sharma, P. et al. 2007. 4-[6-(2-Aminoethyl)naphthalen-2-yl]benzonitriles are potent histamine H3 receptor antagonists with high CNS penetration. *Bioorg. Med. Chem. Lett.* 17:1443–1446.
141. Cowart, M., Black, L., Liu, H. et al. 2007. Optimization of H3 antagonist series for H3 selectivity over the hERG channel. *36th European Histamine Research Soceity Meeting*, Florence, Italy, May 9–13. Abst. O35.
142. Altenbach, R.J., Liu, H., Esbenshade, T.A. et al. 2005. Bicyclic heteroaromatic histamine H3 antagonists: Synthesis, potency, and in vivo profiles of analogs optimized for drug-likeness. *230th ACS National Meeting*, Washington, DC, August 28 to September 1. Abst. MEDI-102.
143. Milicic, I., Browman, K.E., Baranowski, J.L. et al. 2007. Effects of repeated H3 receptor antagonist administration on H3 receptor expression and function in rats. *FASEB J.* 21:A790–A79c.
144. Medhurst, A.D. 2004. Pre-clinical evaluation of novel H3 receptor antagonists. *33th Eur. Histamine Res. Soc. Meeting*, April 28 to May 2, Düsseldorf/Köln, Germany. Abst. O2.
145. GlaxoSmithkline website, 2007, http://www.gsk.com/investors/pp_pipeline_standard.htm.
146. Wilson, D.M. 2005. Discovery of a novel series of potent, orally active histamine H3 receptor antagonists. *Recent Disclosures of Clinical Drug Candidates; Society for Medicines Research Symposium*, London, U.K., December 8.
147. Heightman, T.D. 2005. Knowledge-based high throughput lead generation. *13th RSC-SCI Medicinal Chemistry Symposium*, Cambridge, U.K., September 22.
148. Jin, J., Dhanak, D., Knight, S.D. et al. 2005. Aminoalkoxybenzyl pyrrolidines as novel human urotensin-II receptor antagonists. *Bioorg. Med. Chem. Lett.* 15:3229–3232.
149. Wilson, D.M. 2005. The discovery of a novel series of potent, orally active histamine H3 receptor antagonists. *13th RSC-SCI Medicinal Chemistry Symposium*, Cambridge, U.K., September 22. *delimi.*
150. Dean, D., Apps, J., and Bamford, M. 2006. A novel series of histamine H3 antagonists. *The 19th International Symposium in Medicinal Chemistry (Part IV)*, Istanbul, Turkey. Abst. P247.
151. Bamford, M.J., Dean, D.K., Sehmi, S.S. et al. 2004. WO2004056369A1.
152. Medhurst, A.D., Atkins, A.R., Beresford, I.J. et al. 2007. GSK189254—a novel H3 receptor antagonist that binds to histamine H3 receptors in Alzheimer's disease brain and improves cognitive performance in preclinical models. *J. Pharmacol. Exp. Ther.* 321:1032–1045.
153. Woolley, M., Gartlon, J., and Pemberton, D. 2006. The histamine H3 receptor antagonist GSK189254, improves performance in the rat novel object recognition and attentional set shifting tasks. *BAP Summer Meeting*, 23–26 July, Oxford, U.K. Abst. TE12.
154. Giannoni, P., Passani, M.B., Nosi, D. et al. 2007. Detection of functional heterogeneity of histaminergic neurons in response to GSK189254, a novel H3 receptor antagonist. *36th Eur. Histamine. Res. Soc. Meeting*, May 9–12, 2007, Florence, Italy. Abst. O6.
155. Medhurst, A.D., Briggs, M.A., Bruton, G. et al. 2007. Structurally novel histamine H3 receptor antagonists GSK207040 and GSK334429 improve scopolamine-induced memory impairment and capsaicin-induced secondary allodynia in rats. *Biochem. Pharmacol.* 73:1182–1194.
156. Bamford, M.J., Heightman, T.D., Wilson, D.M. et al. 2005. WO2005087746A1.
157. Bailey, N., Bamford, M.J., Dean, D.K. et al. 2005. WO2005058837A1.

158. Bamford, M.J. and Wilson, D.M. 2007. WO2007025596A1.

159. Orlek, B.S. 2006. Discovery of two new series of histamine H3 receptor antagonists. *17th Symposium on Medicinal Chemistry in Eastern England*, Hatfield, U.K.

160. Johnstone, V. 2006. Design and synthesis of novel histamine H3 antagonists: Potential therapeutics for the treament of alzheimers disease. *The 19th International Symposium in Medicinal Chemistry (Part IV)*. Istanbul, Turkey. Abst. P288.

161. Orlek, B.S. 2006. Discovery of two new series of histamine H3 receptor antagonists. *Abstr. 17th Symposium on Medicinal Chemistry in Eastern England*, Hatfield, U.K.

162. Cooper, I.R., Abberley, L., and Briggs, M. 2006. Novel potent H3 antagonists: Therapeutics for the treatment of dementia including alzheimer's disease. *The 19th International Symposium in Medicinal Chemistry (Part IV)*. Istanbul, Turkey. Abst. P247.

163. Bailey, J.M., Bruton, G., Huxley, A. et al. 2005. WO2005014571A1.

164. Ancliff, R.A., Bamford, M.J., Hodgson, S.T. et al. 2007. WO2007009741A1.

165. Zaragoza, F., Stephensen, H., Knudsen, S.M. et al. 2004. 1-Alkyl-4-acylpiperazines as a new class of imidazole-free histamine H3 receptor antagonists. *J. Med. Chem.* 47:2833–2838.

166. Peschke, B., Bak, S., Hohlweg, R. et al. 2004. Cinnamic amides of (S)-2-(aminomethyl) pyrrolidines are potent H3 antagonists. *Bioorg. Med. Chem.* 12:2603–2616.

167. Peschke, B., Bak, S., Hohlweg, R. et al. 2006. Benzo[b]thiophene-2-carboxamides and benzo[b]furan-2-carboxamides are potent antagonists of the human H3-receptor. *Bioorg. Med. Chem. Lett.* 16:3162–3165.

168. Lau, J.F., Jeppesen, C.B., Rimvall, K. et al. 2006. Ureas with histamine H3-antagonist receptor activity-A new scaffold discovered by lead-hopping from cinnamic acid amides. *Bioorg. Med. Chem. Lett.* 16:5303–5308.

169. Zaragoza, F., Stephensen, H., Peschke, B. et al. 2005. 2-(4-Alkyl-1-piperazinyl)quinolines as a new class of imidazole-free histamine H3 receptor antagonists. *J. Med. Chem.* 48:306–311.

170. Jesudason, C.D., Beavers, L.S., Cramer, J.W. et al. 2006. Synthesis and SAR of novel histamine H3 receptor antagonists. *Bioorg. Med. Chem. Lett.* 16:3415–3418.

171. Beavers, L.S., Gadski, R.A., Hipkind, P.A. et al. 2002. WO2002076925A2.

172. Beavers, L.S., Gadski, R.A., Hipkind, P.A. et al. 2005. WO2005082893A2.

173. Beavers, L.S., Finley, D.R., Gadski, R.A. et al. 2006. WO2006101808A1.

174. Beavers, L.S., Finley, D.R., Finn, T.P. et al. 2005. WO2005097740A1.

175. Beavers, L.S., Gadski, R.A., Jesudason, C.D. et al. 2005. WO2005121080A1.

176. Finley, D.R., Finn, T.P., Hipkind, P.A. et al. 2006. WO2006023462A1.

177. Hipkind, P.A., Takakuwa, T., Jesudason, C.D. et al. 2006. WO2006107661A1.

178. Jesudason, C.D., Beavers, L.S., and Cramer, J.W. 2006. (3-Piperidin-1-ylpropoxy)-tetrahydroisoquinolines and tetra-hydroazepines: A novel series of selective histamine H3 receptor antagonists. *35th Eur. Histamine Res. Soc. Meeting*, Delphi, Greece, Abst. P11.

179. Gadski, R.A., Hipkind, P.A., Jesudason, C.D. et al. 2004. WO2004018432A1.

180. Beavers, L.S., Finley, D.R., Gadski, R.A. et al. 2004. WO2004026837A2.

181. Poissonnet, G., Parmentier, J.-G., and Boutin, J.A. 2006. Rational exploration of structural databases: The case of H3 ligands. *Abstr. 1st Coast to Coast Medicinal and Synthetic Chemistry Symposium*, Torquay, U.K.

182. Goldstein, S., Poissonnet, G., Parmentier, J-G. et al. 2003. EP1275647A1.

183. Desos, P., Cordi, A. and Lestage, P. 2006. WO2006120348A1.

184. Casara, P., Chollet, A.M., Dhainaut, A. et al. 2005. FR2866647A1.

185. Freichel, C., Arthur, S.G., and Hertel, C. 2006. Histamine 3 receptor inverse agonists for the treatment of obesity. Biological and chemical challenges. *35th Eur. Histamine Res. Soc. Meeting,* Delphi, Greece, Abst. P8.

186. Mcarthur, S.G., Hertel, C., Nettekoven, M.H. et al. 2005. WO2005117865A1.

187. Mcarthur, S.G., Hertel, C., Nettekoven, M.H. et al. 2006. US2006084679A1.
188. Nettekoven, M.H., Plancher, J-M., Roche, O. et al. 2006. US2006160855A1.
189. Nettekoven, M.H., Plancher, J-M., Richter, H. et al. 2007. WO2007065820A1.
190. Richter, H.G.F., Adams, D.R., Benardeau, A. et al. 2006. Synthesis and biological evaluation of novel hexahydro-pyrido[3´,2´:4,5]pyrrolo[1,2-a]pyrazines as potent and selective 5-HT2C receptor agonists. *Bioorg. Med. Chem. Lett.* 16:1207–1211.
191. Nettekoven, M. and Roche, O. 2007. WO2007068641A1.
192. Bernardelli, P., Cronin, A.M., Denis, A. et al. 2005. WO2005108384A1.
193. Wlodecki, B. 2006. US2006047114A1.
194. Howard, H.R. and Wlodecki, B. 2005. US2005282811A1.
195. Wager, T.T. and Chandrasekaran, R.Y. 2005. US2005171181A1.
196. Howard, H.R. and Wlodecki, B. 2005. US2005245543A1.
197. Wager, T.T. and Chandrasekaran, R.Y. 2005. US2005171181A1.
198. Strang, R.S., Lunn, G. and Mathias, J.P. 2005. EP1595881A1.
199. Mizutani, T., Nagase, T., Sato, N. et al. 2005. WO2005115993A1.
200. Takahashi, T., Kanatani, A., Tokita, S. et al. 2005. WO2005077953A1.
201. Jitsuoka, M., Sato, N., Tsukahara, D. et al. 2006. WO2006028239A1.
202. Bennani, Y., Anderson, J.T., Wang, J. et al. 2006. WO2006071750A1.
203. Folmer, J., Hunt, S.F., Hamley, P. et al. 2006. WO2006014135A1.
204. Folmer, J., Hunt, S.F., Hamley, P. et al. 2006. WO2006014136A1.
205. Diaz Martin, J.A. and Jimenez Bargueno, M.D. 2005. WO2005118547A1.
206. Diaz Martin, J.A., Escribano Arenales, B. and Martin Escudero Perez, U. 2005. WO2005037810A2.
207. Pringle, W.C., Peterson, J.M., Xie, L. et al. 2006. WO2006089076A2.
208. Xie, L., Ochterski, J.W., Gao, Y. et al. 2007. WO2007016496A2.
209. Aslanian, R., Zhu, X., Tom, W. et al. 2006. Benzimidazole-substituted (3-phenoxypropyl) amines as histamine H3 receptor ligands. *232nd ACS National Meeting*, San Francisco, CA, September 10–14, 2006. Abst. MEDI-501.
210. Aslanian, R.G., Tom, W.C. and Zhu, X. 2006. WO2006078775A1.
211. Aslanian, R.G., Berlin, M.Y., Mangiaracina, P. et al. 2004. WO2004000831A1.
212. Ting, P.C., Aslanian, R.G., Berlin, M.Y. et al. 2004. WO2003103669A1.
213. Celanire, S. and Denonne, F. 2006. WO2006103045A1.
214. Celanire, S., Talaga, P., Leurs, R. et al. 2006. WO2006103057A1.
215. Santora, V.J., Covel, J.A., Hayashi, R. et al. 2007. WO2007061741A2.
216. De Esch, I.J.P., Mills, J.E.J., Perkins, T.D.J. et al. 2001. Development of a pharmacophore model for histamine H3 receptor antagonists, using the newly developed molecular modeling program SLATE. *J. Med. Chem.* 44:1666–1674.
217. De Esch, I.J.P., Timmerman, H., Menge, W.M.P.B. et al. 2000. A qualitative model for the histamine H3 receptor explaining agonistic and antagonistic activity simultaneously. *Archiv der Pharmazie* (Weinheim, Germany) 333:254–260.
218. Ter Laak, A.M., Timmerman, H., Leurs, R. et al. 1995. Modelling and mutation studies on the histamine H1-receptor agonist binding site reveal different binding modes for H1-agonists: Asp116 (TM3) has a constitutive role in receptor stimulation. *J. Comp.-Aided Mol. Design* 9:319–330.
219. Windhorst, A.D., Timmerman, H., Worthington, E.A. et al. 2000. Characterization of the binding site of the histamine H3 Receptor. 2. Synthesis, *in vitro* pharmacology, and QSAR of a series of monosubstituted benzyl analogues of thioperamide. *J. Med. Chem.* 43:1754–1761.
220. Lorenzi, S., Mor, M., Bordi, F. et al. 2005. Validation of a histamine H3 receptor model through structure–activity relationships for classical H3 antagonists. *Bioorg. Med. Chem.* 13:5647–5657.

221. Uveges, A.J., Kowal, D., Zhang, Y. et al. 2002. The role of transmembrane helix 5 in agonist binding to the human H3 receptor. *J. Pharmacol. Exp. Ther.* 301:451–458.

222. Moguilevsky, N., Varsalona, F., Guillaume, J.P. et al. 1995. Pharmacological and functional characterisation of the wild-type and site-directed mutants of the human H1 histamine receptor stably expressed in CHO cells. *J Recept. Signal Transduct. Res* 15:91–102.

223. Leurs, R., Smit, M.J., Tensen, C.P. et al. 1994. Site-directed mutagenesis of the histamine H1-receptor reveals a selective interaction of asparagine207 with subclasses of H1-receptor agonists. *Biochem. Biophys. Res. Commun.* 201:295–301.

224. Gantz, I., DelValle, J., Wang, L.D. et al. 1992. Molecular basis for the interaction of histamine with the histamine H2 receptor. *J. Biol. Chem.* 267:20840–20843.

225. Shin, N., Coates, E., Murgolo, N.J. et al. 2002. Molecular modeling and site-specific mutagenesis of the histamine-binding site of the histamine H4 receptor. *Mol. Pharmacol.* 62:38–47.

226. Visiers, I., Ballesteros, J.A., and Weinstein, H. 2002. Three-dimensional representations of G protein-coupled receptor structures and mechanisms. *Methods Enzymol.* 343:329–371.

227. Morini, G., Comini, M., Rivara, M. et al. 2006. Dibasic non-imidazole histamine H3 receptor antagonists with a rigid biphenyl scaffold. *Bioorg. Med. Chem. Lett.* 16:4063–4067.

228. Stark, H., Sippl, W., Ligneau, X. et al. 2001. Different antagonist binding properties of human and rat histamine H3 receptors. *Bioorg. Med. Chem. Lett.* 11:951–954.

229. Ligneau, X., Morisset, S., Tardivel-Lacombe, J. et al. 2000. Distinct pharmacology of rat and human histamine H3 receptors: Role of two amino acids in the third transmembrane domain. *Br. J. Pharmacol.* 131:1247–1250.

230. Yao, B.B., Hutchins, C.W., Carr, T.L. et al. 2003. Molecular modeling and pharmacological analysis of species-related histamine H3 receptor heterogeneity. *Neuropharmacol.* 44:773–786.

231. Boeckler, F., Lanig, H., and Gmeiner, P. 2005. Modeling the similarity and divergence of dopamine D2-like receptors and identification of validated ligand-receptor complexes. *J. Med. Chem.* 48:694–709.

232. Bockaert, J. and Pin, J.P. 1999. Molecular tinkering of G protein-coupled receptors: An evolutionary success. *EMBO J.* 18:1723–1729.

233. Fahmy, K., Jager, F., Beck, M. et al. 1993. Protonation states of membrane-embedded carboxylic acid groups in rhodopsin and metarhodopsin II: A Fourier-transform infrared spectroscopy study of site-directed mutants. *Proc. Natl Acad. Sci. U.S.A.* 90:10206–10210.

234. Okada, T., Fujiyoshi, Y., Silow, M. et al. 2002. Functional role of internal water molecules in rhodopsin revealed by X-ray crystallography. *Proc. Natl Acad. Sci. U.S.A.* 99:5982–5987.

235. Axe, F.U., Bembenek, S.D., and Szalma, S. 2006. Three-dimensional models of histamine H3 receptor antagonist complexes and their pharmacophore. *J. Mol. Graph. Model.* 24:456–464.

236. Schlegel, B. 2005. The human histamine H3-receptor: A molecular modelling study of a G-protein coupled receptor. Dissertation, Cuvillier Verlag, Göttingen, September 25.

237. Schlegel, B., Stark, H., Sippl, W. et al. 2005. Model of a specific human histamine H3 receptor (hH3R) binding pocket suitable for virtual drug design. *Inflamm. Res.* 54:S50–S51.

238. Narkhede, S.S. and Degani, M.S. 2007. Pharmacophore refinement and 3D-QSAR studies of histamine H3 antagonists. *QSAR Combi. Sci.* 26:744–753.

239. Jansen, F.P., Leurs, R., and Timmerman, H. 1998. Synthesis of radioligands for the histamine H3 receptor. In: *The Histamine H3 Receptor: A Target for New Drugs*. Eds R. Leurs, H. Timmerman, Elsevier, Amsterdam: pp. 127–144.

240. Windhorst, A.D., Leurs, R., Menge, W.M. et al. 1998. Synthesis of radioligands for the histamine H3 receptor. In: *The Histamine H3 Receptor: A Target for New Drugs*. Eds R. Leurs, H. Timmerman, Elsevier, Amsterdam: pp. 139–174.

241. Esbenshade, T.A., Yao, B.B., Witte, D.G. et al. 2005. Use of novel, non-imidazole inverse agonist radioligands to define histamine H3 receptor pharmacology. *Inflamm. Res.* 54:S46–S47.

242. Yao, B.B., Witte, D.G., Miller, T.R. et al. 2006. Use of an inverse agonist radioligand [3H]A-317920 reveals distinct pharmacological profiles of the rat histamine H3 receptor. *Neuropharmacology* 50:468–478.

243. Witte, D.G., Yao, B.B., Miller, T.R. et al. 2006. Detection of multiple H3 receptor affinity states utilizing [3H]A-349821, a novel, selective, non-imidazole histamine H3 receptor inverse agonist radioligand. *Br. J. Pharmacol.* 148:657–670.

244. Barbier, A.J., Berridge, C., Dugovic, C. et al. 2004. Acute wake-promoting actions of JNJ-5207852, a novel, diamine-based H3 antagonist. *Br. J. Pharmacol.* 143:649–661.

245. Airaksinen, A.J., Jablonowski, J.A., van der, M.M. et al. 2006. Radiosynthesis and biodistribution of a histamine H3 receptor antagonist 4-[3-(4-piperidin-1-yl-but-1-ynyl)-[11C]benzyl]-morpholine: Evaluation of a potential PET ligand. *Nucl. Med. Biol.* 33:801–810.

246. Plisson, C. 2006. WO2006072596A1.

247. Cowart, M., Gfesser, G.A., Bhatia, K. et al. 2006. Fluorescent benzofuran histamine H3 receptor antagonists with sub-nanomolar potency. *Inflamm. Res.* 55:S47–S48.

248. Amon, M., Ligneau, X., Camelin, J.C. et al. 2007. Highly potent fluorescence-tagged nonimidazole histamine H3 receptor ligands. *Chem. Med. Chem.* 2:708–716.

249. Keith, C.T., Borisy, A.A., and Stockwell, B.R. 2005. Multicomponent therapeutics for networked systems. *Nat. Rev. Drug Disc.* 4:71–78.

250. Zimmermann, G.R., Lehar, J., and Keith, C.T. 2007. Multi-target therapeutics: When the whole is greater than the sum of the parts. *Drug Disc. Today* 12:34–42.

251. Nakaya, M., Fukushima, Y., Takeuchi, N. et al. 2005. Nasal allergic response mediated by histamine H3 receptors in murine allergic rhinitis. *Laryngoscope* 115:1778–1784.

252. McLeod, R.L., Mingo, G.G., Kreutner, W. et al. 2005. Effect of combined histamine H1 and H3 receptor blockade on cutaneous microvascular permeability elicited by compound 48/80. *Life Sci.* 76:1787–1794.

253. McLeod, R.L., Rizzo, C.A., West, R.E., Jr. et al. 2003. Pharmacological characterization of the novel histamine H3-receptor antagonist N-(3,5-dichlorophenyl)-N'-[[4-(1H-imidazol-4-ylmethyl)phenyl]methyl]urea (SCH 79687). *J. Pharmacol. Exp. Ther.* 305:1037–1044.

254. Taylor-Clark, T. and Foreman, J. 2005. Histamine-mediated mechanisms in the human nasal airway. *Curr. Opin. Pharmacol.* 5:214–220.

255. Fonquerna, S. and Miralpeix, M. 2006. H1 antihistamines: Patent highlights 2000–2005. *Expert Opin. Ther. Pat.* 16:109–117.

256. Anthes, J.C., West, R.E., Hey, J.A. et al. 2004. WO2004066960A2.

257. Cremers, T.IF.H. and Hogg Willigers, S. 2005. WO2005056056A2.

258. Schwartz, J. and Lecomte, J. 2005. WO2005000315A1.

259. Morphy, R., Kay, C., and Rankovic, Z. 2004. From magic bullets to designed multiple ligands. *Drug Disc. Today* 9:641–651.

260. Huls, A., Purand, K., Stark, H. et al. 1996. Diphenylmethyl ethers: Synthesis and histamine H3-receptor antagonist in vitro and in vivo activity. *Bioorg. Med. Chem. Lett.* 6:2013–2018.

261. Aslanian, R., Mutahi, M.W., Shih, N.Y. et al. 2002. Identification of a novel, orally bioavailable histamine H3 receptor antagonist based on the 4-benzyl-(1H-imidazol-4-yl) template. *Bioorg. Med. Chem. Lett.* 12:937–941.

262. Shih, N-Y., Aslanian, R.G., Solomon, D.M. et al. 2002. WO200244141A2.
263. Isensee, K., Amon, M., and Sasse, B. 2007. Novel potent dual histamine H1/H3 receptor antagonists. *36th European Histamine Research Society Meeting*, May 9–12 2007, Florence, Italy. Abst. P33.
264. Tosco, P., Bertinaria, M., Di Stilo, A. et al. 2004. A new class of NO-donor H3-antagonists. *Farmaco* 59:359–371.
265. Tosco, P., Bertinaria, M., Di Stilo, A. et al. 2005. Non-imidazole histamine NO-donor H3-antagonists. *Farmaco* 60:507–512.
266. Tosco, P., Bertinaria, M., Di Stilo, A. et al. 2005. Furoxan analogues of the histamine H3-receptor antagonist imoproxifan and related furazan derivatives. *Bioorg. Med. Chem.* 13:4750–4759.
267. Decker, M. 2007. Recent advances in the development of hybrid molecules/designed multiple compounds with antiamnesic properties. *Mini-Rev. Med. Chem.* 7:221–229.
268. Muñoz-Torrero, D. and Camps, P. 2006. Dimeric and hybrid anti-alzheimer drug candidates. *Curr. Med. Chem.* 13:399–422.
269. Apelt, J., Ligneau, X., Pertz, H.H. et al. 2002. Development of a new class of nonimidazole histamine H3 receptor ligands with combined inhibitory histamine N-methyltransferase activity. *J. Med. Chem.* 45:1128–1141.
270. Apelt, J., Grassmann, S., Ligneau, X. et al. 2005. Search for histamine H3 receptor antagonists with combined inhibitory potency at Nt-methyltransferase: Ether derivatives. *Pharmazie* 60:97–106.
271. Grassmann, S., Apelt, J., Sippl, W. et al. 2003. Imidazole derivatives as a novel class of hybrid compounds with inhibitory histamine N-methyltransferase potencies and histamine H3 receptor affinities. *Bioorg. Med. Chem.* 11:2163–2174.
272. Grassmann, S., Apelt, J., Ligneau, X. et al. 2004. Search for histamine H(3) receptor ligands with combined inhibitory potency at histamine N-methyltransferase: Omega-piperidinoalkanamine derivatives. *Arch. Pharm.* (Weinheim) 337:533–545.
273. Petroianu, G., Arafat, K., Sasse, B.C. et al. 2006. Multiple enzyme inhibitions by histamine H3 receptor antagonists as potential procognitive agents. *Pharmazie* 61:179–182.
274. Horton, J.R., Sawada, K., Nishibori, M. et al. 2005. Structural basis for inhibition of histamine N-methyltransferase by diverse drugs. *J. Mol. Biol.* 353:334–344.
275. Vohora, D., Pal, S.N., and Pillai, K.K. 2005. Modulation of spontaneous alternation performance of mice treated with thioperamide and tacrine in a cross maze task. *Fundam. Clin. Pharmacol.* 19:531–532.
276. Hey, J.A. and Aslanian, R.G. 2002. WO2002072093A2.
277. Gray, J.A. and Roth, B.L. 2006. Developing selectively nonselective drugs for treating CNS disorders. *Drug Discov. Today Ther. Strat.* 3:413–419.
278. Keith, J.M., Gomez, L.A., Letavic, M.A. et al. 2007. Dual serotonin transporter/histamine H3 ligands: Optimization of the H3 pharmacophore. *Bioorg. Med. Chem. Lett.* 17:702–706.
279. Letavic, M.A., Keith, J.M., Jablonowski, J.A. et al. 2007. Novel tetrahydroisoquinolines are histamine H3 antagonists and serotonin reuptake inhibitors. *Bioorg. Med. Chem. Lett.* 17:1047–1051.
280. Keith, J.M., Gomez, L.A., Wolin, R.L. et al. 2007. Pyrrolidino-tetrahydroisoquinolines as potent dual H3 antagonist and serotonin transporter inhibitors. *Bioorg. Med. Chem. Lett.* 17:2603–2607.
281. Letavic, M.A., Keith, J.M., Ly, K.S. et al. 2007. Novel naphthyridines are histamine H3 antagonists and serotonin reuptake transporter inhibitors. *Bioorg. Med. Chem. Lett.* 17:2566–2569.
282. Lin, J.S., Dauvilliers, Y., Arnulf, I. et al. 2008. An inverse agonist of the histamine H_3 receptor improves wakefulness in narcolepsy: studies in orexin-/- mice and patients. Neurobiol. Dis. 30(1):74–83.

283. JP Morgan 24th Annual Healthcare Conference, San Francisco, CA, January 2006, Cephalon website, www.cephalon.com.

284. Merrill Lynch Global Pharmaceutical, Biotechnology and Medical Device Conference, February 2007, Cephalon website, www.cephalon.com.

285. Hunter, J. Neurology, GlaxoSmithKline website, http://www.gsk.com/investors/presentations_webcasts04.htm.

286. Ratti, E. Psychiatry, GlaxoSmithKline website, http://www.gsk.com/investors/presentations_webcasts04.htm.

287. http://www.schizophreniaforum.org/res/trials/all.pdf.

288. Effectiveness of the drug GSK189254 in treating patients with narcolepsy, http://clinicaltrials.gov/show/NCT00366080.

289. A study of GSK189254 and duloxetine in the electrical hyperalgesia model of healthy volunteers, http://clinicaltrials.gov/show/NCT00387413.

290. An imaging study to investigate the distribution of GSK239512 in the brain, http://clinicaltrials.gov/show/NCT00474513.

291. Effects of single doses of GW784568X on allergic rhinitis symptoms in male subjects whilst in an environmental chamber, http://clinicaltrials.gov/show/NCT00404586.

292. Norman, P. 2007. A H3 antagonist for treating allergic rhinitis: A development candidate? *Expert Opin. Ther. Pat.* 17:449–452.

293. McLeod, R.L., Mingo, G.G., Herczku, C. et al. 1999. Combined histamine H1 and H3 receptor blockade produces nasal decongestion in an experimental model of nasal congestion. *Am. J. Rhinol.* 13:391–399.

294. http://www.stanleyresearch.org/Trial/Drug/AwardedTrial.aspx.

295. http://www.schizophreniaforum.org/res/trials/all.pdf.

296. Schwartz, J., Lecomte, J., Raga, M., Sallares, J., Guerrero, M. et al. 2006. WO2006103546A2.

297. Raga, M.M. et al. 2006. WO2006084833A1.

298. Schwartz, J. and Lecomte, J. 2006. WO2006103537A2.

299. Sanofi-Aventis website, http://www.sanofi-aventis.com/rd/portfolio/p_rd_portfolio_snc.asp.

300. Dastmalchi, S., Hamzeh-Mivehroud, M., Ghafourian, T. et al. 2007. Molecular modeling of histamine H3 receptor and QSAR studies on arylbenzofuran derived H3 antagonists. *J. Mol. Graph. Model.* 26(5):834–844.

301. Roche, O. and Rodriguez Sarmiento, R.M. 2007. A new class of histamine H3 receptor antagonists derived from ligand based design. *Bioorg. Med. Chem. Lett.* 17:3670–3675.

302. Del Tredici, A.L., Eskildsen, J., Andersen, C.B. et al. 2007. Identification of histamine H3 receptor antagonists. *FASEB J.* 21:A790–A79d.

303. DiModica, L. 2004. Fixed-combination therapies for the treatment of CNS disorders. Analysis of current trends and future prospects among U.S. physicians and HMOs. *Decision Resour.* November 2004.

304. Mierzwa, R., King, A., Conover, M.A. et al. 1994. Verongamine, a novel bromotyrosine-derived histamine H3-antagonist from the marine sponge Verongula gigantean. *J. Nat. Prod.* 57:175–177.

6 Peripheral Actions and Therapeutic Potential in Periphery

Gabriella Coruzzi and Maristella Adami

CONTENTS

Introduction... 167
Gastrointestinal Tract... 168
    Gastric Acid Secretion... 169
        Histamine H_3 Receptors and *Helicobacter pylori*............................ 171
    Gastric Mucosal Defense.. 173
    Gastrointestinal Motility 174
        Histamine H_3 Receptor Heterogeneity 175
    Intestinal Secretion.. 177
    Intestinal Mucosal Defense 177
        Visceral Pain 177
Cardiovascular System.. 178
    Heart... 178
        Signal-Transducing Pathways 181
    Vessels 181
        Presynaptic Histamine H_3 Receptors 181
        Postsynaptic Histamine H_3 Receptors... 183
Respiratory System 184
Allergy, Inflammation, and Immunity.. 186
Tissue Growth and Carcinogenesis.. 189
Other Peripheral Locations and Functions 189
Histamine H_4 Receptors... 191
Conclusions 191
Acknowledgment 192
References.. 192

INTRODUCTION

The long story of histamine started a century ago when amine was synthesized as a chemical curiosity [1]. Soon afterward, Sir Henry Dale and his colleagues isolated histamine from the ergot and described its major biological actions, including the ability to mimic anaphylaxis [2,3]. Since then, much knowledge has been accumulated concerning the synthesis, storage, metabolism, receptors, and pathophysiological actions of this biogenic amine in central and peripheral tissues. The early recognition of allergic effects of histamine, during antigen challenge, led to the development of H_1 antihistamines for the treatment of allergy [4], whereas the identification of gastric H_2 receptors revolutionized the treatment of acid-related diseases [5]. It is now recognized that the pleiotropic effects of histamine are mediated by two additional types of receptors, namely, H_3 and H_4, which are primarily distributed in central and peripheral tissues, respectively. Although the discovery of histamine H_3 receptors [6] has highlighted the role of histamine as a neurotransmitter (NT) in the central nervous system (CNS), the recently identified H_4 receptor has expanded the knowledge on the role of histamine in inflammation and allergy and has attracted great interest as a target candidate for novel therapeutics [7].

Although the majority of H_3 receptors are located in the brain, they have also been detected in some peripheral tissues, in amounts lower than in the CNS [8–10]. H_3 receptors are primarily localized to nerve terminals of a number of fibers, where they negatively modulate NT release; however, immunohistochemistry and functional studies have also evidenced H_3 receptors on paracrine cells and postjunctional membranes of effector organs [11,12].

The characterization of histamine H_3 receptors has been made possible by the development of the selective agonist (R)α-methylhistamine and the antagonist thioperamide [13], followed by other selective compounds [12,14]; however, since most of the known H_3 receptor ligands also bind to the H_4 receptor [15,16], a major reclassification of H_3 ligands is imperative, to identify H_3-receptor-mediated effects.

In this chapter, we focus on the distribution and functional role of H_3 receptors in peripheral tissues, with particular attention to the gastrointestinal (GI) tract, cardiovascular, respiratory, and immune systems. A brief summary of peripheral effects mediated by the newly discovered H_4 receptor is also given.

GASTROINTESTINAL TRACT

Evidence for a pathophysiological role of histamine in the GI tract is abundant [17–19]. Histamine and histidine decarboxylase (HDC) are widely distributed in the gut, in various storing cells, including mast cells, enterochromaffin-like (ECL) cells, basophils, macrophages, T lymphocytes [17,20], gastrin-producing cells [21], and enteric neurons of the myenteric plexus [22,23]. In the GI tract, histamine exerts pleiotropic effects, which involve different target cells and all four types of receptors identified so far [11,24,25]. Although radioligand-binding studies and immunohistochemistry have detected H_3 receptors in the gut of guinea pigs [8] and rats [9,26], no evidence was provided for the presence of H_3 receptors in the human bowel [27,28].

A number of functional bioassays carried out in experimental animals have demonstrated the role of H_3 receptors in the regulation of gastric acid secretion, intestinal motility, intestinal secretion, and mucosal protection.

GASTRIC ACID SECRETION

The leading role of histamine in the intricate network-regulating acid production was definitely assessed with the discovery of H_2 receptors and the enormous clinical impact of H_2 receptor blockers in the treatment of peptic ulcer disease [5]. In the fundic mucosa, the stimulation of ECL cells to secrete histamine constitutes the major regulatory pathway for the secretion of acid through the parietal cell (Figure 6.1) [29]. The activation of H_2 receptors by histamine increases acid production, gastrin release from G cells, and the cellular size of parietal cells [30,31]. Following the discovery of the H_3 receptor, several research groups have reexamined the role of histamine in the gastric mucosa [11,18,32]. In the rat stomach, H_3 receptor mRNA was detected during embryonic life (E18) and became widely expressed within the adult gastric mucosa [9]; moreover, the presence of this receptor was recently confirmed in the rat gastric fundus by immunohistochemistry [26]. Although a huge amount of data have been accumulated over the past 20 years, the role of H_3 receptors in the regulation of acid production is still enigmatic, because results obtained in the different assays and species are contradictory (Tables 6.1 and 6.2). Inhibitory effects were observed early in conscious cats and dogs against indirect secretory stimuli (2-deoxy-D-glucose, pentagastrin, bombesin, and food), suggesting the occurrence of H_3 receptors on cholinergic nerves or ECL cells. In line with this, a negative

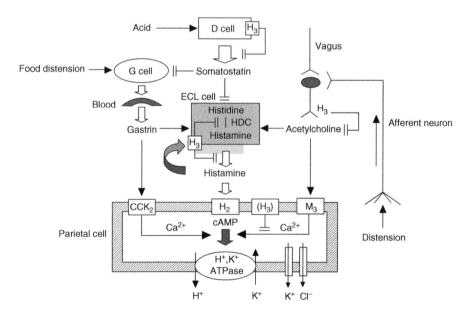

FIGURE 6.1 Scheme illustrating the proposed locations and functions of H_3 receptors in the gastric mucosa, based on literature data concerning different bioassays and species. Inhibitory H_3 receptors mediate opposite effects on acid secretion depending on the cell location; the inhibition of ECL histamine synthesis and secretion and cholinergic neurotransmission limits excess acid production, whereas the inhibition of somatostatin secretion from D cells contributes to the acid stimulatory effects of histamine. (ECL, enterochromaffin-like cells; HDC, histidine decarboxylase; →, stimulation; —||, inhibition.)

TABLE 6.1
Effects of H_3 Receptor Activation on Gastric Acid Secretion (*In Vivo*)

Species	Technique	Agonist	Effect	References
Rat	Pylorus ligation	(R)α-MHA (i.p.)	0	42
		(R)α-MHA (i.c.v.)	↓	43
	GF	N^α-MHA	↑ (i.p., i.g., basal); ↓ (i.c.v., basal)	44
	Anesthetized animal	(R)α-MHA	0 (basal, HA, 2-DG, PGAS)	42
		Immepip	0 (basal, PGAS)	45
		(R)α-MHA	↓ (EVS); 0 (basal, PGAS, BET)	46
		Methimepip	0 (basal)	Adami, unpublished data
Cat	GF	(R)α-MHA	↓ (2-DG); 0 (dimaprit, PGAS)	47
	GF and HP	(R)α-MHA	↓ (food, PGAS); 0 (basal, HA)	48
Dog	GF	(R)α-MHA	↓ (2-DG, PGAS, BBS); 0 (basal, HA)	49–51
		BP 2.94	↓ (2-DG, BBS); 0 (HA)	39

Note: BBS, bombesin; BET, bethanechol; 2-DG, 2-deoxy-D-glucose; EVS, electrical vagal stimulation; GF, gastric fistula; HA, histamine; HP, Heidenhain pouch; i.c.v., intracerebroventricular; i.g., intragastric; i.p., intraperitoneal; N^α-MHA, N^α-methylhistamine; PGAS, pentagastrin; (R)α-MHA, (R)α-methylhistamine; ↓, decrease; 0, no effect; ↑, increase.

Source: Modified from Bertaccini, G., Poli, E., and Coruzzi, G., in *The Histamine H_3 Receptor: A Target for New Drugs*, Elsevier Amsterdam, 1998, 59–111. With permission.

modulation on histamine synthesis and release was observed in several species and in various experimental models (Table 6.3). However, stimulatory effects on acid production following H_3 receptor activation were reported in mouse-, rat-, dog-, and human gastric mucosa, due to H_3 receptor-mediated inhibitory effects on somatostatin secretion from both fundic and antral G cells [33,34]. However, the occurrence of inhibitory H_3 receptors on D cells was not confirmed by other groups in rats [35–37], rabbits [38], or anesthetized dogs [39] (Table 6.3). In the human gastric tumoral cell line HGT1, H_3 receptors were associated with phosphatidyl inositol turnover [40] but not with cAMP levels in human fundic membranes [41].

In conclusion, H_3-receptor-mediated effects in the gastric mucosa appear to depend on the species and the experimental model (*in vivo* versus *in vitro*). It has also to be hypothesized that the use of the dual H_3/H_4 ligands, (R)α-methylhistamine and thioperamide, may contribute to the contradictory data. To support this, recent experiments carried out in the isolated rat gastric fundus with the highly selective agonist methimepip [69] and the nonimidazole H_3 receptor antagonist FUB649 [70] definitely confirmed inhibitory effects on acid production following H_3 receptor activation [54].

TABLE 6.2
Effects of H_3 Receptor Activation on Gastric Acid Secretion (*In Vitro*)

Species	Technique	Agonist	Effect	References
Mouse	Whole stomach	(R)α-MHA	↑(basal)	33
	Gastric glands	(R)α-MHA	0 (basal)	52
Rat	Whole stomach	(R)α-MHA	0 (basal, gastrin)	53
	Gastric fundus	(R)α-MHA	0 (basal, HA, PGAS, ISO)	42
		Methimepip	0 (basal, PGAS); ↓ (EFS)	54
		Immepip	0 (basal, PGAS, EFS)	54
Guinea pig	Gastric fundus	(R)α-MHA	0 (A23187, EFS)	55
		(R)α-MHA	0 (basal)	18
Rabbit	Fundic glands	(R)α-MHA, Imetit	↓ (CARB)	56
	Parietal cells	Nα-MHA	0 (CARB, forskolin)	57
Human	Fundic membranes	(R)α-MHA	0 (adenylate cyclase)	41
	Gastric cell line HGT1	(R)α-MHA	↓ (IP formation)	40

Note: A23187, calcium ionophore A23187; CARB, carbachol; EFS, electrical field stimulation; HA, histamine; IP, inositol phosphate; ISO, isoprenaline; Nα-MHA, Nα-methylhistamine; PGAS, pentagastrin; (R)α-MHA, (R)α-methylhistamine; ↓, decrease; 0, no effect; ↑, increase.

Source: Modified from Bertaccini, G., Poli, E., and Coruzzi, G., in *The Histamine H_3 Receptor: A Target for New Drugs*, Elsevier Amsterdam, 1998, 59–111. With permission.

Histamine H_3 Receptors and *Helicobacter pylori*

Overwhelming evidence supports a casual relationship between *Helicobacter pylori* (*Hp*) infection and the development of peptic ulcer disease and gastric cancer [71]. However, the effects of *Hp* on gastric acid secretion are very complex and can be associated with various acid secretory states, according to the disease conditions (duodenal ulcer, gastric ulcer, or chronic active type B gastritis), the stage of infection (acute versus chronic), or the strain-dependent inhibition of H^+/K^+-ATPase [72]. Recently, an alternative mechanism by which the bacterium might influence acid secretion was proposed, based on the observation that *Hp*-infected, but not healthy, gastric mucosa produces a side-chain methylated histamine derivative, Nα-methylhistamine, which is a potent H_3 receptor agonist [68,73]. Likewise, Nα-methylhistamine was found in the gastric juice of *Hp*-infected individuals but not in that of healthy subjects [30,74]. The activation of inhibitory H_3 receptors on D cells by Nα-methylhistamine may reduce somatostatin secretion and lead to the hypergastrinemia and enhanced acid production, commonly observed in duodenal ulcer patients during *Hp* infection [68,75–77]. In contrast, the activation of inhibitory H_3 receptors on rat fundic ECL cells may reduce histamine synthesis and release [62,63]; to complicate matters, *Hp* lipopolysaccharide was found to stimulate histamine release and ECL cell proliferation in rats, possibly through increased gastrin levels [78]. Originally described as a potent H_2 receptor agonist [79], Nα-methylhistamine became a widely used ligand to investigate H_3-receptor-mediated effects, due to the high affinity at H_3 receptors [80,81]; however, several groups have emphasized the H_2-receptor-mediated effects of Nα-methylhistamine, either at parietal or at G cells

TABLE 6.3

Effects of H_3 Receptor Activation on Neuronal, Endocrine, and Paracrine Mediators of the Gastric Mucosa

Mediator	Effect	Species	Technique	References
Acetylcholine	↓	Rat	Whole stomach *in vitro*	58
Gastrin	↑	Rat	Whole stomach *in vitro*	35
	↑	Rat	Antral segments	34
	0	Rabbit	G cells	30
	0	Cat	*In vivo*	59,60
	0	Dog	*In vivo*	50
	↑	Dog	Antral segments	34
	↑	Human	Antral segments	34
Histamine	↑	Mouse	Whole stomach *in vitro*	33
	↑	Rat	Antral segments	34
	↑	Rat	Fundic segments	61
	↓	Rat	Whole stomach *in vitro*	53,35
	↓	Rat	Purified ECL cells	62–64
	↓	Rabbit	Gastric glands	65
			Fundic cells	66[a]
	↓	Dog	Anesthetized animal	51,67
	↑	Dog	Antral segments	34
	↑	Human	Antral segments	34
Somatostatin	↓	Mouse	Whole stomach *in vitro*	33
	↓	Rat	Antral segments	34
	↓	Rat	Fundic segments	61
	↓	Rat	Whole stomach *in vitro, in vivo*	35–37
	0	Rabbit	Fundic D cells	38
	0	Cat	*In vivo*	60
	↓	Dog	Antral segments	34
	0	Dog	Anesthetized animal	39
	↓	Human	Antral segments	34,68

Note: ECL, enterochromaffin-like cells; ↓, decrease; 0, no effect; ↑, increase.

[a] Histamine synthesis.

Source: Modified from Bertaccini, G., Poli, E., and Coruzzi, G., in *The Histamine H_3 Receptor: A Target for New Drugs*, Elsevier Amsterdam, 1998, 59–111. With permission.

in various animal species, including humans [38,79,82] and in CHO cells expressing human H_2 receptors [83]. These intriguing data may be explained by the interaction of N^α-methylhistamine with both H_2 and H_3 receptors located at different sites in the gastric mucosa (Figure 6.2). Recently, a lower production of inflammatory cytokines (tumor necrosis factor α [TNFα] and interleukin-6 [IL-6]) was observed following *Hp* infection in HDC knockout mice, suggesting a role for histamine in the *Hp*-mediated immune responses [84]. In conclusion, the functional significance of *Hp*-produced N^α-methylhistamine seems to be an additional subject of controversy in the pathophysiology of *Hp* infection.

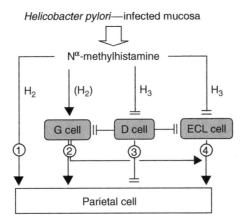

FIGURE 6.2 N^α-methylhistamine produced by *Helicobacter pylori* may influence acid secretion through different pathways: (1) activation of excitatory H_2 receptors on parietal cells; (2) activation of excitatory H_2 receptors on gastrin-producing G cells; (3) activation of inhibitory H_3 receptors on D cells, reducing somatostatin-mediated inhibitory drive on ECL cells, G cells, and parietal cells; (4) activation of inhibitory H_3 receptors on ECL cells, to limit histamine release. (ECL, enterochromaffin-like cells; →, stimulation; ⊣, inhibition.) (*Source*: Modified from Bertaccini, G., Poli, E., and Coruzzi, G., in *The Histamine H_3 Receptor: A Target for New Drugs*, Elsevier Amsterdam, 1998, 59–111. With permission.)

GASTRIC MUCOSAL DEFENSE

The role of histamine in ulcerogenesis is unclear, since both ulcerogenic and gastro-protective effects have been reported following histamine or selective H_1 or H_2 receptor ligands [18]. The discovery of H_3 receptors has highlighted the protective effects of histamine in the gastric mucosa, since a number of reports have suggested an involvement of this receptor in mucosal protection against acute gastric damage induced by absolute ethanol, aspirin, indomethacin, ammonia, and, at a lesser extent, cold/restraint stress [85–90]. Moreover, H_3 receptor activation by N^α-methylhistamine was reported to accelerate the healing of chronic gastric ulcer induced by acetic acid [90].

The mechanisms underlying (R)α-methylhistamine-induced gastroprotection include enhancement of the reepithelization process, migration of pit cells, restitution of the mucosal surface, mucus synthesis [85,91] and HCO_3^- secretion [92], and TGFα production [93]. H_3-receptor-mediated effects were also associated with increased gastric mucosal blood flow [44] and sensory nerve activation. In particular, it was demonstrated in the rat stomach that H_3 receptors, possibly located in sensory neurons, are involved in the gastric mucosal hyperemia that follows disruption of the mucosal barrier [94,95].

More recently, it was shown by our group that (R)α-methylhistamine and the selective H_3 receptor agonist FUB407 [96] display strong proliferative effects in the whole GI tract and, particularly, in the gastric fundus and colon [97,98], confirming previous studies on isolated ECL cells [64]. The activation of gastric mucosal DNA synthesis and cell renewal would account for the rapid process of restitution and repair of superficial mucosal damage [99].

Despite the bulk of data concerning gastroprotection induced by (R)α-methylhistamine and N^α-methylhistamine, more recent findings have challenged the hypothesis

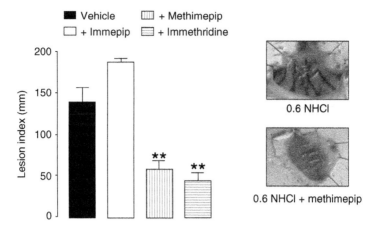

FIGURE 6.3 (See color insert following page 148.) Effects of the dual H_3/H_4 receptor agonist immepip (30 mg/kg s.c.) and the selective H_3 receptor agonists methimepip (30 mg/kg s.c.), and immethridine (30 mg/kg s.c.) on the gastric damage induced by HCl 0.6 N i.g. (■) in the conscious rat. On the ordinate lesion index, values are mean ±SEM from 8–10 rats. **$p < .01$ versus vehicle (saline). (See Morini, G., Grandi, D., Krause, M., Schunack, W., *Inflamm. Res.* 46, S101–S102, 1997 for methodological details.)

that the H_3 receptor subtype is involved: it was shown in our laboratory that the H_3 receptor agonists, imetit and immepip, previously supposed to be more selective than (R)α-methylhistamine, did not protect against HCl-induced gastric lesions in rats [100]. With the advent of H_4 receptors, it has become clear that many H_3 ligands are indeed dual H_3/H_4 receptor agonists or antagonists [101]; thus, a possible gastrolesive effect mediated by H_4 receptors, which masks H_3-receptor-mediated protection, could explain the ineffectiveness of immepip and imetit [102]. This hypothesis was recently confirmed by using the highly selective H_3 receptor agonists, immethridine [103] and methimepip [69], which elicited a strong mucosal protection against HCl-induced gastric damage in conscious rats (Figure 6.3). These results validate the hypothesis that H_3 receptors mediate beneficial effects of histamine in the gastric mucosa.

GASTROINTESTINAL MOTILITY

The effects of histamine on GI contractility involve stimulatory H_1 receptors located on smooth muscle, relaxant H_2 receptors, as well as excitatory H_2 receptors located on cholinergic nerve terminals [24]. Radioligand-binding studies and immunohistochemistry have shown that histamine H_3 receptors are expressed in the small and large intestine of rodents [8,9] and act as prejunctional inhibitory receptors, modulating NT release from intrinsic neurons of the myenteric plexus and the associated neurogenic contractions (Figure 6.4) [11,18]. Inhibitory effects following H_3 receptor activation by N^α-methylhistamine and (R)α-methylhistamine were reported in different areas of the GI tract and in most animal species (Table 6.4). Most data were obtained in the guinea pig ileum, which became the assay of choice for the screening of new selective ligands. In this tissue, H_3 receptor agonists inhibited cholinergic and nonadrenergic, noncholinergic (NANC), as well as adrenergic neurotransmission,

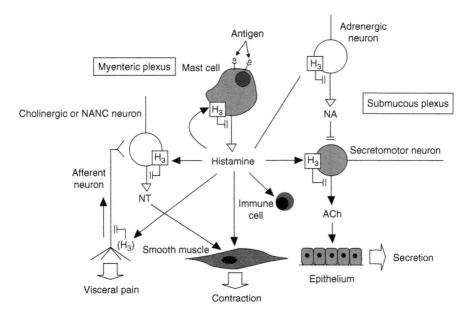

FIGURE 6.4 Scheme illustrating the proposed locations and functions of H_3 receptors in the intestine (H_1 and H_2 receptors are not shown in the figure). Histamine released from activated mast cells may regulate intestinal contractility through inhibitory H_3 receptors located on cholinergic, NANC neurons of the myenteric plexus; moreover, activation of inhibitory H_3 receptors in enteric nerves of the submucous plexus may influence mucosal ion secretion. The role of H_3 receptors in visceral pain and immune function is uncertain. (ACh, acetylcholine; NA, noradrenaline; NT, neurotransmitter; →, stimulation; —|, inhibition.

suggesting a general prejunctional inhibitory mechanism for the regulation of intestinal neural activity, possibly in concert with α_2 adrenoceptors [104,105]. In peripheral neurons of the GI tract, H_3 receptors are coupled to inhibition of Ca^{2+} influx into the nerve terminal through neuronal N-type Ca^{2+} channels and consequent inhibition of NT exocytosis [104,106].

The inhibition of NT release following H_3 receptor activation was not observed in mice [108], rats [110], and rabbits [128]; neither in intact animals nor in isolated assays. Finally, no evidence was found for the occurrence of H_3 receptors on human bowel [27], in line with the lack of H_3 receptor mRNA expression [28].

Histamine H_3 Receptor Heterogeneity

On the basis of the biphasic displacement of the [^{3}H] N^α-methylhistamine binding by thioperamide and burimamide, West et al. [129] suggested the existence of H_3 receptor subtypes, referred to as H_{3A} and H_{3B}. According to this classification, histamine H_3 receptors in the guinea pig ileum would belong to the H_{3A} subtype, functionally identified in other central and peripheral tissues [104,130–133]. However, H_3 receptors different from the H_{3A} or H_{3B} subtype were identified in porcine enterochromaffin cells [134] and in the guinea pig jejunum [135]. At present, the identification of H_3 receptor heterogeneity in functional studies is a great challenge, when considering the existence of interspecies differences in the receptor protein sequences, splice

TABLE 6.4
Effects of H₃ Receptor Activation on Gastrointestinal Motility

Species	Technique	Parameter	Agonist	Effect	References
Mouse	Ileum *in vitro*	EFS-induced contraction (cholinergic)	(R)α-MHA	0	107
	Conscious animal	Intestinal transit	(R)α-MHA, Immepip	↓	107
			Nᵅ-MHA	0	108
Rat	Ileum *in vitro*	EFS-induced contraction (cholinergic)	(R)α-MHA	0	27,109
		SP- or nicotine-induced contraction	HA, (R)α-MHA	0	27
	Conscious animal	Intestinal transit	HA, (R)α-MHA (peripheral)	0	110
Guinea pig	Oesophagus *in vitro*	EFS-induced contraction (cholinergic and NANC)	HA, Nᵅ-MHA	0	111
	Gastric fundus *in vitro*	NANC relaxation	Immepip	0	112
	Duodenum *in vitro*	EFS-induced contraction (cholinergic)	(R)α-MHA, Nᵅ-MHA	↓	81
	Ileum *in vitro*	EFS-induced contraction (cholinergic)	Nᵅ-MHA	↓	80
			(R)α-MHA	↓	111,113–117
			Imetit	↓	103
			Immepip	↓	69,103,117
			Methimepip	↓	69
			Immethridine	↓	103
		NANC-induced contraction	(R)α-MHA	↓	114,118–120
		SP- or nicotine-induced contraction	HA, (R)α-MHA	0	27
		Peristalsis	(R)α-MHA, Immepip	0	121
		Peristalsis	HA, (R)α-MHA	↓	122
	LMMP ileal strips	[³H]-choline release	HA	↓	123,124
			HA, (R)α-MHA	↓	125
		[³H]-NA release	HA, (R)α-MHA	↓	104
	Ileal cells *in vitro*	Basal tone	(R)α-MHA, Immepip	0	126
		ACh-induced contraction	(R)α-MHA, Immepip	↓	126
	Myenteric ganglia	EPSP	HA, Nᵅ-MHA	↓	127
	Colon *in vitro*	EFS-induced contraction (cholinergic)	(R)α-MHA	↓	114
Rabbit	Conscious animal	Myoelectrical activity	(R)α-MHA, immepip	0	128
	Colon *in vitro*	EFS-induced contraction	(R)α-MHA, immepip	0	128
Human	Colon *in vitro*	EFS-induced contraction (cholinergic)	HA, (R)α-MHA	0	27
		SP- or nicotine-induced contraction	HA, (R)α-MHA	0	27

Note: ACh, acetylcholine; EFS, electrical field stimulation; EPSP, excitatory postsynaptic potential; HA, histamine; IPSP, inhibitory postsynaptic potential; LMMP, longitudinal muscle-myenteric plexus; Nᵅ-MHA, Nᵅ-methylhistamine; NA, noradrenaline; NANC, nonadrenergic, noncholinergic; (R)α-MHA, (R)α-methylhistamine; SP, substance P; ↓, decrease; 0, no effect.

variants, receptor oligomerization, constitutive activity, as well as the affinity of H_3 receptor ligands for the histamine H_4 receptor.

Intestinal Secretion

It is increasingly recognized that mucosal mast cells play a key role in the defense against harmful stimuli within the GI tract [19,136,137]. Histamine is one of the key mast cell mediators in orchestrating intestinal defensive programs and works as a paracrine signal to influence ENS function, afferent fibers, epithelium activity, and immune response (Figure 6.4). Once released from enteric mast cells in inflamed bowel or in response to sensitizing antigens, histamine exerts several effects (through activation of H_1 and H_2 receptors), including smooth muscle contractility, enhancement of neuronal excitability in submucosal secretomotor neurons, neurogenic secretory diarrhea and visceral pain, symptoms that are normally associated with gut inflammation, food allergy, or parasitic infections [138,139]. Several reports have suggested that in the guinea pig prejunctional, H_3 receptors exert a negative modulation on secretomotor neurons of the submucous plexus, acting as a *brake mechanism* to prevent excess neural excitation [140–143]. However, unlike the guinea pig, the role of H_3 receptors in the regulation of chloride secretion was not reported in the rat [144], dog [145], pig [146], or human colonic epithelium [147].

Intestinal Mucosal Defense

Increasing evidence has suggested a role for mast cells and histamine, in particular, in the pathogenesis of inflammatory bowel disease (IBD), irritable bowel syndrome (IBS), and food allergies [19,137]. In line with this, histamine levels are elevated in both ulcerative colitis (UC) and Crohn's disease (CD) patients and in allergic enteropathy [148]. Several histamine receptors have been involved in the protective effect of histamine in the intestinal mucosa: H_1 receptor antagonists attenuated the damage induced by acetic acid [149] or by ischemia-reperfusion [150]; H_3 receptor activation by (R)α-methylhistamine reduced the extent of mucosal damage and the increase in myeloperoxidase activity induced in the rat by acetic acid [151]; and the prodrug of (R)α-methylhistamine, compound BP 2.94 [152], protects against the mucosal damage induced in rats by trinitrobenzensulphonic acid (TNBS), a model of human IBD [153]. Finally, the highly selective H_4 receptor antagonist JNJ7777120 ameliorated experimental colitis in rats [25] and prevented ischemia-induced intestinal damage [150]. These findings are too limited to hypothesize possible therapeutic approaches; nevertheless, they indicate the involvement of H_1, H_3, and H_4 receptors in the intestinal mucosal defense.

Visceral Pain

Histamine is an important mediator of visceral hypersensitivity, which is a common feature of functional bowel disorders [154]. It has been recently confirmed in IBS patients that mast cell histamine released by the colonic mucosa can induce visceral hyperalgesia, by exciting nociceptive sensory nerve [155]. Histamine augments the sensory input to the brain by activating H_1 receptors expressed on afferent neurons supplying the small intestine of rats [156] and cats [157]. Prejunctional histamine H_3 receptors have been involved in the histamine-induced discharge of visceral afferents in rat jejunum and in the sensitization of the afferent response to bradykinin [158] but not in rectal allodynia [159].

CARDIOVASCULAR SYSTEM

Histamine induces marked cardiovascular effects, such as hypotension and tachycardia, which are mediated by three types of receptors—H_1, H_2, and H_3—located on the vascular and cardiac cell membranes, and with components of the autonomic nervous system [160,161]. Vascular H_1 receptors are responsible for lowering of blood pressure and increase in vascular permeability, whereas histamine H_2 receptors primarily control heart rate, contractility, and excitability [161].

Although binding experiments and immunohistochemistry showed a very low density of H_3 receptors in the cardiovascular system of rats and guinea pigs [8,9], evidence for a function role of histamine H_3 receptors in the heart has been accumulated over the past years [162–164]. Functional studies have suggested that H_3 receptors are mainly located presynaptically on postganglionic sympathetic nerve fibers, innervating blood vessels and the heart. Their activation leads to the inhibition of noradrenaline release and the associated pressor and cardiostimulatory responses [163,165].

HEART

Early evidence that prejunctional histamine H_3 receptors may modulate sympathetic nerve activity on the heart was provided by Luo et al. [166] who showed a reduction of neurogenic but not myogenic contractions of the isolated guinea pig right atrium following (R)α-methylhistamine. Subsequently, H_3-receptor-mediated inhibition of adrenergic neurotransmission was constantly reported in a number of preparations *in vitro* and *in vivo* (Table 6.5). As observed in other peripheral tissues [167,168], H_3 receptors were also detected in cardiac sensory C fibers, where they modulate the antidromic release of neuropeptides such as calcitonin gene-related peptide (CGRP) and tachykinins (Figure 6.5) [169]. However, no immunohistochemical studies have been performed to test the hypothesis that H_3 receptors are located on peptidergic fibers. Because elevated plasma CGRP levels occur in congestive heart failure, septic shock, and acute myocardial infarction, modulation of CGRP release by H_3 receptors may be clinically relevant. Recently, histamine immunoreactivity was demonstrated in the guinea pig cardiac sympathetic varicosities, where histamine coexists with noradrenaline and is coreleased after neural activation [170]; moreover, the involvement of H_3 receptors in the negative regulation of histamine release from sympathetic nerves has suggested for the first time that H_3 receptors act as autoreceptors also in periphery [170].

The ineffectiveness of H_3 receptor blockers on basal cardiac functions [184] indicate that these receptors are quiescent under physiologic conditions, although amounts of histamine sufficient to activate H_3 receptors are very low in comparison with H_1 or H_2 subtype [197]. In contrast, H_3 receptors become activated during

TABLE 6.5
Effects of H_3 Receptor Activation on Cardiac Function

Species	Technique	Parameter	Effect	References
Mouse $H_3R^{-/-}$ knockout	Whole heart *in vitro*	Ischemia-induced arrhythmias, NA release	↓	171
Rat	Whole heart *in vitro*	Ischemia-induced arrhythmias	↑	172
		48/80- or allergen-induced ACh release	↑	173
		Ischemia-induced NA release	↓	174
		Ischemia-induced NA release	0	175
	Pithed animal	Electrically-evoked tachycardia	↓	176
	Anesthetized animal	Basal heart rate	0	177–179
		Nicotine-evoked tachycardia	↓	180
Guinea pig	Right atrium *in vitro*	EFS-induced inotropic response	↓	166
		EFS-induced NA release	↓	181
		EFS-induced chronotropic response	↓	182,183
		Vagally and sympathetic responses	↓	183
	Left atrium *in vitro*	EFS-induced response, NA release	↓	182
		BK-induced response, CGRP release	↓	169
	Whole heart *in vitro*	Ischemia-induced NA release, arrhythmias	↓	184,185
		Capsaicin-induced response, CGRP release	↓	169
		Hypoxia-induced cardiac depression	↓	186
	Anesthetized animal	Basal heart rate	↓	179,187
		Nicotine-evoked tachycardia	↓	188
		Tachycardia (bulbar stimulation)	↓	189
	Pithed animal	Tachycardia (spinal nerve stimulation)	↓	190
Rabbit	Right atrium *in vitro*	EFS evoked tachycardia	0	183
		Vagal and sympathetic responses	0	183
	Conscious animal	Basal heart rate	↓	179
Dog	Ventricle *in vitro*	EFS-evoked inotropic response	↓	191
	Anesthetized animal	Basal heart rate	0	192
		Sepsis-induced shock	↑	191
		Anaphylactic shock	↑	193
		EFS-induced response, NA release	↓	194
Human	Right atrium *in vitro*	Ischemia-induced NA release	↓	195
	Atrial synaptosomes	K^+-evoked NA release	↓	196
	Pectinate muscles	EFS-induced inotropic response	↓	196

Note: ACh, acetylcholine; BK, bradykinin; CGRP, calcitonin gene-related peptide; EFS, electrical field stimulation; NA, noradrenaline; ↓, decrease; 0, no effect; ↑, increase.

Source: Modified from Bertaccini, G., Poli, E., and Coruzzi, G., in *The Histamine H_3 Receptor: A Target for New Drugs*, Elsevier Amsterdam, 1998, 59–111. With permission.

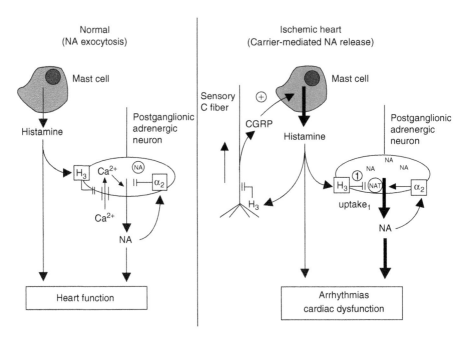

FIGURE 6.5 Proposed locations and functional role of H_3 receptors in normal and ischemic heart, based on data obtained in guinea pig and human heart. H_3 receptors are quiescent and noradrenaline (NA) exocytosis is mainly regulated by α_2 adrenoceptors. During acute and protracted ischemia ATP depletion promotes Na^+ accumulation in sympathetic nerve endings and prevents vesicular NA storage; this forces the reversal of the neuronal uptake$_1$ transporter (NAT) from an inward to an outward direction, and NA is massively released. α_2 adrenoceptor activation further increases NA release. Histamine, released in excess during ischemia, activates H_3 receptors located on sympathetic postganglionic nerve endings, thus reducing NA release and the associated arrhythmic responses. Moreover, prejunctional inhibitory H_3 receptors located on sensory C fibers inhibit the antidromic release of CGRP. (1, signal-transducing pathways following H_3 receptor activation are described in the text; →, stimulation; —|, inhibition.)

cardiac dysfunctions associated with enhanced adrenergic activity, such as myocardial ischemia [184] or sepsis [191]. An increase in mast cell number and histamine content has been reported in the human heart as a result of ischemia; thus, it is conceivable that in the ischemic heart, H_3 receptors are fully activated and modulate not only the exocytotic but also the carrier-mediated NA release, which is predominant during ischemia [184,185,195,198]. Although H_3-receptor-mediated inhibition of NA exocytosis in normal heart is associated with restricted Ca^{2+} entry through N-type Ca^{2+} channels [182,199,200], the mechanism underlying inhibition of carrier-mediated release is less well understood. It has been hypothesized that H_3 receptors inhibit the activity of the Na^+–H^+ exchanger, a transporter that accumulates Na^+ within the myocyte, due to the inversion of NA transporter, and leads to massive NA release (Figure 6.5) [198,201]. The H_3-receptor-mediated reduction of sympathetic overactivity in the ischemic heart may reduce the incidence and duration of ventricular fibrillation during reperfusion, thus providing a protective action against the dysfunctional consequences of prolonged myocardial ischemia [184]. These effects are of potential interest, when considering that the activation of α_2 adrenoceptors during ischemia stimulates, instead of inhibiting, carrier-mediated NA release (Figure 6.5). The relevance of H_3 receptors in the ischemic heart was confirmed in a human model of protracted ischemia [195,196] and in a transgenic line of mice lacking H_3 receptors, which showed a greater severity of reperfusion arrhythmias [202]. All these findings strongly support the concept that H_3 receptor agonists may represent a new strategy to alleviate cardiac dysfunctions during ischemia.

Signal-Transducing Pathways

As observed in other tissues, cardiac H_3 receptors are associated with a pertussis toxin (PTX)-sensitive Gi/Go protein and adenylate cyclase inhibition; decrease in cAMP and protein kinase A (PKA) activity leads to a reduced Ca^{2+} influx through N-type Ca^{2+} channels and decrease in $[Ca^{2+}]i$ necessary for NA exocytosis [182,199,200]. Recently, a novel signal transduction pathway was unravelled in guinea pig cardiac synaptosomes and in a human neuroblastoma cell line stably transfected with H_3 receptors (SH-SY5Y-H3): H_3 receptors are coupled to a G$\beta\gamma$i-mediated activation of the MA_2PK-PLA_2 cascade, culminating in the formation of an arachidonate metabolite, PGE_2, endowed with antiexocytotic properties [203].

Vessels

Histamine has a marked activity on vascular smooth muscle, which has been attributed to the interaction with H_1 and H_2 receptors, located in endothelium and muscle cell [161–163]. The activation of peripheral histamine H_3 receptors elicits cardiovascular responses that are species-dependent and are associated with H_3 receptors located at different sites: (a) adrenergic varicosity, (b) endothelial cells, and (c) smooth muscle cells (Tables 6.6 and 6.7). However, differently from the heart, the pathophysiological significance of H_3 receptors in vascular tissues has not yet been entirely recognized.

Presynaptic Histamine H_3 Receptors

The first evidence for the existence of H_3 receptors in the cardiovascular system was found in the guinea pig mesenteric artery, where histamine attenuated the amplitude of electrically evoked excitatory junction potentials [212]. Subsequently, vascular presynaptic H_3-receptor-mediating inhibition of sympathetic neurotransmission has been identified under *in vitro* conditions in various vascular beds of different animal species, including humans (Table 6.6). As observed in the heart, histamine H_3 receptors may also modulate the release of neuropeptides, such as substance P and tachykinins, from sensory C fibers, thus contributing to the inhibition of vasodilation and plasma protein extravasation during neurogenic inflammation [167,168]. An interaction between H_3 receptors and α_2 adrenoceptors was suggested in some vascular beds, since effects mediated by H_3 receptors were only detectable under α_2 adrenoceptor blockade [204].

TABLE 6.6
Effects of H_3 Receptor Activation on Vascular Functions

Species	Technique	Parameter	Effect	References
Rat	Tail artery *in vitro*	EFS-induced NA release	↓	204
	Vena cava *in situ*	EFS-induced NA release	0	205
	Pithed animal	ES-evoked pressor response	↓	206,207
	Anesthetized animal	Basal arterial pressure	0	177–180
		Basal arterial pressure	↑	208
		Nicotine-induced pressor response	↓	180
		Mesenteric vascular tone	↓	209
	Freely moving animal	NA overflow	↓	210
	Conscious animal	Footshock-induced pressor response	↓	211
Guinea pig	Ileal artery *in vitro*	EFS-induced contraction	↓	212,213
	Pulmonary artery *in vitro*	EFS-evoked NA release	↓	132
	Pithed animal	ES-evoked pressor response	↓	190
	Anesthetized animal	Basal arterial pressure	↓	179,187
		Nicotine-evoked pressor response	↓	188
		ES-evoked pressor response	↓	189
Rabbit	Conscious animal	Basal arterial pressure	↓	179
Dog	Anesthetized animal	Basal arterial pressure	↓	192
			0	194
		Renal perfusion pressure, NA release	↓	192
		Anaphylaxis	0	214
Human	Saphenous vein *in vitro*	EFS-induced NA release	↓	215
		EFS-induced contraction	↓	216

Note: ES, electrical stimulation; EFS, electrical field stimulation; NA, noradrenaline; ↓, decrease; 0, no effect; ↑, increase.

Source: Modified from Bertaccini, G., Poli, E., and Coruzzi, G., in *The Histamine H_3 Receptor: A Target for New Drugs*, Elsevier Amsterdam, 1998, 59–111. With permission.

Histamine H_3 receptors appear to be involved in the basal regulation of vascular tone in guinea pigs, rabbits, dogs, but not in rats. Furthermore, H_3 receptors located on sympathetic nerve endings may be activated by endogenous histamine during hypertensive states, to limit the sympathetic tone in resistance vessels [207]. In line with this, a progressive rise in blood pressure was observed in conscious rats following chronic depletion of histamine stores, as a result of reduced H_3-receptor-mediated inhibition of sympathetic neural activity [234]. A role of H_3 receptors in the cardiovascular collapse during anaphylaxis is debated: in the dog, by reducing the compensatory neural adrenergic stimulation, H_3 receptors activated during antigen challenge were found to contribute to collapse [193]; however, the lack of effect of thioperamide indicated a limited role in anaphylactic shock [214].

Although species differences may explain some controversial findings, the interaction of histaminergic ligands with nonhistaminergic receptors (5-HT, α_1, and α_2) may contribute to the overall effects on vascular functions [135,178,179,220].

TABLE 6.7
Effects of H_3 Receptor Activation in Endothelial or Vascular Smooth Muscle Cells (*In Vitro*)

Species	Tissue	Location	Effect	References
Rat	Aorta	Endothelium	Relaxation	217,218
	Mesenteric artery	Muscle cell	Relaxation[a]	219
	Pulmonary artery	N/A	Contraction[b]	220
	Whole heart	Endothelium	Coronary dilation	221
Guinea pig	Aorta	Endothelium	Relaxation	222
	Whole heart	Endothelium	Coronary dilation	223
Rabbit	Middle cerebral artery	Endothelium	Relaxation	224,225
	Saphenous artery	Muscle cell	$\uparrow$ Ca^{2+} conductance	226
Cat	Pulmonary vessels[c]	N/A	Relaxation	227
	Mesenteric artery[c]	Endothelium	Relaxation	228
Dog	Femoral artery	Muscle cell	No effect	229
Cow	Oviductal artery	Muscle cell	(Contraction)	230
Human	Umbilical vein	Endothelium	No effect on PGI$_2$ release	231
		Endothelium	No effect on eNOS expression	232
	Dorsal penile artery	Muscle cell	Contraction[a]	233

Note: N/A, not available; NO, nitric oxide; eNOS, endothelial nitric oxide synthase; $\downarrow$, decrease; $\uparrow$, increase.

[a] Thioperamide-insensitive.

[b] Prazosin-sensitive.

[c] *In vivo*.

Postsynaptic Histamine H_3 Receptors

The existence of postsynaptic H_3-receptor-mediating smooth muscle relaxation was first demonstrated by Ea-Kim and Oudart [224] in rabbit middle cerebral artery and subsequently confirmed in several vascular beds (Table 6.7). In some districts, the H_3-receptor-mediated relaxation was found to be endothelium dependent, since the effect of (R)α-methylhistamine was inhibited by the mechanical removal of the endothelium, the application of the nitric oxide (NO)-synthase inhibitor, NG-nitro-L-arginine methyl ester (L-NAME), or inhibitors of endothelial-derived hyperpolarizing factor (EDHF) [218,225]. An involvement of H_3 receptors in the control of endothelial functions was not demonstrated in humans [231,232].

Surprisingly, the existence of excitatory H_3 receptors augmenting Ca^{2+} currents was reported in the rabbit saphenus artery [226]; however, the high concentrations of thioperamide employed and the involvement of PTX-insensitive G proteins, instead of the Gi/Go protein found in the heart or in the intestine [106,182] would suggest an anomalous H_3 receptor.

RESPIRATORY SYSTEM

Histamine has several actions in the airway and may be an important mediator in asthma [235]. Besides inducing direct bronchoconstriction and airway plasma leakage through the activation of H_1 receptors, histamine stimulates vagal reflexes and activates sensory C fibers to release peptidergic NTs [235]. H_3 receptors were detected in guinea pig lungs, by radioligand-binding studies [13], and in rat and human alveolar macrophages [236]. However, the main evidence for their role in airway function relies on functional assays, which identified H_3-receptor-mediated effects in different species and experimental models (Table 6.8).

H_3 receptors are located prejunctionally at parasympathetic ganglia, postganglionic cholinergic and NANC nerve endings, and sensory fibers, where they exert an inhibitory control on NT release (Figure 6.6). Furthermore, a postjunctional location of H_3 receptors was reported in guinea pig bronchial epithelium [242] and tracheal muscle [240] (Table 6.8).

Besides regulating airway muscle contractility, H_3 receptors have been involved in the inhibition of NANC-induced microvascular leakage through the reduction of neuropeptide release from sensory C fibers [167]; since mast cells are closely associated with cholinergic and sensory fibers, it has been hypothesized a short regulatory feedback that links histamine and inflammatory neuropeptides. Specifically, histamine stimulates the release of neuropeptides that, besides causing direct vascular effects, cause histamine secretion from mast cells [238]. The activation of inhibitory H_3 receptors on sensory nerves would prevent excess neuropeptide release (Figure 6.6); moreover, an H_3-receptor-mediated negative-feedback regulation on histamine release from mast cells was reported in lung during allergen exposure [243]. Thus, H_3 receptors may act as a safety device in asthmatic diseases to prevent increased bronchospasm, airway permeability, and neurogenic inflammation [168]. This hypothesis, however, was not confirmed in a double-blind crossover study carried out in mild atopic asthmatic subjects; in these patients, (R)α-methylhistamine had no effect on the bronchoconstriction induced by the inhaled irritant sodium metabisulfite [255]. The poor pharmacokinetic of (R)α-methylhistamine or its residual H_1-receptor activity may explain the lack of effect; however, phase II clinical trials with compound BP 2.94, developed by Bioproject and INSERM to improve the bioavailability of (R)α-methylhistamine [256] resulted in negative outcomes in exercise-induced asthma [257]. Other studies in humans have been started by Astra Zeneca with more selective ligands for the treatment of chronic obstructive pulmonary disease (COPD) and asthma [258] and will clarify the therapeutic potential of H_3-receptor agonists in airway disease.

Interesting findings were reported on H_3 receptors and nasal mucosa. H_3 receptor mRNA expression was detected in murine nasal mucosa, and its activation modulated allergic symptoms induced by sensitization with ovalbumin [237]. Histamine, release from activated mast cells during allergic reactions, may contribute to nasal congestion, by activating prejunctional inhibitory H_3 receptors in sympathetic varicosities; this would reduce the adrenergic vascular tone and result in nasal vascular engorgement. In cats, the H_3 receptor antagonist thioperamide led to substantial decongestant activity, comparable with oral sympathomimetics, without altering the systemic blood pressure [250]. In humans, although contrasting findings have been reported on H_3-receptor expression [254,259,260], inhibitory H_3 receptors on sympathetic nerve endings were

TABLE 6.8
Effects of H_3 Receptor Activation in the Airways

Species	Technique	Parameter	Effect	References
Mouse	Conscious animal	OVA-induced nasal allergic symptoms	↓	237
Rat	Lung mast cells	HA synthesis	↓	238
Guinea pig	Nasal mucosa *in vitro*	Vascular tone	0	239
	Trachea *in vitro*	ACh-induced contraction	↓	240
	Bronchi *in vitro*	NANC-induced contraction	↓	241
		Epithelium-dependent relaxation	↑	242
	Trachea *in vitro* Lung *in vitro*	BSA-induced HA synthesis	↓	243
	Pulmonary artery *in vitro*	EFS-induced contraction, NA release	↓	132
	Anesthetized animal	Vagally induced tracheal contraction	↓	244
		NANC-induced AML	↓	167
		Sympathetic inhibition of OVA-induced AML	↓	245
		NANC-induced bronchoconstriction	↓	246
		ES-induced bronchoconstriction	0	247
Rabbit	Heart-lung preparation	Pulmonary edema induced by SP, ACh, and capsaicin	↓	248
	Perfused lung	HA release induced by capsaicin and carbachol	↓	249
Cat	Conscious animal	Nasal congestion	↑	250
Pig	Turbinate strips	EFS-induced vasoconstriction	↓	251
Cattle	Trachea *in vitro*	HA-induced contraction	0	252
	Bronchi *in vitro*	HA-induced contraction	0	252
Human	Bronchi *in vitro*	EFS-induced cholinergic contraction	↓	253
	Turbinate strips	EFS-induced vasoconstriction	↓	254
	Asthmatic patients	MBS-induced bronchoconstriction	0	255

Note: ACh, acetylcholine; AML, airway microvascular leakage; BSA, bovine serum albumin; ES, electrical stimulation; EFS, electrical field stimulation; HA, histamine; MBS, metabisulfite; NA, noradrenaline; NANC, nonadrenergic, noncholinergic; OVA, ovalbumin; SP, substance P; ↑, increase; 0, no effect; ↓, decrease.

Source: Modified from Bertaccini, G., Poli, E., and Coruzzi, G., in *The Histamine H_3 Receptor: A Target for New Drugs*, Elsevier Amsterdam, 1998, 59–111. With permission.

found to regulate vascular tone and nasal patency [254], supporting a potential therapeutic advantage of H_3-receptor antagonists, alone or in association with H_1-receptor antagonists, in the treatment of allergic rhinitis and histamine-dependent nasal congestive disease. Recently, Schering-Plough filed a patent application for combined H_1, H_3, and H_4 receptor blockade as a mean to treat allergic diseases [261].

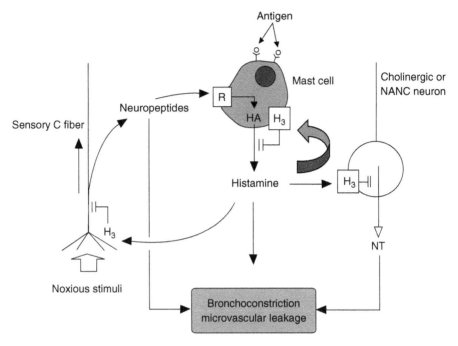

FIGURE 6.6 Proposed locations of histamine H_3 receptors in the airways. Prejunctional H_3 receptors negatively control NT release from cholinergic, NANC, and sensory-C fibers, thus reducing bronchoconstriction and microvascular leakage. ($\rightarrow$, stimulation; $\dashv$, inhibition.)

ALLERGY, INFLAMMATION, AND IMMUNITY

Accumulating evidence has suggested that histamine plays an essential role in inflammation, immediate hypersensitivity reaction, and cellular and humoral immune responses [262–264]. As a preformed mediator, histamine is primarily stored in basophils, mast cells, and in other cellular sources, including platelets, endothelial cells, macrophages, and T cells. Moreover, *neosynthesized* or *nascent* histamine can be produced during the immune response, under the regulatory influence of cytokines [263]. Once released by immunoglobulin E (IgE)-dependent or independent stimuli, histamine exerts multiple regulatory effects that contribute to the pathophysiology of allergic rhinitis, asthma, urticaria, and anaphylactic shock. Specifically, histamine induces vasodilation, increase in vascular permeability, bronchospasm, and pruritus. More recently, it has become evident that histamine exerts less dramatic effects in the immune system and entertains a complex relationship with cytokines, involving both H_1 and H_2 receptors [263]. Although H_1 receptors mediate the classical proinflammatory and allergic effects of histamine, H_2 receptors may be primarily involved in antiinflammatory and immunosuppressive activity [265]. Recently, a key role for H_4 receptors in inflammation and allergy has emerged (see section Histamine H_4 Receptors) and has confirmed that histamine may be an important component of the cytokine network activated during allergic reactions.

Data on the role played by H_3 receptors in the inflammatory and immune responses are limited and intriguing (Table 6.9). H_3 receptor mRNA expression was detected in human alveolar macrophages [236] and in dendritic cells, where, in concert with H_1 receptors, they act as positive stimulants, by increasing antigen-presenting capacity, proinflammatory cytokine (Il-12) production, and Th1 priming activity [266].

TABLE 6.9
Effects of H_3 Receptor Ligands on Inflammatory and Immune Response

Species	Tissue	Parameter	H_3 Ligand	Effect	References
Mouse	Nasal mucosa	Allergic response	(R)α-MHA	↓	237
	Paw	Zymosan-induced edema	BP 2.94	↓	267
		FCA-induced edema and Carrageenan-induced edema	BP 2.94	↓	268
Rat	Peritoneal MC	Anaphylactic	(R)α-MHA	↓	269
		HA release	(R)α-MHA	0	270
		48/80-induced HA release	(R)α-MHA, THIO	0	269
			Nα-MHA, THIO	0	271
		TNFα release	HA	↓	272
		HA release induced by antidromic ES or SP perfusion	(R)α-MHA	↓	273
	Lung MC	HA synthesis	(R)α-MHA	↓	13
	Spleen MC	HA synthesis	(R)α-MHA	↓	238
	Jejunum and thymus MC	HA synthesis	(R)α-MHA	0	238
	Skin, trachea, esophagus, urinary bladder	Capsaicin-induced plasma extravasation	BP 2.94	↓	267
		Neurogenic edema	(R)α-MHA	0	274
Guinea pig	Lung MC/basophils	HA release	(R)α-MHA	↓	235
	Bronchial MC	Allergen-induced HA synthesis	(R)α-MHA THIO	0 ↑	243
Human	Adenoidal MC	HA release	(R)α-MHA THIO	0 ↑	275 275
	Colon MC	HA-induced tryptase release	CLOB	0	276
	Eosinophils	Chemotaxis	HA (R)α-MHA BUR	↑ 0 ↓	277
	Basophils	HA release	(R)α-MHA, THIO	0	278,279

(continued)

TABLE 6.9   (Continued)

Species	Tissue	Parameter	H$_3$ Ligand	Effect	References
	Alveolar macrophages	IL-10 release	(R)α-MHA	↑	236
	Bronchial epithelial cell line BEAS-2B	IL-6, IL-8 production	HA, (R)α-MHA	↑	280
		TNFα/IFNγ-induced production of RANTES and MIG	(R)α-MHA	↓	280
	Monocytes	LPS-induced TNFα release; ICAM-1 expression	(R)α-MHA, THIO	0	281
		LPS-induced IL-18 release	(R)α-MHA, THIO	0	282
		LPS-induced IL-12 release	HA	↓[a]	283
		LPS-induced IL-10 release	HA	↑[a]	283
	B-cell line	IL-10 production	HA, (R)α-MHA	↑	284
	Dendritic cells	Chemotaxis	HA, (R)α-MHA	↑	266

Note: 48/80, compound 48/80; BUR, burimamide; CLOB, clobenpropit; ES, electrical stimulation; FCA, Freund's complete adjuvant; HA, histamine; ICAM-1, intercellular adhesion molecule-1; IFNγ, interferon gamma; IL, interleukin; IODOPH, iodophenpropit; LPS, lipopolysaccharide; MIG, monokine-induced gamma-interferon; MC, mast cell; N^α-MHA, N^α-methylhistamine; (R)α-MHA, (R)α-methylhistamine; RANTES, regulated on activation, normal T-cell expressed, and presumably secreted; SP, substance P; THIO, thioperamide; TNFα, tumor necrosis factor α; ↓, decrease; 0, no effect; ↑, increase.

[a]   Thioperamide-insensitive.

Source: Modified from Bertaccini, G., Poli, E., and Coruzzi, G., in *The Histamine H$_3$ Receptor: A Target for New Drugs*, Elsevier Amsterdam, 1998, 59–111. With permission.

Early data have suggested that H$_3$ receptors located on sensory nerve endings inhibit neurogenic microvascular leakage in the rat paw by prejunctional inhibition of neuropeptide release and have a protective role on neurogenic inflammation [168]. Subsequently, antiinflammatory effects following (R)α-methylhistamine or its pro-drug, compound BP 2.94, were confirmed in mice and rats [267,268,285,286] but not in guinea pigs [287]. Thus, a possible therapeutic use of H$_3$ receptor agonists in the treatment of inflammatory disorders is suggested. If confirmed, the antiinflammatory activity of H$_3$ receptor agonists would have the additional advantage of inducing gastroprotective effects; thus these compounds would represent the prototype of a novel class of gastrosparing nonsteroidal antiinflammatory drugs (NSAIDs). This approach is currently being validated in ongoing clinical trials with compound BP 2.94 [256]. The release of histamine is one of the most important aspects of hista-mine biology; the effect of H$_3$ receptor ligands on histamine release from mast cells is controversial, depending on species, tissue, stimulus, and ligand used (Table 6.9). To date, expression of H_3 receptors has not been demonstrated on human mast cells. It is of interest that Raible et al. [277], by the use of thioperamide, hypothesized the existence of an unusual histamine receptor on human eosinophils, which mediates histamine-induced increase in cytosolic calcium mobilization. It is now recognized that the histamine receptor mediating eosinophil chemotaxis and function belongs exclusively to the H_4 subtype (for review see Ref. 7). Thus, the cross-reactivity of H_3 antagonists with the H_4 receptors may offer an explanation for early data on H_3 receptor expression on peripheral mast cells [272,275].

In conclusion, the role of histamine H_3 receptors in the inflammatory/immune response is still unclear due to the involvement of all four subtypes of histamine receptors and the use of dual H_3/H_4 receptor ligands, namely, (R)α-methylhistamine and thioperamide, as selective pharmacological tools. Highly selective receptor ligands are eagerly awaited to clarify the intricate aspects of histamine pathophysiology in inflammation and immunity.

TISSUE GROWTH AND CARCINOGENESIS

Histamine was long ago proposed to act as a mitogen factor and have a role in carcinogenesis and tumor proliferation [288]. Histamine synthesis is greatly stimulated in rapidly proliferating tissues, such as fetal tissues, in tissues undergoing repair, in human malignant cells, as well as in experimentally induced tumors [265]. Proliferative effects of histamine have been mainly related to H_1-receptor activation, although recently the majority of reports point toward a key role of H_2 receptors [263]. Furthermore, an intracellular site (H_{IC}), distinct from H_1, H_2, and H_3 receptors and linked to P450 enzyme, has been proposed to mediate the growth-promoting effects of histamine [289]. Data concerning the role of H_3 receptors on cell growth are limited; in contrast with the hyperproliferative effects of H_3-receptor agonists, previously described in the GI tract [97], H_3 receptors were found to inhibit rat cholangiocyte growth after bile duct ligation, and the effect was associated with downregulation of cAMP-dependent PKA/ERK1/2/Elk-1 phosphorylation [290]. Recent studies have reported high levels of both H_3 receptor and HDC mRNA within embryonic rat epithelia [9], in AtT-20 cell line from a murine anterior pituitary tumor [291] and in malignant breast cells [292].

OTHER PERIPHERAL LOCATIONS AND FUNCTIONS

Over the past years, radioligand-binding studies and immunohistochemistry have evidenced H_3 receptors in a number of other peripheral tissues; moreover, an array of effects have been reported following H_3-receptor ligand administration (Table 6.10). However, reports are anecdotal and mostly based on the effects of *historical* compounds; thus, the involvement of H_3 receptors needs confirmation. H_3 receptors have been identified in several tissues of the rat, including brown adipose tissue [293], liver [9], cochlea [294], skin [9,10], and pancreas of guinea pig [8]. In humans, H_3 receptor mRNA was detected in the nasal mucosa [260] but not in the skin [295].

TABLE 6.10
Effects of H$_3$ Receptor Ligands in Other Peripheral Tissues

Tissue	Species	Ligand	Parameter	Effect	References
Skin	Mouse	THIO	Pruritus	↑	296
		(R)α-MHA		↓	
		CLOB, IODOPH	Scratching behavior	↑	297
		N^α-MHA, THIO	Barrier repair	0	298
		CLOB, IODOPH	Vascular permeability	↑	286
		(R)α-MHA	Vascular permeability	↓	285
	Rat	(R)α-MHA	HA release from MC	↓	13,273
	Guinea pig	THIO, CLOB	Vascular permeability	↓	287
	Cat	(R)α-MHA	ES-evoked sudomotor response	↓	299
	Human	(R)α-MHA	Wheal, flare	↑ (H$_1$)	300
Iris	Rat	(R)α-MHA	ES-induced midriasis	↓	301
	Rabbit	HA	EFS-induced miosis	↓	302
	Cat	(R)α-MHA	ES-induced midriasis	↓	303
	Human	HA	EFS-induced miosis	↓	302
	Cow	THIO	Iris dilator muscle tone	0	304
Retina	Pig	(R)α-MHA	EFS-evoked NA release	↓	305
Ciliary muscle	Human	THIO	Muscle tone	0	306
Cornea	Cow	THIO	Ca^{2+} mobilization	0	307
Pancreas	Guinea pig	(R)α-MHA	EFS-induced amylase secretion	↓	308
Liver	Rat	BP 2.94	CCl$_4$-induced toxicity	↓	309
Gallbladder	Guinea pig	(R)α-MHA	EFS-induced contraction	0	310
Adrenals	Cow	THIO, CLOB	Steroidogenesis	↓[a]	311
		(R)α-MHA	cAMP	0	312
Detrusor	Human	(R)α-MHA	Ca^{2+} mobilization	↑	313
Bladder	Human	(R)α-MHA	Sphincter tone	↑	314
Vas deferens	Rat	HA	EFS-induced NA release	↓	315
		(R)α-MHA	EFS-induced contraction	0	316
	Guinea pig	(R)α-MHA	NA release	↓	317
Corpus cavernosum	Rabbit	(R)α-MHA, THIO	NA-induced contraction	0	318
Uterus	Mouse	(R)α-MHA	EFS-induced NA release	0	319
		HA	Muscle tone	↓	320
	Swine	N^α-MHA	EFS-induced contraction	0	321
Mammary gland	Mouse	FUB 181[b]	Milk secretion	↑	322
Platelets	Rat	(R)α-MHA	5-HT uptake	0	323

Note: cAMP, adenosine 3′,5′-monophosphate; CCl$_4$, carbon tetrachloride; CLOB, clobenpropit; ES, electrical stimulation; EFS, electrical field stimulation; 5-HT, 5-hydroxytryptamine; HA, histamine; IODOPH, iodophenpropit; MC, mast cell; NA, noradrenaline; N^α-MHA, N^α-methyhistamine; (R)α-MHA, (R)α-methylhistamine; SP, substance P; THIO, thioperamide; ↑, increase; 0, no effect; ↓, decrease.

[a]   P450 site.

[b]   H$_3$ receptor selective antagonist.

Source: Modified from Bertaccini, G., Poli, E., and Coruzzi, G., in *The Histamine H$_3$ Receptor: A Target for New Drugs*, Elsevier Amsterdam, 1998, 59–111. With permission.

The effects reported in the skin after H_3-receptor ligand administration seem attractive; in a guinea pig model of urticaria, combined administration of H_1- and H_3-receptor antagonists attenuated 48/80-induced inflammatory skin responses to a greater extent than either H_1 or H_3 antagonist alone [287]. However, the activation of H_3 receptors reduced scratching behavior in mice [296,297] and inhibited the release of neuropeptides and the associated neurogenic inflammation [285]. These findings led to hypothesize that the H_3 receptor may become a novel target for the treatment of allergic skin disease such as urticaria and pruritus.

HISTAMINE H_4 RECEPTORS

Following the elucidation of the human genoma, the histamine H_4 receptor has been recently cloned by several independent groups [7,15,101]. It is a G-protein-coupled receptor that, conversely from H_3 subtype, is nearly absent in the brain and is preferentially expressed in peripheral tissues, particularly in bone marrow and immunocompetent cells such as eosinophils, T lymphocytes, and dendritic cells. Moderate expression was found in spleen, thymus, small and large intestine, and heart. The use of the first highly selective antagonist, compound JNJ7777120 [324], has provided consistent evidence that H_4 receptor is involved in the inflammatory and immune responses elicited by histamine; specifically, this receptor mediates the chemoattractant properties of histamine, including recruitment of eosinophils, alteration in cell shape, mast cells chemotaxis, and upregulation of adhesion molecule expression. The antiinflammatory and antiallergic effects of H_4 receptor antagonists observed in various *in vitro* and *in vivo* models have opened a new window for therapeutic approaches in inflammation and allergy [7]. Furthermore, H_4 receptor blockade has been recently associated with protective effects against ischemia-reperfusion injury in the liver [325], against TNBS-induced colitis in rats [25] and indomethacin-induced gastric lesions in rats [102]. In addition, the possibility that the newly discovered H_4 receptor mediates excitatory effects of histamine in the stomach was recently suggested in rats [102]. The prospect of a therapeutic application of H_4 receptor antagonists in pathological GI disorders looks very promising.

CONCLUSIONS

In the past years, histamine research has received a new impetus from the discovery of H_3 and, more recently, H_4 receptors and has tremendously increased our knowledge on the role of histamine in health and disease. However, the multiple locations of H_3 receptors in the same tissue, along with the other histamine receptor subtypes, and the interaction of H_3-receptor ligands with the H_4 receptor, make this knowledge fragmentary, and still difficult to understand the functional significance of H_3 receptors in periphery. As a result, although strong indications exist for a therapeutic use of H_3-receptor ligands in CNS disorders, their therapeutic potential in periphery is still uncertain. Nevertheless, experimental animal data would suggest a future therapeutic application of H_3 ligands in GI disorders, myocardial ischemia, hypertension, asthma, and nasal congestion; it is noteworthy that in most tissues these receptors seem to be quiescent under physiological conditions and gain importance during pathological states, suggesting a lack of interference with basal functions. However, the limited availability of human data precludes any definite conclusion, and H_3 ligands still remain *orphan drugs* in search of a disease, at least in periphery.

Finally, the recent discovery of the H_4 receptor, although opening a new field of investigation in inflammation and allergy, has contributed to make histamine pharmacology in the periphery more complex than previously thought. Thus, the understanding of the functional role of H_3 and H_4 receptors in periphery will represent a great challenge for future research.

ACKNOWLEDGMENT

The authors thank Silvana Spaggiari for the excellent help in preparing the manuscript.

REFERENCES

1. Windaus, A., and Vogt, W. 1907. Synthese des imidazolyl athylamins. *Ber. Dtsch. Chem. Ges.* 40:3691–3695.
2. Dale, H.H., and Laidlaw, P.P. 1910. The physiological action of beta-imidazolylethylamine. *J. Physiol.* 41:318–344.
3. Dale, H.H., and Laidlaw, P.P. 1919. Histamine shock. *J. Physiol.* 52:355–390.
4. Bovet, D., and Staub, A.M. 1937. Action protectrice des ethers phenoliques an cours de l'intoxications histaminique. *CR Soc. Biol.* (Paris) 124:547–549.
5. Black, J.W., Duncan, W., Durant, C., Ganellin, C.R., and Parsons, M.E. 1972. Definition and antagonism of histamine H_2 receptors. *Nature* 236:385–390.
6. Arrang, J.M., Garbarg, M., and Schwartz, J.C. 1983. Auto-inhibition of brain histamine release mediated by a novel class (H_3) of histamine receptors. *Nature* 302:832–837.
7. Zhang, M., Thurmond, R.L., and Dunford, P.J. 2007. The histamine H_4 receptor: a novel modulator of inflammatory and immune disorders. *Pharmacol. Ther.* 113:594–606.
8. Korte, A., Myers, J., Shih, N.Y., Egan, R.W., and Clark, M.A. 1990. Characterization and tissue distribution of H_3 histamine receptors in guinea pigs by N^α-methylhistamine. *Biochem. Biophys. Res. Commun.* 168:979–986.
9. Héron, A., Rouleau, A., Cochois, V., Pillot, C., Schwartz, J.C., and Arrang, J.M. 2001. Expression analysis of the histamine H_3 receptor in developing rat tissues. *Mech. Dev.* 105:167–173.
10. Cannon, K.E., Chazot, P.L., Hann, V., Shenton, F., Hough, L.B., and Rice, F.L. 2007. Immunohistochemical localization of histamine H_3 receptors in rodent skin, dorsal root ganglia, superior cervical ganglia, and spinal cord: potential antinociceptive targets. *Pain* 129:76–92.
11. Bertaccini, G., Poli, E., and Coruzzi, G. 1998. Functional role of the histamine H_3 receptor in peripheral tissues. In *The Histamine H_3 Receptor: A Target for New Drugs*, eds. R. Leurs, and H. Timmerman, pp. 59–111. Amsterdam: Elsevier.
12. Leurs, R., Bakker, R.A., Timmerman, H., and de Esch, I.J. 2005. The histamine H_3 receptor: from gene cloning to H_3 receptor drugs. *Nat. Rev. Drug Discov.* 4:107–120.
13. Arrang, J.M., Garbarg, M., Lancelot, J. et al. 1987. Highly potent and selective ligands for histamine H_3 receptors. *Nature* 327:117–123.
14. Stark, H., Arrang, J.M., Ligneau, X. et al. 2001. The histamine H_3 receptor and its ligands. *Progr. Med. Chem.* 38:279–308.
15. Jablonowski, J.A., Carruthers, N.I., and Thurmond, R.L. 2004. The histamine H_4 receptor and potential therapeutic use for H_4 ligands. *Mini-Rev. Med. Chem.* 4:993–1000.
16. Gbahou, F., Vincent, L., Humbert-Claude, M., Tardivel-Lacombe, J., Chabret, C., and Arrang, J.M. 2006. Compared pharmacology of human histamine H_3 and H_4 receptors: structure-activity relationships of histamine derivatives. *Br. J. Pharmacol.* 147:744–754.

17. Rangachari, P.K. 1992. Histamine: mercurial messenger in the gut. *Am. J. Physiol.* 262:G1–G13.
18. Coruzzi, G., Poli, E., Morini, G., and Bertaccini, G. 2000. The histamine H_3 receptor. In *Molecular Targets for Drug Development: GI Diseases*, eds. T.S. Gaginella, and A. Guglietta, pp. 239–267. Totowa: Humana Press.
19. Wood, J.D. 2006. Histamine, mast cells, and the enteric nervous system in the irritable bowel syndrome, enteritis, and food allergies. *Gut* 55:445–447.
20. Häkanson, R., and Sundler, F. 1991. Histamine-producing cells in the stomach and their role in the regulation of acid secretion. *Scand. J. Gastroenterol.* 180 (Suppl.):88–94.
21. Hunyady, B., Zolyomi, A., Hoffman, B.J., and Mezey, E. 1998. Gastrin-producing endocrine cells: a novel source of histamine in the rat stomach. *Endocrinology* 139:4404–4415.
22. Ekblad, E., Wahlestedt, C., Hakanson, R., Sundler, F., Watanabe, T., and Wada, H. 1985. Is histamine a neurotransmitter in the gut? Evidence from histidine decarboxylase immunocytochemistry. *Acta Physiol. Scand.* 123:225–227.
23. Panula, P., Kaartinen, M., Macklin, M., and Costa, E. 1985. Histamine-containing peripheral neuronal and endocrine systems. *J. Histochem. Cytochem.* 33:933–941.
24. Bertaccini, G., and Coruzzi, G. 1992. Histamine receptors in the digestive system. In *The Histamine Receptor*, eds. J.C. Schwartz, and H.L. Haas, pp. 183–230. New York: Wiley-Liss.
25. Varga, C., Horvath, K., Berko, A., Thurmond, R.L., Dunford, P.J., and Whittle, B.J. 2005. Inhibitory effects of histamine H_4 receptor antagonists on experimental colitis in the rat. *Eur. J. Pharmacol.* 522:130–138.
26. Chazot, P., Shenton, F., Schunack, W., Grandi, D., and Morini, G. 2007. Influence of (R)-α-methylhistamine on the histamine H_3 receptor in the rat gastrointestinal tract. *Inflamm. Res.* 56 (Suppl. 1):S1–S2.
27. Hemedah, M., Loiacono, R., Coupar, I.M., and Mitchelson, F.J. 2001. Lack of evidence for histamine H_3 receptor function in rat ileum and human colon. *Naunyn-Schmiedeberg's Arch. Pharmacol.* 363:133–138.
28. Sander, L.E., Lorentz, A., Sellge, G. et al. 2006. Selective expression of histamine receptors H_1R, H_2R, and H_4R, but not H_3R, in the human intestinal tract. *Gut* 55:498–504.
29. Lindström, E., Chen, D., Norlen, P., Andersson, K., and Hakanson, R. 2001. Control of gastric acid secretion: the gastrin-ECL cell-parietal cell axis. *Comp. Biochem. Physiol. A Mol. Integr. Physiol.* 128:505–514.
30. Bliss, P.W., Healey, Z.V., Arebi, N., and Calam, J. 1999. $N^α$-methylhistamine and histamine stimulate gastrin release from rabbit G-cells via histamine H_2-receptors. *Aliment. Pharmacol. Ther.* 13:1669–1674.
31. Aihara, T., Nakamura, E., Amagase, K. et al. 2003. Pharmacological control of gastric acid secretion for the treatment of acid-related peptic disease: past, present, and future. *Pharmacol. Ther.* 98:109–127.
32. Schubert, M.L. 2000. Gastric secretion. *Curr. Opin. Gastroenterol.* 16:463–468.
33. Vuyyuru, L., and Schubert, M.L. 1997. Histamine, acting via H_3 receptors, inhibits somatostatin and stimulates acid secretion in isolated mouse stomach. *Gastroenterology* 113:1545–1552.
34. Vuyyuru, L., Schubert, M.L., Harrington, L., Arimura, A., and Makhlouf, G.M. 1995. Dual inhibitory pathways link antral somatostatin and histamine secretion in human, dog, and rat stomach. *Gastroenterology* 109:1566–1574.
35. Badò, A., Moizo, L., Laigneau, J.P., Delwaide, J., and Lewin, M.J. 1994. H_3-receptor regulation of vascular gastrin and somatostatin releases by the isolated rat stomach. *Yale J. Biol. Med.* 67:113–121.
36. Kaneko, H., Konagaya, T., and Kusugami, K. 2002. *Helicobacter pylori* and gut hormones. *J. Gastroenterol.* 37:77–86.

37. Konagaya, T., Kusugami, K., Yamamoto, H., Kaneko, H., Nagai, H., and Mitsuma, T. 1998. Effect of histamine on thyrotropin-releasing hormone and somatostatin secretion in rat stomach. *Hepatogastroenterology* 45:567–572.

38. Beales, I.L., and Calam, J. 1998. The histamine H_3 receptor agonist N^α-methylhistamine produced by *Helicobacter pylori* does not alter somatostatin release from cultured rabbit fundic D-cells. *Gut* 43:176–181.

39. Soldani, G., Bertini, S., Rouleau, A., Schwartz, J.C., and Coruzzi, G. 1999. Gastric antisecretory effects of compound BP 2-94: a histamine H_3-receptor agonist prodrug. *Dig. Dis. Sci.* 44:2380–2385.

40. Cherifi, Y., Pigeon, C., Le Romancer, M., Badò, A., Reyl-Desmars, F., and Lewin, M.J. 1992. Purification of a histamine H_3 receptor negatively coupled to phosphoinositide turnover in the human gastric cell line HGT1. *J. Biol. Chem.* 267:25315–25320.

41. Gespach, C., Fagot, D., and Emami, S. 1989. Pharmacological control of the human gastric histamine H_2 receptor by famotidine: comparison with H_1, H_2 and H_3 receptor agonists and antagonists. *Eur. J. Clin. Invest.* 19:1–10.

42. Coruzzi, G., Adami, A., and Bertaccini, G. 1992. Histamine H_3 receptors are not involved in the regulation of rat gastric secretion. *Pharmacology* 44:190–195.

43. Barocelli, E., Ballabeni, V., Chiavarini, M., and Impicciatore, M. 1995. R-α-methylhistamine-induced inhibition of gastric acid secretion in pylorus-ligated rats via central histamine H_3-receptors. *Br. J. Pharmacol.* 115:1326–1330.

44. Kwiecien, S., Brzozowski, T., Konturek, P.C. et al. 2001. Effect of central and peripheral actions of histamine and its metabolite N-α methyl histamine on gastric secretion and acute gastric lesions. *J. Physiol. Pharmacol.* 52:625–638.

45. Coruzzi, G., Morini, G., Adami, M., and Grandi, D. 2001. Role of histamine H_3 receptors in the regulation of gastric functions. *J. Physiol. Pharmacol.* 52:539–553.

46. Ballabeni, V., Calcina, F., Bosetti, M. et al. 2002. Different role of the histamine H_3-receptor in vagal-, bethanecol-pentagastrin-induced gastric acid secretion in anaesthetized rats. *Scand. J. Gastroenterol.* 137:754–758.

47. Coruzzi, G., Bertaccini, G., and Schwartz, J.C. 1991. Evidence that histamine H_3 receptors are involved in the control of gastric acid secretion in the conscious cat. *Naunyn-Schmiedeberg's Arch. Pharmacol.* 343:225–227.

48. Badò, A., Hervatin, F., and Lewin, M.J. 1991. Pharmacological evidence for histamine H_3 receptor in the control of gastric acid secretion in cats. *Am. J. Physiol.* 260:G631–G635.

49. Soldani, G., Mengozzi, G., Intorre, L., De Giorgi, G., Coruzzi, G., and Bertaccini, G. 1993. Histamine H_3 receptor-mediated inhibition of gastric acid secretion in conscious dogs. *Naunyn-Schmiedeberg's Arch. Pharmacol.* 347:61–65.

50. Soldani, G., Intorre, L., Bertini, S., Luchetti, E., Coruzzi, G., and Bertaccini, G. 1994. Regulation of gastric acid secretion by histamine H_3 receptors in the dog: an investigation into the site of action. *Naunyn-Schmiedeberg's Arch. Pharmacol.* 350:218–223.

51. Soldani, G., Garbarg, M., Intorre, L., Bertini, S., Rouleau, A., and Schwartz, J.C. 1996. Modulation of pentagastrin-induced histamine release by histamine H_3 receptors in the dog. *Scand. J. Gastroenterol.* 31:631–638.

52. Muller, M.J., Padol, I., and Hunt, R.H. 1993. Acid secretion in isolated murine gastric glands: classification of histaminergic and cholinergic receptors. *Gastroenterology* 104 (Suppl.):A151.

53. Sandvik, A.K., Lewin, M.J., and Waldum, H.L. 1989. Histamine release in the isolated vascularly perfused stomach of the rat: regulation by autoreceptors. *Br. J. Pharmacol.* 96:557–562.

54. Adami, M., Coruzzi, G., Guaita, E., Schunack, W., Kitbunnadaj, R., and Timmerman, H. 2004. Neuronal histamine H_3 receptors mediate antisecretory effects in the rat. *Inflamm. Res.* 53 (Suppl. 1):S25–S26.

55. Stanovnik, L., and Logonder-Mlinsek, M. 1996. Mast cell histamine in gastric secretion-a study on the isolated portion of a guinea pig stomach. *Pflugers Arch.* 431 (Suppl. 2): R219–R220.
56. Badò, A., Laigneau, J.P., Moizo, L., Cherifi, Y., and Lewin, M.J. 1995. H_3-receptor activation inhibits cholinergic stimulation of acid secretion in isolated rabbit fundic glands. *J. Pharmacol. Exp. Ther.* 275:1099–1103.
57. Beales, I.L., and Calam, J. 1997. Effect of N^αmethylhistamine on acid secretion in isolated cultured rabbit parietal cells: implications for *Helicobacter pylori* associated gastritis and gastric physiology. *Gut* 40:14–19.
58. Yokotani, K., Murakami, Y., Okada, S., Wang, M., and Nakamura, K. 2000. Histamine H_3 receptor-mediated inhibition of endogenous acetylcholine release from the isolated, vascularly perfused rat stomach. *Eur. J. Pharmacol.* 392:23–29.
59. Badò, A., Dubrasquet, M., and Lewin, M.J. 1990. Evidence of histamine H_3 receptors in the stomach: physiological role in gastric acid regulation. *Gastroenterology* 98(Suppl.): A17.
60. Sobhani, I., Canedo, S., Alchepo, B. et al. 2002. Putative effect of *Helicobacter pylori* and gastritis on gastric acid secretion in cat. *Am. J. Physiol.* 282:G727–G734.
61. Vuyyuru, L., Harrington, L., Arimura, A., and Schubert, M.L. 1997. Reciprocal inhibitory paracrine pathways link histamine and somatostatin secretion in the fundus of the stomach. *Am. J. Physiol.* 273:G106–G111.
62. Prinz, C., Kajimura, M., Scott, D.R., Mercier, F., Helander, H.F., and Sachs, G. 1993. Histamine secretion from rat enterochromaffinlike cells. *Gastroenterology* 105:449–461.
63. Kidd, M., Tang, L.H., Miu, K., Lawton, G.P., Sandor, A., and Modlin, I.M. 1996. Autoregulation of enterochromaffin-like cell histamine secretion via the histamine 3 receptor subtype. *Yale J. Biol. Med.* 69:9–19.
64. Modlin, I.M., Lawton, G.P., Tang, L.H., Miu, K., and Schwartz, J.C. 1995. Histamine-3 receptor modulation of ECL histamine secretion and DNA synthesis. *Gastroenterology* 108:A992.
65. Badò, A., Moizo, L., Laigneau, J.P., and Lewin, M.J. 1992. Pharmacological characterization of histamine H_3 receptors in isolated rabbit gastric glands. *Am. J. Physiol.* 262: G56–G61.
66. Hollande, F., Bali, J.P., and Magous, R. 1993. Autoregulation of histamine synthesis through H_3 receptors in isolated fundic mucosal cells. *Am. J. Physiol.* 265:G1039–G1044.
67. Payne, N.A., and Gerber, J.G. 1997. Effect of adenosine and histamine receptor stimulation on canine histamine release to pentagastrin. *Digestion* 58:352–360.
68. Courillon-Mallet, A., Launay, J.M., Roucayrol, A.M. et al. 1995. *Helicobacter pylori* infection: physiopathologic implication of N^α-methylhistamine. *Gastroenterology* 108:959–966.
69. Kitbunnadaj, R., Hashimoto, T., Poli, E. et al. 2005. N-substituted piperidinyl alkyl imidazoles: discovery of methimepip as a potent and selective histamine H_3 receptor agonist. *J. Med. Chem.* 48:2100–2107.
70. Meier, G., Apelt, J., Reichert, U. et al. 2001. Influence of imidazole replacement in different structural classes of histamine H_3-receptor antagonists. *Eur. J. Pharm. Sci.* 13:249–259.
71. Marshall, B.J., and Warren, J.R. 1984. Unidentified curved bacilli in the stomach of patients with gastritis and peptic ulceration. *Lancet* 1:1311–1315.
72. Howden, C.W. 1996. Clinical expressions of *Helicobacter pylori* infection. *Am. J. Med.* 100:27S-32S.
73. Wessler, S., Hocher, M., Fischer, W. et al. 2000. *Helicobacter pylori* activates the histidine decarboxylase promoter through a mitogen-activated protein kinase pathway independent of pathogenicity island-encoded virulence factors. *J. Biol. Chem.* 275:3629–3636.

74. Murray, S., Taylor, G.W., Karim, Q.N., Bliss, P., and Calam, J. 2000. N α-methylhistamine: association with *Helicobacter pylori* infection in humans and effects on gastric acid secretion. *Clin. Chim. Acta* 301:181–192.

75. El-Omar, E., Penman, I., Dorrian, C.A., Ardill, J.E.S., and McColl, K.E.L. 1993. Eradicating *Helicobacter pylori* infection lowers gastrin mediated acid secretion by two thirds in patients with duodenal ulcer. *Gut* 34:1060–1065.

76. Queiroz, D.M., Mendes, E.N., Rocha, G.A. et al. 1993. Effect of *Helicobacter pylori* eradication on antral gastrin- and somatostatin-immunoreactive cell density and gastrin and somatostatin concentrations. *Scand. J. Gastroenterol.* 28:858–864.

77. McGowan, C.C., Cover, T.L., and Blaser, M.J. 1996. *Helicobacter pylori* and gastric acid: biological and therapeutic implications. *Gastroenterology* 110:926–938.

78. Kidd, M., Miu, K., Tang, L.H. et al. 1997. *Helicobacter pylori* lipopolysaccharide stimulates histamine release and DNA synthesis in rat enterochromaffin-like cells. *Gastroenterology* 113:1110–1117.

79. Bertaccini, G., Cavaggioni, A., Zappia, L., and Mossini, F. 1973. Action of some N$^{\alpha}$-methyl derivatives of histamine on gastric secretion of the rat. *Pharmacol. Res. Commun.* 5:71–80.

80. Trzeciakowski, J.P. 1987. Inhibition of guinea pig ileum contractions mediated by a class of histamine receptors resembling the H_3 subtype. *J. Pharmacol. Exp. Ther.* 243:874–880.

81. Coruzzi, C., Poli, E., and Bertaccini, G. 1991. Histamine receptors in isolated guinea pig duodenal muscle: H_3 receptors inhibit cholinergic neurotransmission. *J. Pharmacol. Exp. Ther.* 258:325–331.

82. Konturek, P.C., Konturek, S.J., Sito, E. et al. 2001. Luminal N$^{\alpha}$-methylhistamine stimulates gastric acid secretion in duodenal ulcer patients *via* releasing gastrin. *Eur. J. Pharmacol.* 412:181–185.

83. Saitoh, T., Fukushima, Y., Otsuka, H. et al. 2002. Effects of N-α-methyl-histamine on human H_2 receptors expressed in CHO cells. *Gut* 50:786–789.

84. Klausz, G., Buzas, E., Scharek, P. et al. 2004. Effects of *Helicobacter pylori* infection on gastric inflammation and local cytokine production in histamine-deficient (histidine decarboxylase knock-out) mice. *Immunol. Lett.* 94:223–228.

85. Morini, G., Grandi, D., and Bertaccini, G. 1995. (R)-α-methylhistamine inhibits ethanol-induced gastric lesions in the rat: involvement of histamine H_3 receptors? *Digestion* 56:145–152.

86. Palitzsch, K.D., Morales, R.E., Kronauge, J.F. et al. 1995. Effect of histamine on haemorrhagic mucosal lesions is related to vascular permeability in rats: studies with histamine, H_1-, H_2- and H_3-agonists and bradykinin. *Eur. J. Gastroenterol. Hepatol.* 7:447–453.

87. Belcheva, A., Marazova, K., Lozeva, V., and Schunack, W. 1997. Effects of (R)-α-methylhistamine and its prodrug BP 2.94 on gastric mucosal lesions in cold/restraint stressed rats. *Inflamm. Res.* 46 (Suppl. 1):S113–S114.

88. Morini, G., Grandi, D., Krause, M., and Schunack, W. 1997. Gastric mucosal injury by nonsteroidal anti-inflammatory drugs is reduced by (R)-α-methylhistamine and its prodrugs in the rat. *Inflamm. Res.* 46(Suppl. 1):S101–S102.

89. Warzecha, Z., Dembinski, A., Brzozowski, T. et al. 2000. Gastroprotective effect of histamine and acid secretion on ammonia-induced gastric lesions in rats. *Scand. J. Gastroenterol.* 35:916–924.

90. Konturek, P.C., Nikiforuk, A., Brzozowski, T. et al. 2004. Effect of N-α-methylhistamine on ulcer healing in rats. *Inflamm. Res.* 53(Suppl. 1):S27–S28.

91. Morini, G., Grandi, D., Arcari, M.L., Galanti, G., and Bertaccini, G. 1997. Histological effect of (R)-α-methylhistamine on ethanol damage in rat gastric mucosa: influence on mucus production. *Dig. Dis. Sci.* 42:1020–1028.

92. Coruzzi, G., Gambarelli, E., and Bertaccini, G. 1996. Stimulatory effect of (R)α-methylhistamine on duodenal HCO_3^- secretion in anaesthetized rats. *Ital. J. Gastroenterol.* 28:520–522.

93. Konturek, P.C., Brzozowski, T., Gaca, P. et al. 2005. Histamine and its metabolite N-α-methyl histamine accelerate ulcer healing in rats: role of H_3 receptors, sensory nerves and TGFα. XXXIVth Meeting of the Histamine Research Society, Bled, Slovenija.

94. Rydning, A., Lyng, O., Adamsen, B.L., Falkmer, S., Sandvik, A.K., and Gronbech, J.E. 2001. Mast cells are involved in the gastric hyperemic response to acid back diffusion via release of histamine. *Am. J. Physiol. Gastrointest. Liver Physiol.* 280:G1061–G1069.

95. Pawlik, W.W., Obuchowicz, R., Pawlik, M.W. et al. 2004. Histamine H_3 receptors modulate reactive hyperemia in rat gut. *J. Physiol. Pharmacol.* 55:651–661.

96. Sasse, A., Stark, H., Reidemeister, S. et al. 1999. Novel partial agonists for the histamine H_3 receptor with high *in vitro* and *in vivo* activity. *J. Med. Chem.* 42:4269–4274.

97. Morini, G., Grandi, D., and Schunack, W. 2002. Ligands for histamine H_3 receptors modulate cell proliferation and migration in rat oxyntic mucosa. *Br. J. Pharmacol.* 137:237–244.

98. Grandi, D., Schunack, W., and Morini, G. 2006. Epithelial cell proliferation is promoted by the histamine H_3 receptor agonist (R)-α-methylhistamine throughout the rat gastrointestinal tract. *Eur. J. Pharmacol.* 538:141–147.

99. Dembinski, A., Warzecha, Z., Ceranowicz, P. et al. 2005. Role of capsaicin-sensitive nerves and histamine H_1, H_2, and H_3 receptors in the gastroprotective effect of histamine against stress ulcers in rats. *Eur. J. Pharmacol.* 508:211–221.

100. Morini, G., Timmerman, H., Schunack, W., and Grandi, D. 2002. Agonists for the histamine H_3-receptor differ in their gastroprotective activity in the rat. *Inflamm. Res.* 51(Suppl. 1):S75–S76.

101. de Esch, I.J., Thurmond, R.L., Jongejan, A., and Leurs, R. 2005. The histamine H_4 receptor as a new therapeutic target for inflammation. *Trends Pharmacol. Sci.* 26:462–469.

102. Coruzzi, G., Adami, M., Guaita, E., de Esch, I.J.P., and Leurs, R. 2006. Gastric effects of the histamine H_4 receptor antagonists JNJ7777120 and VUF6002. XXXVth Meeting of the European Histamine Research Society, Delphi, Greece.

103. Kitbunnadaj, R., Zuiderveld, O.P., Christophe, B. et al. 2004. Identification of 4-(1H-imidazol-4(5)-ylmethyl)pyridine (immethridine) as novel, potent, and highly selective histamine H_3 receptor agonist. *J. Med. Chem.* 47:2414–2417.

104. Blandizzi, C., Tognetti, M., Colucci, R., and Del Tacca, M. 2000. Histamine H_3 receptors mediate inhibition of noradrenaline release from intestinal sympathetic nerves. *Br. J. Pharmacol.* 129:1387–1396.

105. Poli, E., Pozzoli, C., and Bertaccini, G. 1997. Interaction between histamine H_3 receptors and other prejunctional receptor systems in the isolated guinea pig duodenum. *J. Pharmacol. Exp. Ther.* 281:393–399.

106. Poli, E., Pozzoli, C., Coruzzi, G., and Bertaccini, G. 1994. Signal transducing mechanisms coupled to histamine H_3 receptors and $α_2$ adrenoceptors in the guinea pig duodenum: possible involvement of N-type Ca^{2+} channels. *J. Pharmacol. Exp. Ther.* 270:788–794.

107. Pozzoli, C., Todorov, S., Schunack, W., Timmerman, H., Coruzzi, G., and Poli, E. 2002. Role of histamine H_3 receptors in control of mouse intestinal motility *in vivo* and *in vitro*: comparison with $α_2$-adrenoceptors. *Dig. Dis. Sci.* 47:1065–1072.

108. Oishi, R., Adachi, N., and Saeki, K. 1993. $N^α$-methylhistamine inhibits intestinal transit in mice by central histamine H_1 receptor activation. *Eur. J. Pharmacol.* 237:155–159.

109. Poli, E., Pozzoli, C., and Coruzzi, G. 2001. Role of histamine H_3 receptors in the control of gastrointestinal motility. An overview. *J. Physiol. Paris* 95:67–74.

110. Fargeas, M.J., Fioramonti, J., and Bueno, L. 1989. Involvement of different receptors in the central and peripheral effects of histamine on intestinal motility in the rat. *J. Pharm. Pharmacol.* 41:534–540.

111. Hemedah, M., and Mitchelson, F. 1997. Comparison of the effects of histamine and N$^\alpha$-methylhistamine on neuronal function in the guinea-pig oesophagus and ileum. *J. Pharm. Pharmacol.* 49:1217–1221.

112. Todorov, S., Pozzoli, C., Zamfirova, R., and Poli, E. 2003. Prejunctional modulation of non-adrenergic non-cholinergic (NANC) inhibitory responses in the isolated guinea-pig gastric fundus. *Neurogastroenterol. Motil.* 15:299–306.

113. Hew, R.W., Hodgkinson, C.R., and Hill, S.J. 1990. Characterization of histamine H$_3$-receptors in guinea-pig ileum with H$_3$-selective ligands. *Br. J. Pharmacol.* 101:621–624.

114. Leurs, R., Brozius, M.M., Smit, M.J., Bast, A., and Timmerman, H. 1991. Effects of histamine H$_1$-, H$_2$- and H$_3$-receptor selective drugs on the mechanical activity of guinea-pig small and large intestine. *Br. J. Pharmacol.* 102:179–185.

115. Perez-Garcia, C., Morales, L., and Alguacil, L.F. 1998. Histamine H$_3$ receptor desensitization in the guinea-pig ileum. *Eur. J. Pharmacol.* 341:253–256.

116. Lee, J.J., and Parsons, M.E. 2000. Signaling mechanisms coupled to presynaptic A$_1$- and H$_3$-receptors in the inhibition of cholinergic contractile responses of the guinea pig ileum. *J. Pharmacol. Exp. Ther.* 295:607–613.

117. Poli, E., Menozzi, A., Pozzoli, C. et al. 2004. Functional characterization of the novel histamine H$_3$ receptor agonist, VUF 5810, on the guinea-pig isolated ileum. *Inflamm. Res.* 53 (Suppl. 1):S77–S78.

118. Lees, G.M., and Steel, M.C. 1990. Histamine H$_3$-receptor-mediated inhibition of cholinergic and non-adrenergic, non-cholinergic neuro-effector transmission in guinea-pig isolated ileum. *Eur. J. Pharmacol.* 183:1145.

119. Menkveld, G.J., and Timmerman, H. 1990. Inhibition of electrically-evoked contractions of guinea-pig ileum preparations mediated by the histamine H$_3$ receptor. *Eur. J. Pharmacol.* 186:343–347.

120. Taylor, S.J., and Kilpatrick, G.J. 1992. Characterization of histamine-H$_3$ receptors controlling non-adrenergic non-cholinergic contractions of the guinea pig isolated ileum. *Br. J. Pharmacol.* 105:667–674.

121. Poli, E., and Pozzoli, C. 1997. Histamine H$_3$ receptors do not modulate reflex-evoked peristaltic motility in the isolated guinea-pig ileum. *Eur. J. Pharmacol.* 327:49–56.

122. Izzo, A.A., Costa, M., Mascolo, N., and Capasso, F. 1998. The role of histamine H$_1$, H$_2$ and H$_3$ receptors on enteric ascending synaptic transmission in the guinea pig ileum. *J. Pharmacol. Exp. Ther.* 287:952–957.

123. Poli, E., Coruzzi, G., and Bertaccini, G. 1991. Histamine H$_3$ receptors regulate acetylcholine release from the guinea pig ileum myenteric plexus. *Life Sci.* 48:PL63–PL68.

124. Yau, W.M., and Youther, M.L. 1993. Selective inhibition of acetylcholine release from myenteric plexus by histamine$_3$ receptor activation. *Gastroenterology* 104(Suppl.):A605.

125. Blandizzi, C., Colucci, R., Tognetti, M., De Polis, B., and Del Tacca, M. 2001. H$_3$ receptor-mediated inhibition of intestinal acetylcholine release: pharmacological characterization of signal transduction pathways. *Naunyn-Schmiedeberg's Arch. Pharmacol.* 363:193–202.

126. Bertaccini, G., Morini, G., Coruzzi, G., and Schunack, W. 2000. Histamine H$_3$ receptors in the guinea pig ileum: evidence for a postjunctional location. *J. Physiol. Paris* 94:1–4.

127. Tamura, K., Palmer, J.M., and Wood, J.D. 1988. Presynaptic inhibition produced by histamine at nicotinic synapses in enteric ganglia. *Neuroscience* 25:171–179.

128. Pozzoli, C., Poli, E., Costa, A., and De Ponti, F. 1997. Absence of histamine H$_3$ receptors in the rabbit colon: species difference. *Gen. Pharmacol.* 28:217–221.

129. West, R.E., Zweig, A., Shih, N.Y., Siegel, M.I., Egan, R.W., and Clark, M.A. 1990. Identification of two H$_3$ histamine receptor subtypes. *Mol. Pharmacol.* 38:610–613.

130. Schlicker, E., Kathmann, M., Reidemeister, S., Stark, H., and Schunack, W. 1994. Novel histamine H$_3$ receptor antagonists: affinities in an H$_3$ receptor binding assay and potencies in two functional H$_3$ receptor models. *Br. J. Pharmacol.* 112:1043–1048.

131. Kathmann, M., Schlicker, E., Detzner, M., and Timmerman, H. 1993. Nordimaprit, homodimaprit, clobenpropit and imetit: affinities for H_3 binding sites and potencies in a functional H_3 receptor model. *Naunyn-Schmiedeberg's Arch. Pharmacol.* 348:498–503.

132. Rizzo, C.A., Tozzi, S., Monahan, M.E., and Hey, J.A. 1995. Pharmacological characterization of histamine H_3 receptors in isolated guinea pig pulmonary artery and ileum. *Eur. J. Pharmacol.* 294:329–335.

133. Harper, E.A., Shankley, N.P., and Black, J.W. 1999. Evidence that histamine homologues discriminate between H_3-receptors in guinea-pig cerebral cortex and ileum longitudinal muscle myenteric plexus. *Br. J. Pharmacol.* 128:751–759.

134. Schwörer, H., Reimann, A., Ramadori, G., and Racke, K. 1994. Characterization of histamine H_3 receptors inhibiting 5-HT release from porcine enterochromaffin cells: further evidence for H_3 receptor heterogeneity. *Naunyn-Schmiedeberg's Arch. Pharmacol.* 350:375–379.

135. Leurs, R., Kathmann, M., Vollinga, R.C., Menge, W.M., Schlicker, E., and Timmerman, H. 1996. Histamine homologues discriminating between two functional H_3 receptor assays. Evidence for H_3 receptor heterogeneity? *J. Pharmacol. Exp. Ther.* 276:1009–1015.

136. Bauer, O., and Razin, E. 2000. Mast cell-nerve interactions. *News Physiol. Sci.* 15:213–218.

137. Penissi, A.B., Rudolph, M.I., and Piezzi, R.S. 2003. Role of mast cells in gastrointestinal mucosal defense. *Biocell* 27:163–172.

138. Cooke, H.J., and Reddix, R.A. 1994. Neural regulation of intestinal electrolyte transport. In *Physiology of the Gastrointestinal Tract*, ed. L.R. Johnson, pp. 2083–2132. New York: Raven Press.

139. Wood, J.D. 2004. Enteric neuroimmunophysiology and pathophysiology. *Gastroenterology* 127:635–657.

140. Cooke, H.J., and Wang, Y.Z. 1994. H_3 receptors: modulation of histamine-stimulated neural pathways influencing electrogenic ion transport in the guinea pig colon. *J. Auton. Nerv. Syst.* 50:201–207.

141. Frieling, T., Cooke, H.J., and Wood, J.D. 1994. Neuroimmune communication in the submucous plexus of guinea pig colon after sensitization to milk antigens. *Am. J. Physiol.* 267:G1087–G1093.

142. Liu, S., Xia, Y., Hu, H., Ren, J., Gao, C., and Wood, J.D. 2000. Histamine H_3 receptor-mediated suppression of inhibitory synaptic transmission in the submucous plexus of guinea-pig small intestine. *Eur. J. Pharmacol.* 397:49–54.

143. Liu, S., Hu, H.Z., Gao, N. et al. 2003. Neuroimmune interactions in guinea pig stomach and small intestine. *Am. J. Physiol.* 284:G154–G164.

144. Schultheiss, G., Hennig, B., Schunack, W., Prinz, G., and Diener. M. 2006. Histamine-induced ion secretion across rat distal colon: involvement of histamine H_1 and H_2 receptors. *Eur. J. Pharmacol.* 546:161–170.

145. Rangachari, P.K., and Prior, T. 1994. Functional subtyping of histamine receptors on the canine proximal colonic mucosa. *J. Pharmacol. Exp. Ther.* 271:1016–1026.

146. Ahrens, F., Gabel, G., Garz, B., and Aschenbach, J.R. 2003. Histamine-induced chloride secretion is mediated via H_2-receptors in the pig proximal colon. *Inflamm. Res.* 52:79–85.

147. Keely, S.J., Stack, W.A., O'Donoghue, D.P., and Baird, A.W. 1995. Regulation of ion transport by histamine in human colon. *Eur. J. Pharmacol.* 279:203–209.

148. Raithel, M., Matek, M., Baenkler, H.W., Jorde, W., and Hahn, E.G. 1995. Mucosal histamine content and histamine secretion in Crohn's disease, ulcerative colitis and allergic enteropathy. *Int. Arch. Allergy Immunol.* 108:127–133.

149. Nosalova, V., Ondrejickova, O., and Pecivova, J. 1999. Effects of histamine H_1 antagonist dithiaden on acetic acid-induced colitis in rats. *Physiol. Rev.* 48:65–72.

150. Tsunada, S., Fujimoto, K., Gotoh, Y. et al. 1994. Role of histamine receptors in intestinal repair after ischemia-reperfusion in rats. *Gastroenterology* 107:1297–1304.
151. Nosalova, V., Cerna, S., Schunack, W., Grandi, D., and Coruzzi, G. 2001. Effects of (R)α-methylhistamine on experimental colitis. *Inflamm. Res.* 50(Suppl 2):S108–S109.
152. Krause, M., Rouleau, A., Stark, H., Garbarg, M., Schwartz, J.C., and Schunack, W. 1996. Structure–activity relationships of novel azomethine prodrugs of the histamine H_3-receptor agonist (R)-α-methylhistamine: from alkylaryl to substituted diaryl derivatives. *Pharmazie* 51:720–726.
153. Coruzzi, G., Poli, E., Pozzoli, C. et al. 2002. Effect of BP 2.94, a histamine H_3-receptor agonist prodrug, on different models of colitis. *Inflamm. Res.* 51(Suppl. 1):S31–S32.
154. Perdue, M.H., Chung, M., and Gall, D.G. 1984. Effect of intestinal anaphylaxis on gut function in the rat. *Gastroenterology* 86:391–397.
155. Barbara, G., Wang, B., Stanghellini, V. et al. 2007. Mast-cell-dependent excitation of visceral-nociceptive sensory neurons in irritable bowel sindrome. *Gastroenterology* 132:26–37.
156. Kreis, M.E., Jiang, W., Kirkup, A.J., and Grundy, D. 2002. Co-sensitivity of vagal mucosal to histamine and 5-HT in the rat jejunum. *Am. J. Physiol.* 283:G612–G617.
157. Fu, L.W., Pan, H.L., and Longhurst, J.C. 1997. Endogenous histamine stimulates ischemically sensitive abdominal visceral afferents through H_1 receptors. *Am. J. Physiol.* 273:H2726–H2737.
158. Brunsden, A.M., and Grundy, D. 1999. Sensitization of visceral afferents to bradykinin in rat jejunum *in vitro*. *J. Physiol.* 521:517–527.
159. Coelho, A.M., Fioramonti, J., and Bueno, L. 1998. Mast cell degranulation induces delayed rectal allodynia in rats: role of histamine and 5-HT. *Dig. Dis. Sci.* 43:727–737.
160. McNeill, J.H. 1984. Histamine and the heart. *Can. J. Physiol. Pharmacol.* 62:720–726.
161. Levi, R., Rubin, L.E., and Gross, S.S. 1991. Histamine in cardiovascular function and dysfunction: recent developments. In *Handbook Experimental Pharmacology 97: Histamine and Histamine Antagonists,* ed. B. Uvnas, pp. 347–383. Berlin: Springer.
162. Göthert, M., Garbarg, M., Hey, J.A., Schlicker, E., Schwartz, J.C., and Levi, R. 1995. New aspects of the role of histamine in cardiovascular function: identification, characterization, and potential pathophysiological importance of H_3 receptors. *Can. J. Physiol. Pharmacol.* 73:558–564.
163. Malinowska, B., Godlewski, G., and Schlicker, E. 1998. Histamine H_3 receptors. General characterization and their function in the cardiovascular system. *J. Physiol. Pharmacol.* 49:191–211.
164. Levi, R., and Smith, N.C. 2000. Histamine H_3-receptors: a new frontier in myocardial ischemia. *J. Pharmacol. Exp. Ther.* 292:825–830.
165. Levi, R., Rubin, L.E., and Gross, S.S. 1991. Histamine in cardiovascular function and dysfunction: recent developments. In *Handbook Experimental Pharmacology 97, Histamine and Histamine Antagonist,* ed. B. Uvnas, pp. 347–383. Berlin: Springer.
166. Luo, X.X., Tan, Y.H., and Sheng, B.H. 1991. Histamine H_3-receptors inhibit sympathetic neurotransmission in guinea pig myocardium. *Eur. J. Pharmacol.* 204:311–314.
167. Ichinose, M., Belvisi, M.G., and Barnes, P.J. 1990. Histamine H_3-receptors inhibit neurogenic microvascular leakage in airways. *J. Appl. Physiol.* 68:21–25.
168. Ohkubo, T., Shibata, M., Inoue, M., Kaya, H., and Takahashi, H. 1995. Regulation of substance P release mediated *via* prejunctional histamine H_3 receptors. *Eur. J. Pharmacol.* 273:83–88.
169. Imamura, M., Smith, N.C.E., Garbarg, M., and Levi, R. 1996. Histamine H_3-receptors-mediated inhibition of calcitonin gene-related peptide release from cardiac C-fibers. *Circ. Res.* 78:863–869.
170. Li, M., Hu, J., Chen, Z. et al. 2006. Evidence for histamine as a neurotransmitter in the cardiac sympathetic nervous system. *Am. J. Physiol.* 291:H45–H51.

171. Koyama, M., Heerdt, P.M., and Levi, R. 2003. Increased severity of reperfusion arrhythmias in mouse hearts lacking histamine H_3-receptors. *Biochem. Biophys. Res. Commun.* 306:792–796.

172. Maggi, M.B., and Curtis, M.J. 1994. The antiarrhythmic effects of thioperamide in isolated rat heart. *Br. J. Pharmacol.* 113:179P.

173. Fuder, H., Ries, P., and Schwartz, P. 1994. Histamine and serotonin released from the rat perfused heart by compound 48/80 or by allergen challenge influence noradrenaline or acetylcholine exocytotic release. *Fundam. Clin. Pharmacol.* 8:477–490.

174. Yamamoto, S., Tamai, I., Takaoka, M., and Matsumura, Y. 2004. Role of histamine H_3 receptors during ischemia/reperfusion in isolated rat hearts. *J. Cardiovasc. Pharmacol.* 43:353–357.

175. Mazenot, C., Durand, A., Ribuot, C., Demenge, P., and Godin-Ribuot, D. 1999. Histamine H_3-receptor stimulation is unable to modulate noradrenaline release by the isolated rat heart during ischaemia-reperfusion. *Fundam. Clin. Pharmacol.* 13:455–460.

176. Malinowska, B., and Schlicker, E. 1993. Identification of endothelial H_1, vascular H_2 and cardiac presynaptic H_3 receptors in the pithed rat. *Naunyn-Schmiedeberg's Arch. Pharmacol.* 347:55–60.

177. Hegde, S.S., Chan, P., and Eglen, R.M. 1994. Cardiovascular effects of R-α-methylhistamine, a selective histamine H_3 receptor agonist, in rats: lack of involvement of histamine H_3 receptors. *Eur. J. Pharmacol.* 251:43–51.

178. Coruzzi, G., Gambarelli, E., Bertaccini, G., and Timmerman, H. 1995. Cardiovascular effects of selective agonists and antagonists of histamine H_3 receptors in the anaesthetized rat. *Naunyn-Schmiedeberg's Arch. Pharmacol.* 351:569–575.

179. McLeod, R.L., Gertner, S.B., and Hey, J.A. 1994. Species differences in the cardiovascular responses to histamine H_3 receptor activation. *Eur. J. Pharmacol.* 259:211–214.

180. Oudart, N., Javellaud, J., and Ea Kim, L. 1995. A histamine H_3-agonist attenuates the cardiovascular response to nicotine in rats. *Pharmacol. Res.* 31(Suppl.):250.

181. Luo, X.X., Wen, A.D., Guo, Z.A., and Tan, Y.H. 1996. Direct evidence for histamine H_3 receptor-mediated inhibition of norepinephrine release from sympathetic terminals of guinea pig myocardium. *Acta Pharmacol. Sin.* 17:425–428.

182. Endou, M., Poli, E., and Levi, R. 1994. Histamine H_3-receptor signaling in the heart: possible involvement of G_i/G_o proteins and N-type Ca^{2+} channels. *J. Pharmacol. Exp. Ther.* 269:221–229.

183. Charles, J., Angus, J.A., and Wright, C.E. 2003. Central endogenous histamine modulates sympathetic outflow through H_3 receptors in the conscious rabbit. *Br. J. Pharmacol.* 139:1023–1031.

184. Imamura, M., Poli, E., Omoniyi, A.T., and Levi, R. 1994. Unmasking of activated histamine H_3-receptors in myocardial ischemia: their role as regulators of exocytotic norepinephrine release. *J. Pharmacol. Exp. Ther.* 271:1259–1266.

185. Imamura, M., Lander, H.M., and Levi, R. 1996. Activation of histamine H_3-receptors inhibits carrier-mediated norepinephrine release during protracted myocardial ischemia. *Circ. Res.* 78:475–481.

186. Akagi, M., Hamada, K., Nishioka, E., Fukuishi, N., and Akagi, R. 1995. Role of histamine H_3 receptor on hypoxia-reoxygenation induced cardiac dysfunction in guinea pigs. *Meth. Find. Exp. Clin. Pharmacol.* 17:30–35.

187. Ea-Kim, L., Javellaud, J., and Oudart, N. 1993. Histamine H_3 agonist decreases arterial blood pressure in the guinea-pig. *J. Pharm. Pharmacol.* 45:929–931.

188. Ea-Kim, L., Javellaud, J., and Oudart, N. 1996. Reduction of the pressor response to nicotine in the guinea pig by a histamine H_3 agonist is attenuated by an inhibitor of nitric oxide synthesis. *J. Cardiovasc. Pharmacol.* 27:607–613.

189. Hey, J.A., del Prado, M., Egan, R.W., Kreutner, W., and Chapman, R.W. 1992. Inhibition of sympathetic hypertensive responses in the guinea-pig by prejunctional histamine H_3 receptors. *Br. J. Pharmacol.* 107:347–351.

190. Hutchison, R.W., and Hey, J.A. 1994. Pharmacological characterization of the inhibitory effect of (R)-α-methylhistamine on sympathetic cardiopressor responses in the pithed guinea-pig. *J. Auton. Pharmacol.* 14:393–402.

191. Li, X., Eschun, G., Bose, D. et al. 1998. Histamine H_3 activation depresses cardiac function in experimental sepsis. *J. Appl. Physiol.* 85:1693–1701.

192. Yamasaki, T., Tamai, I., and Matsumura, Y. 2001. Activation of histamine H_3 receptors inhibits renal noradrenergic neurotransmission in anesthetized dogs. *Am. J. Physiol.* 280:R1450–R1456.

193. Chrusch, C., Sharma, S., Unruh, H. et al. 1999. Histamine H_3 receptor blockade improves cardiac function in canine anaphylaxis. *Am. J. Respir. Crit. Care Med.* 160:1142–1149.

194. Mazenot, C., Ribuot, C., Durand, A., Joulin, Y., Demenge, P., and Godin-Ribuot, D. 1999. *In vivo* demonstration of H_3-histaminergic inhibition of cardiac sympathetic stimulation by R-α-methyl-histamine and its prodrug BP 2.94 in the dog. *Br. J. Pharmacol.* 126:264–268.

195. Hatta, E., Yasuda, K., and Levi, R. 1997. Activation of histamine H_3 receptors inhibits carrier-mediated norepinephrine release in a human model of protracted myocardial ischemia. *J. Pharmacol. Exp. Ther.* 283:494–500.

196. Imamura, M., Seyedi, N., Lander, H.M., and Levi, R. 1995. Functional identification of histamine H_3-receptors in the human heart. *Circ. Res.* 77:206–210.

197. Hill, S.J., Ganellin, C.R., Timmerman, H. et al. 1997. International Union of Pharmacology. XIII. Classification of histamine receptors. *Pharmacol. Rev.* 49:253–278.

198. Schomig, A. 1990. Catecholamines in myocardial ischemia. Systematic and cardiac release. *Circulation* 82:13–22.

199. Silver, R.B., Poonwasi, K.S., Seyedi, N., Wilson, S.J., Lovenberg, T.W., and Levi, R. 2002. Decreased intracellular calcium mediates the histamine H_3-receptor-induced attenuation of norepinephrine exocytosis from cardiac sympathetic nerve endings. *Proc. Natl Acad. Sci. U.S.A.* 99:501–506.

200. Seyedi, N., Mackins, C.J., Machida, T., Reid, A.C., Silver, R.B., and Levi, R. 2005. Histamine H_3-receptor-induced attenuation of norepinephrine exocytosis: a decreased protein kinase A activity mediates a reduction in intracellular calcium. *J. Pharmacol. Exp. Ther.* 312:272–280.

201. Silver, R.B., Mackins, C.J., Smith, N.C. et al. 2001. Coupling of histamine H_3 receptors to neuronal Na^+/H^+ exchange: a novel protective mechanism in myocardial ischemia. *Proc. Natl Acad. Sci. U.S.A.* 98:2855–2859.

202. Koyama, M., Seyedi, N., Fung-Leung, W.P., Lovenberg, T.W., and Levi, R. 2003. Norepinephrine release from the ischemic heart is greatly enhanced in mice lacking histamine H_3 receptors. *Mol. Pharmacol.* 63:378–382.

203. Levi, R., Seyedi, N., and Schafer, U. 2007. Histamine H_3-receptor signalling in cardiac sympathetic nerves: identification of a novel $MAPK$-PLA_2-COX-PGE_2-EP_3R pathway. *Biochem. Pharmacol.* 73:1146–1156.

204. Godlewski, G., Malinowska, B., Schlicker, E., and Bucher, B. 1997. Identification of histamine H_3-receptors in the tail artery from normotensive and spontaneously hypertensive rats. *J. Cardiovasc. Pharmacol.* 29:801–807.

205. Schneider, D., Schlicker, E., Malinowska, B., and Molderings, G. 1991. Noradrenaline release in the rat vena cava is inhibited by y-aminobutyric acid *via* $GABA_B$ receptors but not affected by histamine. *Br. J. Pharmacol.* 104:478–482.

206. Malinowska, B., and Schlicker, E. 1991. H_3 receptor-mediated inhibition of the neurogenic vasopressor response in pithed rats. *Eur. J. Pharmacol.* 205:307–310.

207. Godlewski, G., Malinowska, B., Buczko, W., and Schlicker, E. 1997. Inhibitory H_3 receptors on sympathetic nerves of the pithed rat: activation by endogenous histamine and operation in spontaneously hypertensive rats. *Naunyn-Schmiedeberg's Arch. Pharmacol.* 355:261–266.
208. Räntfors, J., and Cassuto, J. 2003. Role of histamine receptors in the regulation of edema and circulation postburn. *Burns* 29:769–777.
209. Obuchowicz, R., Pawlik, M.W., Brzozowski, T., Konturek, S.J., and Pawlik, W.W. 2004. Involvement of central and peripheral histamine H_3 receptors in the control of the vascular tone and oxygen uptake in the mesenteric circulation of the rat. *J. Physiol. Pharmacol.* 55:255–267.
210. Smit, J., Coppes, R.P., van Tintelen, E.J.J., Roffel, A.F., and Zaagsma, J. 1997. Prejunctional histamine H_3-receptors inhibit electrically evoked endogenous noradrenaline overflow in the portal vein of freely moving rats. *Naunyn-Schmiedeberg's Arch. Pharmacol.* 355:256–260.
211. Acuña, Y., Mathison, Y., Campos, H.A., and Israel, A. 1998. Thioperamide, a histamine H_3-receptor blocker, facilitates vasopressor response to footshocks. *Inflamm. Res.* 47:109–114.
212. Ishikawa, S., and Sperelakis, N. 1987. A novel class H_3 of histamine receptors on perivascular nerve terminals. *Nature* 327:158–160.
213. Beyak, M., and Vanner, S. 1995. Histamine H_1 and H_3 vasodilator mechanisms in the guinea pig ileum. *Gastroenterology* 108:712–718.
214. Mink, S., Becker, A., Sharma, S., Unruh, H., Duke, K., and Kepron, W. 1999. Role of autacoids in cardiovascular collapse in anaphylactic shock in anaesthetized dogs. *Cardiovasc. Res.* 43:173–182.
215. Molderings, G.J., Weissenborn, G., Schlicker, E., Likungu, J., and Gothert, M. 1992. Inhibition of noradrenaline release from the sympathetic nerves of the human saphenous vein by presynaptic histamine H_3 receptors. *Naunyn-Schmiedeberg's Arch. Pharmacol.* 346:46–50.
216. Valentine, A.F., Rizzo, C.A., Rivelli, M.A., and Hey, J.A. 1999. Pharmacological characterization of histamine H_3 receptors in human saphenous vein and guinea pig ileum. *Eur. J. Pharmacol.* 366:73–78.
217. Djuric, D.M., and Andjelkovic, I.Z. 1995. The evidence for histamine H_3 receptor-mediated endothelium-dependent relaxation in isolated rat aorta. *Mediators Inflammation* 4:217–221.
218. Djuric, D.M., Nesic, M.T., and Andjelkovic, I.Z. 1996. Endothelium-dependent relaxation of rat aorta to a histamine H_3 agonist is reduced by inhibitors of nitric oxide synthase, guanylate cyclase and Na^+, K^+-ATPase. *Mediators Inflammation* 5:69–74.
219. Adeagbo, A.S., and Oriowo, M.A. 1998. Histamine receptor subtypes mediating hyperpolarization in the isolated perfused rat mesenteric pre-arteriolar bed. *Eur. J. Pharmacol.* 347:237–244.
220. Lau, W.H., Kwan, Y.W., Au, A.L., and Cheung, W.H. 2003. An *in vitro* study of histamine on the pulmonary artery of the Wistar-Kyoto and spontaneously hypertensive rats. *Eur. J. Pharmacol.* 470:45–55.
221. Kostic, M.M., and Jakovljevic, V.L.J. 1996. Role of histamine in the regulation of coronary circulation. *Physiol. Res.* 45:297–303.
222. Rosic, M., Collis, C.S., Anjelkovic, I.Z., Segal, M.B., Djuric, D., and Zlokovic, B.V. 1991. The effects of (R) α-methyl histamine on the isolated guinea pig aorta. *Agents Actions* 33(Suppl.):283–287.
223. Pierpaoli, S., Marzocco, C., Bello, M.G., Schunack, W., Mannaioni, P.F., and Masini, E. 2003. Histaminergic receptors modulate the coronary vascular response in isolated guinea pig hearts. Role of nitric oxide. *Inflamm. Res.* 52:390–396.

224. Ea-Kim, L., and Oudart, N. 1988. A highly potent and selective H$_3$ agonist relaxes rabbit middle cerebral artery, *in vitro. Eur. J. Pharmacol.* 150:393–396.

225. Ea-Kim, L., Javellaud, J., and Oudart, N. 1992. Endothelium-dependent relaxation of rabbit middle cerebral artery to a histamine H$_3$-agonist is reduced by inhibitors of nitric oxide and prostacyclin synthesis. *Br. J. Pharmacol.* 105:103–106.

226. Oike, M., Kitamura, K., and Kuriyama, H. 1992. Histamine H$_3$-receptor activation augments voltage-dependent Ca^{2+} current via GTP hydrolysis in rabbit saphenous artery. *J. Physiol.* 448:133–152.

227. Neely, C.F., Matot, I., Haile, D., Nguyen, J., and Batra, V. 1995. Tone-dependent responses of histamine in feline pulmonary vascular bed. *Am. J. Physiol.* 268:H653–H661.

228. Champion, H.C., and Kadowitz, P.J. 1998. R-(-)-α-methyl-histamine has nitric oxide-mediated vasodilator activity in the mesenteric vascular bed of the cat. *Eur. J. Pharmacol.* 343:209–216.

229. Arai, M., and Chiba, S. 1999. Endothelium-dependent vasodilatation mechanisms by histamine in simian but not in canine femoral arterial branches. *J. Auton. Pharmacol.* 19:267–273.

230. Martinez, A.C., Novella, S., Raposo, R., Recio, P., Labadia, A., and Costa, G. 1997. Histamine receptors in isolated bovine oviductal arteries. *Eur. J. Pharmacol.* 326:163–173.

231. Bull, H.A., Courtney, P.F., Rustin, M.H., and Dowd, P.M. 1992. Characterization of histamine receptor sub-types regulating prostacyclin release from human endothelial cells. *Br. J. Pharmacol.* 107:276–281.

232. Li, H., Burkhardt, C., Heinrich, U.R., Brausch, I., Xia, N., and Forstermann, U. 2003. Histamine upregulates gene expression of endothelial nitric oxide synthase in human vascular endothelial cells. *Circulation* 107:2348–2354.

233. Martinez, A.C., Prieto, D., and Raposo, R. 2000. Endothelium-independent relaxation induced by histamine in human dorsal penile artery. *Clin. Exp. Pharmacol. Physiol.* 27:500–507.

234. Campos, H.A., Acuña, Y., Magaldi, L., and Israel, A. 1996. Alpha-fluoromethylhistidine, an inhibitor of histamine biosynthesis causes arterial hypertension. *Naunyn-Schmiedeberg's Arch. Pharmacol.* 354:627–632.

235. Barnes, P.J. 1992. Histamine receptors in the respiratory tract. In *The Histamine Receptor*, eds. J.C. Schwartz, and H.L. Haas, pp. 253–270. New York: Wiley-Liss.

236. Sirois, J., Menard, G., Moses, A.S., and Bissonnette, E.Y. 2000. Importance of histamine in the cytokine network in the lung through H$_2$ and H$_3$ receptors: stimulation of IL-10 production. *J. Immunol.* 164:2964–2970.

237. Nakaya, M., Fukushima, Y., Takeuchi, N., and Kaga, K. 2005. Nasal allergic response mediated by histamine H$_3$ receptors in murine allergic rhinitis. *Laryngoscope* 115:1778–1784.

238. Dimitriadou, V., Rouleau, A., Dam Trung Tuong, M. et al. 1994. Functional relationship between mast cells and C-sensitive nerve fibers evidenced by histamine H$_3$-receptor modulation in rat lung and spleen. *Clin. Sci.* 87:151–163.

239. Bockman, C.S., and Zeng, W. 2002. Histamine receptor type coupled to nitric oxide-induced relaxation of guinea-pig nasal mucosa. *Auton. Autacoid Pharmacol.* 22:269–276.

240. Cardell, L.O., and Edvinsson, L. 1994. Characterization of the histamine receptors in the guinea-pig lung: evidence for relaxant histamine H$_3$ receptors in the trachea. *Br. J. Pharmacol.* 111:445–454.

241. Burgaud, J.L., and Oudart, N. 1993. Effect of an histaminergic H$_3$ agonist on the non-adrenergic non-cholinergic contraction in guinea-pig perfused bronchioles. *J. Pharm. Pharmacol.* 45:955–958.

242. Burgaud, J.L., and Oudart, N. 1993. Bronchodilatation of guinea-pig perfused bronchioles induced by the H_3-receptor for histamine: role of epithelium. *Br. J. Pharmacol.* 109:960–966.

243. Allen, M.C., Graham, P., and Morris, G. 1996. Histamine forming capacity (HFC) and its modulation by H_3 receptor ligands in a model of bronchial hyper-responsiveness. *Inflamm. Res.* 45:118–122.

244. Ichinose, M., Stretton, C.D., Schwartz, J.C., and Barnes, P.J. 1989. Histamine H_3-receptors inhibit cholinergic neurotransmission in guinea-pig airways. *Br. J. Pharmacol.* 97:13–15.

245. Danko, G., Hey, J.A., Egan, R.W., Kreutner, W., and Chapman, R.W. 1994. Histamine H_3 receptors inhibit sympathetic modulation of airway microvascular leakage in allergic guinea pigs. *Eur. J. Pharmacol.* 254:283–286.

246. Ichinose, M., and Barnes, P.J. 1989. Histamine H_3-receptors modulate nonadrenergic noncholinergic neural bronchoconstriction in guinea-pig *in vivo. Eur. J. Pharmacol.* 174:49–55.

247. Hey, J.A., del Prado, M., Egan, R.W., Kreutner, W., and Chapman, R.W. 1992. (R)-α-methylhistamine augments neural, cholinergic bronchospasm in guinea pigs by histamine H_1-receptor activation. *Eur. J. Pharmacol.* 211:421–426.

248. Delaunois, A., Gustin, P., Garbarg, M., and Ansay, M. 1995. Modulation of acetylcholine, capsaicin and substance P effects by histamine H_3 receptors in isolated perfused rabbit lungs. *Eur. J. Pharmacol.* 277:243–250.

249. Nemmar, A., Delaunois, A., Beckers, J.F., Sulon, J., Bloden, S., and Gustin, P. 1999. Modulatory effect of imetit, a histamine H_3 receptor agonist, on C-fibers, cholinergic fibers and mast cells in rabbit lungs in vitro. *Eur. J. Pharmacol.* 371:23–30.

250. McLeod, R.L., Mingo, G.G., Herczku, C. et al. 1999. Combined histamine H_1 and H_3 receptor blockade produces nasal decongestion in an experimental model of nasal congestion. *Am. J. Rhinol.* 13:391–399.

251. Varty, L.M., and Hey, J.A. 2002. Histamine H_3 receptor activation inhibits neurogenic sympathetic vasoconstriction in porcine nasal mucosa. *Eur. J. Pharmacol.* 452:339–345.

252. Jolly, S., and Desmecht, D. 2003. Functional identification of epithelial and smooth muscle histamine-dependent relaxing mechanisms in the bovine trachea, but not in bronchi. *Comp. Biochem. Physiol. C Toxicol. Pharmacol.* 134:91–100.

253. Ichinose, M., and Barnes, P.J. 1989. Inhibitory histamine H_3-receptors on cholinergic nerves in human aiways. *Eur. J. Pharmacol.* 163:383–386.

254. Varty, L.M., Gustafson, E., Laverty, M., and Hey, J.A. 2004. Activation of histamine H_3 receptors in human nasal mucosa inhibits sympathetic vasoconstriction. *Eur. J. Pharmacol.* 484:83–89.

255. O'Connor, B.J., Lecomte, J.M., and Barnes, P.J. 1993. Effect of an inhaled histamine H_3-receptor agonist on airway responses to sodium metabisulphite in asthma. *Br. J. Clin. Pharmacol.* 35:55–57.

256. Fozard, J.R. 2000. BP-294 Ste Civile Bioprojet. *Curr. Opin. Investig. Drugs* 1:86–89.

257. Celanire, S., Wijtmans, M., Talaga, P., Leurs, R., and de Esch, I.J. 2005. Keynote review: histamine H_3 receptor antagonists reach out for the clinic. *Drug Discov. Today* 10:1613–1627.

258. Burns, S., and Hamley, P. 2005. Imidazol derivatives of piperidine as histamine antagonists. WO2005014579.

259. Uddman, R., Moller, S., Cardell, L.O., and Edvinsson, L. 1999. Expression of histamine H_1 and H_2 receptors in human nasal mucosa. *Acta Otolaryngol.* 119:588–591.

260. Nakaya, M., Takeuchi, N., and Kondo, K. 2004. Immunohistochemical localization of histamine receptor subtypes in human inferior turbinates. *Ann. Otol. Rhinol. Laryngol.* 113:552–557.

261. Anthes, J.C., West, R.E., Hey, J.A., and Aslanian, R.G. 2005. Combination of H_1, H_3 and H_4 receptor antagonists for treatment of allergic and non-allergic pulmonary inflammation, congestion and allergic rhinitis in my patent list. US2005090527.

262. Falus, A. 1994. Inflammation: the role of histamine. In *Histamine and Inflammation*, ed. A. Falus, pp. 63–77. Georgetown: Landes, R.G. Co.

263. Schneider, E., Rolli-Derkinderen, M., Arock, M., and Dy, M. 2002. Trends in histamine research: new functions during immune responses and hematopoiesis. *Trends Immunol.* 23:255–263.

264. Tanaka, S., and Ichikawa, A. 2006. Recent advances in molecular pharmacology of the histamine systems: immune regulatory roles of histamine produced by leukocytes. *J. Pharmacol. Sci.* 101:19–23.

265. Bartholeyns, J., and Fozard, J.R. 1985. Role of histamine in tumor development. *Trends Pharmacol. Sci.* 6:123–125.

266. Idzko, M., La Sala, A., Ferrari, D. et al. 2002. Expression and function of histamine receptors in human monocyte-derived dendritic cells. *J. Allergy Clin. Immunol.* 109:839–846.

267. Rouleau, A., Garbarg, M., Ligneau, X. et al. 1997. Bioavailability, antinociceptive and antiinflammatory properties of BP 2-94, a histamine H_3-receptor agonist prodrug. *J. Pharmacol. Exp. Ther.* 281:1085–1094.

268. Rouleau, A., Stark, H., Schunack, W., and Schwartz, J.C. 2000. Anti-inflammatory and antinociceptive properties of BP 2-94, a histamine H_3-receptor agonist prodrug. *J. Pharmacol. Exp. Ther.* 295:219–225.

269. Kohno, S., Nakao, S., Ogawa, K., Yamamura, H., Nabe, T., and Ohata, K. 1994. Possible participation of histamine H_3-receptors in the regulation of anaphylactic histamine release from isolated rat peritoneal mast cells. *Jpn. J. Pharmacol.* 66:173–180.

270. Stenton, G.R., and Lau, H.Y. 1997. Effects of histamine agonists and antagonists on rat peritoneal mast cells. *Inflamm. Res.* 46(Suppl. 1):S15–S16.

271. Rozniecki, J.J., Letourneau, R., Sugiultzoglu, M., Spanos, C., Gorbach, J., and Theoharides, T.C. 1999. Differential effects of histamine 3 receptor-active agents on brain, but not peritoneal, mast cell activation. *J. Pharmacol. Exp. Ther.* 290:1427–1435.

272. Bissonnette, E.Y. 1996. Histamine inhibits tumor necrosis factor α release by mast cells through H_2 and H_3 receptors. *Am. J. Respir. Cell. Mol. Biol.* 14:620–626.

273. Ohkubo, T., Shibata, M., Inoue, M., Kaya, H., and Takahashi, H. 1994. Autoregulation of histamine release via the histamine H_3 receptor on mast cells in the rat skin. *Arch. Int. Pharmacodyn.* 328:307–314.

274. Brain, S.D., Newbold, P., and Kajekar, R. 1995. Modulation of the release and activity of neuropeptides in the microcirculation. *Can. J. Physiol. Pharmacol.* 73:995–998.

275. Bent, S., Fehling, U., Braam, U., and Schmutzler, W. 1991. The influence of H_1-, H_2- and H_3-receptors on the spontaneous and ConA induced-histamine release from human adenoidal mast cells. *Agents Actions* 33:67–70.

276. He, S.H., Xie, H., and Fu, Y.L. 2005. Inhibition of tryptase release from human colon mast cells by histamine receptor antagonists. *Asian. Pac. J. Allergy Immunol.* 23:35–39.

277. Raible, D.G., Lenahan, T., Fayvilevich, Y., Kosinski, R., and Schulman, E.S. 1994. Pharmacological characterization of a novel histamine receptor on human eosinophils. *Am. J. Respir. Crit. Care Med.* 149:1506–1511.

278. Tedeschi, A., Lorini, M., Arquati, M., and Miadonna, A. 1991. Regulation of histamine release from human basophil leucocytes: role of H_1, H_2 and H_3 receptors. *Allergy* 46:626–631.

279. Kleine-Tebbe, J., Schramm, J., Bolz, M., Lipp, R., Schunack, W., and Kunkel, G. 1990. Influence of histamine H_3-antagonists on human leukocytes. *Agents Actions* 30:137–139.

280. Muller, T., Myrtek, D., Bayer, H. et al. 2006. Functional characterization of histamine receptor subtypes in a human bronchial epithelial cell line. *Int. J. Mol. Med.* 18:925–931.
281. Morichika, T., Takahashi, H.K., Iwagaki, H. et al. 2003. Histamine inhibits lipopolysaccharide-induced tumor necrosis factor-α production in an intercellular adhesion molecule-1- and B7.1-dependent manner. *J. Pharmacol. Exp. Ther.* 304:624–633.
282. Takahashi, H.K., Iwagaki, H., Mori, S., Yoshino, T., Tanaka, N., and Nishibori, M. 2004. Histamine inhibits lipopolysaccharide-induced interleukin (IL)-18 production in human monocytes. *Clin. Immunol.* 112:30–34.
283. Elenkov, I.J., Webster, E., Papanicolaou, D.A., Fleisher, T.A., Chrousos, G.P., and Wilder, R.L. 1998. Histamine potently suppresses human IL-12 and stimulates IL-10 production via H_2 receptors. *J. Immunol.* 161:2586–2593.
284. Kimata, H., Fujimoto, M., Ishioka, C., and Yoshida, A. 1996. Histamine selectivity enhances human immunoglobulin E (IgE) and IgG4 production induces by anti-CD58 monoclonal antibody. *J. Exp. Med.* 184:357–364.
285. Poveda, R., Fernández-Dueñas, V., Fernández, A., Sánchez, S., Puig, M., and Planas, E. 2006. Synergistic interaction between fentanyl and the histamine H_3 receptor agonist (R)α-methylhistamine, on the inhibition of nociception and plasma extravasation in mice. *Eur. J. Pharmacol.* 541:53–56.
286. Hossen, M.A., Fujii, Y., Sugimoto, Y., Kayasuga, R., and Kamei, C. 2003. Histamine H_3 receptors regulate vascular permeability changes in the skin of mast cell-deficient mice. *Int. Immunopharmacol.* 3:1563–1568.
287. McLeod, R.L., Mingo, G.G., Kreutner, W., and Hey, J.A. 2005. Effect of combined histamine H_1 and H_3 receptor blockade on cutaneous microvascular permeability elicited by compound 48/80. *Life Sci.* 76:1787–1794.
288. Kahlson, G., Rosengren, E., and Steinhardt, C. 1963. Histamine-forming capacity of multiplying cells. *J. Physiol. London.* 169:487–498.
289. LaBella, F.S., and Brandes, L.J. 2000. Interaction of histamine and other bioamines with cytochrome P450: implications for cell growth modulation and chemoprevention by drugs. *Cancer Biol.* 10:47–53.
290. Francis, H., Franchitto, A., Ueno, Y. et al. 2007. H_3 histamine receptor agonist inhibits biliary growth of BDL rats by downregulation of the cAMP-dependent PKA/ERK$_{1/2}$/ELK-1 pathway. *Lab. Invest.* 87:473–487.
291. Clark, M.A., Korte, A., Myers, J., and Egan, R.W. 1992. High affinity histamine H_3 receptors regulate ACTH release by AtT-20 cells. *Eur. J. Pharmacol.* 210:31–35.
292. Medina, V., Cricco, G., Nunez, M. et al. 2006. Histamine-mediated signaling processes in human malignant mammary cells. *Cancer Biol. Ther.* 5:1462–1471.
293. Karlstedt, K., Ahman, M.J., Anichtchik, O.V., Soinila, S., and Panula, P. 2003. Expression of the H_3 receptor in the developing CNS and brown fat suggests novel roles for histamine. *Mol. Cell. Neurosci.* 24:614–622.
294. Azuma, H., Sawada, S., Takeuchi, S., Higashiyama, K., Kakigi, A., and Takeda, T. 2003. Expression of mRNA encoding the H_1, H_2 and H_3 histamine receptors in the rat cochlea. *Neuroreport.* 14:423–425.
295. Lippert, U., Artuc, M., Grutzkau, A. et al. 2004. Human skin mast cells express H_2 and H_4, but not H_3 receptors. *J. Invest. Dermatol.* 123:116–123.
296. Sugimoto, Y., Iba, Y., Nakamura, Y., Kayasuga, R., and Kamei, C. 2004. Pruritus-associated response mediated by cutaneous histamine H_3 receptors. *Clin. Exp. Allergy* 34:456–459.
297. Hossen, M.A., Inoue, T., Shinmei, Y., Fujii, Y., Watanabe, T., and Kamei, C. 2006. Role of substance P on histamine H_3 antagonist-induced scratching behavior in mice. *J. Pharmacol. Sci.* 100:297–302.

298. Ashida, Y., Denda, M., and Hirao, T. 2001. Histamine H_1 and H_2 receptor antagonists accelerate skin barrier repair and prevent epidermal hyperplasia induced by barrier disruption in a dry environment. *J. Invest. Dermatol.* 116:261–265.

299. Koss, M.C. 1994. Histamine H_3 receptor activation inhibits sympathetic-cholinergic responses in cats. *Eur. J. Pharmacol.* 257:109–115.

300. Kavanagh, G.M., Sabroe, R.A., Greaves, M.W., and Archer, C.B. 1998. The intradermal effects of the H_3 receptor agonist (R)α-methylhistamine in human skin. *Br. J. Dermatol.* 138:622–626.

301. Yu, Y., Kawarai, M., and Koss, M.C. 2001. Histamine H_3 receptor-mediated inhibition of sympathetically evoked mydriasis in rats. *Eur. J. Pharmacol.* 419:55–59.

302. Yoshitomi, T., Ishikawa, H., Haruno, I., and Ishikawa, S. 1995. Effect of histamine and substance P on the rabbit and human iris sphincter muscle. *Graefe's Arch. Clin. Exp. Ophthalmol.* 233:181–185.

303. Koss, M.C., and Hey, J.A. 1993. Prejunctional inhibition of sympathetically evoked pupillary dilation in cats by activation of histamine H_3 receptors. *Naunyn-Schmiedeberg's Arch. Pharmacol.* 348:141–145.

304. Kamei, C.H. 1996. Effects of histamine and related compounds on the bovine iris dilator. *Methods Find. Exp. Clin. Pharmacol.* 18:273–278.

305. Schlicker, E., Schunack, W., and Gothert, M. 1990. Histamine H_3 receptor-mediated inhibition of noradrenaline release in pig retina discs. *Naunyn-Schmiedeberg's Arch. Pharmacol.* 342:497–501.

306. Markwardt, K.L., Magnino, P.E., and Pang, I.H. 1997. Histamine induced contraction of human ciliary muscle cells. *Exp. Eye Res.* 64:713–717.

307. Crawford, K.M., MacCallum, D.K., and Ernst, S.A. 1992. Histamine H_1 receptor-mediated Ca^{2+} signaling in cultured bovine corneal endothelial cells. *Invest. Ophthalmol. Vis. Sci.* 33:3041–3049.

308. Jennings, L.J., Salido, G.M., Pariente, J.A., Davison, J.S., Singh, J., and Sharkey, K.A. 1996. Control of exocrine secretion in the guinea-pig pancreas by histamine H_3 receptors. *Can. J. Physiol. Pharmacol.* 74:744–752.

309. Valcheva-Kuzmanova, S.V., Popova, P.B., Krasnaliev, I.J., Galunska, B.T., Belcheva, A., and Schunack, W. 2004. Protective effect of BP 2-94, a histamine H_3-receptor agonist prodrug, in a model of carbon tetrachloride-induced hepatotoxicity in rats. *Folia Med. (Plovdiv)* 46:36–41.

310. Jennings, L.J., Salido, G.M., Pozo, M.J. et al. 1995. The source and action of histamine in the isolated gallbladder. *Inflamm. Res.* 44:447–453.

311. LaBella, F.S., Queen, G., Glavin, G., Durant, G., Stein, D., and Brandes, L.J. 1992. H_3 receptor antagonists, thioperamide, inhibits adrenal steroidogenesis and histamine binding to adrenocortical microsomes and binds to cytochrome P450. *Br. J. Pharmacol.* 107:161–164.

312. Marley, P.D., Thomson, K.A., Jachno, K., and Johnston, M.J. 1991. Histamine-induced increases in cyclic AMP levels in bovine adrenal medullary cells. *Br. J. Pharmacol.* 104:839–846.

313. Neuhaus, J., Weimann, A., Stolzenburg, J.U., Dawood, W., Schwalenberg, T., and Dorschner, W. 2006. Histamine receptors in human detrusor smooth muscle cells: physiological properties and immunohistochemical representation of subtypes. *World J. Urol.* 24:202–209.

314. Neuhaus, J., Oberbach, A., Schwalenberg, T., and Stolzenburg, J.U. 2006. Cultured smooth muscle cells of the human vesical sphincter are more sensitive to histamine than are detrusor smooth muscle cells. *Urology* 67:1086–1092.

315. Vassilev, P., Staneva-Stoytcheva, D., and Mutafova-Yambolieva, V. 1991. Do H_3-receptors participate in the effects of histamine on electrically-evoked contractions of rat vas deferens? *Gen. Pharmacol.* 22:643–645.

316. Poli, E., Todorov, S., Pozzoli, C., and Bertaccini, G. 1994. Presynaptic histamine H_2 receptors modulate the sympathetic nerve transmission in the isolated rat vas deferens; no role for H_3-receptors. *Agents Actions* 42:95–100.

317. Luo, X.X., and Tan, Y.H. 1994. Presynaptic histamine H_1- and H_3-receptors modulate sympathetic neurotransmission in isolated guinea pig vas deferens. *Acta Pharmacol. Sin.* 15:60–64.

318. Kim, Y.C., Davies, M.G., Lee, T.H., Hagen, P.O., and Carson, C.C. 1995. Characterization and function of histamine receptors in corpus cavernosum. *J. Urol.* 153:506–510.

319. Montesino, H., Villar, M., Vega, E., and Rudolph, M.I. 1995. Histamine, a neuromodulator of noradrenergic transmission in uterine horns from mice in diestrus. *Biochem. Pharmacol.* 50:407–411.

320. Rubio, E., Navarro-Badenes, J., Palop, V., Morales-Olivas, F.J., and Martinez-Mir, I. 1999. The effects of histamine on the isolated mouse uterus. *J. Auton. Pharmacol.* 19:281–289.

321. Kitazawa, T., Shishido, H., Sato, T., and Taneike, T. 1997. Histamine mediates the muscle layer-specific responses in the isolated swine myometrium. *J. Vet. Pharmacol. Ther.* 20:187–197.

322. Wagner, W., Ichikawa, A., Tanaka, S., Panula, P., and Fogel, W.A. 2003. Mouse mammary epithelial histamine system. *J. Physiol. Pharmacol.* 54:211–223.

323. Pawlak, D., Malinowska, B., Wollny, T., Godlewski, G., and Buczko, W. 1996. Lack of specific influence of histamine and histamine H_1, H_2 and H_3 receptor ligands on the serotonin uptake and release in rat blood platelets. *Pol. J. Pharmacol.* 48:615–620.

324. Thurmond, R.L., Desai, P.J., Dunford, P.J. et al. 2004. A potent and selective histamine H_4 receptor antagonist with anti-inflammatory properties. *J. Pharmacol. Exp. Ther.* 309:404–413.

325. Adachi, N., Liu, K., Motoki, A., Nishibori, M., and Arai, T. 2006. Suppression of ischemia/reperfusion liver injury by histamine H_4 receptor stimulation in rats. *Eur. J. Pharmacol.* 544:181–187.

Section C

Therapeutic Potential in Central Nervous System Disorders

7 Cognitive Functions, Attention-Deficit Hyperactivity Disorders, and Alzheimer's Disease

Maria Beatrice Passani, Patrizio Blandina,
Kaitlin E. Browman, and Gerard B. Fox

CONTENTS

Introduction..213
Attention-Deficit Hyperactivity Disorder 214
    Disease State..214
    Therapeutic Options and Considerations 216
    Theories of Disease Basis..217
    Rationale for H_3 Receptor Antagonist Efficacy 217
    Experimental Disease Models and Preclinical Data..........................218
Alzheimer's Disease 222
    Disease State..222
    Therapeutic Options and Considerations 223
    Theories of Disease Basis..224
    Rationale for H_3 Receptor Antagonist Efficacy 225
    Experimental Disease Models and Preclinical Data..........................227
Potential Future Directions..230
Conclusions 230
Acknowledgment 230
References...231

INTRODUCTION

Attention-deficit hyperactivity disorder (ADHD) and Alzheimer's disease (AD) are debilitating neurological disorders that affect patients at both ends of the age spectrum. Patients with ADHD often exhibit behavioral heterogeneity for symptoms such as inattention, impulsivity, and hyperactivity, which can complicate diagnosis. Thus, it is likely that many children, adolescents, and adults remain untreated. Of those who are treated, the most efficacious drugs currently available are stimulants, which have been used for many decades. Unfortunately, there are numerous side effects associated with the use of stimulants, and there is a general reluctance to treat children with such drugs. For these reasons, this field is currently focused on identifying nonstimulant alternatives that have equal or better efficacy. Since the etiology of ADHD is unknown, a number of different approaches have been investigated, largely focusing on ways to improve cognitive domains affected in ADHD, such as attention. The histaminergic system in the central nervous system (CNS) is implicated in the control of wakefulness, and strong preclinical evidence suggests that blockade of histamine H_3 receptors can increase wakefulness, decrease impulsivity, and improve attention as well as other cognitive domains.

These observations have encouraged investigators to broaden the scope for identifying potential clinical uses for H_3 receptor antagonists from ADHD to also include treating cognitive impairments associated with schizophrenia (see Chapter 9) and AD. With respect to the latter, profound deficits across multiple cognitive domains are the hallmark of this devastating and ultimately fatal disease, particularly in the aging population. Although many investigators are focused on exciting disease-modifying approaches that target underlying pathology first recognized over 100 years ago, there will remain a clear need to improve the function of Alzheimer's patients, and it is likely that disease-modifying treatments will be augmented by palliative treatments that will improve quality of life. Unfortunately, most current treatments offer at best only partial remittance from the relentless deterioration of the brain and cognitive faculties. Histamine H_3 receptor antagonists represent an exciting potential advance in this regard since, unlike many other neurotransmitter receptors in the brain, expression of H_3 receptors is maintained in Alzheimer's patients offering the potential to broadly improve cognitive functioning.

In this chapter, we explore the disease state and known disease basis for both ADHD and AD. In addition, we summarize best-available disease models and then focus on the potential for H_3 receptor antagonists to treat these disorders, where there is a significant unmet medical need.

ATTENTION-DEFICIT HYPERACTIVITY DISORDER

Disease State

ADHD, as defined by the *Diagnostic and Statistical Manual of Mental Disorders*, Fourth Edition, Text Revision (DSM-IV TR), is diagnosed using behavioral criteria. Behavioral heterogeneity among ADHD sufferers complicates the diagnosis and makes it difficult to establish its prevalence. The main characteristics of ADHD include a continual pattern of inattention and hyperactivity–impulsivity, and can be classified into three different subtypes (see Table 7.1 for details): (a) predominantly inattentive, (b) predominantly hyperactive–impulsive (hyperactivity without inattention), or (c) combined [1]. The condition arises before the age of seven and frequently persists through adolescence and into adulthood, although the behavioral features of the condition vary at different ages. Children with the hyperactive–impulsive subtype usually develop symptoms of ADHD by 4 years of age, with significant difficulties contributing to academic challenges by the age of eight. In contrast, children with the inattentive subtype tend to develop difficulties later, with a typical age

TABLE 7.1

Examples of Criteria for ADHD Taken from the DSM-IV-TR

ADHD Type	Examples of Criteria Taken from the DSM-IV-TR[a]
Inattention	Often fails to give close attention to details or makes careless mistakes in schoolwork, work, or other activities
	Often has difficulty sustaining attention in tasks or play activity
	Often does not seem to listen when spoken to directly
	Often does not follow through on instructions and fails to finish schoolwork, chores, or duties in the workplace (not due to oppositional behavior or failure to understand instructions)
	Often has difficulty organizing tasks and activities
	Often avoids, dislikes, or is reluctant to engage in tasks that require sustained mental effort (such as schoolwork or homework)
	Often looses things necessary for tasks or activities (e.g., toys, school assignments, pencils, books, or tools)
	Often easily distracted by extraneous stimuli
	Often forgetful in daily activities
Hyperactivity	Often fidgets with hands or feet or squirms in seat
	Often leaves seat in classroom or in other situations in which remaining seated is expected
	Often runs about or climbs excessively in situations in which it is inappropriate (in adolescents or adults, may be limited to subjective feelings of restlessness)
	Often has difficulty playing or engaging in leisure activities quietly
	Often *on the go* or often acts as if *driven by a motor*
	Often talks excessively
Impulsivity	Often blurts out answers before questions have been completed
	Often has difficulty awaiting turn
	Often interrupts or intrudes on others (e.g., butts into conversations or games)

[a] ADHD predominantly inattentive type—this subtype is used if six (or more) symptoms of inattention (but fewer than six symptoms of hyperactivity–impulsivity) have persisted for at least 6 months; ADHD predominantly hyperactive–impulsive type—this subtype should be used if six (or more) symptoms of hyperactivity–impulsivity (but fewer than six of inattention) have persisted for at least 6 months; ADHD combined type—this subtype should be used if six (or more) symptoms of inattention and six (or more) symptoms of hyperactivity–impulsivity have persisted for at least 6 months.

of presenting with noticeable difficulties ~9–10 years of age. In adolescence, the hyperactive and impulsive symptoms may become less evident, but the problems with inattention often persist.

It can be difficult to estimate worldwide prevalence rates, as all countries do not use the DSM-IV TR criteria. In Europe, the *International Classification of Disease* manual (ICD-10) is more frequently used, leading to a much lower rate of diagnosis and a more severe population being treated. In the United States, ADHD is the most common neurobehavioral disorder of childhood and is among the most prevalent chronic health conditions affecting school-aged children. ADHD accounts for 30–50% of all referrals for child mental health services in the United States [1], comprising the majority of the economic cost of childhood mental disorders.

Although it is generally accepted that ADHD persists into adulthood (for a review see Ref. 2), there is less of a consensus on the best diagnostic criteria suitable for diagnosing adults with ADHD. As children approach adulthood, a number of developmental changes occur, and diagnostic criteria are not currently identifying how the subtypes change during this transition period. Furthermore, adult diagnostic criteria currently rely on symptomology identified in younger populations and likely do not adequately capture all adults with ADHD. In general, there are three approaches for diagnosing adult ADHD: the Wender Utah criteria, the DSM-IV criteria, and laboratory assessments (see Ref. 2). Although the DSM-IV criteria have been used (successfully) in diagnosing adult ADHD, the scale is likely not the most appropriate for diagnosing adults. Other scales that have been validated include the Adult Self-Report Scale (ASRS), developed in conjunction with the World Health Organization (http://www.med.nyu.edu/psych/assets/adhdscreener.pdf) and the Conners Adult ADHD Rating Scale (CAARS), comprising self-reports and observer ratings, and provide normative data for comparison.

THERAPEUTIC OPTIONS AND CONSIDERATIONS

The primary pharmacological treatments for ADHD are the stimulants and, in particular, methylphenidate (Ritalin, Ritalin LA, Ritalin SR, Concerta, Focalin, Methylin, Methylin ER, Metadate ER, and Metadate CD) and amphetamine (Adderall, Adderall XR, Dexedrine, Dexedrine Spansule, and DesxtroStat) [1,3,4]. Stimulants are estimated to be effective in 70% of adolescents and appear to improve both cognitive deficits and general behavior [3,5]. Common short-term adverse effects such as appetite suppression, sleep disturbances, and abdominal pain [4,5] are reported with the stimulant class. Longer-term adverse effects are still debated, with reports suggesting motor tic development as well as some height/weight decreases among adolescents with ADHD [4,6].

The first nonstimulant therapy designed for ADHD, Strattera™ (atomoxetine) is also the first product launched for the treatment of adults with ADHD. Atomoxetine is not a scheduled drug, and lacks methylphenidatelike drug reinforcement properties in monkeys [7]. The efficacy of atomoxetine is not generally considered to be better than methylphenidate, although in one clinical report [8], atomoxetine was reported to have better effects on inattentive symptoms compared to the hyperactive–impulsive symptoms, which would be consistent with a noradrenergic mechanism of action. Side effects observed with atomoxetine are an extension of its pharmacology (e.g., elevated blood pressure, urinary dysfunction) or to those of the primary metabolite (4-OH-atomoxetine) that shows modest affinity [9] for several opioid receptors (e.g., constipation or other GI disturbances). Short-term side effects may include sedation, appetite suppression, nausea, vomiting, and headaches. In contrast to the stimulants, some emerging longer-term side effect data suggest that normal growth in height and weight is found with atomoxetine treatment [10].

The third line of therapy for ADHD, antidepressants and antihypertensive therapies, is used less frequently than stimulants, but can be effective. These drugs are sometimes used in combination with stimulants in patients with comorbid symptoms. Commonly used agents are tricyclics (TCAs), buproprion, or α-adreno-ceptor agonists (clonidine, guanfacine, etc.). The therapeutic limitations of these diverse compounds include weight loss; sleep disturbances; abuse liability and social stigma of stimulants; and the cardiovascular side effects and less-well-defined efficacy of atomoxetine, TCAs, or α-adrenergic agents. Concerns regarding the safety of these medications, particularly in children, have limited their use.

THEORIES OF DISEASE BASIS

Controversy has historically surrounded the status of ADHD as a genuine medical condition. Evidence that ADHD is found in different cultures with a genetic component has underscored the value of designating ADHD as a medical disorder [11]. Typically, research into mechanisms underlying ADHD has focused on the dopaminergic system, at least in part because efficacious treatments can act on this monoaminergic system. As a result, candidate gene searches have focused on the dopaminergic system (for a review of pharmacogenomic ADHD studies see Ref. 12). Genes associated with ADHD include the dopamine transporter (DAT1), dopamine D2 (DRD2)\D4 (DRD4) and D5 receptor (DRD5) subtypes, and the dopa-β-*hydroxylase* gene (DBH) [12].

Evidence has also supported an association between ADHD and the cholinergic system. ADHD is associated with prenatal exposure to nicotine [13], and mice lacking the β2 subunit of the nicotininc acetylcholine receptor show hyperactivity, inattention, and impulsivity [14]. An intron mutation in the gene coding for the α4 subunit of neuronal nicotinic receptors (NNRs) was associated with ADHD characterized by severe inattention. Although the functional consequence of this mutation is unknown, the location is suggestive of effects on pre-mRNA stability or splicing [15].

Meta-analyses have also implicated polymorphisms in the genes coding for SNAP-25 (a presynaptic plasma membrane protein with an integral role in synaptic transmission) and the serotonin transporter with ADHD. SNAP-25 forms a complex with syntaxin 1a and synaptic vesicle proteins such as VAMP-2 (synaptobrevin 2) and synaptotagmin, which mediates calcium-dependent exocytosis of neurotransmitter from the synaptic vesicle into the synaptic cleft [16]. High levels of SNAP-25 have been found in regions such as the hippocampus, neocortex, thalamus, substantia nigra, and cerebellum. In a recent study of 93 ADHD nuclear families in Ireland, significant increased preferential transmission of the SNAP-25 polymorphism Ddel allele 1 was found [17]. In a separate study of Canadian families with ADHD, significant increased preferential transmission of the SNAP-25 polymorphism Ddel allele 2 was found [18]. Additional haplotype analysis of SNAP-25 implicates SNAP-25 in the etiology of ADHD.

Although the exact mechanism underlying ADHD is unknown, imaging studies suggest that ADHD appears to be associated with decreased activity of the prefrontal cortex; an observation consistent with the impaired attention and executive function characteristic of the disease (for a review see Ref. 11).

RATIONALE FOR H₃ RECEPTOR ANTAGONIST EFFICACY

Cognition is a complex phenomenon involving the integration of multiple neurological and behavioral activities among which arousal and attention are crucial conditions for responding to behavioral and cognitive challenges [19]. Increasing evidence supports a fundamental role of the neuronal histamine system and, in particular, of histamine H_3 receptors as modulator of the sleep–wake cycle and cognitive processes [20]. Histaminergic neurons fire tonically and specifically during wakefulness [21] and control cortical activation, a salient sign of wakefulness [20,22]. This effect is achieved both directly, through excitatory interactions with cholinergic corticopetal neurons originating from the nucleus basalis magnocellularis [23] and the substantia innominata [24], and indirectly, through thalamo- and hypothalamo-cortical circuitries activation [25]. The importance of histamine in arousal is supported by the nature of the interactions between histamine and orexin neurons, which have a crucial role in sleep regulation [26–28]. The histamine deficiency shown in narcoleptic dogs [29] and the observation that histidine decarboxylase-knockout (KO) mice are unable to remain awake when high vigilance is required [30] confirm that histamine seems to be required to maintain arousal. Histidine decarboxylase-KO mice lack histamine, since this enzyme is determinant of neuronal histamine production [31,32]. Since arousal is a prerequisite for other brain functions such as learning and memory, histamine thus can have an important indirect influence on cognitive processing.

There is also much evidence suggesting that the histaminergic system may also influence biological processes underlying learning and memory directly [20,33]. Numerous observations support the complexity of the brain histamine system at the levels of histamine-containing neurons, H_3 receptors, interactions of H_3 receptors with signal transduction pathways, and the diversity of neurotransmitters whose synthesis and release are modulated by H_3 receptors. Neuronal heterogeneity likely contributes to the diversity of H_3 receptor function through autoreceptor or heteroreceptor control of neurotransmitter release, as demonstrated for acetylcholine and noradrenaline in the rat cortex and hippocampus and dopamine in the rat prefrontal cortex. Furthermore, the H_3 receptor shows functional constitutive activity, polymorphisms in humans and rodents with a differential distribution of splice variants in the CNS, and potential coupling to different intracellular signal transduction mechanisms. Despite the genetic, pharmacological, and functional complexity of the H_3 receptor, the histamine system as a challenging and promising therapeutic target to control cognitive disorders.

EXPERIMENTAL DISEASE MODELS AND PRECLINICAL DATA

There are many advantages in developing animal models of ADHD, including results from a simpler system may be easier to interpret, treatment groups can be genetically homogeneous, and testing environments can be tightly controlled. Ideally, animal models should resemble the clinical disorder, including etiology, pathophysiology, behavioral phenotype, and response to clinically efficacious pharmacological treatments. One of the most widely accepted animal models of ADHD is the spontaneous hypertensive rat (SHR), a strain that was originally developed from Wistar Kyoto (WKY) rats in Japan more than 40 years ago (for a recent review see Ref. 34). When selecting for hypertension, hyperactivity was also observed. SHRs exhibit many behavioral features of ADHD, including hyperactivity, inattention, and impulsivity. Hyperactivity in the SHR strain is dependent on the test environment, with disturbances compared to control rat strains observed in unfamiliar environments and more modest hyperactivity observed in the home cage (see Ref. 35). Attentional deficits are observed as increased percentage of errors in operant tasks, whereas impulsivity is observed as the inability of SHRs to delay a response to obtain a larger reward. Response inhibition and cognitive function are also impaired in the SHR in a 5-trial inhibitory avoidance paradigm [36] and 5-CSRTT [37] when compared with age- and sex-matched controls from other rat strains. These aspects of behavioral dysfunction correspond to the clinical symptoms of hyperactivity, impulsivity, and inattention/cognitive impairment, as described earlier. Thus, the SHR is a good model for studying multiple facets of ADHD, as they offer good face validity for the human disorder (Table 7.2).

TABLE 7.2
Summary of Animal Models/Assays of ADHD

Animal Model	Basic Description	References
SHR	The most widely accepted animal model of ADHD is the SHR, a strain that was originally developed from WKY rats more than 40 years ago. When selecting for hypertension, hyperactivity was also observed. Since then, the SHR has been studied extensively from face, predictive, and construct validity perspectives.	34
DAT KO mouse	The DAT KO mouse shows about a 300-fold decrease in the rate of clearance of extracellular DA due to the lack of the gene that encodes DAT-1. These KO mice also show evidence of hyperactivity and other behavioral abnormalities similar to those observed in patients with ADHD.	38,39
Synaptosome associated protein of 25 kDa (SNAP-25, coloboma mutant)	The coloboma mutation arose from neutron irradiation mutagenesis studies, producing a deletion on chromosome 2 that disrupted coding of four known genes for the proteins phospholipase β1 and β4, jagged 1, and SNAP-25. Coloboma mice display impulsivity and impaired inhibition. Spontaneous hyperactivity was reduced by d-amphetamine but not methylphenidate.	40–44
6-Hydroxydopamine (6-OHDA) lesions	Exposure of rat pups to 6-OHDA selectively lesions DA projections to the frontal cortex, resulting in an age-dependent increase in spontaneous locomotor activity and cognitive impairment. Impulsivity is not present in 6-OHDA-lesioned rats, and as such these rats may be useful models for understanding hyperactivity in ADHD.	35
Dorsal prefrontal cortex (dPFC) lesions	Lesions of the prefrontal cortex impair regulation of attention and impulsivity as well as working memory. Attentional deficits can be attenuated by amphetamine.	45,46
Environmental toxins	Chronic exposure to lead or polychlorinated biphenyls can cause motor hyperactivity as well as cognitive impairment and impulsivity in rodents. Methylphenidate and amphetamine may ameliorate some of these symptoms in mice, but these models have not been well characterized.	35

(continued)

TABLE 7.2   (Continued)

Animal Model	Basic Description	References
Neonatal hypoxia	Anoxia in perinatal humans is a risk factor for developing ADHD. In rats, neonatal hypoxia produces behavioral symptoms similar to those observed in clinical ADHD, such as age-related hyperactivity and deficits in cognitive functioning.	35
In utero exposure	Nicotine—mice exposed to prenatal nicotine show increased spontaneous locomotion.	47
	Alcohol—rats exposed prenatally to ethanol show attentional deficits and decreased activity of dopamine neurons. Methylphenidate administration normalizes dopamine neuron activity.	48,49
Thyroid hormone receptor transgenic animals	Transgenic mice expressing TRβ1 (a human mutant thyroid receptor) display characteristic symptoms of ADHD, including inattention, hyperactivity, and deficiency in a delayed reward procedure.	50
5-CSRTT; selection of poor performers	In the 5-CSRTT procedure, some rats are generally poor performers. This subset of rats was improved on some measures by treatment with methylphenidate.	51

Note: 5-CSRTT, 5-choice serial reaction time test; DA, dopamine; TRH, thyroid hormone receptor.

In terms of construct validity, the behavioral alterations observed in the SHR are believed to have a genetics-based etiology, consistent with human genetic studies. Studies in humans are consistent with the widely held belief that hypofunction of the mesocortical dopaminergic system contributes to the main symptoms of ADHD. For example, in three genomewide scans, the DAT1 candidate gene was linked to ADHD symptomatology [52]. In SHR, the DAT is overexpressed in the striatum. Cholinergic function is also disrupted in SHRs, with decreases in the expression of NNRs containing the α4 subunit observed in multiple brain regions, especially the frontal cortex in prehypertensive juvenile SHRs [53–55].

The SHR also offers predictive validity, that is, compounds efficacious in treating the human disorder are also efficacious in this animal model. For example, juvenile SHRs, which do not exhibit the potential confound of hypertension that develops later in the adult SHR, respond to stimulant drugs that are clinically efficacious for treating ADHD, such as methylphenidate (Ritalin®). Locomotor hyperactivity and decreased delayed reinforcement in SHRs are reportedly attenuated in a dose-related manner by low doses of methylphenidate [56,57], whereas impaired spontaneous alternation behavior in the Y maze, which may be gender-specific (worse in male rats), was restored by methylphenidate treatment [57]. Similarly, increased impulsivity assessed in an elevated plus maze was also lowered by methylphenidate [57], although it is difficult to dissociate this from potential anxiety-related measures. Impaired response inhibition/attention in 5-TIA is effectively reversed by doses of methylphenidate [36] producing plasma levels (~4 to 17 ng/mL) similar to those efficacious in the clinic (~8 to 10 ng/mL). Similarly, nonstimulants with different mechanisms, such as the NNR agonist, ABT-418, that are effective in clinical trials for ADHD [58] also reverse impairments in response inhibition/attention in 5-TIA [36] at efficacious plasma levels consistent between SHRs (3.5 ng/mL) and humans (8–30 ng/mL). This is an important point since novel nonstimulant drugs represent an important new area of focus for ADHD research [59]. Furthermore, in adults with ADHD, nicotine administration improves cognitive function and behavioral inhibition to a level at least as comparable with methylphenidate [60]. Nicotine also reverses behavioral impairments in SHRs tested in the Y maze, an effect that is blocked by the $\alpha4\beta2$ NNR antagonists, mecamylamine, and dihydro-β-erythroidine [61]. SHRs are also reportedly sensitive to D-amphetamine, demonstrating reduced motor activity and impulsiveness [35].

From the early 1980s, histamine H_3 receptor antagonists containing an imidazole moiety, such as ciproxifan, thioperamide, and clobenpropit, were developed and subsequently evaluated across a range of behavioral tests in various rodent strains, including the SHR. These compounds were efficacious across a number of different cognitive domains, including attention. Although these first-generation drugs served as early reference standards, imidazole-ring containing ligands are not suitable compounds to develop as drugs in humans since they are associated with inhibition of cytochrome P450 enzymes, potentially leading to drug–drug interactions. In addition, the affinity of some compounds such as thioperamide for the human H_3 receptor is low when compared to the rodent receptor [62,63]. However, the successful cloning and functional expression of the histamine H_3 receptors from various species over the past 10 years [64] has greatly facilitated efforts to identify nonimidazole-based small molecule antagonists. Investigators at Abbott Laboratories have demonstrated improved cognitive performance in the 5-TIA model in SHRs following administration of potent and selective antagonists such as ABT-239 [65] and other nonimidazole- [36,65–67] and imidazole-based [36,66] H_3 receptor antagonists. Investigators at Johnson & Johnson have also shown significant improvements in a 7-TIA variant of this model of ADHD in SHRs with the nonimidazole H_3 antagonist, JNJ-180181457 [68].

Although inattention and impulsivity are key symptoms of ADHD and SHR models fulfill important characteristics of ADHD including measures of attention and impulsivity, these terms are quite general and are often used loosely. For example, the cognitive domain of *attention* covers a number of processes including selective and divided attention, vigilance, and distractibility. Impulsivity, often operationally defined as a failure to stop a response, has been linked to increased probability of suicide, gambling, drug abuse, and aggression. Consequently, there is much interest in modeling aspects of attention and impulsivity preclinically as specifically as possible, to aid in the development of novel, nonstimulant therapies for ADHD. In humans, the continuous performance test (CPT) has been used for more than 50 years as a diagnostic tool for measuring attention in humans. A rodent analog of the CPT has been developed, the 5-choice continuous performance task (5-CSRTT), in which separate measures of selective attention, impulsivity, motivation, and motor function can be obtained [69]. The 5-CSRTT relies on visual cues that predict a food reward that is delivered only when the rodent correctly chooses the location of a short duration (typically less than 1 s during testing) light stimulus. Sustained attention can be operationalized using this task by measuring the percent of correct or incorrect choices or the number of missed responses over a test session. Impulsivity is typically measured by assessing the number of responses between trials. Other variables such as latency to respond or the number of missed responses are also collected and can provide information on motor function. The 5-CSRTT can also be conducted in nonhuman primates [70], although research using monkeys in this regard lags considerably behind that conducted in rodents.

Although the clinically used ADHD drug, methylphenidate, shows efficacy in the 5-CSRTT, one of the best-studied pharmacological effects is with nicotine. In preclinical studies in rats, acute nicotine administration increased response accuracy, reduced omission errors, and decreased reaction time [71]. Nicotine has also demonstrated efficacy in adults with ADHD in the CPT, providing additional potential predictive validity with this task. An early study with the imidazole-based histamine H_3 receptor antagonist, ciproxifan, demonstrated an effect on attention measures, observed when demands on attention were increased [72]. However, other investigators demonstrated a failure of the H_3 receptor antagonist, thioperamide, to reverse a scopolamine-induced attention deficit [73]. To address this issue, investigators at Wyeth and Abbott Laboratories collaborated to demonstrate that ciproxifan had a main effect to reduce premature responding, a measure of impulsivity, in studies conducted independently at both research sites [74]. In addition, Wyeth investigators found that ciproxifan could improve accuracy, a measure of attention, when task conditions were made more difficult under conditions of variable stimulus duration. Nicotine, used as a comparator and positive control in these studies, significantly improved accuracy and reduced errors of omission (reflecting improved attention and vigilance) but had no effect on impulsivity.

Histamine H_3 receptor antagonists are currently under evaluation in a number of clinical studies, including ADHD studies, where clinical outcome will ultimately determine not only the predictive value of these models for this target but also the potential of H_3 antagonists as fully efficacious, nonstimulant treatments for ADHD.

ALZHEIMER'S DISEASE

DISEASE STATE

AD, the most common form of dementia, is a progressive and devastating illness that robs the affected individual of the ability to learn, reason, remember recent events, and ultimately communicate and perform daily activities. This gradual decline in memory and multiple cognitive domains is also frequently accompanied by additional noncognitive behavioral symptoms such as agitation, anxiety, hallucinations, and delusions. As a disease of the elderly, Alzheimer's currently affects more than 15–20 million people worldwide [75] with a prevalence of up to 10% in patients aged above 65 and increasing to ~50% in patients aged 85 or older. Every 72 s someone in the United States is diagnosed with AD. By the year 2050, it is estimated that this will increase to one person developing AD every 33 s. The costs to society are enormous ($150 billion annually in the United States alone and an estimated $248 billion globally) and are projected to double by 2050. As the world population continues to age, without effective intervention, it is likely that AD will become the most critical and overwhelming health problem for developed countries this century. For further information on this topic, see *Alzheimer's Disease Facts and Figures*, published by the Alzheimer's Association (2007) (www.alz.org).

Diagnosis of AD is based largely on symptoms and neurological examination since there are no reliable diagnostic biomarkers. Currently, there are two main sets of diagnostic criteria that are used by clinicians to define a diagnosis of AD: DSM-IV-TR and The National Institute of Neurological and Communicative Disorders and Stroke-Alzheimer's Disease and Related Disorder Association (NINDS-ADRDA) [76]. Using the latter classification system, AD can be considered as possible, probable, or definite. A possible or probable diagnosis can be made while the patient is still living, whereas a definitive diagnosis is not possible until histopathological examination, usually postmortem. Accurate diagnosis using these criteria is usually made ~80 to 90% of the time. However, recent advances in neuroimaging techniques, notably positron emission tomography (PET) with tracers that bind pathology thought to underlie AD (see next section) or that delineate hypometabolism associated with pathology promise to improve these figures in the future [77,78].

Mild cognitive impairment (MCI), characterized by subtle loss in cognitive function greater than the decline found in normal aging in otherwise healthy subjects, is frequently considered prodromal to AD. Indeed, an estimated 10–15% of patients diagnosed with MCI will convert to AD every year [79], reaching a total of ~80% within 6 years [79]. In comparison, the annual conversion rate in the normal elderly population is ~1 to 2% [80]. Early detection of MCI may therefore afford a good opportunity for therapeutic intervention aimed at preventing the conversion to AD or at slowing down the process. However, because there is no accepted definition of MCI yet, it can be difficult to compare across studies due to the range of diagnostic criteria adopted. Neuroimaging may help with diagnosis and monitoring of treatment efficacy in the future: recent studies using PET [81] and MRI [82] have successfully identified MCI noninvasively in small patient populations, although much work is needed in this area to bring these findings into everyday clinical use.

THERAPEUTIC OPTIONS AND CONSIDERATIONS

Perhaps the single-most influential event driving the symptomatic treatment of AD was the initial formulation of the *cholinergic hypothesis* almost 30 years ago [83,84]. Simply stated, the dysfunction of cholinergic neurons in AD brain areas known to be important in cognitive function contributes substantially to the cognitive decline observed in AD and with advanced age [85]. This hypothesis implied that treatment strategies that could improve cholinergic function should ameliorate cognitive impairments associated with AD and aging (today, this might be described as MCI). As a direct result, we now have a total of five drugs that are approved for the treatment of cognitive symptoms in AD: tacrine (Cognex), donepezil (Aricept), rivastigmine (Exelon), galantamine (Reminyl), and memantine (Namenda) (and numerous other medications may be used for the treatment of comorbidities as described earlier). The first four of these are acetyylcholinesterase inhibitors, which increase available acetylcholine levels by blocking the enzyme that catalyzes the breakdown of this neurotransmitter; all four are approved for the palliative treatment of mild to moderate AD. The last, memantine, is a noncompetitive N-methyl-D-aspartate (NMDA) receptor antagonist, whose mechanism of action is not understood. Memantine is approved for the palliative treatment of moderate to severe AD. However, despite the availability of these drugs, there remains a significant unmet need in the treatment of AD. Although cholinesterase inhibitors and memantine described earlier can have beneficial effects, only modest improvements in 30–50% of patients are seen for a limited time period (typically <6–12 months). This may be because, with continued progression of the disease, there are fewer sources of acetylcholine left to modulate due to ongoing neurodegeneration. Side effects such as diarrhea, nausea, and insomnia further limit the use of these drugs, and there is a clear need for new approaches to provide greater relief from the debilitating cognitive symptoms. Histamine H_3 receptor blockade with selective antagonists or inverse agonists is currently attracting a lot of attention as a potential new source of palliative treatment for AD that has the potential to retain efficacy for longer periods with minimal side effects (see later sections).

The unmet need in AD treatment extends beyond drugs that provide greater symptomatic relief with fewer side effects, to treatments that will ultimately slow, halt, or reverse the progression of the disease. Unfortunately, there are currently no effective treatments approved in this regard. This is not for want of trying, and there are numerous agents in preclinical and clinical development employing various approaches. These include neuronal nicotinic acetylcholine receptor agonists ($\alpha 7$ and $\alpha 4 \beta 2$ agonists), RAGE antagonists, β and γ secretase inhibitors, anti-Aβ antibodies (nonspecific or soluble oligomer-specific), and histamine H_3 receptor antagonists—all of which may offer the potential for disease-modifying efficacy through differing mechanisms. Demonstration of such efficacy will be a difficult task, given the slowly progressing nature of AD, but should it be possible, the rewards will be worth the challenge. Importantly, should a means of halting the pathogenesis of AD be identified, there will remain a clear need for more effective palliative treatments since this is what will ultimately determine the functional outcome on Alzheimer's patients' daily lives.

THEORIES OF DISEASE BASIS

AD is named after the German physician, Dr. Alois Alzheimer, who in 1906 described unusual pathology in a recently deceased patient that he associated with cognitive decline over the previous 5 years. The symptoms he described did not fit any known diagnostic criteria at that time and the unknown disorder soon appeared in the medical literature as *Alzheimer's disease*. AD is characterized by a significant degeneration of cortical neurons and a marked atrophy of the cerebral cortex, pathology that was originally noted by Dr. Alzheimer (see Ref. 86 for a recent review). Modern imaging techniques such as volumetric MRI have mapped this decline longitudinally in the same patients with familial AD from presymptomatic and prodromal stages to clinical progression of the disease [87]. These high-resolution images collected over a period of up to 11 years can be assembled effectively into time-lapse information and clearly illustrate the profound loss of cortical gray matter, particularly in temporal and parietal regions and gradually encompassing much of the frontal cortex—regions critical for intact cognitive and executive functioning. In fact, these studies from the laboratories of Nick Fox and others [88] demonstrate that volumetric MRI focused on assessing tissue loss in the medial temporal lobe or hippocampus is sensitive enough to detect significant changes 3 years before clinical diagnosis and can predict future cognitive decline with a high degree of specificity.

One hundred years after Dr. Alzheimer's first description of his new disease, neuroimaging techniques such as those described earlier help us to understand that cerebral atrophy reflects the progression of AD. However, two additional features of the unusual pathology identified by Dr. Alzheimer, which would ultimately be known as *tangles* and *plaques*, are now also hallmark pathological features of the disease. Neurofibrillary tangles are intracellular fibrils composed of paired helical filaments linked by hyperphosphorylated tau protein. Tangles are present in axons and dendrites, which can lead to dystrophic neurites in the extracellular space, often associated with amyloid beta plaques [89]. Since tau is a microtubule-associated protein, the presence of tangles leads to a disruption of the neuronal cytoskeleton, which is responsible for maintaining the structural and functional integrity of the neuron. Plaques are known to be formed as a consequence of amyloid beta overproduction from a high molecular weight precursor protein called amyloid beta precursor protein (APP). Through sequential proteolytic cleavage by two enzyme secretases (β and γ secretase), amyloid beta peptides of varying lengths are produced. The two species of most interest contain 40 (Aβ1-40) or 42 (Aβ1-42) amino acids. The latter species, Aβ1-42, is more prone to aggregation into insoluble plaques and is elevated in AD, suggesting a clinical role in the pathophysiology of AD [90]. This led to the *amyloid cascade hypothesis*, proposed by Hardy and Higgins [91], which posited that deposition of Aβ1-42 into plaques is a key initial event leading to AD. Later researchers began to target removal of Aβ1-42 amyloid plaques with antibody-based approaches as a potential disease-modifying approach [92,93]. In addition to deposition of amyloid beta into plaques extracellularly, amyloid beta is also found in the cerebrovasculature and can cause cerebral amyloid angiopathy. In addition, emerging evidence from transgenic mice and human Alzheimer's patients suggests that amyloid beta can accumulate intracellularly or even within mitochondria, both of which may lead to progression of AD (see Ref. 94 for a recent review).

Intensive research in recent years has now revealed that the clinical symptoms of AD are not directly correlated with the deposition of amyloid plaques or the formation of intracellular tangles; instead neurodegeneration and loss of synaptic connections between neurons appear to better correlate with clinical progression. This has led to a flurry of activity targeting neurotoxic soluble Aβ oligomers [95–98] or more specific soluble Aβ globulomers [99] with vaccination or passive immunization approaches in slowing disease progression and improving symptoms. Several clinical trials are currently investigating such approaches, and time will tell whether these will be productive or not (see next section).

RATIONALE FOR H₃ RECEPTOR ANTAGONIST EFFICACY

The progressive decline in cognitive functioning characteristic of AD is linked to neuropathological changes across a number of brain regions and involves dysfunction of multiple neurotransmitter systems, is described earlier. Histamine

H_3 receptor antagonists represent an exciting potential advance in this regard since neuronal histamine levels are decreased in the temporal cortex of brains from individuals diagnosed with AD, which may contribute to the cognitive decline either directly or through the cholinergic system [100]. Thus, development of drugs that increase histaminergic activity in affected brain regions have been proposed to have potential utility in treating AD. This is supported by recent work by Medhurst et al. [101] at GlaxoSmithKline, who demonstrated for the first time that H_3 receptor expression remains prevalent in medial temporal cortex samples from patients diagnosed with AD, including in subjects with severe late stages of the disease. This is an important point since other drug targets often decline with the increased neurodegeneration that accompanies the relentless progression of Alzheimer's.

Much of the preclinical basic research in this area has focused on improving performance in variations of cognition assays that measure aspects of different cognitive domains affected in AD. For example, an early study demonstrated that i.c.v. administration of histamine can facilitate social memory, an effect that was mimicked by the H_3 receptor antagonist, thioperamide [102]. Conversely, an inhibitor of the neuronal synthesis of histamine, α-fluoromethylhistidine, prolonged recognition time, as did the H_3 receptor agonist, immepip. It was concluded from these studies that the histaminergic system facilitates short-term social memory [102]. Social recognition memory in rats relies on the ability of rodents to use olfactory cues to recall a social interaction with a conspecific juvenile, and social recognition in AD patients is frequently impaired. More recently, selective nonimidazole H_3 receptor antagonists developed at Johnson & Johnson and Abbott Laboratories facilitated short-term social recognition memory in adult rats [68,103,104], and ABT-239 was able to restore recognition memory in aged rats to a level equivalent to performance of a younger adult [65]. Similarly, other groups have used a novel-object recognition model in rodents to assess short-term memory; this time for a familiar versus an unfamiliar object placed in a test arena (instead of a familiar versus an unfamiliar juvenile rat in social recognition). This is relevant to AD since short-term memory is also impaired early in the disease course. Using this test, colleagues at GlaxoSmithKline and BioProjet demonstrated improved recognition memory with the selective H_3 receptor antagonists GSK189254 [101] and BF2.649 [105]. GSK189254 was effective in attenuating temporal-based deficits in naïve rats (i.e., reducing the *forgetting* associated with the passing of time), whereas BF2.649 improved similar performance in naïve mice as well as attenuating scopolamine-induced learning deficits in a similar test in mice.

Another assay that is commonly used to assess cognitive function preclinically is the passive avoidance (sometimes referred to as inhibitory avoidance) test, which assesses longer-term memory consolidation. In a mouse model of premature senescence, early work demonstrated that impaired memory in a step-through passive avoidance paradigm could be reversed with the H_3 receptor antagonist, thioperamide [106]. In additional passive avoidance and object recognition tests, pretreatment with H_3 agonists impaired performance, implying a role for H_3 receptors in acquisition rather than recall, since posttreatment had no effect [107]. Interestingly, the H_3 receptor antagonists, clobenpropit and thioperamide, were both able to prevent scopolamine-induced amnesia, implying a potential utility for H_3 receptor antagonists in neurodegenerative disorders such as Alzheimer's where cholinergic function is impaired. Similarly, the H_3 receptor antagonists GSK189254, GSK207040, and GSK334429 reversed scopolamine-induced amnesia in rats [101,108]. These findings are consistent with observations of reduced brain ACh levels following H_3 receptor agonist administration [109] and increased brain ACh levels following administration of H_3 receptor antagonists [65,101,105]. Furthermore, H_3 receptor KO mice are not sensitive to scopolamine disruption of performance in the passive avoidance test, supporting an important role for H_3 receptors in modulating cholinergic function important for this cognitive domain [110].

Explicit spatial memory is impaired in AD, and H_3 receptor antagonists have shown efficacy in reversing deficits in preclinical animal tests of spatial learning and memory. For example, the H_3 receptor antagonist, GSK189254, improved spatial learning and memory in aged rats using a hidden platform version of the water maze [101], whereas ciproxifan, thioperamide, and ABT-239 reduced scopolamine-induced errors in discriminating the location of a fixed, compared to a floating, escape platform using a two-choice discrimination version of the water maze [65,111]. Furthermore, i.c.v. injection of histamine or thioperamide ameliorated memory impairment induced by scopolamine in an eight-arm radial maze in rats [112]. In another spatial memory task, the Barnes maze, mice lacking H_3 receptors, showed improved spatial learning and memory [113], and ciproxifan attenuated scopolamine-induced impairment in the Barnes maze [111], consistent with the concept that blockade of H_3 receptors can enhance spatial reference memory. The effect of thioperamide on consolidation and recall mechanisms of place recognition memory were also studied in rats using a two-trial delayed comparison paradigm in a Y-maze. Interestingly, thioperamide enhanced memory retention when administered postacquisition, but did not affect rat performance when injected 45 min before the trial testing [114]. Finally, in rats treated with MK801 (NMDA receptor antagonist), clobenpropit improved spatial memory retention in a radial maze test [115].

EXPERIMENTAL DISEASE MODELS AND PRECLINICAL DATA

Standard laboratory rodents such as mice and rats do not generally develop neurodegenerative pathology typical of AD. However, when aged to ~2 years, older rats and mice do exhibit impaired performance across a range of cognitive domains that are affected in AD. During the earlier stages of the human disease, impaired recent memory formation is most pronounced and is usually the impetus for the patient to seek medical help. Recent memory can be measured relatively easily in the rodent, although extra attention to detail is usually required when running the same tests in older rodents. Aged rats exhibit impaired short-term or social memory as measured in versions of object recognition or social recognition tests; these impairments can be reversed with pharmacological treatments including drugs such as donepezil (used clinically to relieve early symptoms in AD) as well as H_3 receptor antagonists such as ABT-239 [65]. Owing to the difficulty in obtaining and maintaining an aged rodent colony, similar tests are often run in mature adult rats (typically 4–6 months old), with the assumption that improvements in recent memory will translate to the aged or disease state. Cholinesterase inhibitors (e.g., tacrine, donepezil) and H_3 receptor antagonists (e.g., GSK189254, ciproxifan) have shown efficacy in such models [101,104]. During later stages of AD, patients typically exhibit moderate to severe impairments in cognitive function, practically across all cognitive domains. Aged rats also exhibit impairment across a range of cognitive tests such as impaired spatial navigation as assessed in tests such as the Barnes maze or water maze; impaired long-term memory as evident in tests such as inhibitory avoidance and water maze; and impaired attention in tests such as the five-choice serial reaction time task. Although some of these impairments can be reversed with drugs used clinically in the palliative treatment of AD, many critics still regard these models as insufficient to make a case for potential efficacy in AD and instead take the *preponderance of evidence* approach when deciding which compounds to bring forward for development.

In contrast to rodents, aged nonhuman primates do show both behavioral and neuropathological abnormalities that resemble those found in aged humans and patients with AD. In macaques, these include progressive cognitive impairments at the end of the second decade of life (average lifespan ~37–40 years) as well as a decline in cholinergic (and other neurotransmitter) function, evidence of diffuse amyloid beta plaques in cortical tissue, amyloid deposits in the cerebrovasculature, dystrophic neurites, and neurodegeneration (see Refs 116 and 117 for review). Palliative therapies such as donepezil that show some benefit in human AD also show some benefit in improving cognitive function in aged monkeys. Of note, the modest benefit afforded by donepezil in monkeys can be limited to certain populations as in humans with AD (e.g., differential response of female and male aged macaques [>20 years] that exhibit impaired performance in a delayed matching to sample [DMTS] task) [118]. Variations of delayed response tasks such as DMTS are most frequently employed in nonhuman primates since it is possible to measure cognitive domains relevant for human aging and AD such as recent memory and attention. Importantly, similar tasks are employed to assess cognitive function in human AD patients, so that translation from aged nonhuman primate to aged humans and AD patients is possible [119]. However, because aged monkeys are rare and often cost-prohibitive for many investigators, it is important to also have small animal models of AD. In recent years, this has led to an explosion of interest in transgenic mouse (and rat) models.

Several genetic mutations have been identified as causative in familial AD, and over the past 10 years our understanding of the underlying pathology of AD has been aided through the development of numerous transgenic mouse models that exhibit some of the key behavioral and pathological features of the disease. As a consequence, investigators have attempted to evaluate potential therapeutic approaches to intervene in the progression of this disease as well as more advanced palliative treatments compared to currently approved drugs. However, owing to the complex relationship between pathology and behavior in these mice and indeed in AD, this has been fraught with many difficulties, particularly with respect to reliability and interpretation. Furthermore, characterization of transgenic mice has been hampered by intellectual property issues, and as a result, it is often difficult to compare data across laboratories. Despite the number of transgenic lines and crosses that have been described [120–122], none recapitulates all aspects of AD, possibly because

AD takes decades to develop in humans, and the lifespan of rodent may be too short. Nevertheless, several transgenic lines do model subsets of the pathology, and some of the more popular ones are now discussed.

AD-relevant transgenic models can be broadly classified into mice that model the amyloid beta pathology or mice that model the tangle (tau) pathology, although some lines have been designed in an attempt to model both. Of the mice modeling, the amyloid beta pathology, perhaps one of the best known, is the commercially available Tg2576 mouse [123], which overexpresses the human APP Swedish mutation. This line exhibits amyloid plaques from 9 to 12 months of age onward in key brain regions such as the hippocampus, entorhinal, and frontal cortex as well as increased levels of soluble amyloid beta oligomers and vascular amyloid. No neurodegeneration is evident; however, and in our hands, these mice have proven very difficult to work with in behavioral studies of cognitive function. Thus, although useful, the Tg2576 line is an incomplete model of AD. Other popular mice modeling amyloid beta pathology include APP/Lo London mutation, APP23 Swedish mutation, and the PDAPP Indiana mutation (see Ref. 121 for a review). Intriguingly, a relatively recent transgenic line, the so-called triple transgenic model of AD (3 × Tg-AD), exhibits plaques and tangles as well as intracellular amyloid beta and synaptic dysfunction [124]. This line incorporates the Tg2576 Swedish mutation as well as human tau and presenillin (PS1) mutations. Reversible behavioral deficits are reported for 3 × Tg-AD mice as well as many of the others mentioned earlier, but it is difficult to rigorously and independently validate these data. Transgenic lines modeling tau pathology (e.g., JNPL3) or amyloid and tau pathology (e.g., TAPP) exhibit tangles in spinal cord and brainstem and suffer from marked motor disturbances and are not generally suitable for cognitive testing. An exception to this is the 3 × Tg-AD mouse line, exhibiting cognitive impairment that correlates with intraneuronal amyloid beta, which precedes extracellular Aβ deposition as plaques and the subsequent increase in tau pathology [94]. Similarly, the APP/tau line develops amyloid deposits, neurofibrillary tangles, neuronal loss, as well as cognitive impairment.

In addition to the use of aged animals and transgenic mice, Alzheimer's researchers have long used lesion models to try to reproduce cognitive and cholinergic deficits observed in the human disease. Cholinergic neurons within the basal forebrain nuclei are found alongside various noncholinergic neurons, and nonselective lesions of all neuron types within this area lead to disruptions of cognitive functioning across a number of behavioral tasks including the water maze. In contrast, selective lesions to the basal forebrain cholinergic neurons using the immunotoxin, 192 IgG-saporin, which kills neurons expressing p75 nerve growth factor receptors, does not have much effect on water maze performance in mature rats and has only moderate impairing effects in aged rats [125]. Pharmacological reversal of such lesions has been challenging. For example, the nicotinic agonist, ABT-418, failed to improve measures of sustained attention in a rat-operant task in 192 IgG-saporin-lesioned rats, whereas it readily improved performance in sham-operated rats [126].

To the best of our knowledge, no data assessing the effects of H_3 receptor antagonists have been published in nonhuman primate or rodent transgenic models of AD. With respect to primate models, this may be related to the difficulties inherent in conducting such studies or the potential differences in splice variants of H_3 receptors found in monkey versus human and rodent brain tissues [127]. With regard to transgenic models, this may be because of the difficulties encountered in obtaining sufficient numbers of commercially available animals or with the (largely unpublished but well-recognized) difficulties associated with assessing behavioral function in such animals. However, at the XXXV annual meeting of the European Histamine Research Society (May 10–13, 2006, Delphi, Greece), Ning and colleagues from Wyeth presented data suggesting increased neuronal H_3 receptor expression in brains of Tg2576 mice, which overexpress the Swedish mutation of APP. Furthermore, scopolamine-induced amnesia for contextual memory in these mice was reversed by the H_3 receptor antagonist, ciproxifan, supporting the potential utility for H_3 receptor antagonists for the treatment of AD.

POTENTIAL FUTURE DIRECTIONS

The H_3 histaminergic field awaits with interest the results of ongoing clinical studies to determine whether blockade of these receptors can deliver efficacy in various disease states such as ADHD, Alzheimer's, and schizophrenia. Although evidence of improved daily function as a consequence of relieving symptoms in these diseases will be a key step forward, there is also a slow recognition that modulation of H_3 receptors may have potential disease altering effects. For example, H_3 receptors have been linked to neuroprotective mechanisms in the developing hippocampus [128] and in hibernating hamsters [129] as well as playing a potential role in ischemia-reperfusion pathology in the rat brain [130]. The potential for symptom and disease-altering effects through modulation of H_3 receptors, if supported by additional evidence, thus represents an exciting area for further research. Additional work to develop hybrid molecules that concomitantly block H_3 receptors plus an additional pharmacology (e.g., also inhibit cholinesterases) also represents an interesting new approach to the treatment of AD that is attracting some attention [131].

CONCLUSIONS

Research in the H_3 histaminergic field has come a long way in the past decade, and clear preclinical evidence exists for efficacy of H_3 receptor antagonists in animal models of ADHD or of cognitive domains relevant for ADHD and AD. Importantly, we have finally reached the stage where H_3 receptor antagonists are also being evaluated in clinical trials for safety and efficacy across a range of neurological disorders including ADHD and AD. The results of these clinical trials are eagerly awaited with the hope that drugs targeting histamine H_3 receptors will be as efficacious and successful as predecessor drugs targeting H_1 and H_2 receptors for their respective disease indications.

ACKNOWLEDGMENT

The authors thank Lawrence Black for help with the preparation of this manuscript.

REFERENCES

1. Chung, B., Suzuki, A.R. and Mcgough, J.J. 2002. New drugs for treatment of attention-deficit/hyperactivity disorder. *Expert Opin Emerg Drugs* 7: 269–276.
2. Mcgough, J.J. and Barkley, R.A. 2004. Diagnostic controversies in adult attention deficit hyperactivity disorder. *Am J Psychiatry* 161: 1948–1956.
3. Biederman, J., Spencer, T. and Wilens, T. 2004. Evidence-based pharmacotherapy for attention-deficit hyperactivity disorder. *Int J Neuropsychopharmacol* 7: 77–97.
4. Wolraich, M.L., Wibbelsman, C.J., Brown, T.E., Evans, S.W., Gotlieb, E.M., Knight, J.R., Ross, E.C., Shubiner, H.H., Wender, E.H. and Wilens, T. 2005. Attention-deficit/hyperactivity disorder among adolescents: a review of the diagnosis, treatment, and clinical implications. *Pediatrics* 115: 1734–1746.
5. Evans, S.W., Pelham, W.E., Smith, B.H., Bukstein, O., Gnagy, E.M., Greiner, A.R., Altenderfer, L. and Baron-Myak, C. 2001. Dose-response effects of methylphenidate on ecologically valid measures of academic performance and classroom behavior in adolescents with ADHD. *Exp Clin Psychopharmacol* 9: 163–175.
6. Greenhill, L.L., Pliszka, S., Dulcan, M.K., Bernet, W., Arnold, V., Beitchman, J., Benson, R.S., Bukstein, O., Kinlan, J., Mcclellan, J., Rue, D., Shaw, J.A. and Stock, S. 2002. Practice parameter for the use of stimulant medications in the treatment of children, adolescents, and adults. *J Am Acad Child Adolesc Psychiatry* 41(2 Suppl): 26S–49S.
7. Wee, S. and Woolverton, W.L. 2004. Evaluation of the reinforcing effects of atomoxetine in monkeys: comparison to methylphenidate and desipramine. *Drug Alcohol Depend* 75: 271–276.
8. Michelson, D., Adler, L., Spencer, T., Reimherr, F.W., West, S.A., Allen, A.J., Kelsey, D., Wernicke, J., Dietrich, A. and Milton, D. 2003. Atomoxetine in adults with ADHD: two randomized, placebo-controlled studies. *Biol Psychiatry* 53: 112–120.
9. Creighton, C.J., Ramabadran, K., Ciccone, P.E., Liu, J., Orsini, M.J. and Reitz, A.B. 2004. Synthesis and biological evaluation of the major metabolite of atomoxetine: elucidation of a partial kappa-opioid agonist effect. *Bioorg Med Chem Lett* 14: 4083–4085.
10. Michelson, D., Allen, A.J., Busner, J., Casat, C., Dunn, D., Kratochvil, C., Newcorn, J., Sallee, F.R., Sangal, R.B., Saylor, K., West, S., Kelsey, D., Wernicke, J., Trapp, N.J. and Harder, D 2002. Once-daily atomoxetine treatment for children and adolescents with attention deficit hyperactivity disorder: a randomized, placebo-controlled study. *Am J Psychiatry* 159: 1896–1901.
11. Faraone, S.V. and Biederman, J. 1998. Neurobiology of attention-deficit hyperactivity disorder. *Biol Psychiatry* 44: 951–958.
12. Mcgough, J.J. 2005. Attention-deficit/hyperactivity disorder pharmacogenomics. *Biol Psychiatry* 57: 1367–1373.
13. Mick, E., Biederman, J., Faraone, S.V., Sayer, J. and Kleinman, S. 2002. Case-control study of attention-deficit hyperactivity disorder and maternal smoking, alcohol use, and drug use during pregnancy. *J Am Acad Child Adolesc Psychiatry* 41: 378–385.
14. Granon, S. and Changeux, J.P. 2006. Attention-deficit/hyperactivity disorder: a plausible mouse model? *Acta Paediatr* 95: 645–649.
15. Todd, R.D., Lobos, E.A., Sun, L.W. and Neuman, R.J. 2003. Mutational analysis of the nicotinic acetylcholine receptor alpha 4 subunit gene in attention deficit/hyperactivity disorder: evidence for association of an intronic polymorphism with attention problems. *Mol Psychiatry* 8: 103–108.
16. Bark, C., Bellinger, F.P., Kaushal, A., Mathews, J.R., Partridge, L.D. and Wilson, M.C. 2004. Developmentally regulated switch in alternatively spliced SNAP-25 isoforms alters facilitation of synaptic transmission. *J Neurosci* 24: 8796–8805.

17. Brophy, K., Hawi, Z., Kirley, A., Fitzgerald, M. and Gill, M. 2002. Synaptosomal-associated protein 25 (SNAP-25) and attention deficit hyperactivity disorder (ADHD): evidence of linkage and association in the Irish population. *Mol Psychiatry* 7: 913–917.
18. Barr, C.L., Feng, Y., Wigg, K., Bloom, S., Roberts, W., Malone, M., Schachar, R., Tannock, R. and Kennedy, J.L. 2000. Identification of DNA variants in the SNAP-25 gene and linkage study of these polymorphisms and attention-deficit hyperactivity disorder. *Mol Psychiatry* 5: 405–409.
19. Cahill, L. and Mcgaugh, J.L. 1995. A novel demonstration of enhanced memory associated with emotional arousal. *Conscious Cogn* 4: 410–421.
20. Passani, M.B., Lin, J.S., Hancock, A., Crochet, S. and Blandina, P. 2004. The histamine H_3 receptor as a novel therapeutic target for cognitive and sleep disorders. *Trends Pharmacol Sci* 25: 618–625.
21. Sakai, K., Mansari, M.E., J-S, L., Zhang, J. and Mercier, G.V. 1990. The posterior hypothalamus in the regulation of wakefulness and paradoxical sleep. In *The Diencephalon and Sleep*, ed. M. Mancia, pp. 171–198. Raven Press: New York.
22. Lin, J.S. 2000. Brain structures and mechanisms involved in the control of cortical activation and wakefulness, with emphasis on the posterior hypothalamus and histaminergic neurons. *Sleep Med Rev* 4: 471–503.
23. Cecchi, M., Passani, M.B., Bacciottini, L., Mannaioni, P.F. and Blandina, P. 2001. Cortical acetylcholine release elicited by stimulation of histamine H_1 receptors in the nucleus basalis magnocellularis: a dual-probe microdialysis study in the freely moving rat. *Eur J Neurosci* 13: 68–78.
24. Lin, J.S., Sakai, K. and Jouvet, M. 1994. Hypothalamo-preoptic histaminergic projections in sleep–wake control in the cat. *Eur J Neurosci* 6: 618–625.
25. Lin, J.S., Hou, Y., Sakai, K. and Jouvet, M. 1996. Histaminergic descending inputs to the mesopontine tegmentum and their role in the control of cortical activation and wakefulness in the cat. *J Neurosci* 16: 1523–1537.
26. Mignot, E., Taheri, S. and Nishino, S. 2002. Sleeping with the hypothalamus: emerging therapeutic targets for sleep disorders. *Nat Neurosci* 5 (Suppl): 1071–1075.
27. Huang, Z.L., Qu, W.M., Li, W.D., Mochizuki, T., Eguchi, N., Watanabe, T., Urade, Y. and Hayaishi, O. 2001. Arousal effect of orexin A depends on activation of the histaminergic system. *Proc Natl Acad Sci USA* 98: 9965–9970.
28. Eriksson, K.S., Sergeeva, O., Brown, R.E. and Haas, H.L. 2001. Orexin/hypocretin excites the histaminergic neurons of the tuberomammillary nucleus. *J Neurosci* 21: 9273–9279.
29. Nishino, S., Fujiki, N., Ripley, B., Sakurai, E., Kato, M., Watanabe, T., Mignot, E. and Yanai, K. 2001. Decreased brain histamine content in hypocretin/orexin receptor-2 mutated narcoleptic dogs. *Neurosci Lett* 313: 125–128.
30. Parmentier, R., Ohtsu, H., Djebbara-Hannas, Z., Valatx, J.L., Watanabe, T. and Lin, J.S. 2002. Anatomical, physiological, and pharmacological characteristics of histidine decarboxylase knock-out mice: evidence for the role of brain histamine in behavioral and sleep–wake control. *J Neurosci* 22: 7695–7711.
31. Green, J.P., Prell, G.D., Khandelwal, J.K. and Blandina, P. 1987. Aspects of histamine metabolism. *Agents Actions* 22: 1–15.
32. Kollonitsch, J., Perkins, L.M., Patchett, A.A., Doldouras, G.A., Marburg, S., Duggan, D.E., Maycock, A.L. and Aster, S.D. 1978. Selective inhibitors of biosynthesis of aminergic neurotransmitters. *Nature* 274: 906–908.
33. Passini, M.B., Bacciottini, L., Mannaioni, P.F. and Blandina, P. 2000. Central histaminergic system and cognition. *Neurosci Biobehav Rev* 2000: 107–113.
34. Russell, V.A. 2007. Neurobiology of animal models of attention-deficit hyperactivity disorder. *J Neurosci Methods* 161: 185–198.

35. Sagvolden, T., Russell, V.A., Aase, H., Johansen, E.B. and Farshbaf, M. 2005. Rodent models of attention-deficit/hyperactivity disorder. *Biol Psychiatry* 57: 1239–1247.

36. Fox, G.B., Pan, J.B., Esbenshade, T.A., Bennani, Y.L., Black, L.A., Faghih, R., Hancock, A.A. and Decker, M.W. 2002. Effects of histamine H(3) receptor ligands GT-2331 and ciproxifan in a repeated acquisition avoidance response in the spontaneously hypertensive rat pup. *Behav Brain Res* 131: 151–161.

37. De Bruin, N.M., Kiliaan, A.J., De Wilde, M.C. and Broersen, L.M. 2003. Combined uridine and choline administration improves cognitive deficits in spontaneously hypertensive rats. *Neurobiol Learn Mem* 80: 63–79.

38. Gainetdinov, R.R., Wetsel, W.C., Jones, S.R., Levin, E.D., Jaber, M. and Caron, M.G. 1999. Role of serotonin in the paradoxical calming effect of psychostimulants on hyperactivity. *Science* 283: 397–401.

39. Jones, S.R., Gainetdinov, R.R., Jaber, M., Giros, B., Wightman, R.M. and Caron, M.G. 1998. Profound neuronal plasticity in response to inactivation of the dopamine transporter. *Proc Natl Acad Sci* 95: 4029–4034.

40. Hess, E.J., Collins, K.A., Copeland, N.G., Jenkins, N.A. and Wilson, M.C. 1994. Deletion map of the coloboma (Cm) locus on mouse chromosome 2. *Genomics* 21: 257–261.

41. Hess, E.J., Collins, K.A. and Wilson, M.C. 1996. Mouse model of hyperkinesis implicates SNAP-25 in behavioral regulation. *J Neurosci* 16: 3104–3111.

42. Hess, E.J., Jinnah, H.A., Kozak, C.A. and Wilson, M.C. 1992. Spontaneous locomotor hyperactivity in a mouse mutant with a deletion including the Snap gene on chromosome 2. *J Neurosci* 12: 2865–2874.

43. Bruno, K.J., Freet, C.S., Twining, R.C., Egami, K., Grigson, P.S. and Hess, E.J. 2007. Abnormal latent inhibition and impulsivity in coloboma mice, a model of ADHD. *Neurobiol Dis* 25: 206–216.

44. Wilson, M.C. 2000. Coloboma mouse mutant as an animal model of hyperkinesis and attention deficit hyperactivity disorder. *Neurosci Biobehav Rev* 24: 51–57.

45. Dalley, J.W., Cardinal, R.N. and Robbins, T.W. 2004. Prefrontal executive and cognitive functions in rodents: neural and neurochemical substrates. *Neurosci Biobehav Rev* 28: 771–784.

46. Chudasama, Y., Nathwani, F. and Robbins, T.W. 2005. D-amphetamine remediates attentional performance in rats with dorsal prefrontal lesions. *Behav Brain Res* 158: 97–107.

47. Paz, R., Barsness, B., Martenson, T., Tanner, D. and Allan, A.M. 2007. Behavioral teratogenicity induced by nonforced maternal nicotine consumption. *Neuropsychopharmacology* 32: 693–699.

48. Hausknecht, K.A., Acheson, A., Farrar, A.M., Kieres, A.K., Shen, R.Y., Richards, J.B. and Sabol, K.E. 2005. Prenatal alcohol exposure causes attention deficits in male rats. *Behav Neurosci* 119: 302–310.

49. Xu, C. and Shen, R.Y. 2001. Amphetamine normalizes the electrical activity of dopamine neurons in the ventral tegmental area following prenatal ethanol exposure. *J Pharmacol Exp Ther* 297: 746–752.

50. Siesser, W.B., Zhao, J., Miller, L.R., Cheng, S.Y. and Mcdonald, M.P. 2006. Transgenic mice expressing a human mutant beta1 thyroid receptor are hyperactive, impulsive, and inattentive. *Genes Brain Behav* 5: 282–297.

51. Puumala, T., Ruotsalainen, S., Jakala, P., Koivisto, E., Riekkinen, P., Jr. and Sirvio, J. 1996. Behavioral and pharmacological studies on the validation of a new animal model for attention deficit hyperactivity disorder. *Neurobiol Learn Mem* 66: 198–211.

52. Heiser, P., Friedel, S., Dempfle, A., Konrad, K., Smidt, J., Grabarkiewicz, J., Herpertz-Dahlmann, B., Remschmidt, H. and Hebebrand, J. 2004. Molecular genetic aspects of attention-deficit/hyperactivity disorder. *Neurosci Biobehav Rev* 28: 625–641.

53. Hernandez, C.M., Hoifodt, H. and Terry, A.V., Jr. 2003. Spontaneously hypertensive rats: further evaluation of age-related memory performance and cholinergic marker expression. *J Psychiatry Neurosci* 28: 197–209.
54. Terry, A.V., Jr., Hernandez, C.M., Buccafusco, J.J. and Gattu, M. 2000. Deficits in spatial learning and nicotinic-acetylcholine receptors in older, spontaneously hypertensive rats. *Neuroscience* 101: 357–368.
55. Gattu, M., Terry, A.V., Jr., Pauly, J.R. and Buccafusco, J.J. 1997. Cognitive impairment in spontaneously hypertensive rats: role of central nicotinic receptors. Part II. *Brain Res* 771: 104–114.
56. Sagvolden, T., Metzger, M.A., Schiorbeck, H.K., Rugland, A.L., Spinnangr, I. and Sagvolden, G. 1992. The spontaneously hypertensive rat (SHR) as an animal model of childhood hyperactivity (ADHD): changed reactivity to reinforcers and to psychomotor stimulants. *Behav Neural Biol* 58: 103–112.
57. Ueno, K.I., Togashi, H., Mori, K., Matsumoto, M., Ohashi, S., Hoshino, A., Fujita, T., Saito, H., Minami, M. and Yoshioka, M. 2002. Behavioural and pharmacological relevance of stroke-prone spontaneously hypertensive rats as an animal model of a developmental disorder. *Behav Pharmacol* 13: 1–13.
58. Wilens, T.E., Biederman, J., Spencer, T.J., Bostic, J., Prince, J., Monuteaux, M.C., Soriano, J., Fine, C., Abrams, A., Rater, M. and Polisner, D. 1999. A pilot controlled clinical trial of ABT-418, a cholinergic agonist, in the treatment of adults with attention deficit hyperactivity disorder. *Am J Psychiatry* 156: 1931–1937.
59. Pataki, C.S., Feinberg, D.T. and Mcgough, J.J. 2004. New drugs for the treatment of attention-deficit/hyperactivity disorder. *Expert Opin Emerg Drugs* 9: 293–302.
60. Levin, E.D., Conners, C.K., Silva, D., Canu, W. and March, J. 2001. Effects of chronic nicotine and methylphenidate in adults with attention deficit/hyperactivity disorder. *Exp Clin Psychopharmacol* 9: 83–90.
61. Ueno, K., Togashi, H., Matsumoto, M., Ohashi, S., Saito, H. and Yoshioka, M. 2002. Alpha4beta2 nicotinic acetylcholine receptor activation ameliorates impairment of spontaneous alternation behavior in stroke-prone spontaneously hypertensive rats, an animal model of attention deficit hyperactivity disorder. *J Pharmacol Exp Ther* 302: 95–100.
62. Ligneau, X., Morisset, S., Tardivel-Lacombe, J., Gbahou, F., Ganellin, C.R., Stark, H., Schunack, W., Schwartz, J.-C. and Arrang, J.M. 2000. Distinct pharmacology of rat and human histamine H_3 receptors; role of two amino acids in the third transmembrane domain. *Br J Pharmacol* 131: 1247–1250.
63. Tardivel-Lacombe, J., Rouleau, A., Heron, A., Morisset, S., Pillot, C., Cochois, V., Schwartz, J.C. and Arrang, J.M. 2000. Cloning and cerebral expression of the guinea pig histamine H_3 receptor: evidence for two isoforms. *Neuroreport* 11: 755–759.
64. Lovenberg, T.W., Roland, B.L., Wilson, S.J., Jiang, X., Pyati, J., Huvar, A., Jackson, M.R. and Erlander, M.G. 1999. Cloning and functional expression of the human histamine H_3 receptor. *Mol Pharmacol* 55: 1101–1107.
65. Fox, G.B., Esbenshade, T.A., Pan, J.B., Radek, R.J., Krueger, K.M., Yao, B.B., Browman, K.E., Buckley, M.J., Ballard, M.E., Komater, V.A., Miner, H., Zhang, M., Faghih, R., Rueter, L.E., Bitner, R.S., Drescher, K.U., Wetter, J., Marsh, K., Lemaire, M., Porsolt, R.D., Bennani, Y.L., Sullivan, J.P., Cowart, M.D., Decker, M.W. and Hancock, A.A. 2005. Pharmacological properties of ABT-239 [4-(2-{2-[(2R)-2-Methylpyrrolidinyl]ethyl}-benzofuran-5-yl)benzonitrile]: II. Neurophysiological characterization and broad preclinical efficacy in cognition and schizophrenia of a potent and selective histamine H_3 receptor antagonist. *J Pharmacol Exp Ther* 313: 176–190.
66. Curtis, M.P., Dwight, W., Pratt, J., Cowart, M., Esbenshade, T.A., Krueger, K.M., Fox, G.B., Pan, J.B., Pagano, T.G., Hancock, A.A., Faghih, R. and Bennani, Y.L. 2004.

D-amino acid homopiperazine amides: discovery of A-320436, a potent and selective non-imidazole histamine H(3)-receptor antagonist. *Arch Pharm* (Weinheim) 337: 219–229.

67. Esbenshade, T.A., Fox, G.B., Krueger, K.M., Baranowski, J.L., Miller, T.R., Kang, C.H., Denny, L.I., Witte, D.G., Yao, B.B., Pan, J.B., Faghih, R., Bennani, Y.L., Williams, M. and Hancock, A.A. 2004. Pharmacological and behavioral properties of A-349821, a selective and potent human histamine H_3 receptor antagonist. *Biochem Pharmacol* 68: 933–945.

68. Bonaventure, P., Letavic, M., Dugovic, C., Wilson, S., Aluisio, L., Pudiak, C., Lord, B., Mazur, C., Kamme, F., Nishino, S., Carruthers, N. and Lovenberg, T. 2007. Histamine H_3 receptor antagonists: from target identification to drug leads. *Biochem Pharmacol* 73: 1084–1096.

69. Robbins, T.W. 2002. The 5-choice serial reaction time task: behavioural pharmacology and functional neurochemistry. *Psychopharmacology* (Berl) 163: 362–380.

70. Taffe, M.A., Davis, S.A., Yuan, J., Schroeder, R., Hatzidimitriou, G., Parsons, L.H., Ricaurte, G.A. and Gold, L.H. 2002. Cognitive performance of MDMA-treated rhesus monkeys: sensitivity to serotonergic challenge. *Neuropsychopharmacology* 27: 993–1005.

71. Stolerman, I.P., Mirza, N.R., Hahn, B. and Shoaib, M. 2000. Nicotine in an animal model of attention. *Eur J Pharmacol* 393: 147–154.

72. Ligneau, X., Lin, J., Vanni-Mercier, G., Jouvet, M., Muir, J.L., Ganellin, C.R., Stark, H., Elz, S., Schunack, W. and Schwartz, J. 1998. Neurochemical and behavioral effects of ciproxifan, a potent histamine H_3 receptor antagonist. *J Pharmacol Exp Ther* 287: 658–666.

73. Kirkby, D.L. and Higgins, G.A. 1998. Characterization of perforant path lesions in rodent models of memory and attention. *Eur J Neurosci* 10: 823–838.

74. Day, M., Pan, J.B., Buckley, M.J., Cronin, E., Hollingsworth, P.R., Hirst, W.D., Navarra, R., Sullivan, J.P., Decker, M.W. and Fox, G.B. 2007. Differential effects of ciproxifan and nicotine on impulsivity and attention measures in the 5-choice serial reaction time test. *Biochem Pharmacol* 73: 1123–1134.

75. Caselli, R.J., Beach, T.G., Yaari, R. and Reiman, E.M. 2006. Alzheimer's disease a century later. *J Clin Psychiatry* 67: 1784–1800.

76. Mckhann, G., Drachman, D., Folstein, M., Katzman, R., Price, D. and Stadlan, E.M. 1984. Clinical diagnosis of Alzheimer's disease: report of the NINCDS-ADRDA work group under the auspices of department of health and human services task force on Alzheimer's disease. *Neurology* 34: 939–944.

77. Edison, P., Archer, H.A., Hinz, R., Hammers, A., Pavese, N., Tai, Y.F., Hotton, G., Cutler, D., Fox, N., Kennedy, A., Rossor, M. and Brooks, D.J. 2007. Amyloid, hypometabolism, and cognition in Alzheimer disease: an [11C]PIB and [18F]FDG PET study. *Neurology* 68: 501–508.

78. Rowe, C.C., Ng, S., Ackermann, U., Gong, S.J., Pike, K., Savage, G., Cowie, T.F., Dickinson, K.L., Maruff, P., Darby, D., Smith, C., Woodward, M., Merory, J., Tochon-Danguy, H., O'keefe, G., Klunk, W.E., Mathis, C.A., Price, J.C., Masters, C.L. and Villemagne, V.L. 2007. Imaging beta-amyloid burden in aging and dementia. *Neurology* 68: 1718–1725.

79. Petersen, R.C., Doody, R., Kurz, A., Mohs, R.C., Morris, J.C., Rabins, P.V., Ritchie, K., Rossor, M., Thal, L. and Winblad, B. 2001. Current concepts in mild cognitive impairment. *Arch Neurol* 58: 1985–1992.

80. Petersen, R.C., Smith, G.E., Waring, S.C., Ivnik, R.J., Tangalos, E.G. and Kokmen, E. 1999. Mild cognitive impairment: clinical characterization and outcome. *Arch Neurol* 56: 303–308.

81. Kemppainen, N.M., Aalto, S., Wilson, I.A., Nagren, K., Helin, S., Bruck, A., Oikonen, V., Kailajarvi, M., Scheinin, M., Viitanen, M., Parkkola, R. and Rinne, J.O. 2007. PET amyloid ligand [11C]PIB uptake is increased in mild cognitive impairment. *Neurology* 68: 1603–1606.

82. Davatzikos, C., Fan, Y., Wu, X., Shen, D. and Resnick, S.M. 2006. Detection of prodromal Alzheimer's disease via pattern classification of MRI. *Neurobiol Aging* Dec 13, 29: 523–524.

83. Coyle, J.T., Price, D.L. and Delong, M.R. 1983. Alzheimer's disease: a disorder of cortical cholinergic innervation. *Science* 219: 1184–1190.

84. Bartus, R.T., Dean, R.L., 3rd, Beer, B. and Lippa, A.S. 1982. The cholinergic hypothesis of geriatric memory dysfunction. *Science* 217: 408–414.

85. Terry, A.V., Jr. and Buccafusco, J.J. 2003. The cholinergic hypothesis of age and Alzheimer's disease-related cognitive deficits: recent challenges and their implications for novel drug development. *J Pharmacol Exp Ther* 306: 821–827.

86. Samanta, M.K., Wilson, B., Santhi, K., Kumar, K.P. and Suresh, B. 2006. Alzheimer disease and its management: a review. *Am J Ther* 13: 516–526.

87. Ridha, B.H., Barnes, J., Bartlett, J.W., Godbolt, A., Pepple, T., Rossor, M.N. and Fox, N.C. 2006. Tracking atrophy progression in familial Alzheimer's disease: a serial MRI study. *Lancet Neurol* 5: 828–834.

88. Rusinek, H., De Santi, S., Frid, D., Tsui, W.H., Tarshish, C.Y., Convit, A. and De Leon, M.J. 2003. Regional brain atrophy rate predicts future cognitive decline: 6-year longitudinal MR imaging study of normal aging. *Radiology* 229: 691–696.

89. Lee, V.M. and Trojanowski, J.Q. 1992. The disordered neuronal cytoskeleton in Alzheimer's disease. *Curr Opin Neurobiol* 2: 653–656.

90. Hardy, J. and Selkoe, D.J. 2002. The amyloid hypothesis of Alzheimer's disease: progress and problems on the road to therapeutics. *Science* 297: 353–356.

91. Hardy, J.A. and Higgins, G.A. 1992. Alzheimer's disease: the amyloid cascade hypothesis. *Science* 256: 184–185.

92. Schenk, D. 2002. Amyloid-beta immunotherapy for Alzheimer's disease: the end of the beginning. *Nat Rev Neurosci* 3: 824–828.

93. Schenk, D., Barbour, R., Dunn, W., Gordon, G., Grajeda, H., Guido, T., Hu, K., Huang, J., Johnson-Wood, K., Khan, K., Kholodenko, D., Lee, M., Liao, Z., Lieberburg, I., Motter, R., Mutter, L., Soriano, F., Shopp, G., Vasquez, N., Vandevert, C., Walker, S., Wogulis, M., Yednock, T., Games, D. and Seubert, P. 1999. Immunization with amyloid-beta attenuates Alzheimer-disease-like pathology in the PDAPP mouse. *Nature* 400: 173–177.

94. Laferla, F.M., Green, K.N. and Oddo, S. 2007. Intracellular amyloid-beta in Alzheimer's disease. *Nat Rev Neurosci* 8: 499–509.

95. Klein, W.L. 2002. Abeta toxicity in Alzheimer's disease: globular oligomers (ADDLs) as new vaccine and drug targets. *Neurochem Int* 41: 345–352.

96. Klein, W.L. 2002. ADDLs & protofibrils—the missing links? *Neurobiol Aging* 23: 231–235.

97. Lesne, S., Koh, M.T., Kotilinek, L., Kayed, R., Glabe, C.G., Yang, A., Gallagher, M. and Ashe, K.H. 2006. A specific amyloid-beta protein assembly in the brain impairs memory. *Nature* 440: 352–357.

98. Safe, S.H. 1994. Polychlorinated biphenyls (PCBs): environmental impact, biochemical and toxic responses, and implications for risk assessment. *Crit Rev Toxicol* 24: 87–149.

99. Barghorn, S., Nimmrich, V., Striebinger, A., Krantz, C., Keller, P., Janson, B., Bahr, M., Schmidt, M., Bitner, R.S., Harlan, J., Barlow, E., Ebert, U. and Hillen, H. 2005. Globular amyloid beta-peptide oligomer—a homogenous and stable neuropathological protein in Alzheimer's disease. *J Neurochem* 95: 834–847.

100. Panula, P., Rinne, J., Kuokkanen, K., Eriksson, K.S., Sallmen, T., Kalimo, H. and Relja, M. 1998. Neuronal histamine deficit in Alzheimer's disease. *Neuroscience* 82: 993–997.
101. Medhurst, A.D., Atkins, A.R., Beresford, I.J., Brackenborough, K., Briggs, M.A., Calver, A.R., Cilia, J., Cluderay, J.E., Crook, B., Davis, J.B., Davis, R.K., Davis, R.P., Dawson, L.A., Foley, A.G., Gartlon, J., Gonzalez, M.I., Heslop, T., Hirst, W.D., Jennings, C., Jones, D.N., Lacroix, L.P., Martyn, A., Ociepka, S., Ray, A., Regan, C.M., Roberts, J.C., Schogger, J., Southam, E., Stean, T.O., Trail, B.K., Upton, N., Wadsworth, G., Wald, J.A., White, T., Witherington, J., Woolley, M.L., Worby, A. and Wilson, D.M. 2007. GSK189254, a novel H_3 receptor antagonist that binds to histamine H_3 receptors in Alzheimer's disease brain and improves cognitive performance in preclinical models. *J Pharmacol Exp Ther* 321: 1032–1045.
102. Prast, H., Argyriou, A. and Philippu, A. 1996. Histaminergic neurons facilitate social memory in rats. *Brain Res.* 734: 316–318.
103. Cowart, M., Gfesser, G.A., Browman, K.E., Faghih, R., Miller, T.R., Milicic, I., Baranowski, J.L., Krueger, K.M., Witte, D.G., Molesky, A.L., Komater, V.A., Buckley, M.J., Diaz, G.J., Gagne, G.D., Zhou, D., Deng, X., Pan, L., Roberts, E.M., Diehl, M.S., Wetter, J.M., Marsh, K.C., Fox, G.B., Brioni, J.D., Esbenshade, T.A. and Hancock, A.A. 2007. Novel heterocyclic-substituted benzofuran histamine H_3 receptor antagonists: in vitro properties, drug-likeness, and behavioral activity. *Biochem Pharmacol* 73: 1243–1255.
104. Fox, G.B., Pan, J.B., Radek, R.J., Lewis, A.M., Bitner, R.S., Esbenshade, T.A., Faghih, R., Bennani, Y.L., Williams, M., Yao, B.B., Decker, M.W. and Hancock, A.A. 2003. Two novel and selective nonimidazole H_3 receptor antagonists A-304121 and A-317920: II. In vivo behavioral and neurophysiological characterization. *J Pharmacol Exp Ther* 305: 897–908.
105. Ligneau, X., Perrin, D., Landais, L., Camelin, J.C., Calmels, T.P., Berrebi-Bertrand, I., Lecomte, J.M., Parmentier, R., Anaclet, C., Lin, J.S., Bertaina-Anglade, V., La Rochelle, C.D., D'aniello, F., Rouleau, A., Gbahou, F., Arrang, J.M., Ganellin, C.R., Stark, H., Schunack, W. and Schwartz, J.C. 2007. BF2.649 [1-{3-[3-(4-Chlorophenyl)propoxy]-propyl}piperidine, hydrochloride], a nonimidazole inverse agonist/antagonist at the human histamine H_3 receptor: preclinical pharmacology. *J Pharmacol Exp Ther* 320: 365–375.
106. Meguro, K., Yanai, K., Sakai, N., Sakurai, E., Maeyama, K., Sasaki, H. and Watanabe, T. 1995. Efects of thioperamide, a histamine H_3 antagonist, on the step-through passive avoidance response and histidine decarboxylase activity in senescence-accelerated mice. *Pharmacol Biochem Behav* 50: 321–325.
107. Giovannini, M.G., Bartolini, L., Bacciottini, L., Greco, L. and Blandina, P. 1999. Effects of H_3 receptor agonists and antagonists on cognitive performance and scopolamine-induced amnesia. *Behav Brain Res* 104: 147–155.
108. Medhurst, A.D., Briggs, M.A., Bruton, G., Calver, A.R., Chessell, I., Crook, B. et al. 2007. Structurally novel histamine H_3 receptor antagonists GSK207040 and GSK334429 improve scopolamine-induced memory impairment and capsaicin-induced secondary allodynia in rats. *Biochem Pharmacol* 73: 1182–1194.
109. Blandina, P., Giorgetti, M., Bartolini, L., Cecchi, M., Timmerman, H., Leurs, R., Pepeu, G. and Giovanni, M.G. 1996. Inhibition of cortical acetylcholine release and cognitive performance by histamine H_3 receptor activation in rats. *Br J Pharmacol* 119: 1656–1664.
110. Toyota, H., Dugovic, C., Koehl, M., Laposky, A.D., Weber, C., Ngo, K., Wu, Y., Lee, D.H., Yanai, K., Sakurai, E., Watanabe, T., Liu, C., Chen, J., Barbier, A.J.,

Turek, F.W., Fung-Leung, W.P. and Lovenberg, T.W. 2002. Behavioral characterization of mice lacking histamine H(3) receptors. *Mol Pharmacol* 62: 389–397.

111. Komater, V.A., Buckley, M.J., Browman, K.E., Pan, J.B., Hancock, A.A., Decker, M.W. and Fox, G.B. 2005. Effects of histamine H₃ receptor antagonists in two models of spatial learning. *Behav Brain Res* 159: 295–300.

112. Chen, Z. and Kamei, C. 2000. Facilitating effects of histamine on spatial memory deficit induced by scopolamine in rats. *Acta Pharmacol Sin* 21: 814–818.

113. Rizk, A., Curley, J., Robertson, J. and Raber, J. 2004. Anxiety and cognition in histamine H₃ receptor-/-mice. *Eur J Neurosci* 19: 1992–1996.

114. Orsetti, M., Ferretti, C., Gamalero, R. and Ghi, P. 2002. Histamine H₃ receptor blockade in the rat nucleus basalis magnocellularis improves place recognition memory. *Psychopharmacology* 159: 133–137.

115. Huang, Y.W., Hu, W.W., Chen, Z., Zhang, L.S., Shen, H.Q., Timmerman, H., Leurs, R. and Yanai, K. 2004. Effect of the histamine H₃-antagonist clobenpropit on spatial memory deficits induced by MK-801 as evaluated by radial maze in Sprague–Dawley rats. *Behav Brain Res* 151: 287–293.

116. Borchelt, D.R.E.A. 1997. Animal models relevant to Alzheimer's disease. In *Pharmacological Treatment of Alzheimer's Disease,* eds. J.D. Brioni and M.W. Decker, pp. 315–327, Wiley: Hoboken, NJ.

117. Bartus, R.T. 2000. On neurodegenerative diseases, models, and treatment strategies: lessons learned and lessons forgotten a generation following the cholinergic hypothesis. *Exp Neurol* 163: 495–529.

118. Buccafusco, J.J., Jackson, W.J., Stone, J.D. and Terry, A.V. 2003. Sex dimorphisms in the cognitive-enhancing action of the Alzheimer's drug donepezil in aged Rhesus monkeys. *Neuropharmacology* 44: 381–389.

119. Squire, L.R., Zola-Morgan, S. and Chen, K.S. 1988. Human amnesia and animal models of amnesia: performance of amnesic patients on tests designed for the monkey. *Behav Neurosci* 102: 210–221.

120. Mcgowan, E., Eriksen, J. and Hutton, M. 2006. A decade of modeling Alzheimer's disease in transgenic mice. *Trends Genet* 22: 281–289.

121. Sankaranarayanan, S. 2006. Genetically modified mice models for Alzheimer's disease. *Curr Top Med Chem* 6: 609–627.

122. Eriksen, J.L. and Janus, C.G. 2007. Plaques, tangles, and memory loss in mouse models of neurodegeneration. *Behav Genet* 37: 79–100.

123. Hsiao, K.K. 1995. Understanding the biology of beta-amyloid precursor proteins in transgenic mice. *Neurobiol Aging* 16: 705–706.

124. Oddo, S., Caccamo, A., Shepherd, J.D., Murphy, M.P., Golde, T.E., Kayed, R., Metherate, R., Mattson, M.P., Akbari, Y. and Laferla, F.M. 2003. Triple-transgenic model of Alzheimer's disease with plaques and tangles: intracellular Abeta and synaptic dysfunction. *Neuron* 39: 409–421.

125. Bannon, A.W., Curzon, P., Gunther, K.L. and Decker, M.W. 1996. Effects of intraseptal injection of 192-IgG-saporin in mature and aged long-evans rats. *Brain Res* 718: 25–36.

126. Mcgaughy, J., Decker, M.W. and Sarter, M. 1999. Enhancement of sustained attention performance by the nicotinic acetylcholine receptor agonist ABT-418 in intact but not basal forebrain-lesioned rats. *Psychopharmacology* 144: 175–182.

127. Yao, B.B., Sharma, R., Cassar, S., Esbenshade, T.A. and Hancock, A.A. 2003. Cloning and pharmacological characterization of the monkey histamine H₃ receptor. *Eur J Pharmacol* 482: 49–60.

128. Kukko-Lukjanov, T.K., Soini, S., Taira, T., Michelsen, K.A., Panula, P. and Holopainen, I.E. 2006. Histaminergic neurons protect the developing hippocampus from kainic acid-induced neuronal damage in an organotypic coculture system. *J Neurosci* 26: 1088–1097.

129. Canonaco, M., Madeo, M., Alo, R., Giusi, G., Granata, T., Carelli, A., Canonaco, A. and Facciolo, R.M. 2005. The histaminergic signaling system exerts a neuroprotective role against neurodegenerative-induced processes in the hamster. *J Pharmacol Exp Ther* 315: 188–195.

130. Lozada, A., Munyao, N., Sallmen, T., Lintunen, M., Leurs, R., Lindsberg, P.J. and Panula, P. 2005. Postischemic regulation of central histamine receptors. *Neuroscience* 136: 371–379.

131. Petroianu, G., Arafat, K., Sasse, B.C. and Stark, H. 2006. Multiple enzyme inhibitions by histamine H_3 receptor antagonists as potential procognitive agents. *Pharmazie* 61: 179–182.

8 Sleep Disorders

Jonathan E. Shelton, Timothy W. Lovenberg, and Christine Dugovic

CONTENTS

Introduction 241
    The Sleep/Wake Cycle 242
    The Function of the Sleep/Wake Cycle 244
    Underlying Processes of the Sleep/Wake Cycle 245
    Biochemical and Physiological Mechanisms That Control
        the Sleep/Wake Cycle 246
H_3 Receptor and the Sleep/Wake Cycle 247
    The Role of Histamine in the Regulation of the Sleep/Wake Cycle 247
    H_3 Receptor Agonists and Sleep Induction and Promotion 251
    H_3 Receptor Antagonists as Wake-Promoting Agents 251
    Comparative Electroencephalogram Spectral Study with H_3 Receptor
        Antagonists versus Psychostimulants 254
    Utilizing Transgenic Models to Define the Role of H_3 Receptor
        in Sleep/Wake Regulation 256
    H_3 Receptor Antagonism Combined with Selective Serotonin Reuptake
        Inhibitor 258
Indications for H_3 Receptor Antagonists in Sleep/Wake Disorders 261
    Excessive Daytime Sleepiness 261
    Narcolepsy 262
    Sleep Apnea 265
    Idiopathic Hypersomnia 267
Summary 267
References 268

INTRODUCTION

For several decades, scientists have investigated mechanisms that regulate the sleep/ wake cycle. Only recently, however, have we started to learn that the regulation of the active wake phase and a sleep period is more than merely passive. In fact, the control of when an individual sleeps and when he/she is awake is extremely complex and requires communication among several brain regions and the periphery through the release of various neurotransmitters and peptides [1]. The derangement of one

or more of these physiological processes can result in a number of sleep disturbances such as insomnia, sleep apnea, circadian rhythm disorders, narcolepsy, and
parasomnias. Current research has also demonstrated that disruptions in the sleep/
wake cycle can result in not only a disruption in the normal sleep pattern but also
negatively influence other physiological systems within the body including metabolism, cardiovascular, and the ability to defend against pathogens [2–5]. Owing to the
extensive implications of ensuring the correct quantity and quality of sleep, it has
become necessary to develop pharmacological intervention to correct disruptions in
the regulation of the sleep/wake cycle. Recent pharmacological research has given
rise to a number of agents including hypnotics that promote somnolence and also the
development of wake-promoting agents including modafinil and the histamine
H_3 receptor antagonists that hold promise to combat the alterations in sleep and
arousal. The present review will focus on H_3 receptor antagonists as promising clinical candidates for the treatment of daytime sleepiness.

THE SLEEP/WAKE CYCLE

Sleep was once believed to be a static process where the brain shuts down during
the night, and in the morning, the central processes are aroused so that an individual
can assume daily activities. This axiom was discredited, however, with the birth of
modern sleep research that was built around the invention of the electroencephalogram (EEG) to measure brain activity. By placing a series of electrical leads on
specific areas of the human scalp, a computer is able to record both subtle and obvious changes in brain activity throughout the various states of vigilance. Today, to
accurately identify each sleep/wake state, sleep studies are routinely performed by
coupling the brain activity measured with the EEG with an electrooculogram (EOG)
for recording eye movements and an electromyogram (EMG) for the assessment of
muscle activity. Using this triad (EEG, EMG, EOG) for polysomnography, sleep was
shown not to be static, but a very dynamic process consisting of various vigilance
states that cycle in an ultradian fashion. The first state is termed *wake* and is defined
as a state of arousal in which brain activity can alternate between a desynchronized
pattern consisting of low voltage, fast EEG waveforms, and a pattern that is sinu-
soidal in which alpha waves are the primary frequency (8–13 Hz) (Figure 8.1a).
In addition, the EMG will display prominent tonic activity as the individual moves,
whereas the EOG will also report movement in the ocular region as the eyes scan the
visual field and relay environmental cues to the brain. The second vigilance state is
referred to nonrapid eye movement (NREM) sleep. This state of sleep actually comprises four defined stages that represent the progression from a light sleep to deeper
more intense sleep as the night progresses. While an individual transitions into these
deeper stages of NREM, brain activity decreases and, therefore, the EEG switches
from a desynchronous, mixed alpha frequency in stage 1 to intense high-amplitude
delta waveforms (0.5–5 Hz) with no EMG activity (stage 4) (Figure 8.1a). The third
state of the sleep/wake cycle is rapid eye movement (REM) sleep. During this stage,
the EEG will switch back to low-voltage, theta-frequency (4–8 Hz) waveform with
relatively no activity recorded in the EMG except for small twitches that can occur
(Figure 8.1a). In addition, the EOG will detect bursts of activity as the eyes actuate

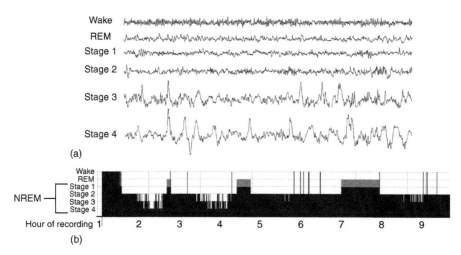

FIGURE 8.1 (a) Polysomnographic traces depicting the various waveforms that are characteristic of a specific state of vigilance. While awake, the fast frequency alpha (8–13 Hz) waveform predominates the EEG spectrum. As the individual starts to fall asleep, these high frequency desynchronous waveforms in the aroused state give rise to a mixed slower frequency in stages 1 and 2 and finally delta waves (0.5–5 Hz) that are the hallmarks of stages 3 and 4 of NREM sleep. The third vigilance state is referred to as REM sleep and is characterized by the appearance of waveforms in the theta frequency (4–8 Hz). (b) Hypnogram illustrating the transition between the various states of vigilance under optimal conditions in the human during the night. Approximately 20–30 min will elapse from the time an individual lies down in bed until he/she begins to fall asleep and enter the early stages of NREM sleep. The transition between stages 1 and 2 can occur very rapidly. As sleep progresses during the early part of the night, the lighter stages of NREM eventually give rise to deeper, more intense sleep during stages 3 and 4. At ~2 to 2.5 h after the induction of sleep, short episodes of REM will begin to appear. As the night continues, the deeper sleep occurring during stages 3 and 4 will diminish, and the frequency and duration of REM sleep episodes will increase. In addition, during the latter portions of the night, an individual will experience more frequent arousals.

in different directions. Under ideal sleep conditions, the ultradian transition between one episode of REM to the next will occur approximately every 90 min [6]. As the sleep cycle progresses throughout the night, the frequency of stages 3 and 4 of NREM sleep diminishes and gives rise to more frequent episodes of stage 2 NREM and REM sleep (Figure 8.1b). In addition to the readouts from the EEG, EMG, and EOG, sleep studies may also be coupled to additional monitors to measure heart and respiratory rate, a sensor to measure blood oxygen saturation, and also leads to monitor if an individual masticates during sleep. Using these polysomnographic traces as a guide, an investigator will visually assign states of vigilance to a defined period of time utilizing criteria first proposed by Rechtschaffen and Kales in a book titled *A Manual of Standardized Terminology, Techniques, and Scoring System for Sleep Stages of Human Subject*. Once these records are scored, several parameters related to the sleep/wake cycle including latency to NREM and REM sleep and also the architecture and consolidation of the various sleep stages can be assessed.

While these measurements can be useful to measure the quantity and relative quality of sleep, delta power (also referred to as slow wave activity) is calculated to assess the intensity of NREM sleep. From the very early days of sleep research, the prevalence of large slow waves in the delta frequency band (0.5–5 Hz) during the latter stage of NREM sleep was apparent on the EEG trace. These early sleep studies noted that as an individual progressed into stages 3 and 4 of NREM sleep and the brain waves recorded by the EEG transitioned from higher-frequency, low-amplitude to slower-frequency, high-amplitude delta waves, the ability to arouse the individual from slumber became increasingly difficult. Therefore, the correlation between the intensity and depth of sleep and the appearance of the delta waveforms was established. Subsequent mathematical analysis revealed that to calculate an index of sleep intensity, a power spectra analysis of NREM and REM sleep is performed by the transformation of the recorded digital signal into a frequency domain by a fast Fourier transformation. By examining not only the frequency but also the amplitude of each waveform, the intensity (as an index of quality) of sleep can be determined. Therefore, the assignment of the vigilance state (to calculate the duration of wake, NREM, or REM) and spectral analysis of the EEG waveforms are not mutually exclusive approaches, but rather complementary, and aid sleep researchers in determining both the quantity and quality of sleep for an individual.

THE FUNCTION OF THE SLEEP/WAKE CYCLE

Given the heterogenous state of the sleep/wake cycle, supplying an answer to the simple question as to why an organism sleeps is very complex, and several theories have been proposed. The first theory postulates that sleep is essential for an organism to conserve energy [7]. During sleep, the basal metabolic rate will decrease between 5 and 25% when compared to energy consumption during the waking hours [8]. Another theory is that sleep is needed for the restoration and repair of both peripheral and central processes [7]. During stages 3 and 4 of NREM sleep, the growth hormone signaling cascade is initiated and the amplified signal results in increased protein synthesis and cell mitosis [9]. Also, sleep may be needed to maintain an active immune defense against invading pathogens [3,10,11]. In severe chronic sleep restriction conditions, Rechtschaffen and colleagues [10] demonstrated that sleep-restricted rats were more prone to infection when compared to controlled nonsleep-deprived rats. In the most extreme sleep-deprived protocol, extended periods (~2 weeks) devoid of sleep resulted in death due to depleted host defense [12,13]. Accordingly, sleep may be represented as a state in which physiological systems (immune, metabolic) undergo growth, rejuvenation, and repair. Therefore, the true nature as to why an organism sleeps may be to ensure the survival of organism through the integration of all of these theories.

Additional theories highlight the importance of REM sleep. One theory supports the link between REM sleep and behavior. REM-centric sleep deprivation during the early years of development can result in behavioral maladjustments, lasting sleep fragmentation, and alteration in neuron survival [14,15]. In addition, several studies have emphasized the relationship between REM sleep and spatial and procedural memory consolidation, whereas slow wave sleep (stages 3 and 4) of NREM sleep is important in tasks involving declarative memory [16,17]. Another study has reported improved performance on perceptual or motor task following sleep [18]. However, the underlying mechanisms demonstrating a direct connection between sleep and memory are still under investigation. The results of these investigations will help to clarify how the various stages of sleep shape brain plasticity.

UNDERLYING PROCESSES OF THE SLEEP/WAKE CYCLE

The general view of sleep regulation is that two main processes are integrated to control the amount and timing of sleep [19]. The first process is related to the homeostatic mechanism (referred to as Process S) that dictates the overall drive to sleep and is a function of prior waking. Therefore, in an ideal situation, an individual is accruing sleep debt with each passing hour that he or she is awake. However, during the night, sleep drive normalizes as the person sleeps and compensates for the accumulated sleep debt experienced during the waking hours. Conversely, because sleep is under homeostatic regulation and will therefore try to maintain an average, sleep drive is diminished as a person sleeps and the sleep debt is paid. To examine how an organism responds to disruptions in the homeostatic process, researchers can vastly enhance sleep pressure by extending the time spent awake through various manipulations (e.g., total sleep deprivation or partial sleep restriction). Once sleep restriction is terminated and the subject is allowed to resume an undisturbed sleep period, the investigator can then measure the duration and slow wave activity of NREM sleep during the recovery period to assess the homeostat. Prolonged sleep restriction periods will be followed by an increased duration of NREM sleep that is accompanied by elevation in the slow wave activity of the recovery sleep.

The second process that interacts with Process S to regulate the sleep/wake cycle is timing (Process C) [19]. Throughout the day, an organism will experience cycles with peaks and troughs of activity (and inactivity) that can occur at various intervals. These cycles can be relatively short and range from a few seconds or hours (ultradian), ~24 h (diurnal), or a year (circannual). Owing to these temporal influences, various physiological systems within an organism will undergo various periods of peaks and troughs. For example, body temperature is not fixed at 37°C. Core body temperature will fluctuate between a peak during the mid-afternoon and obtain its nadir in early morning. A similar diurnal pattern can be measured with blood pressure and respiratory rate as well as a number of hormones including cortisol, prolactin, and leptin [20,21]. There are two important features to diurnal rhythms. The first is that the endogenous rhythm will occur even in the absence of environmental exogenous cues (i.e., light, food), which is also referred to as *zeitgebers* (German for "time giver"). Application of these cues to an individual will thus entrain the diurnal cycle. Entrainment to the 24-h cycle occurs when the cycle is reset due to signals from a *zeitgeber*. The second aspect is that even under free running conditions and, therefore, an absence of these inputs, the rhythm will exhibit a cycle of ~24 h or circadian (from the Latin *circa* for "approximately" and dies "day"). The persistence of a circadian rhythm in the absence of environmental cues provides evidence that circadian rhythms arise from an endogenous pacemaker that is independent of the environment.

The principal mammalian circadian clock resides within an area of the rostral hypothalamus termed the *suprachiasmatic nucleus* (SCN), which receives input from the retina [22,23]. In 1970s, a series of experiments demonstrated that damage to the SCN could disrupt and eventually destroy endocrine and behavioral circadian rhythms in rodents [24–26]. Rhythms were restored, however, when the SCN from a donor was transplanted into an animal with an ablated SCN [27]. Results of these studies helped to define the role of the mammalian SCN as the master circadian pacemaker. However, with the SCN lesion, it was shown that the overall amount of the sleep and wake does not significantly change, but the normal 24-h rhythm is no longer present.

Thus, the sleep/wake cycle is predominantly regulated by the integration of two mechanisms: Process S (homeostatic) and Process C (circadian). The circadian component influences sleep by integrating it to the time of day and behaves like an endogenous clock that can run in the presence or absence of external cues. The homeostatic component is related to the duration of wake [19,28]. Therefore, the longer an individual is awake, the higher the sleep drive. The accumulation or dissipation of sleep pressure resides in the interaction between the two components. For a diurnal species, Process S accrues during the day and diminishes during the rest period. The circadian Process C for sleep propensity, however, obtains its peak during the latter portion of the night. Thus, the diurnal animal will experience the onset of sleep when the greatest separation between Processes S and C occurs.

BIOCHEMICAL AND PHYSIOLOGICAL MECHANISMS THAT CONTROL THE SLEEP/WAKE CYCLE

The nuts and bolts of how an individual progresses from a state of arousal to NREM and, eventually, REM sleep are complex. Insight into a potential arousal pathway arose from the work of von Economo in which he identified patients who slept excessively (~20 h/day) due to a form of encephalitis. Further investigation by von Economo [29] revealed that this excessive sleep was due to lesions located between the midbrain and the diencephalon. These findings coupled with the reports from Moruzzi and Magoun helped to conceptualize the idea of arousal pathway(s) located within the brain [30].

Reports from a number of subsequent studies helped to identify the brain regions that are responsible in promoting wake. This arousal pathway was shown to originate from two routes with the first pathway emerging from the pedunculopontine (PPT) and laterodorsal tegmental (LDT) nuclei located in the pons. Within these brain regions, clusters of neurons synthesize and secrete the neurotransmitter acetylcholine. The activity of these cells is highest during wake and REM sleep, whereas they remain quiescent during NREM sleep when brain activity is diminished. During wake, this arousal signal is then transmitted from the brain stem to the reticular formation in the thalamus and then subsequently relayed onto the cortex.

The second arousal pathway circumvents the thalamus and relies on the input from several distinct brain regions located within the brain stem and lateral hypothalamus to communicate with the cerebral cortex. This pathway is located within the locus coeruleus that releases norepinephrine, the tuberomammillary nucleus (TMN) (histamine), A10 nuclei (dopamine), the dorsal, and medial raphe nuclei (serotonin). In addition, the arousal signal emanating from these areas is further reinforced by neurons in the hypothalamus that secrete the peptides such as orexin (also referred to as hypocretin).

During the active period, orexin is synthesized by a cluster of neurons within the posterior lateral hypothalamus as prepro-orexin peptide that is eventually cleaved by the enzyme convertase that liberates two peptides, orexin-A and orexin-B. Orexin-A can bind to either the G-protein-coupled orexin-1 or orexin-2 receptor, whereas orexin-B has only an affinity for the orexin-2 receptor. These receptors have specific localizations within areas of the brain that regulate sleep and wake including the TMN (orexin-2), LC (orexin-1), or the raphe, LDT, PPT that express both the orexin-1 and orexin-2 receptors. The result of orexin activation of these postsynpatic receptors is the release of wake-promoting neurotransmitters (i.e., histamine, acetylcholine, serotonin, norepinephrine) [31–33]. In turn, the release of these neurotransmitters inhibits the activity of the sleep centers within a distinct region of the lateral preoptic area of the hypothalamus termed the *ventral lateral preoptic* (VLPO) area [1,33].

During the natural rest period, however, the tonus of the orexin neurons is low. Without the orexin input to drive arousal, the transition into sleep will occur due to activation of a cluster of neurons located within the VLPO. Animal studies have reported that ablation of this area results in ~50% decrease in NREM and REM sleep [34]. Further neuroanatomical studies have identified clusters of inhibitory neurons within the VLPO that are most active during the sleep phase [35–37]. The terminals of these neurons located within the LC and TMN release the inhibitory neurotransmitters γ-aminobutyric acid (GABA) and galanin and therefore diminish the release of norepinephrine, serotonin, and histamine, respectively (Figure 8.2) [37,38].

H₃ RECEPTOR AND THE SLEEP/WAKE CYCLE

THE ROLE OF HISTAMINE IN THE REGULATION OF THE SLEEP/WAKE CYCLE

Approximately one century ago, Dale and his colleagues [39–41] isolated histamine from a common mold, ergot. Following the identification of this small molecule, subsequent research by Lewis in 1924 reported that the release of histamine resulted in the classical allergic *triple response* consisting of immediate red spots due to vasodilation, development of the wheal or localized swelling, and reflex of the nerve terminals resulting in flare [42]. The identification of histamine as a potential mediator of this immune response resulted in the development of the first generation of antihistamines such as phenbenzamine and mepyramine. Interestingly, the administration of this class of compounds not only alleviated the acute allergic inflammatory response, but also reported the drowsiness and somnolence [43]. With the identification of histamine as a mediator of central processes in the brain during the 1980s, it became apparent that disruption of the histaminergic signal might mediate the sedative effects of these compounds [44–46].

In tissues of the central nervous system, the synthesis and metabolism of the neurotransmitter histamine is regulated by the activity of major two enzymes. Histidine decarboxylase (HDC) is responsible for the metabolic conversion of the

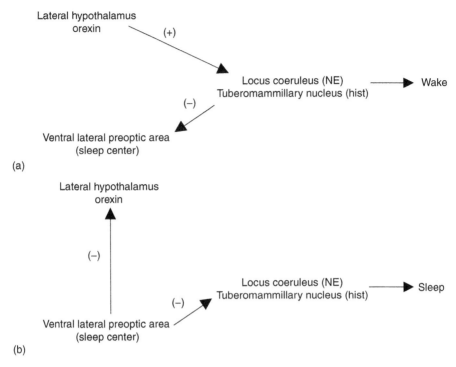

FIGURE 8.2 (a) Central regulation of neurochemical pathways that promote wake. During the light phase of a diurnal species, the tonus of the orexin neurons is elevated. The increased release of the orexin peptide during the active period results in activation of wake-promoting areas of the brain including the LC that releases the catecholamine norepinephrine and the TMN that releases histamine. The activation of the LC and the TMN results in a bimodal pathway leading to arousal. The first is to sequester the sleep centers localized within the VLPO, and the second is to activate arousal pathways in higher brain centers such as the cortex. (b) Activation of sleep centers within the VLPO that promotes sleep. During the night, however, the activity of the orexin neurons is diminished due to the influence of the inhibitory neuromodulators GABA and galanin released from nerve terminals emanating from the sleep centers within the VLPO. In addition, the VLPO inhibits the arousal promoting areas within the LC and the TMN. The net effect of these actions is to promote sleep.

essential amino acid precursor, L-histidine to histamine. To counteract the release and subsequent increase in histamine concentration, a second enzyme, histamine-N-methyltransferase inactivates histamine by methylating the imidazole ring. Once synthesized in the brain, histamine can act at the synaptic cleft by binding to a number of its receptors. Histamine receptor subtypes 1 and 2 (H_1 and H_2) are located on postsynaptic neurons and are responsible for relaying the histaminergic signal to downstream targets. The third type of histamine receptor (H_3) is predominantly an autoreceptor located presynaptically on histamine neurons and is involved in regulating the secretion of histamine into the synaptic space. On binding to the ligand, the H_3 receptor diminishes the release of histamine through an intracellular signaling cascade involving G_i proteins [47]. The H_3 receptor is also located on other neurons and modulates the release of various neurotransmitters including acetylcholine, norepinephrine, serotonin, dopamine, and GABA [48].

Histaminergic neurons are localized within the TMN and surrounding posterior hypothalamic area. These neurons send projections to a number of brain regions that are known to promote wake including corticothalamic and hypothalamic tracts, pons and the locus coeruleus to stimulate the release of wake-promoting neurotransmitters including dopamine, serotonin, norepinephrine, and acetylcholine [49]. Electrophysiological studies have reported that these neurons are tonically active during wake [50,51]. However, as brain activity starts to diminish as an organism starts to transition from wake to sleep, the output signal of these neurons become quiescent during NREM and REM sleep because of the diminished orexin signal and release of the inhibitory neurotransmitter GABA from terminals whose perikarya originate from the VLPO [50,51].

During the mid to late 1980s, results from a series of studies that involved disrupting histamine synthesis in both rodents and felines helped establish a direct link between histamine and the regulation of the sleep/wake cycle. The irreversible inhibitor of HDC, α-fluoromethylhistidine, was injected intraperitoneally at 50 mg/kg into rats during the light phase (the normal sleep/rest period for the rat, a nocturnal species). This had the effect of decreasing histamine synthesis, and the most striking observation from this study was that the time spent awake was dramatically reduced. This decrease in wake duration was paralleled with an increased time spent in NREM and REM sleep [52,53]. In cats, the peripheral or central administration of α-fluoromethylhistidine contributed to an increase in deep slow wave sleep at the expense of wake, whereas light sleep and REM sleep were unaffected by the administration of the compound [54]. In contrast, when the compound SKF-91488, an inhibitor of histamine-N-methyltransferase, which increases histamine concentration by inhibiting its metabolic inactivation, was injected centrally in the cat, a significant increase in wake was recorded [54].

Genetic manipulation of the histaminergic signal has also provided insight as to the role of histamine in the regulation of the sleep/wake cycle. Cortical EEG sleep studies utilizing mice that lack the gene for HDC reported an increase in REM sleep duration in the light phase and an alteration in the theta frequency band during wake when compared to wild-type (WT) controls [55]. In addition, HDC knockout (KO) mice exhibited decreased latency to NREM sleep after being subjected to a stimulus such as a novel environment [55]. In this study, the investigators demonstrated that the peripheral injection of α-fluoromethylhistidine, an inhibitor of the HDC to WT mice paralleled the decrease of wake observed in the HDC KO mice [55]. The administration of this compound to the HDC KO mice did not alter their sleep/wake cycle [55]. These results demonstrate that histamine is needed to maintain wake, so that the organism can adapt to behavioral adversity.

In addition, pharmacological manipulation of the histaminergic signal was utilized to identify receptor subtypes that regulate the sleep/wake cycle. Intracerebroventricular administration of the agonist for the postsynaptic H_1 receptor, 2-thiazolyethylamine, increased time spent awake in a dose-dependent manner with a concomitant decrease in both NREM and REM sleep in rats [56,57]. In contrast, peripheral administration of brain-penetrant antagonists of the H_1 receptor, pyrilamine and diphenhydramine, decreased wake and increased NREM sleep [56]. Further evidence that the H_1 receptor is involved in regulating the sleep/wake cycle was confirmed by first injecting 2-thiazolyethylamine with subsequent administration of pyrilamine, thus negating the sleep-promoting effect of the agonist [56]. Similar soporific effects were recorded with both the peripheral and central administration of the H_1 antagonist mepyramine in the cat [54].

To identify the mechanism that results in sedation following H_1 receptor antagonist administration, an EEG spectral analysis study was performed after the administration of the H_1 receptor antagonists diphenhydramine, pyrilamine, and cyproheptadine. Starting at 30 min postinjection and continuing for the remainder of the study, the compounds resulted in an EEG pattern that was indicative of drowsiness (increased slow wave activity as recorded from the frontal cortex). The sedative effect invoked by the H_1 receptor antagonists was diminished following pretreatment with the histamine precursor, histidine, and the acetylcholinesterase inhibitor physostigmine, whereas serotonin was without effect [58]. These findings demonstrate that the alterations in the delta and theta bands recorded from the rat frontal cortex elicited by the H_1 receptor antagonists are due to modulation of both histaminergic and cholinergic signal transmission.

The genetic and pharmacological identity of the H_3 receptor remained elusive until the seminal work originating from the Schwartz laboratory at the INSERM in France. In 1983, utilizing tissue isolated from the cortical region of the rat, it was demonstrated that once histamine was released from the presynaptic nerve terminal, the neurotransmitter could then feedback on a novel class of histamine receptor and inhibit its own release from the nerve terminal [59]. The autoreceptor was pharmacologically different from the two previously described histamine receptors (H_1 and H_2). Therefore, this novel class of histamine receptor identified by Schwartz and his colleagues was termed H_3.

The genetic identity of this novel receptor was not determined until 1998. By searching for homology of expressed sequence tag databases, a partial clone (GPCR97) was identified. This particular receptor exhibited significant homology to monoamine receptors previously reported. Subsequent molecular studies revealed the identity of GPCR97 to be the H_3 receptor [60]. Neuroanatomical investigation was able to localize these receptors to various areas of the brain known to regulate the sleep/wake cycle and behavioral and cognition including the striatum, hippocampus, amygdala, thalamus, and cortex [61,62].

In addition to its role as an autoreceptor regulating histamine, the H_3 receptor also acts as a heteroreceptor on nonhistamine containing neurons (acetylcholine, norepinephrine, serotonin, dopamine, and GABA) [48]. Because the H_3 receptor is a negative modulator of arousal-promoting neurotransmitters (i.e., acetylcholine, norepinephrine, serotonin), it was hypothesized that inhibiting the action of the receptor through specific antagonists might increase wake, and conversely, activation of the receptor might promote sleep. Utilizing electrophysiological techniques, specific neurons in the posterior hypothalamus were recorded during various states of vigilance in freely moving cats. From these studies, two main clusters of neurons were reported [63]. The first set resided within the TMN and surrounding areas and were sensitive to H_3 receptor manipulation. The tonus of these neurons was specific to wake such that as the animals transitioned from wake to light sleep, the action potentials recorded from these neurons dramatically decreased. Finally, as cats entered deeper stages of NREM and REM sleep, these neurons became quiescent. Administration of the H_3 receptor antagonist ciproxifan significantly elevated the firing rate of these neurons, whereas injection of the H_3 receptor agonists imetit or α-methylhistamine significantly decreased the discharge rate of these neurons. The authors noted that the discharge rate from a second group of neurons localized within the TMN and surrounding areas occurred primarily during wake. However, these neurons were insensitive to the activation or inhibition of the H_3 receptor [63]. These published accounts highlight the complex physiological, pharmacological, and anatomical link between H_3 receptor modulations and wake and sleep promotion.

H_3 Receptor Agonists and Sleep Induction and Promotion

Several studies have evaluated the sleep-inducing and sleep-promoting effects of various H_3 receptor agonists. Administration of BP-2.94 (20 and 30 mg/kg, p.o.) to rats significantly increased total time spent sleeping by ~30 min [64]. An increase in time spent in NREM sleep was responsible for the augmentation of total sleep time. This discrepancy when compared to vehicle was at the expense of both wake and REM sleep following administration of BP-2.94 to Wistar rats. The compound did not possess sleep-inducing effects since the time to the onset of NREM and REM sleep was comparable between BP-2.94 and vehicle. Interestingly, these sleep-promoting effects do not translate across other H_3 receptor agonists. Injection of the high-affinity H_3 receptor agonist immepip (5 and 10 mg/kg, i.p.) to rats did not significantly impact any of the sleep/wake parameters. Only a small, yet significant, decrease in the latency to NREM sleep was noted [64]. The lack of an effect of immepip was surprising since similar doses of the compound elicited a sustained decrease (~60 to 70%) in histamine concentration as measured through microdialysis from the frontal cortex in Sprague–Dawley rats [65]. With the uncertain efficacy of H_3 receptor agonists promoting and inducing sleep, studies to develop compounds that activate the H_3 receptor have diminished over the years.

H_3 Receptor Antagonists as Wake-Promoting Agents

Owing to the heterogenic nature of the H_3 receptor, developing specific antagonists to elevate concentrations of arousal promoting neurotransmitters such as histamine, acetylcholine, norepinephrine, and serotonin became an attractive target for developing wake-promoting agents. Early development of H_3 receptor antagonists was restricted to compounds that were derived from the structure of histamine and contained a 2-substituted imidazole moiety (Figure 8.3). These compounds (thioperamide, ciproxifan, and proxyfan) demonstrated efficacy by significantly increasing the time spent awake in rats [66]. However, these imidazole-containing H_3 receptor antagonists had several limitations that made them poor candidates for drug development. The imidazole-based structure severely hinders penetration of these compounds across the blood–brain barrier, therefore, limiting their centrally mediated efficacy. Also, these compounds inhibit the cytochrome P450 enzymes that can result in potential interactions with other drugs [67]. On the basis of the limitations of the imidazole containing

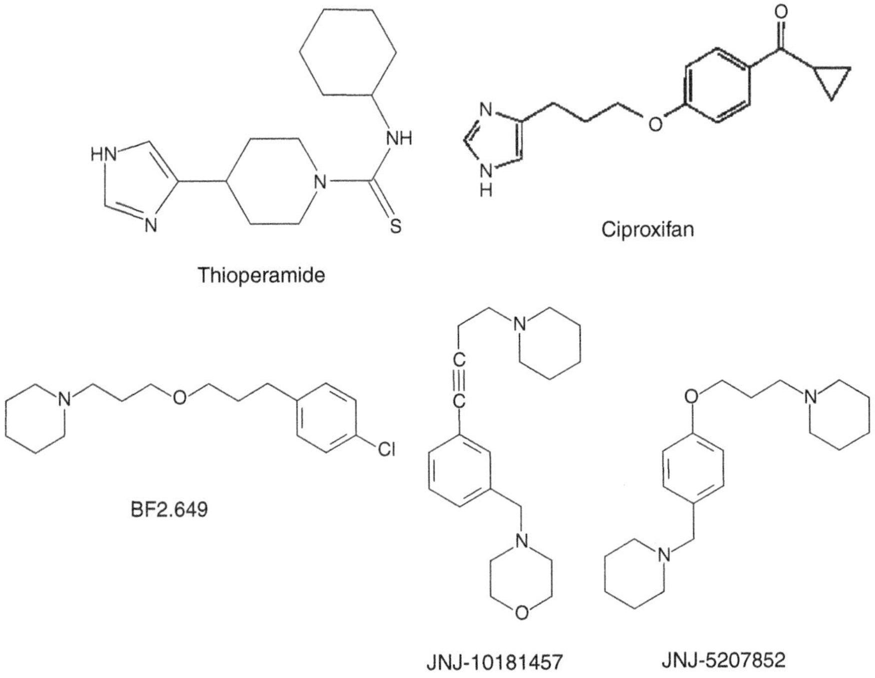

Thioperamide

Ciproxifan

BF2.649

JNJ-10181457   JNJ-5207852

FIGURE 8.3   Chemical structures of H$_3$ receptor ligands.

H$_3$ receptor antagonists, recent medicinal chemistry approaches have been utilized to develop compounds with greater selectivity and fewer limitations.

Recently, several nonimidazole-containing H$_3$ receptor antagonists have been described. One such compound, BF2.649 (Figure 8.3), has been disclosed to be in phase II clinical trials. *In vitro* analysis of this compound confirmed that BF2.649 is a potent competitive antagonist for the H$_3$ receptor (K_i = 0.16 nM) as well as an inverse agonist (EC$_{50}$ = 1.5 nM) [68]. Further studies reported that BF2.649 also increased concentrations of dopamine and acetylcholine in rat prefrontal cortex and elevated concentrations of histamine metabolic by-products in mouse brain, confirming the inhibition of the H$_3$ receptor by BF2.649 [69]. *In vivo,* BF2.649 demonstrated a potent wake-promoting effect in cats [68].

Johnson & Johnson Pharmaceutical Research and Development, L.L.C. has also characterized various H$_3$ receptor antagonists. One of the better-characterized compounds is JNJ-10181457 (shown in Figure 8.3). *In vitro* analysis revealed that JNJ-10181457 exhibited a high affinity for binding to the human H$_3$ receptor (K_i = ~1 nM). Further investigation demonstrated that following oral administration, JNJ-10181457 (10 mg/kg) crossed the blood–brain barrier and gave 85% occupancy of the H$_3$ receptor [70].

To compare the wake promoting effects of thioperamide, ciproxifan, BF-2.649, and JNJ-10181457, all compounds were subcutaneously injected at 10 mg/kg at 2 h into the light (i.e., sleep phase) in Sprague–Dawley rats implanted with EEG/EMG electrodes (Figure 8.4). The remaining 10 h of the light phase were recorded, and

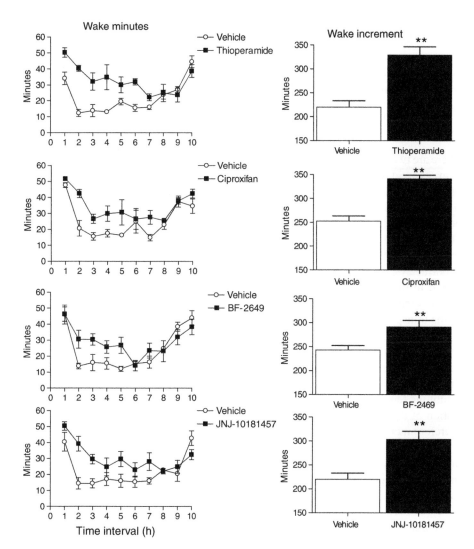

FIGURE 8.4 Wake promotion induced by various H_3 receptor inverse agonists and antago- nists. Thioperamide, Ciproxifan, BF-2649, and JNJ-10181457 were subcutaneously admin- istered (10 mg/kg) 2 h after the onset of the light phase into male Sprague–Dawley rats implanted with EEG/EMG electrodes. The following 10 h were recorded and visually scored as wake, NREM, or REM. The increased time spent awake was calculated for each rat and expressed in 1-h intervals. In addition, the increment in wake was averaged over the 10-h recording period. Data are reported as mean $\pm$ SEM ($n = 3$–5/compound), and statistical significance was determined through the comparison of vehicle versus compound treatment by paired t-test (**$p < .01$).

the resulting polysomnographic traces were visually scored so that states of vigi- lance could be assigned. Of the four compounds injected, thioperamide exhibited the most potent wake-promoting effect, significantly increasing the time spent awake by 109 min. The duration of the increased wake was ~7 h after injection of thioperamide. Equipotent in their ability to increase wake were ciproxifan and JNJ-10181457 (+89 and +84 min, respectively). The duration of the wake-promoting effect was comparable to thioperamide (~7 h) for these two compounds. The least potent of the four compounds in promoting wake was BF-2.649. The increase in wake was 48 min, and the duration was ~5 h (Figure 8.4).

COMPARATIVE ELECTROENCEPHALOGRAM SPECTRAL STUDY WITH H₃ RECEPTOR ANTAGONISTS VERSUS PSYCHOSTIMULANTS

There are two commonly prescribed stimulants to promote arousal for such indications as excessive daytime sleepiness (EDS) in narcolepsy and attention-deficit hyperactivity disorder (ADHD) [71]. The first drug is the prescription psychostimulant amphetamine (Adderall®), which increases the time spent awake by binding to the monoamine transporters and increasing extracellular levels of the biogenic amines dopamine, norepinephrine, and serotonin. Amphetamine is a racemic mix with D-amphetamine acting primarily on the dopaminergic systems, while L-amphetamine activates the norepinephrine system [72]. The primary stimulant effects of amphetamine, however, are linked to the enhanced dopaminergic activity in the mesolimbic area in the brain. Hence, amphetamine also binds to the dopamine transporter and blocks the ability of the transporter to extinguish the elevated dopamine levels from the synaptic space [73,74]. In addition, amphetamine increases the efflux of dopamine from the intracellular space by reverse transport through the dopamine transporter [75,76].

The second compound commonly prescribed to alleviate ADHD and daytime drowsiness due to narcolepsy is methylphenidate (Ritalin®). This drug works by inhibiting the activity of the dopamine and norepinephrine transporters, the concentration of these biogenic amines drastically increase within the synaptic space and therefore increase the wake-promoting signal.

To assess the differences on EEG spectral activity elicited by the H₃ receptor antagonists (JNJ-6379490 and thioperamide) versus psychostimulants (methylphenidate and amphetamine), a series of experiments were performed on male Wistar rats chronically implanted with EEG/EMG electrodes. The H₃ receptor antagonists (JNJ-6379490 [10 mg/kg], thioperamide [10 mg/kg]), or psychostimulants (methylphenidate [10 mg/kg], and amphetamine [2.5 mg/kg]) or vehicle were subcutaneously administered to rats ($n = 8$–10/group) at 2 h after the onset of the light phase (the natural sleep period for nocturnal species such as the rat). At 30 and 60 min after the injection, rats were transferred to the recording chamber and a series of 10-min recording sessions of EEG and EMG were performed during the vigilant state of wake.

Fast Fourier Transformation performed spectral analysis of the EEG on each of the 10-min EEG recording periods. The power densities in each of the five predetermined frequency bands (delta: 1.2–4 Hz, theta: 4.2–8 Hz, alpha: 8.2–12 Hz, beta-1: 12.2–20 Hz, and beta-2: 20.2–30 Hz) of power spectra were averaged over all artifact-free epochs during the 10-min sampling and were expressed as percent of baseline values (obtained from a 10-min recording period before drug administration). Statistical significance of the baseline-vehicle and baseline-drug treatment comparisons was assessed by means of the Wilcoxon signed-rank test ($*p < .05$, $**p < .01$).

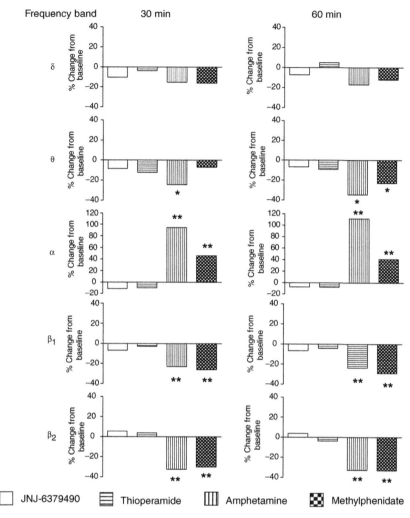

FIGURE 8.5 Comparative study on the effects of the H₃ receptor antagonists JNJ-5207852 and thioperamide, and the psychostimulants methylphenidate and amphetamine on EEG power spectral activity in awake rats. The experiments were carried out on male adult Wistar rats chronically implanted with EEG/EMG electrodes. Following an adaptation period, pharmacological tests were initiated by subcutaneously administering JNJ-5207852 (10 mg/kg), thioperamide (10 mg/kg), methylphenidate (10 mg/kg), amphetamine (2.5 mg/kg), and vehicle (saline) ($n = 8$–10 per dose) at 2 h after the onset of the light phase. Thirty minutes after injection, a series of 10-min recording sessions were performed during the state of wake at 30 and 60 min after treatment. Spectral analysis of the EEG using the fast Fourier transform was performed on each of the EEG recording periods. The densities for the following frequency bands (delta [δ]: 1.2–4 Hz, theta [θ]: 4.2–8 Hz, alpha [α]: 8.2–12 Hz, beta-1 [β_1]: 12.2–20 Hz, and beta-2 [β_2]: 20.2–30 Hz) of the power spectra were averaged over artifact-free epochs and were expressed as percent change from baseline values. Data are reported as mean ± SEM and statistical significance of the vehicle–compound comparisons was assessed by means of the Wilcoxon signed-rank test (*$p < .05$, **$p < .01$).

As illustrated in Figure 8.5, methylphenidate and amphetamine induced a pronounced increase of the power density in the alpha band and a reduction of the power in all the other frequency bands (delta, theta, beta-1, and beta-2). This effect was immediate and was present across the entire experimental paradigm. These alterations in EEG activity are indicative of an enhancement of alertness. However, the increase in alpha power, which was particularly prominent after amphetamine treatment, reflected the marked increase in locomotor activity due to the activation of the dopaminergic system.

In contrast, the H_3 receptor antagonists JNJ-6379490 and thioperamide did not produce any alteration of the EEG power spectral activity over the entire experimental procedure in awake rats. Although all the tested compounds are wake-promoting agents (i.e., producing a higher percentage of waking behavior) as observed in the rat spontaneous sleep/wake cycle, the H_3 receptor antagonists, unlike methylphenidate and amphetamine, leave the EEG signal intact during wake, thus preserving the qualitative aspect of vigilance. Interestingly, H_3 receptor antagonists do not affect EEG spectral power within the 1–30 Hz band (Figure 8.5). However, H_3 receptor antagonists did increase the γ band (30–60 Hz) in animals [55] that is related to attention and memory in humans [77].

UTILIZING TRANSGENIC MODELS TO DEFINE THE ROLE OF H_3 RECEPTOR IN SLEEP/WAKE REGULATION

Establishing the connection between histaminergic signaling through the H_3 receptor and the sleep/wake cycle was facilitated by the development of the H_3 KO mouse. This transgenic mouse line was founded when a genetic cassette containing the neomycin resistance gene was introduced into the embryonic stem cells to delete the DNA encoding the H_3 receptor. After confirming the successful elimination of the H_3 receptor in these cells by polymerase chain reaction (PCR), embryonic stem cells with the confirmed deleted gene were injected into embryos to generate chimeric mice. Stable transgenic mouse lines were established by backcrossing these chimeric mice with C57Bl/6J female mice [78].

To understand how the elimination of the H_3 receptor gene influences the sleep/wake cycle, an EEG study was conducted [78]. For this study, 3-month-old H_3 KO and WT littermates were implanted with EEG and EMG electrodes. To identify a potential role for the H_3 receptor on circadian rhythms and levels of spontaneous activity, locomotor activity was measured through an implantable telemetry device located within the peritoneal cavity of each mouse. During the light phase (normal sleep period for mice), there were no detectable changes in activity (Figure 8.6a,b). However, during the 12 h of the dark (active) phase, there was a reduction in spontaneous locomotor activity in the H_3 KO mouse (6393 ± 1714 activity counts) when compared to WT counterparts (8950 ± 1073 activity counts) (Figure 8.6b). This decrease in activity during the dark phase translated to an overall trend to diminish the circadian locomotor activity pattern over the 24-h recording period. Interestingly, the decrease in spontaneous locomotor activity translated to a slight yet nonsignificant decrease in the amount of time spent awake in the H_3 KO when compared to WT counterparts during the first 6 h of the dark phase. However, the overall change in wake was not significant for the remaining 6 h of the dark and 12 h of the

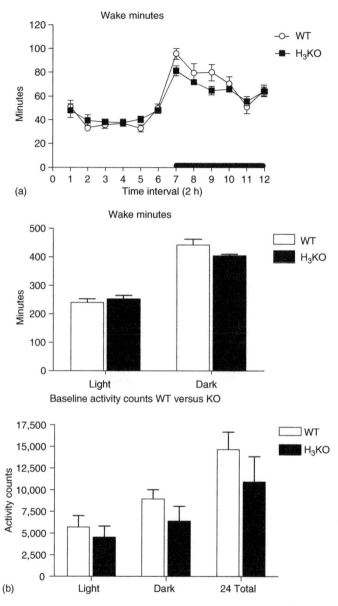

FIGURE 8.6 (a) Profile of the sleep/wake cycle in H_3 KO and WT mice. Polysomnographic traces were recorded for 24 h in H_3 KO ($n = 7$) and WT ($n = 8$) mice implanted with EEG/ EMG electrodes and visually scored as wake, NREM, or REM. Differences in the diurnal distribution of time spent awake were analyzed over the entire recording and reported in 2-h intervals or in 12-h bins (mean ± SEM) that corresponded to 12 h of light or dark. (b) Decreased locomotor activity in the H_3 KO mice during the 12 h of the dark (active) phase when compared to WT counterparts. To assess alterations in locomotor activity between the two genotypes, spontaneous locomotor activity was obtained from telemetric devices implanted into the intraperitoneal cavity of H_3 KO ($n = 8$) and WT ($n = 11$). Baseline activity counts were averaged (mean ± SEM) during the 12 h of light and dark and for the total 24 h.

light phase (Figure 8.6a). NREM and REM sleep amounts were not affected over the 24-h recording period (data not shown).

The decrease in spontaneous activity and subsequent decrease in wake during the first 6 h of the dark phase would appear to be counterintuitive since the H_3 receptor autoregulates the release of histamine through presynaptic inhibition. Therefore, removing the presynaptic inhibition of the H_3 receptor should, in theory, result in elevated levels of histamine within the synaptic cleft, thereby promoting arousal through the H_1 receptor located on the postsynaptic membrane. However, the H_3 KO mouse displays a significant decrease in locomotor activity during the dark phase that would suggest an alternate hypothesis. This surprising finding could be explained by a couple of different mechanisms. To compensate for the elevated histamine levels, there may be a subsequent decrease in the expression of the postsynaptic H_1 receptor. However, binding densities of the H_1 receptor in WT and H_3 KO were comparable [70]. Another plausible explanation arose from a recent study that reported a decrease in histamine concentrations within the brains of H_3 KO mice. To avoid the effects of chronic elevation of histamine in H_3 KO mice, a secondary mechanism may compensate by altering the turnover rate for histamine. However, further investigation is needed to understand how histamine production and metabolism evolve during the development of an organism.

To confirm the role of the H_3 receptor in promoting arousal states, the H_3 receptor antagonists, thioperamide and JNJ-5207852, were administered to WT and H_3 KO mice at light onset. During the first 2 h after injection in WT mice, both compounds resulted in a significant increase in the time spent awake (thioperamide: +32 min, $p < .05$, JNJ-5207852: +23 min, $p < .05$) (Figure 8.7). The increase in wake duration was mirrored by a decrease in NREM sleep, whereas the duration of REM sleep remained intact (data not shown). Neither compound influenced wake or total sleep time when administered to the H_3 KO mice. These data confirm the wake-promoting effects of thioperamide and JNJ-5207852 and verify the important role for the H_3 receptor in mediating arousal.

Further investigation demonstrated that the wake-promoting effect of H_3 receptor antagonists is dependent on the actions of the H_1 receptor. The sleep/wake patterns in H_1 receptor KO mice are relatively comparable to their WT controls. However, the potent wake promotion measured with the H_3 receptor antagonist ciproxifan is totally abolished in the H_1 receptor KO mice. In a parallel fashion, coadministration of the H_1 receptor antagonist pyrilamine completely blocked the wake promotion of ciproxifan in WT mice, therefore highlighting the critical role of coupling the H_3 and H_1 receptors to promote arousal [79].

H_3 Receptor Antagonism Combined with Elective Serotonin Reuptake Inhibitor

Clinical depression is a psychiatric disorder affecting ~340 million people worldwide and is characterized by a mental state of extreme sadness, melancholy, and despair [80]. Episodes of depression can occur as an acute, isolated event or a recurrent phenomenon that can arise throughout the lifetime of an individual. One prominent feature in depressed individuals is a disruption in the regulation of the sleep/wake cycle. These sleep disturbances can manifest in various ways such as

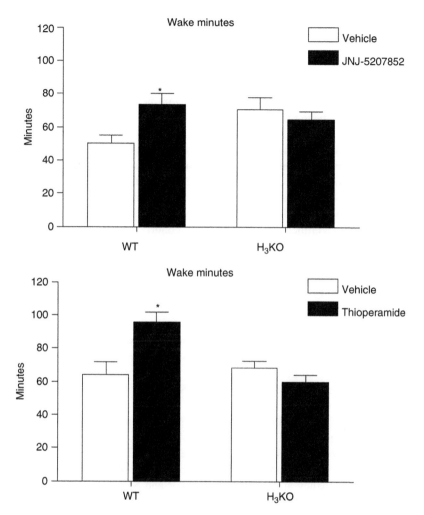

FIGURE 8.7   H$_3$ KO mice are immune to the wake-promoting effects of the H$_3$ receptor antagonists. H$_3$ KO ($n = 7$) and WT ($n = 6$) mice were subcutaneously injected with JNJ-5207852 (10 mg/kg) or thioperamide (10 mg/kg) and the following 2 h were recorded and visually scored as wake, NREM, or REM. Data were calculated as difference in minutes between vehicle and compound administration within genotype and reported as mean ± SEM. Statistical significance was determined by two-way ANOVA followed by a Bonferroni post hoc test (*$p < .05$).

insomnia, decreased time to the onset of REM sleep, and an extended duration of REM sleep [81]. Interestingly, one outcome of treatment with antidepressants is to reverse these alterations in REM sleep [81].

Selective serotonin reuptake inhibitors (SSRIs) are the most prescribed antidepressant drugs to combat depression. By blocking the action of the presynaptic serotonin reuptake transporter (SERT), these drugs elevate serotonin concentrations within the synaptic space. The effectiveness of SSRIs is hindered by a slow onset of action (at least 2 weeks), and they fail to address the fatigue that is often associated with depression. To alleviate the lethargy associated with depression, physicians will prescribe stimulants as adjunct therapy to the regular course of antidepressant therapy [82,83]. However, owing to the enhanced release of dopamine occurring after the administration of stimulants such as amphetamine or methylphenidate, several adverse events have been reported with these drugs including tachycardia, hypertension, the potential for abuse, and behavioral modifications [84]. Modafinil is the most recent prescribed wake-promoting agent with little effect on dopaminergic activity in the striatum and therefore with low abuse potential; however, its mechanism of action is still unclear. Modafinil is currently prescribed for the treatment of EDS associated with narcolepsy, sleep apnea, and shift work sleep disorders [85]. Recently, its efficacy has been reported in the treatment of daytime fatigue and lethargy associated with depression. In a clinical study with a small cohort of depressed patients, adjunct therapy utilizing a low dose of modafinil in combination with classical antidepressants accelerated the therapeutic action as evidenced by improved scores on the Hamilton rating scale for depression [82,86]. In addition, reducing fatigue associated with the depression was also responsive to this adjunct therapy [82,86].

Recent studies have identified additional classes of molecules and targets (i.e., H_3 receptor antagonists) that promote wakefulness without the common adverse side effects associated with the use of stimulants and also exhibit a known mechanism of action unlike modafinil. Johnson & Johnson Pharmaceutical Research and Development, L.L.C. has developed a molecule with a dual mechanism of action that encompasses the antidepressant effects of an SSRI with the wake promotion of an H_3 receptor antagonist.

In particular, JNJ-28583867 exhibits a high affinity for the H_3 receptor (K_i = 10.6 nM) and also SERT (K_i = 3.7 nM). Further binding studies revealed that JNJ-28583867 was 30-fold more selective for SERT as compared to the norepinephrine or dopamine transporters. *Ex vivo* analysis of the compound resulted in a maximal occupancy at both the H_3 receptor and SERT at ~1 h following the subcutaneous administration of 1 mg/kg of JNJ-28583867. When 3 mg/kg of this compound was injected into rats, serotonin levels in the frontal cortex significantly increased by approximately eightfold when compared to basal levels as measured by microdialysis. Although not as potent as for NET (K_i = 121.0 nM) or DAT (K_i = 102.3 nM), JNJ-28583867 induced a modest increase in both norepinephrine and dopamine concentrations within the frontal cortex [87].

To determine *in vivo* efficacy for JNJ-28583867, the compound was subcutaneously injected (0.3, 1, and 3 mg/kg) into male Sprague–Dawley rats chronically implanted with EEG/EMG electrodes for the polysomnographic determination of the states of vigilance. The data reported in Table 8.1 illustrate the response of various sleep/wake parameters to JNJ-28583867 for 8 h after compound injection at 2 h after light onset. Administration of JNJ-28583867 significantly prolonged the onset to NREM sleep at the highest dose (3 mg/kg) by increasing onset time to 182 min compared to 25 min in vehicle-treated animals ($p < .01$), whereas the latency to REM sleep was already delayed at the doses of 1 and 3 mg/kg. At 1 mg/kg, the duration of REM sleep was decreased dramatically by 87% and the highest dose of

TABLE 8.1

Latency to NREM and REM Sleep and Duration of the Vigilance States Following Administration of JNJ-28583867

Latency (min)	JNJ-28583867 (mg/kg)			
	Vehicle	0.3	1	3
NREM	25 ± 3	25 ± 4	43 ± 8	182 ± 32**
REM	55 ± 8	72 ± 13	371 ± 59**	554 ± 43**

Duration (min)	JNJ-28583867 (mg/kg)			
	Vehicle	0.3	1	3
Wake	195 ± 12	190 ± 11	265 ± 18*	362 ± 29**
NREM	237 ± 10	254 ± 12	208 ± 16	116 ± 28**
REM	49 ± 6	36 ± 2	6 ± 3**	2 ± 1**

Note: Values are mean ± SEM ($n = 5$ rats) during the first 8 h after injection. Statistical significance was determined through the comparison of vehicle versus compound treatment by repeated measures one-way analysis of variance, (ANOVA) with Dunnett's multiple comparison post hoc test (*$p < .05$, **$p < .01$).

3 mg/kg almost abolished REM sleep. A significant decrease in NREM sleep was only observed at the highest dose of 3 mg/kg. The decrease in NREM and REM sleep following JNJ-28583867 administration was paralleled by a dose-dependent increase in time spent in wake.

In summary, administration of JNJ-28583867 potently suppressed REM sleep during the 8-h recording period at both the 1 and 3 mg/kg doses. The highest dose (3 mg/kg) exerted a significant wake-promoting effect that inversely correlated with a concomitant decrease in the time spent in NREM sleep. A dual mechanism of action (H_3 receptor antagonism and the inhibition of SERT) for JNJ-28583867 is supported by the fact that REM sleep was potently suppressed at a low dose (1 mg/kg), whereas the effect on NREM sleep was not observed until the highest dose of 3 mg/kg. Therefore, results of the EEG study show that JNJ-28583867 was entirely consistent with its neurochemistry since it combined the REM-suppressing effects of a SERT inhibitor with the wake promotion of an H_3 receptor antagonist. Furthermore, this combination may offer a therapeutic advantage by addressing both the fatigue and the REM sleep changes associated with an antidepressant.

INDICATIONS FOR H_3 RECEPTOR ANTAGONISTS IN SLEEP/WAKE DISORDERS

EXCESSIVE DAYTIME SLEEPINESS

EDS is common in individuals experiencing sleep disturbances. Ramifications of EDS include adverse effects on alertness, vigilance, and cognition. EDS can range from short microsleep episodes to uncontrollable sleep attacks. Over time, this

TABLE 8.2
Potential Therapeutic Indications for H₃ Receptor Antagonists

EDS associated with
Narcolepsy (and associated cataplexy)
Idiopathic hypersomnia
Obstructive sleep apnea
Circadian rhythm disorders: shift work, jet lag

Impaired alertness and cognition associated with
Psychiatric disorders: ADHD, depression, schizophrenia
Neurological disorders: Parkinson's disease, Alzheimer's disease

Chronic fatigue syndrome (CFS) associated with
Fibromyalgia, rheumatoid arthritis, multiple sclerosis, cancer

condition increases the risk of making errors and accidents and severely impairs social and working functioning. EDS is associated with many disorders including narcolepsy, obstructive sleep apnea, and idiopathic hypersomnia that accounts for 80% of these individuals (Table 8.2).

NARCOLEPSY

Narcolepsy is one of the most studied of the disorders of primary somnolence. However, the etiology of this sleep disorder remains a mystery. Recent epidemiological investigation has reported that the rate of occurrence of narcolepsy is ~1 in 2000 individuals and is primarily characterized by extended periods of EDS [88]. This sleep disruption can be accompanied by a number of additional disorders related to the inappropriate intrusion of REM sleep into wake including cataplexy (muscle atonia) in ~40% of narcoleptic patients and also hypnagogic hallucinations and sleep paralysis. The occurrence of EDS by itself or in combination with hypnagogic hallucinations or sleep paralysis is the primary reporting symptom in the majority of narcoleptic individuals. In addition to the alterations in REM sleep components, patients will often experience extensive fragmented sleep patterns during the night. The onset of narcolepsy can occur during the early stages of adulthood; however, there are incidences of narcolepsy beginning as early as childhood and as late as 30–40 years of age. Owing to the enormous repercussion on the sleep/wake rhythm, quality of life is negatively influenced [88].

The etiology for narcolepsy remains unknown. However, recent data have reported a link between narcolepsy-cataplexy and disruption in orexin signaling [33]. The orexin family of peptides is first transcribed as a prepro-orexin peptide. Following enzymatic cleavage of the precursor peptide, two daughter peptides are formed. The first is a 33 amino acid polypeptide chain called orexin-A, whereas the second (orexin-B) is a shorter peptide of 28 amino acids. Neurons responsible for the synthesis of the orexin peptides are localized within the lateral hypothalamus. Projections emanating from the perikarya terminate at several distinct regions within the brain including basal forebrain, LDT, PPT, TMN, LC, raphe nuclei, and

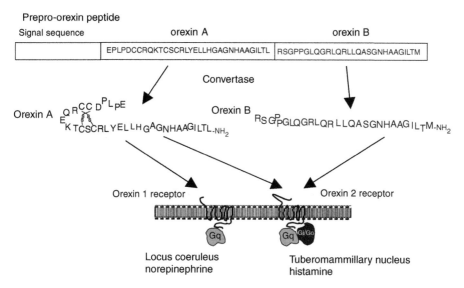

Prepro-orexin peptide

Signal sequence

orexin A

orexin B

FIGURE 8.8 Illustration depicting orexin-signaling pathways. Within the lateral hypothalamus, orexin neurons synthesize the progenitor peptide, prepro-orexin. This precursor is then cleaved through the actions of a convertase enzyme into the daughter peptides, orexin A and B. Orexin A comprises 33 amino acids and is highlighted by the presence of two disulfide bridges. Orexin B, however, is shorter in length at 28 amino acids. Once liberated from prepro-orexin, orexin A can bind to either of the G-protein-coupled receptors (orexin 1 or 2 receptor). Orexin 1 receptors are localized to areas involved in catecholamine release such as the LC, whereas orexin 2 receptors are found in the TMN and help to modulate histamine release. Unlike orexin A, orexin B is more discriminate and will bind specifically to the orexin 2 receptor.

VTA. From these axon terminals, the prepro-orexin, and subsequent orexin-A and orexin-B are secreted. Orexin-A displays an affinity for either of the two orexin receptors (OX_1R or OX_2R). In contrast, orexin-B will only bind to the OX_2R. There exists some overlap in the distribution of these two receptors (VTA, raphe nuclei, LDT, PPT). However, some differences in the expression between the two do exist (LC-OX_1R, TMN-OX_2R) (Figure 8.8) [89,90].

Following an extensive genetic linkage analysis, only one case of narcolepsy could be connected to a mutation in the sequence of DNA that encodes the prepro-orexin peptide [91]. Owing to the sporadic incidence of narcolepsy within the population, the lack of inheritance of the disease was predictable. Instead, the level of orexin in cerebrospinal fluid (CSF) is low or even under detectable limits in the majority of narcoleptic individuals [92,93]. Autopsy studies have confirmed a deficiency in the expression of the orexin peptide in the brain obtained from narcoleptics [91,94]. Further investigation reported that the number of orexin-producing neurons within the posterior and tuberomammillary hypothalamic region were decreased [94].

Recent experiments have demonstrated that the histaminergic system is one of the important executive systems of the orexin signaling to promote arousal. Centrally administered orexin to WT mice increases the time spent awake. This wake-promoting effect was negated in the H_1 receptor KO mouse and reduced following pretreatment with the H_1 receptor antagonist pyrilamine in WT mice [95]. Subsequent investigation has reported that orexin excites histaminergic TMN neurons through OX_2 receptors [96,97], suggesting that the wake-promoting action of orexin is mediated by histaminergic activation through OX_2 receptors. These studies provide evidence of a functional interaction between histaminergic and orexin systems.

Owing to the functional association between orexin and the initiation of the histamine signal, a reduced histaminergic tone may result in EDS in human (reduction in histamine concentration in CSF) and canine (decreased brain histamine content) narcolepsy [98,99]. H_3 receptor antagonists such as thioperamide have been shown to significantly enhance waking in the orexin/ataxin-3 mouse narcoleptic model, demonstrating that H_3 antagonists can counteract the sleepiness associated with the disrupted hypocretin system observed in narcolepsy [70]. Therefore, H_3 receptor antagonists that enhance histamine tone may serve as an effective therapy for the treatment of EDS in narcolepsy.

There are two classifications of narcolepsy in canines. The first is the familial form that arises from a mutation in the OX_2R. The phenotype appears to be solely the result of the mutated receptor since orexin peptide levels within the CSF and the numbers of neurons responsible for the production of orexin are comparable between narcoleptic canines and those that are unaffected [100,101]. The second form of canine narcolepsy occurs sporadically. Dissimilar from the inherited version of the disorder, the sporadic form occurs due to a loss of orexin neurons from the hypothalamic region, resulting in drastically reduced concentrations of orexin within the CSF [101]. Importantly, H_3 receptor antagonists were able to reduce the cataplexy in narcoleptic Dobermans [70].

In mice, there are two mutations that accurately mirror the human narcolepsy-cataplexy (i.e., difficulty in maintaining wake, intrusion of REM sleep during wake and cataplexy). The first translatable model is the product of the deletion of the gene that encodes the prepro-orexin peptide (orexin KO) [102]. The second transgenic line was engineered to induce the destruction of orexin-producing neurons as the animal ages (orexin/ataxin-3 mouse) [103]. Investigators have also examined how the targeted disruption in the genes encoding the two orexin receptors influence states of vigilance. A narcoleptic phenotype has been recorded in mice lacking the OX_2 receptor. However, behavioral and EEG studies suggest that this form of narcolepsy is relatively mild as compared to the narcolepsy observed in orexin KO mice [100,104,105]. Interestingly, a narcoleptic phenotype was not documented in the OX_1R KO mouse. Instead, there is a marked fragmentation of sleep [106]. Only when the double KO of the two receptors was developed, did an overt narcoleptic disorder was observed [102].

Currently, EDS is treated with stimulants. All pharmacological compounds currently used for their wake-promoting effects, such as dextroamphetamine and methylphenidate enhance dopaminergic neurotransmission. Common central adverse effects associated with the use of stimulants include headaches, irritability, tremors, insomnia, and anoxeria. These wake-promoting agents can also alter peripheral physiology, resulting in hypertension and cardiac palpitations. In addition, a narcoleptic individual may develop tolerance to these arousal-stimulating medications [107,108]. Also, these medications carry a potential for abuse and therefore are scheduled prescribed drugs. Furthermore, there is a risk for rebound somnolence once the treatment has been terminated [107–109].

Recently, another type of wake-promoting agent has shown to be efficacious in combating EDS. Modafinil is a wake-promoting drug whose mechanism of action is still relatively unknown. However, certain studies have reported that modafinil may promote wake through various means including inhibiting the release of the inhibitory neurotransmitter GABA by altering serotonergic transmission, activating wake centers within the brain, and enhancing the concentrations of dopamine and norepinephrine by inhibiting their reuptake within the synaptic cleft [109–113]. Modafinil holds an advantage over traditional stimulants because it lacks the adverse events associated with dextroamphetamine and methylphenidate [114]. The half-life of modafinil in the human is ~12 to 15 h, which makes this drug ideal for administering once a day to promote arousal [115]. Therefore, several studies have detailed the effectiveness of using modafinil in the treatment of EDS and sleep disorders that manifest in EDS. Adverse effects associated with modafinil administration include headache and nausea [116].

As an adjunct therapy, drugs that mainly enhance noradrenergic neurotransmission such as the tricyclic antidepressants clomipramine or imipramine are prescribed due to their potent REM suppressant effects. The consequence is a reduction in cataplectic attacks and REM-related symptoms associated with narcolepsy; however, these drugs possess no or modest wake-promoting effects [99]. One drawback to these drugs is their negative impact on cholinergic neurotransmission. Other antidepressants such as venlafaxine (a potent inhibitor of serotonin and norepinephrine uptake and weak inhibitor of the uptake of dopamine) and atomoxetine (a highly specific norepinephrine uptake inhibitor) also possess anticataplectic activity and are generally more tolerated than the tricyclics [99].

The most recent addition to the therapeutic regimen to counteract narcolepsy is sodium oxybate (gamma-hydroxybutyrate [GHB]) that consolidates sleep and significantly reduces the sleep fragmentation commonly observed in narcoleptic patients [117,118]. In addition, recent clinical trials have reported a dose-dependent decrease in the number of cataplectic events over a 12-month period and subjective measures of sleepiness [119,120]. Interestingly, the mechanism of action responsible for the improvement of EDS and reduction in cataplexy with sodium oxybate treatment is not yet elucidated.

Sleep Apnea

Sleep apnea syndrome (SAS) is characterized by frequent, repetitive disruptions in respiration during sleep, resulting in excessive arousal from sleep. Consequences of the arrested breathing during sleep can manifest in EDS and impaired cognitive processes such as learning and memory consolidation [121–125]. In addition to the alteration in neural physiology and behavior, peripheral organ systems are adversely affected, resulting in increased cardiovascular, renal, hepatic, and respiratory morbidity and mortality and metabolic disturbances [126,127].

The mechanisms instigating the pathological modifications to respiration give rise to the two main classifications of sleep apnea. The first type termed *obstructive sleep apnea syndrome* (OSAS) is the result of an upper airway obstruction due to either abnormal anatomy or failure of the neck muscles to preserve the patency of the upper airway during sleep. The resulting cessation of respiration (apnea) or hypoventilation (hypopnea) during sleep gives rise to decreased saturated blood oxygen levels (hypoxemia) and increased arterial carbon dioxide (hypercapnia) [128–130]. With termination of the apneic episode, an arousal occurs as the individual struggles to regain his/her breath and resume a normal respiratory rate (respiratory effort-related arousals, RERAs) [131]. Owing to these frequent awakenings, an individual with sleep apnea struggles to achieve the deeper levels of NREM sleep (stages 3 and 4), and therefore, a fully restorative sleep during the night is often unobtainable. The daytime ramifications for the lack of restorative sleep can manifest as EDS, impaired cognition, and loss of concentration [121–125].

One common risk factor among individuals with OSAS is an elevated body mass [132,133]. A correlation exists between the body mass of an individual and the severity of the OSAS. Therefore, as the body mass index of an individual increases, the severity of OSAS increases in a parallel fashion [132]. In addition, obesity can result in excess deposition of fat pads around the neck and upper airway [134,135]. Therefore, the circumference of the neck is also a corollary with the development and severity of OSAS. Additional common risk factors for the development of OSAS include anatomical derangements (i.e., enlarged tonsils and adenoids), edema, and snoring [131]. Recent epidemiological studies have identified ApoE epsilon 4 as a potential familial component for OSAS [136–138].

The treatment for OSAS varies depending on individual need and compliance. The most common form of diminishing the number of apneic events is continuous positive airway pressure (CPAP). On diagnosis of OSAS, an individual will be fitted with a special nasal mask that is connected to a CPAP machine through tubing. The CPAP machine consists of a small air pump that administers continuous positive air pressure to the nasal and upper airway passages to keep these respiratory passages open. Although the benefits of CPAP to alleviate OSAS are well documented, adverse effects have arisen with the use of this treatment including compliance, dry mouth, claustrophobia, nasal congestion, and arousal from sleep [139–141]. An additional treatment for OSAS includes dental appliances to mechanically expand the opening to the upper airway. However, side effects (increased salivation, nasal dryness, and compliance) with the oral appliances also exist [142]. Finally, surgical measures are also undertaken to combat the collapse of the upper airway passages by removing portions of the soft palate and uvula and by advancing the lower jaw [143,144]. The benefits of these surgeries are limited due to the invasiveness of the procedures and moderate rates of success (~30 to 50%) [145].

The second major classification is termed *central sleep apnea syndrome* (CSAS). This form is characterized by the frequent, repetitive respiratory disturbances without an apparent upper airway obstruction. Therefore, instead of blockage or collapse of the airway, the apneic event evolves from a diminished respiratory signal emanating from the central processes that regulate the rate of respiration [146]. In comparison with OSAS, the consequence of CSAS is frequent episodes of hypoxemia accompanied by frequent arousals. Also, in a similar fashion, individuals experiencing CSAS will have severe daytime consequences from the recurring awakenings from sleep. These daytime manifestations include EDS and impaired cognition [131].

Owing to patient compliance issues with both CPAP and oral appliances, the EDS that manifests as part of sleep apnea is often not corrected and results in the administration of stimulants [147]. Pharmacological therapy involving stimulants in individuals with sleep apnea results in a slightly significant improvement in EDS [147]. In recent years, modafinil (or the R-isoform of modafinil, armodafinil) has become the pharmacotherapy of choice to combat the daytime drowsiness that results from the decreased sleep quality due to apneic events [148–150].

IDIOPATHIC HYPERSOMNIA

The manifestations of idiopathic hypersomnia will greatly vary from individual to individual. Roth et al. [151] described the most common form referred to as poly-symptomatic, which is characterized by EDS, prolonged napping, extended noctur-nal sleep (>12 h), and signs of *sleep drunkenness* on awakening. The second major form consists primarily of EDS and is labeled as monosymptomatic [152]. A diag-nosis of idiopathic hypersomnia is pronounced for an individual when he/she does not meet the diagnostic criteria for more *traditional* sleep disorders such as a lack of REM intrusion into wake (narcolepsy-cataplexy) and recurrent interruptions in respiration during sleep (sleep apnea). The study of idiopathic hypersomnia has been severely hampered by a lack of an adequate animal model to mimic the symptoms of the disorder. In addition, the pathophysiology of idiopathic hypersomnia is still elu-sive. One study has reported a decrease in the concentration of monoamines (mainly norepinephrine) in the CSF of idiopathic hypersomnia individuals [153–155]. Recent genetic analysis has hinted to a hereditary component but due to the small number of cohorts of individuals with idiopathic hypersomnia and their relatives, an accurate assessment as to the mode of inheritance is difficult [156].

The treatment for idiopathic hypersomnia includes a regimen of stimulants such as dextroamphetamine and methylphenidate. The use of stimulants, however, is usu-ally less effective in alleviating the symptoms of idiopathic hypersomnia and also less well tolerated when compared to stimulant treatment regimens in narcolepsy. One study has also demonstrated that modafinil is efficacious in combating the EDS associated with this disorder [157,158].

SUMMARY

The sleep/wake cycle is regulated by a homeostatic and a circadian component that interact with each other to maintain the physiological amounts and timing of the sleep/ wake states. A number of neurotransmitters and neuromodulators exert a specific control on each of the vigilance states. Therefore, an impairment in either physiolog-ical or biochemical mechanisms will result in sleep/wake disorders. Histaminergic neurons, which originate in the tuberomammilary nuclei and project throughout the brain, play an important role in arousal mechanisms, and histamine H_3 receptors are involved in this process by an inhibitory control of histamine release and synthesis. Indeed, the pharmacological blockade of presynaptic H_3 receptors promotes wake-fulness, whereas their stimulation produces sedation. The development of specific H_3 receptor antagonists has become a very attractive strategy in the treatment of daytime sleepiness associated with various conditions (narcolepsy, obstructive sleep apnea, and shift work sleep disorders) and impaired alertness and cognition associated with a number of psychiatric disorders such as ADHD and schizophrenia or neurodegenerative disorders.

REFERENCES

1. Saper, C.B., Scammell, T.E., and Lu, J. 2005. Hypothalamic regulation of sleep and circadian rhythms. *Nature* 437: 1257–1263.
2. Miller, M.A. and Cappuccio, F.P. 2007. Inflammation, sleep, obesity and cardiovascular disease. *Curr Vasc Pharmacol* 5: 93–102.
3. Zager, A., Andersen, M.L., Ruiz, F.S., Antunes, I.B., and Tufik, S. 2007. Effects of acute and chronic sleep loss on immune modulation of rats. *Am J Physiol Regul Integr Comp Physiol* 293: R504–R509.
4. Knutson, K.L., Spiegel, K., Penev, P., and Van Cauter, E. 2007. The metabolic consequences of sleep deprivation. *Sleep Med Rev* 11: 163–178.
5. Irwin, M.R., Wang, M., Campomayor, C.O., Collado-Hidalgo, A., and Cole, S. 2006. Sleep deprivation and activation of morning levels of cellular and genomic markers of inflammation. *Arch Intern Med* 166: 1756–1762.
6. Roth, T. 2004. Characteristics and determinants of normal sleep. *J Clin Psychiatry* 65(Suppl 16): 8–11.
7. Siegel, J.M. 2005. Clues to the functions of mammalian sleep. *Nature* 437: 1264–1271.
8. Fraser, R. and Nordin, B.E. 1955. The basal metabolic rate during sleep. *Lancet* 268: 532–533.
9. Goldenberg, N. and Barkan, A. 2007. Factors regulating growth hormone secretion in humans. *Endocrinol Metab Clin North Am* 36: 37–55.
10. Benca, R.M., Kushida, C.A., Everson, C.A., Kalski, R., Bergmann, B.M., and Rechtschaffen, A. 1989. Sleep deprivation in the rat: VII. Immune function. *Sleep* 12: 47–52.
11. Dickstein, J.B. and Moldofsky, H. 1999. Sleep, cytokines and immune function. *Sleep Med Rev* 3: 219–228.
12. Rechtschaffen, A., Gilliland, M.A., Bergmann, B.M., and Winter, J.B. 1983. Physiological correlates of prolonged sleep deprivation in rats. *Science* 221: 182–184.
13. Everson, C.A., Bergmann, B.M., and Rechtschaffen, A. 1989. Sleep deprivation in the rat: III. Total sleep deprivation. *Sleep* 12: 13–21.
14. Majumdar, S. and Mallick, B.N. 2005. Cytomorphometric changes in rat brain neurons after rapid eye movement sleep deprivation. *Neuroscience* 135: 679–690.
15. Mirmiran, M., Scholtens, J., van de Poll, N.E., Uylings, H.B., van der Gugten, J., and Boer, G.J. 1983. Effects of experimental suppression of active (REM) sleep during early development upon adult brain and behavior in the rat. *Brain Res* 283: 277–286.
16. Smith, C. 1995. Sleep states and memory processes. *Behav Brain Res* 69: 137–145.
17. Dotto, L. 1996. Sleep stages, memory and learning. *CMAJ* 154: 1193–1196.
18. Fenn, K.M., Nusbaum, H.C., and Margoliash, D. 2003. Consolidation during sleep of perceptual learning of spoken language. *Nature* 425: 614–616.
19. Borbely, A.A. 1982. A two process model of sleep regulation. *Hum Neurobiol* 1: 195–204.
20. Schoeller, D.A., Cella, L.K., Sinha, M.K., and Caro, J.F. 1997. Entrainment of the diurnal rhythm of plasma leptin to meal timing. *J Clin Invest* 100: 1882–1887.
21. Wehr, T.A. 1998. Effect of seasonal changes in daylength on human neuroendocrine function. *Horm Res* 49: 118–124.
22. Kita, H. and Oomura, Y. 1982. An anterograde HRP study of retinal projections to the hypothalamus in the rat. *Brain Res Bull* 8: 249–253.

23. Kawano, H., Decker, K., and Reuss, S. 1996. Is there a direct retina-raphe-suprachiasmatic nucleus pathway in the rat? *Neurosci Lett* 212: 143–146.

24. Mosko, S.S. and Moore, R.Y. 1979. Neonatal ablation of the suprachiasmatic nucleus. Effects on the development of the pituitary-gonadal axis in the female rat. *Neuroendocrinology* 29: 350–361.

25. Mouret, J., Coindet, J., Debilly, G., and Chouvet, G. 1978. Suprachiasmatic nuclei lesions in the rat: alterations in sleep circadian rhythms. *Electroencephalogr Clin Neurophysiol* 45: 402–408.

26. Gray, G.D., Söderstein, P., Tallentire, D., and Davidson, J.M. 1978. Effects of lesions in various structures of the suprachiasmatic-preoptic region on LH regulation and sexual behavior in female rats. *Neuroendocrinology* 25: 174–191.

27. Vogelbaum, M.A., Galef, J., and Menaker, M. 1993. Factors determining the restoration of circadian behavior by hypothalamic transplants. *J Neural Transplant Plast* 4: 239–256.

28. Tobler, I.I., Franken, P., Trachsel, L., and Borbély, A.A. 1992. Models of sleep regulation in mammals. *J Sleep Res* 1: 125–127.

29. von Economo, C.V. 1930. Sleep as a problem of localization. *J Nervous Mental Disord* 71: 249–259.

30. Moruzzi, G. and Magoun, H.W. 1949. Brain stem reticular formation and activation of the EEG. *J Neuropsychiatry Clin Neurosci* 7: 251–267.

31. Sakurai, T. 2005. Roles of orexin/hypocretin in regulation of sleep/wakefulness and energy homeostasis. *Sleep Med Rev* 9: 231–241.

32. Sakurai, T., Amemiya, A., Ishii, M. et al. 1998. Orexins and orexin receptors: a family of hypothalamic neuropeptides and G protein-coupled receptors that regulate feeding behavior. *Cell* 92: 696.

33. Sakurai, T. 2007. The neural circuit of orexin (hypocretin): maintaining sleep and wakefulness. *Nat Rev Neurosci* 8: 171–181.

34. Lu, J., Greco, M.A., Shiromani, P., and Saper, C.B. 2000. Effect of lesions of the ventrolateral preoptic nucleus on NREM and REM sleep. *J Neurosci* 20: 3830–3842.

35. Chou, T.C., Bjorkum, A.A., Gaus, S.E., Lu, J., Scammell, T.E., and Saper, C.B. 2002. Afferents to the ventrolateral preoptic nucleus. *J Neurosci* 22: 977–990.

36. Lu, J., Bjorkum, A.A., Xu, M., Gaus, S.E., Shiromani, P.J., and Saper, C.B. 2002. Selective activation of the extended ventrolateral preoptic nucleus during rapid eye movement sleep. *J Neurosci* 22: 4568–4576.

37. Gaus, S.E., Strecker, R.E., Tate, B.A., Parker, R.A., and Saper, C.B. 2002. Ventrolateral preoptic nucleus contains sleep-active, galaninergic neurons in multiple mammalian species. *Neuroscience* 115: 285–294.

38. Sherin, J.E., Elmquist, J.K., Torrealba, F., and Saper, C.B. 1998. Innervation of histaminergic tuberomammillary neurons by GABAergic and galaninergic neurons in the ventrolateral preoptic nucleus of the rat. *J Neurosci* 18: 4705–4721.

39. Schild, H.O. 1976. Dale and the development of pharmacology. Lecture given at Sir Henry Dale centennial symposium, Cambridge, September 17–19, 1975. *Br J Pharmacol* 56: 3–7.

40. Dale, H.H. and Laidlaw, P.P. 1910. The physiological action of b-iminazolylethylamine. *J Physiol* 41: 318–344.

41. Dale, H.H. and Laidlaw, P.P. 1919. Histamine shock. *J Physiol* 52: 355–390.

42. Lewis, T. 1927. *Local Means of Producing the Triple Response in the Blood Vessels of Human Skin and Their Response*, Chapter 4, pp. 46–64, Shaw and Son, London.

43. Reiner, P.B. and Kamondi, A. 1994. Mechanisms of antihistamine-induced sedation in the human brain: H1 receptor activation reduces a background leakage potassium current. *Neuroscience* 59: 579–588.

44. Brown, R.E., Stevens, D.R., and Haas, H.L. 2001. The physiology of brain histamine. *Prog Neurobiol* 63: 637–672.

45. Schwartz, J.C., Pollard, H., and Quach, T.T. 1980. Histamine as a neurotransmitter in mammalian brain: neurochemical evidence. *J Neurochem* 35: 26–33.
46. Haas, H. and Panula, P. 2003. The role of histamine and the tuberomamillary nucleus in the nervous system. *Nat Rev Neurosci* 4: 121–130.
47. Endou, M., Poli, E., and Levi, R. 1994. Histamine H_3 receptor signaling in the heart: possible involvement of Gi/Go proteins and N-type Ca^{++} channels. *J Pharmacol Exp Ther* 269: 221–229.
48. Schlicker, E., Malinowska, B., Kathmann, M., and Göthert, M. 1994. Modulation of neurotransmitter release via histamine H3 heteroreceptors. *Fundam Clin Pharmacol* 8: 128–137.
49. Pollard, H., Moreau, J., Arrang, J.M., and Schwartz, J.C. 1993. A detailed autoradiographic mapping of histamine H3 receptors in rat brain areas. *Neuroscience* 52: 169–189.
50. Lin, J.S. 2000. Brain structures and mechanisms involved in the control of cortical activation and wakefulness, with emphasis on the posterior hypothalamus and histaminergic neurons. *Sleep Med Rev* 4: 471–503.
51. Takahashi, K., Lin, J.S., and Sakai, K. 2006. Neuronal activity of histaminergic tuberomammillary neurons during wake–sleep states in the mouse. *J Neurosci* 26: 10292–10298.
52. Monti, J.M., D'Angelo, L., Jantos, H., and Pazos, S. 1988. Effects of a-fluoromethylhistidine on sleep and wakefulness in the rat. Short note. *J Neural Transm* 72: 141–145.
53. Kiyono, S., Seo, M.L., Shibagaki, M., Watanabe, T., Maeyama, K., and Wada, H. 1985. Effects of alpha-fluoromethylhistidine on sleep–waking parameters in rats. *Physiol Behav* 34: 615–617.
54. Lin, J.S., Sakai, K., and Jouvet, M. 1988. Evidence for histaminergic arousal mechanisms in the hypothalamus of cat. *Neuropharmacology* 27: 111–122.
55. Parmentier, R., Ohtsu, H., Djebbara-Hannas, Z., Valatx, J.L., Watanabe, T., and Lin, J.S. 2002. Anatomical, physiological, and pharmacological characteristics of histidine decarboxylase knock-out mice: evidence for the role of brain histamine in behavioral and sleep-wake control. *J Neurosci* 22: 7695–7711.
56. Monti, J.M., Pellejero, T., and Jantos, H. 1986. Effects of H1- and H_2 histamine receptor agonists and antagonists on sleep and wakefulness in the rat. *J Neural Transm* 66: 1–11.
57. Monti, J.M. 1993. Involvement of histamine in the control of the waking state. *Life Sci* 53: 1331–1338.
58. Kaneko, Y., Shimada, K., Saitou, K., Sugimoto, Y., and Kamei, C. 2000. The mechanism responsible for the drowsiness caused by first generation H1 antagonists on the EEG pattern. *Methods Find Exp Clin Pharmacol* 22: 163–168.
59. Arrang, J.M., Garbarg, M., and Schwartz, J.C. 1983. Auto-inhibition of brain histamine release mediated by a novel class (H3) of histamine receptor. *Nature* 302: 832–837.
60. Lovenberg, T.W., Roland, B.L., Wilson, S.J., et al. 1999. Cloning and functional expression of the human histamine H3 receptor. *Mol. Pharmacol.* 55: 1101–1107.
61. Pillot, C., Heron, A., Cochois, V., et al. 2002. A detailed mapping of the histamine H(3) receptor and its gene transcripts in rat brain. *Neuroscience* 114: 173–193.
62. Schwartz, J.C., Arrang, J.M., Garbarg, M., and Korner, M. 1986. Properties and roles of the three subclasses of histamine receptors in brain. *J Exp Biol* 124: 203–224.
63. Vanni-Mercier, G., Gigout, S., Debilly, G., and Lin, J.S. 2003. Waking selective neurons in the posterior hypothalamus and their response to histamine H_3 receptor ligands: an electrophysiological study in freely moving cats. *Behav Brain Res* 144: 227–241.
64. Monti, J.M., Jantos, H., Ponzoni, A., and Monti, D. 1996. Sleep and waking during acute histamine H3 agonist BP 2.94 or H3 antagonist carboperamide (MR 16155) administration in rats. *Neuropsychopharmacology* 15: 31–35.
65. Lamberty, Y., Margineanu, D.G., Dassesse, D., and Klitgaard, H. 2003. H3 agonist immepip markedly reduces cortical histamine release, but only weakly promotes sleep in the rat. *Pharmacol Res* 48: 193–198.

66. Monti, J.M., Jantos, H., Boussard, M., Altier, H., Orellana, C., and Olivera, S. 1991. Effects of selective activation or blockade of the histamine H3 receptor on sleep and wakefulness. *Eur J Pharmacol* 205: 283–287.
67. Celanire, S., Wijtmans, M., Talaga, P., Leurs, R., and de Esch, I.J. 2005. Keynote review: histamine H3 receptor antagonists reach out for the clinic. *Drug Discov Today* 10: 1613–1627.
68. Ligneau, X., Perrin, D., Landais, L., et al. 2007. BF2.649 [1-{3-[3-(4-Chlorophenyl)propoxy]propyl}piperidine, hydrochloride], a nonimidazole inverse agonist/antagonist at the human histamine H3 receptor: preclinical pharmacology. *J Pharmacol Exp Ther* 320: 365–375.
69. Ligneau, X., Landais, L., Perrin, D., et al. 2007. Brain histamine and schizophrenia: potential therapeutic applications of H_3 receptor inverse agonists studied with BF2.649. *Biochem Pharmacol* 73: 1215–1224.
70. Bonaventure, P., Letavic, M., Dugovic, C., et al. 2007. Histamine H3 receptor antagonists: from target identification to drug leads. *Biochem Pharmacol* 73: 1084–1096.
71. Arnsten, A.F. 2006. Stimulants: therapeutic actions in ADHD. *Neuropsychopharmacology* 31: 2376–2383.
72. Fleckenstein, A.E., Volz, T.J., Riddle, E.L., Gibb, J.W., and Hanson, G.R. 2007. New insights into the mechanism of action of amphetamines. *Annu Rev Pharmacol Toxicol.* 47: 681–698.
73. Horn, A.S., Cuello, A.C., and Miller, R.J. 1974. Dopamine in the mesolimbic system of the rat brain: endogenous levels and the effects of drugs on the uptake mechanism and stimulation of adenylate cyclase activity. *J Neurochem* 22: 265–270.
74. Yehuda, S. and Wurtman, R.J. 1975. Dopaminergic neurons in the nigro-striatal and mesolimbic pathways: mediation of specific effects of D-amphetamine. *Eur J Pharmacol* 30: 154–158.
75. Sulzer, D., Maidment, N.T., and Rayport, S. 1993. Amphetamine and other weak bases act to promote reverse transport of dopamine in ventral midbrain neurons. *J Neurochem* 60: 527–535.
76. Khoshbouei, H., Wang, H., Lechleiter, J.D., Javitch, J.A., and Galli, A. 2003. Amphetamine-induced dopamine efflux. A voltage-sensitive and intracellular Na^+-dependent mechanism. *J Biol Chem* 278: 12070–12077.
77. Jensen, O., Kaiser, J., and Lachaux, J.P. 2007. Human gamma-frequency oscillations associated with attention and memory. *Trends Neurosci* 30: 317–324.
78. Toyota, H., Dugovic, C., Koehl, M., et al. 2002. Behavioral characterization of mice lacking histamine H(3) receptors. *Mol Pharmacol* 62: 389–397.
79. Huang, Z.L., Mochizuki, T., Qu, W.M., et al. 2006. Altered sleep–wake characteristics and lack of arousal response to H3 receptor antagonist in histamine H1 receptor knockout mice. *Proc Natl Acad Sci* USA 103: 4687–4692.
80. Jané-Llopis, E., Hosman, C., Jenkins, R., and Anderson, P. 2003. Predictors of efficacy in depression prevention programmes: meta-analysis. *Br J Psychiatry* 183: 384–397.
81. Sharpley, A.L. and Cowen, P.J. 1995. Effect of pharmacologic treatments on the sleep of depressed patients. *Biol Psychiatry* 37: 85–98.
82. Menza, M.A., Kaufman, K.R., and Castellanos, A. 2000. Modafinil augmentation of antidepressant treatment in depression. *J Clin Psychiatry* 61: 378–381.
83. Kaufman, K.R., Menza, M.A., and Fitzsimmons, A. 2002. Modafinil monotherapy in depression. *Eur Psychiatry* 17: 167–169.
84. Ling, W., Rawson, R., Shoptaw, S., and Ling, W. 2006. Management of methamphetamine abuse and dependence. *Curr Psychiatry Rep* 8: 345–354.
85. Prommer, E. 2006. Modafinil: is it ready for prime time? *J Opioid Manag* 2: 130–136.
86. DeBattista, C., Doghramji, K., Menza, M.A., Rosenthal, M.H., and Fieve, R.R. 2003. Modafinil in depression study group. Adjunct modafinil for the short-term treatment of fatigue and sleepiness in patients with major depressive disorder: a preliminary double-blind, placebo-controlled study. *J Clin Psychiatry* 64: 1057–1064.

87. Letavic, M.A., Keith, J.M., Ly, K.S., et al. 2007. Novel naphthyridines are histamine H3 antagonists and serotonin reuptake transporter inhibitors. *Bioorg Med Chem Lett* 17: 2566–2569.
88. Nishino, S. 2007. Clinical and neurobiological aspects of narcolepsy. *Sleep Med* 8: 373–399.
89. Baumann, C.R. and Bassetti, C.L. 2005. Hypocretins (orexins): clinical impact of the discovery of a neurotransmitter. *Sleep Med Rev* 9: 253–268.
90. Baumann, C.R. and Bassetti, C.L. 2005. Hypocretins (orexins) and sleep–wake disorders. *Lancet Neurol* 4: 673–682.
91. Peyron, C., Faraco, J., Rogers, W., et al. 2000. A mutation in a case of early onset narcolepsy and a generalized absence of hypocretin peptides in human narcoleptic brains. *Nat Med* 6: 991–997.
92. Mignot, E., Lammers, G.J., Ripley, B., et al. 2002. The role of cerebrospinal fluid hypocretin measurement in the diagnosis of narcolepsy and other hypersomnias. *Arch Neurol* 59: 1553–1562.
93. Krahn, L.E., Pankratz, V.S., Oliver, L., Boeve, B.F., and Silber, M.H. 2002. Hypocretin (orexin) levels in cerebrospinal fluid of patients with narcolepsy: relationship to cataplexy and HLA DQB1*0602 status. *Sleep* 25: 733–736.
94. Thannickal, T.C., Siegel, J.M., Nienhuis, R., and Moore, R.Y. 2003. Pattern of hypocretin (orexin) soma and axon loss, and gliosis, in human narcolepsy. *Brain Pathol* 13: 340–351.
95. Huang, Z.L., Qu, W.M., Li, W.D., et al. 2001. Arousal effect of orexin A depends on activation of the histaminergic system. *Proc Natl Acad Sci* 98: 9965–9970.
96. Eriksson, K.S., Sergeeva, O., Brown, R.E., and Haas, H.L. 2001. Orexin/hypocretin excites the histaminergic neurons of the tuberomammillary nucleus. *J Neurosci* 21: 9273–9279.
97. Yamanaka, A., Tsujino, N., Funahashi, H., et al. 2002. Orexins activate histaminergic neurons via the orexin 2 receptor. *Biochem Biophys Res Commun* 290: 1237–1245.
98. Nishino, S., Fujiki, N., Ripley, B., et al. 2001. Decreased brain histamine content in hypocretin/orexin receptor-2 mutated narcoleptic dogs. *Neurosci Lett* 313: 125–128.
99. Mignot, E. and Nishino, S. 2005. Emerging therapies in narcolepsy-cataplexy. *Sleep* 28: 754–763.
100. Lin, L., Faraco, J., Li, R., et al. 1999. The sleep disorder canine narcolepsy is caused by a mutation in the hypocretin (orexin) receptor 2 gene. *Cell* 98: 365–376.
101. Ripley, B., Fujiki, N., Okura, M., Mignot, E., and Nishino, S. 2001. Hypocretin levels in sporadic and familial cases of canine narcolepsy. *Neurobiol Dis* 8: 525–534.
102. Chemelli, R.M., Willie, J.T., Sinton, C.M., et al. 1999. Narcolepsy in orexin knockout mice: molecular genetics of sleep regulation. *Cell* 98: 437–451.
103. Hara, J., Beuckmann, C.T., Nambu, T., et al. 2001. Genetic ablation of orexin neurons in mice results in narcolepsy, hypophagia, and obesity. *Neuron* 30: 345–354.
104. Willie, J.T., Chemelli, R.M., Sinton, C.M., et al. 2003. Distinct narcolepsy syndromes in orexin receptor-2 and orexin null mice: molecular genetic dissection of non-REM and REM sleep regulatory processes. *Neuron* 38: 715–730.
105. Aldrich, M.S. and Reynolds, P.R. 1999. Narcolepsy and the hypocretin receptor 2 gene. *Neuron* 23: 625–626.
106. Sakurai, T. 2005. Reverse pharmacology of orexin: from an orphan GPCR to integrative physiology. *Regul Pept* 126: 3–10.
107. Mitler, M.M. 1994. Evaluation of treatment with stimulants in narcolepsy. *Sleep* 17(Suppl 8): S103–S106.
108. Mitler, M.M. and Hayduk, R. 2002. Benefits and risks of pharmacotherapy for narcolepsy. *Drug Saf* 25: 791–809.
109. Thorpy, M. 2007. Therapeutic advances in narcolepsy. *Sleep Med* 8: 427–440.

110. Wisor, J.P. and Eriksson, K.S. 2005. Dopaminergic-adrenergic interactions in the wake promoting mechanism of modafinil. *Neuroscience* 132: 1027–1034.
111. Wisor, J.P., Nishino, S., Sora, I., Uhl, G.H., Mignot, E., and Edgar, D.M. 2001. Dopaminergic role in stimulant-induced wakefulness. *J Neurosci* 21: 1787–1794.
112. Tanganelli, S., Pérez de la Mora, M., Ferraro, L., et al. 1995. Modafinil and cortical gamma-aminobutyric acid outflow. Modulation by 5-hydroxytryptamine neurotoxins. *Eur J Pharmacol* 273: 63–71.
113. Tanganelli, S., Fuxe, K., Ferraro, L., Janson, A.M., and Bianchi, C. 1992. Inhibitory effects of the psychoactive drug modafinil on gamma-aminobutyric acid outflow from the cerebral cortex of the awake freely moving guinea-pig. Possible involvement of 5-hydroxytryptamine mechanisms. *Naunyn Schmiedebergs Arch Pharmacol* 345: 461–465.
114. Ferraro, L., Antonelli, T., O'Connor, W.T., Tanganelli, S., Rambert, F.A., and Fuxe, K. 1997. Modafinil: an antinarcoleptic drug with a different neurochemical profile to d-amphetamine and dopamine uptake blockers. *Biol Psychiatry* 42: 1181–1183.
115. Robertson, P., Jr. and Hellriegel, E.T. 2003. Clinical pharmacokinetic profile of modafinil. *Clin Pharmacokinet* 42: 123–137.
116. Mitler, M.M., Harsh, J., Hirshkowitz, M., and Guilleminault, C. 2000. Long-term efficacy and safety of modafinil (PROVIGIL((R))) for the treatment of excessive daytime sleepiness associated with narcolepsy. *Sleep Med* 1: 231–243.
117. Broughton, R. and Mamelak, M. 1979. The treatment of narcolepsy-cataplexy with nocturnal gamma-hydroxybutyrate. *Can J Neurol Sci* 6: 1–6.
118. Broughton, R. and Mamelak, M. 1980. Effects of nocturnal gamma-hydroxybutyrate on sleep/waking patterns in narcolepsy-cataplexy. *Can J Neurol Sci* 7: 23–31.
119. Scharf, M.B., Brown, D., Woods, M., Brown, L., and Hirschowitz, J. 1985. The effects and effectiveness of gamma-hydroxybutyrate in patients with narcolepsy. *J Clin Psychiatry* 46: 222–225.
120. Lammers, G.J., Arends, J., Declerck, A.C., Ferrari, M.D., Schouwink, G., and Troost, J. 1993. Gammahydroxybutyrate and narcolepsy: a double-blind placebo-controlled study. *Sleep* 16: 216–220.
121. Verstraeten, E. 2007. Neurocognitive effects of obstructive sleep apnea syndrome. *Curr Neurol Neurosci Rep* 7: 161–166.
122. Nowak, M., Kornhuber, J., and Meyrer, R. 2006. Daytime impairment and neurodegeneration in OSAS. *Sleep* 29: 1521–1530.
123. Felmet, K.A. and Petersen, M. 2006. Obstructive sleep apnea and cognitive dysfunction. *JAAPA* 19: 16–20.
124. Black, J.E., Brooks, S.N., and Nishino, S. 2004. Narcolepsy and syndromes of primary excessive daytime somnolence. *Semin Neurol* 24: 271–282.
125. Day, R., Gerhardstein, R., Lumley, A., Roth, T., and Rosenthal, L. 1999. The behavioral morbidity of obstructive sleep apnea. *Prog Cardiovasc Dis* 41: 341–354.
126. Vgontzas, A.N., Bixler, E.O., and Chrousos, G.P. 2005. Sleep apnea is a manifestation of the metabolic syndrome. *Sleep Med Rev* 9: 211–224.
127. Vgontzas, A.N., Bixler, E.O., and Chrousos, G.P. 2003. Metabolic disturbances in obesity versus sleep apnoea: the importance of visceral obesity and insulin resistance. *J Intern Med* 254: 32–44.
128. Malhotra, A. and White, D.P. 2002. Obstructive sleep apnoea. *Lancet* 360: 237–245.
129. Prisant, L.M., Dillard, T.A., and Blanchard, A.R. 2006. Obstructive sleep apnea syndrome. *J Clin Hypertens* 8: 746–750.
130. Provini, F., Vetrugno, R., Lugaresi, E., and Montagna, P. 2006. Sleep-related breathing disorders and headache. *Neurol Sci* 27(Suppl 2): S149–S152.
131. Banno, K. and Kryger, M.H. 2007. Sleep apnea: clinical investigations in humans. *Sleep Med* 8: 400–426.

132. Peppard, P.E., Young, T., Palta, M., Dempsey, J., and Skatrud, J. 2000. Longitudinal study of moderate weight change and sleep-disordered breathing. *JAMA* 284: 3015–3021.

133. Young, T., Peppard, P.E., and Gottlieb, D.J. 2002. Epidemiology of obstructive sleep apnea: a population health perspective. *Am J Respir Crit Care Med* 165: 1217–1239.

134. Davies, R.J., Ali, N.J., and Stradling, J.R. 1992. Neck circumference and other clinical features in the diagnosis of the obstructive sleep apnoea syndrome. *Thorax* 47: 101–105.

135. Davies, R.J. and Stradling, J.R. 1990. The relationship between neck circumference, radiographic pharyngeal anatomy, and the obstructive sleep apnoea syndrome. *Eur Respir J* 3: 509–514.

136. Redline, S. and Tishler, P.V. 2000. The genetics of sleep apnea. *Sleep Med Rev* 4: 583–602.

137. Palmer, L.J., Buxbaum, S.G., Larkin, E., et al. 2003. A whole-genome scan for obstructive sleep apnea and obesity. *Am J Hum Genet* 72: 340–350.

138. Redline, S., Tishler, V., Tosteson, T.D., et al. 1995. The familial aggregation of obstructive sleep apnea. *Am J Respir Crit Care Med* 151(3 Pt 1): 682–687.

139. Nino-Murcia, G., McCann, C.C., Bliwise, D.L., Guilleminault, C., and Dement, W.C. 1989. Compliance and side effects in sleep apnea patients treated with nasal continuous positive airway pressure. *West J Med* 150: 165–169.

140. Pépin, J.L., Leger, P., Veale, D., Langevin, B., Robert, D., and Lévy, P. 1995. Side effects of nasal continuous positive airway pressure in sleep apnea syndrome. Study of 193 patients in two French sleep centers. *Chest* 107: 375–381.

141. Hoffstein, V., Viner, S., Mateika, S., and Conway, J. 1992. Treatment of obstructive sleep apnea with nasal continuous positive airway pressure. Patient compliance, perception of benefits, and side effects. *Am Rev Respir Dis* 145(4 Pt 1): 841–845.

142. Fritsch, K.M., Iseli, A., Russi, E.W., and Bloch, K.E. 2001. Side effects of mandibular advancement devices for sleep apnea treatment. *Am J Respir Crit Care Med* 164: 813–818.

143. Li, K.K. 2005. Surgical therapy for obstructive sleep apnea syndrome. *Semin Respir Crit Care Med* 26: 80–88.

144. Sher, A.E. 2002. Upper airway surgery for obstructive sleep apnea. *Sleep Med Rev* 6: 195–212.

145. Sher, A.E., Schechtman, K.B., and Piccirillo, J.F. 1996. The efficacy of surgical modifications of the upper airway in adults with obstructive sleep apnea syndrome. *Sleep* 19: 156–177.

146. Sleep-related breathing disorders in adults: recommendations for syndrome definition and measurement techniques in clinical research. The Report of an American academy of sleep medicine task force. *Sleep* 1999: 22: 667–689.

147. Veasey, S.C., Guilleminault, C., Strohl, K.P., Sanders, M.H., Ballard, R.D., and Magalang, U.J. 2006. Medical therapy for obstructive sleep apnea: a review by the Medical therapy for obstructive sleep apnea task force of the standards of practice committee of the American academy of sleep medicine. *Sleep* 29: 1036–1044.

148. Black, J.E. and Hirshkowitz, M. 2005. Modafinil for treatment of residual excessive sleepiness in nasal continuous positive airway pressure-treated obstructive sleep apnea/hypopnea syndrome. *Sleep* 28: 464–471.

149. Schwartz, J.R., Hirshkowitz, M., Erman, M.K., and Schmidt-Nowara, W. 2003. Modafinil as adjunct therapy for daytime sleepiness in obstructive sleep apnea: a 12-week, open-label study. *Chest* 124: 2192–2199.

150. Roth, T., White, D., Schmidt-Nowara, W., et al. 2006. Effects of armodafinil in the treatment of residual excessive sleepiness associated with obstructive sleep apnea/hypopnea syndrome: a 12-week, multicenter, double-blind, randomized, placebo-controlled study in nCPAP-adherent adults. *Clin Ther* 28: 689–706.

151. Roth, B., Nevsimalova, S., and Rechtschaffen, A. 1972. Hypersomnia with "sleep drunkenness". *Arch Gen Psychiatry* 26: 456–462.
152. Billiard, M. 1996. Idiopathic hypersomnia. *Neurol Clin* 14: 573–582.
153. Faull, K.F., Thiemann, S., King, R.J., and Guilleminault, C. 1986. Monoamine interactions in narcolepsy and hypersomnia: a preliminary report. *Sleep* 9(1 Pt 2): 246–249.
154. Montplaisir, J., de Champlain, J., Young, S.N., et al. 1982. Narcolepsy and idiopthic hypersomnia: biogenic amines and related compounds in CSF. *Neurology* 32: 1299–1302.
155. Faull, K.F., Guilleminault, C., Berger, P.A., and Barchas, J.D. 1983. Cerebrospinal fluid monoamine metabolites in narcolepsy and hypersomnia. *Ann Neurol* 13: 258–263.
156. Nevsimalova, S. and Roth, B. 1972. Genealogical study of hypersomnia and narcolepsy. *Cesk Neurol Neurochir* 35: 1–8.
157. Bastuji, H. and Jouvet, M. 1988. Successful treatment of idiopathic hypersomnia and narcolepsy with modafinil. *Prog Neuropsychopharmacol Biol Psychiatry* 12: 695–700.
158. Billiard, M. and Dauvilliers, Y. 2001. Idiopathic hypersomnia. *Sleep Med Rev* 5: 349–358.

9 Obesity

*Timothy A. Esbenshade, Michael E. Brune,
and Marina I. Strakhova*

CONTENTS

Introduction 277
Current Approaches to the Treatment of Obesity 278
Role of Histamine in Feeding and Weight Regulation 278
Role of Histamine Receptors in Feeding and Weight Regulation 279
  Histamine H_1 Receptor 280
  Histamine H_3 Receptor 281
Histaminergic Genetic Modifications and Weight Regulation 282
Preclinical Antiobesity Effects of H_3 Receptor Antagonists 285
  Imidazole-Based H_3 Receptor Antagonists 285
  Nonimidazole-Based H_3 Receptor Antagonists 289
Challenges and Promises of Clinical Utility of H_3 Receptor
  Antagonists for the Treatment of Obesity 292
Conclusions 296
Acknowledgments 296
References 297

INTRODUCTION

Since the development of classical antihistamines such as diphenhydramine and fexofenadine, which target the histamine H_1 receptor for the treatment of allergic reactions, histamine receptors have long remained attractive drug targets. Ranitidine and famotidine are histamine H_2 receptor antagonists that inhibit gastric acid secretion through histamine H_2 receptor blockade and remain to this day effective treatments for the amelioration of heartburn and gastric ulcers. Tremendous number of patients have benefited from both histamine H_1 and H_2 receptor antagonists that have been very successful therapeutic agents with very good safety margins (many of these agents are now over-the-counter) and great commercial success. Thus, given the remarkable success of these two classes of histamine receptors and the central role of the more recently described H_3 receptor in the modulation of the release of neurotransmitters (see Chapter 4) involved in cognition, sleep, and homeostasis, academic and industrial laboratories have expended considerable effort to discover and develop potent and selective H_3 receptor antagonists to treat disorders of

(1) cognition (see Chapters 7 and 11) such as attention-deficit hyperactivity disorder (ADHD), Alzheimer's disease, and schizophrenia; (2) sleep (see Chapter 8) such as hypersomnia and narcolepsy; and (3) homeostasis such as obesity. This chapter will briefly review the role of histamine and the H_3 receptor in feeding and weight regulation, and the reader is referred to several, excellent recent reviews [1–4] that provide a more comprehensive overview of the role of histamine and histamine receptors in feeding behavior and maintenance of body weight. Much of this chapter will focus on recent preclinical advances in H_3 receptor antagonist research directed at developing compounds to treat obesity and associated metabolic dysfunction, including the description of the antiobesity properties of these compounds and the challenges and promises associated with this therapeutic approach.

CURRENT APPROACHES TO THE TREATMENT OF OBESITY

Obesity is a global health crisis that results from poor diet and lack of sufficient physical activity that contributes to a number of pathologies including hypertension, coronary heart disease, diabetes, stroke, and cancer [1,5,6]. Remarkably, over the past 20 years, in Europe and North America, the rates of obesity have more than doubled, and at present, over 50% of the adult population is considered overweight or obese [5]. The impact of the morbidity and mortality associated with obesity on health care cost is also expected to rise with the increased incidence of obesity. Thus, there is considerable interest in developing pharmacotherapies to combat obesity. However, despite numerous efforts by pharmaceutical companies to develop such drugs, at present there are only two drugs approved for long-term treatment of obesity in the United States and a third awaiting FDA approval, each with different targets reflecting the etiological complexity of this disease. These prescription drugs include orlistat (Xenical®), sibutramine (Meridia®), and rimonobant (Acomplia®). Orlistat is a lipase inhibitor that functions peripherally in the gut to inhibit intestinal fat absorption. In contrast, both sibutramine, a nonselective norepinephrine/serotonin/dopamine reuptake inhibitor with appetite suppressant and satiety enhancer activity, and rimonobant, a CB_1 cannabinoid receptor antagonist that has shown promising weight loss effects in clinical trials, act centrally to mediate their effects [5]. A number of molecular targets, including those involved in the orexin/leptin pathways, have been extensively explored, and there remain other potential pharmacological sites to be investigated as potential antiobesity targets. Given the critical involvement of the histaminergic system in feeding and weight homeostatic mechanisms to be described later, targets involving this system, including the H_3 receptor, remain an attractive choice for further drug discovery efforts.

ROLE OF HISTAMINE IN FEEDING AND WEIGHT REGULATION

Histamine has been known for a long time to play a critical role in homeostatic regulatory functions such as the control of food consumption and body weight regulation in animals [1,2]. A number of fine reviews have detailed the important neurotransmitter actions of histamine within the central nervous system (CNS) [7,8] (see also Chapter 3), and that this neurotransmitter plays a role in various physiological functions including feeding and weight homeostasis. The cell bodies of histamine synthesizing neurons are localized to the hypothalamic tuberomammillary nucleus and project throughout the CNS to regions including two hypothalamic regions known to regulate food consumption, the paraventricular nucleus, and ventromedial hypothalamus [7,9]. These histaminergic neurons are apparently heterogeneous, perhaps representing functionally distinct neurons [10] that project throughout the CNS [8,9,11] to differentially activate the diverse regulatory pathways ranging from cognition to sleep to feeding and weight homeostasis mediated by histamine [12].

Direct evidence for the involvement of histamine in food intake can be derived from the finding that food consumption and body weight are significantly decreased in both diet-induced obese and diabetic (*db/db*) mice and body fat weight, *ob* gene expression, and serum leptin concentration are also reduced upon the central infusion of histamine [13]. Additionally, food intake is also decreased in rats upon the oral and systemic administration of histidine (histamine precursor), an effect blocked by the coadministration of α-fluoromethyl-histidine, an inhibitor of histidine decarboxylase (HDC) that converts histidine into histamine [14,15]. Histamine also plays an important role in modulating meal size and duration, where it has been shown that the speed of meal consumption was decreased by histamine depletion in the mesencephalic trigeminal sensory nucleus, but meal size and duration was increased by histamine depletion in the ventromedial hypothalamic satiety center [16].

Neuronal input to hypothalamic histamine neurons originates from cortical, septal, and other hypothalamic areas [8]. Histaminergic neuronal function can be regulated by a number of neurotransmitters, including some with defined feeding/weight-regulating mechanisms such as orexin [17] as well as serotonin, glutamate, acetylcholine, and galanin [1,8,18]. The well-established association between orexin and CNS histaminergic systems clearly illustrates the linkage between these two systems in regulating sleep and feeding/weight gain, where orexin deficiency manifests itself with decreased brain histamine content and narcolepsy in dogs [19] and abdominal obesity in narcoleptic humans [20].

Another hormonal/histaminergic system interaction thought to be involved in regulating food consumption is that with the adipocyte-derived hormone, leptin. Evidence for this interaction include the finding of highly elevated serum leptin levels in the presence of deficient histamine synthesis in HDC knockout mice [21,22] and reduced levels of hypothalamic histamine and *tele*-methylhistamine in obese (*ob/ob*) and *db/db* mice [23]. Administration of leptin to *ob/ob* mice increased histamine turnover [23] and decreased food consumption [24]. One can envision increasingly more complex interactions between hormones, receptors, neurotransmitters, and neuronal pathways with the histaminergic system in the regulation of feeding and weight homeostasis, some of which are further detailed in the following sections.

ROLE OF HISTAMINE RECEPTORS IN FEEDING AND WEIGHT REGULATION

As indicated earlier, histamine has been shown to have a demonstrable effect on reducing food consumption and weight gain. Histamine is known to be able to activate all four subtypes (H_1, H_2, H_3, and H_4) of the G-protein-coupled histamine receptors, each of which exhibits distinct expression patterns as well as molecular, pharmacological, and signaling properties [25]. The reader is referred to Chapter 4 for further description of the properties of these receptors. The two most prominent histamine receptors involved in feeding/weight regulation based on scientific data to date are the H_1 and H_3 receptors, and for the purposes of this discussion and to illustrate several rather simple concepts in an otherwise very complex system, the role of these two histamine receptors will be elucidated here, again keeping in mind that the interaction of other neurotransmitters and neuronal pathways may influence the effects mediated by these receptors.

HISTAMINE H_1 RECEPTOR

In the human CNS, H_1 receptors are highly expressed in limbic and neocortical areas and localized to postsynaptic neurons [7]. These receptors play an important regulatory role in the sleep–wake cycle and in the maintenance of attention and vigilance [26]. Indeed, central penetrating H_1 receptor antagonists such as diphenhydramine induce sedation, whereas selective H_1 agonists can augment alertness and vigilance. With respect to regulating feeding responses, activation of ventrolateral posterior hypothalamic H_1 receptors inhibits the consumption of food, whereas this effect is blocked by H_1 receptor antagonists [7]. In another study examining the effects of the direct injection of the H_1 antagonist chlorpheniramine into the paraventricular nucleus, feeding was increased [27]. In addition, H_1 receptor blockade by chlorpheniramine or pyrilamine greatly attenuated the anorectic effects of amylin in rats [28]. In another direct injection study, when histamine was administered directly into the lateral ventricle of agouti yellow obese mice, both body weight and food consumption were decreased, but this effect was negated if the H_1 receptor was ablated in these mice [29]. Although another study failed to show blockade of histidine-induced feeding effects by chlorpheniramine [14], the authors did suggest that the doses may have been sedating, which may have decreased feeding or led to other nonspecific effects involving other neurotransmitter systems that could have impacted food consumption.

Interestingly, it has been recently proposed that antagonism of H_1 receptors by a number of antipsychotic drugs that demonstrate high affinity for these receptors may contribute to weight gain, elevation of lipids, and increased diabetes risk associated with these drugs [30,31]. Further extension of this hypothesis to studies in histamine H_1 receptor knockout mice showed that H_1 antagonists as well as high H_1 receptor affinity atypical antipsychotics such as clozapine and olanzapine failed to induce hypothalamic AMP kinase phosphorylation and activation, a central marker linked to weight gain [32]. However, it should also be noted that no genetic linkage between histaminergic receptor polymorphisms and obesity has been detected [33].

Although centrally active and selective H_1 agonists may make attractive antiobesity agents, none have been identified to date. However, betahistine, an H_1 receptor partial agonist/H_3 receptor antagonist [34], has been demonstrated to inhibit food consumption in rats and goats [35,36]. Interestingly, betahistine was coadministered with the atypical antipsychotic olanzapine in a small number of schizophrenic patients for 6 weeks, and although the patients gained weight, the authors concluded that a larger study was warranted since the degree of weight gain was not clinically significant [37].

HISTAMINE H$_3$ RECEPTOR

The histamine H$_3$ receptor is predominantly expressed in the rodent CNS, with high levels of mRNA and receptor-binding sites detected in cortical areas as well as in other brain regions innervated by histaminergic neurons including the hypothalamus, hippocampus, nucleus accumbens, and striatum, [7,38]. Importantly from a therapeutic drug discovery perspective, the human brain also appears to highly express H$_3$ receptors based on autoradiographic and expression data [39]. In contrast to H$_1$ receptors, H$_3$ receptors are localized presynaptically and can function as autoreceptors to modulate the synthesis and release of histamine and as heteroreceptors to modulate the release of other neurotransmitters such as acetylcholine, norepinephrine, dopamine, serotonin, and others (see Figure 9.1) [7,11,40], which may also play a role in weight regulation and feeding. Additionally, the H$_3$ receptor is known to play a role in sleep/wake regulation as well as in cognitive functioning, prompting extensive drug discovery efforts in the effort to make H$_3$ receptor antagonists for the treatment of disorders of sleep (narcolepsy) and cognition (ADHD, Alzheimer's disease, schizophrenia)—topics that are comprehensively covered in Chapters 5, 7, 8, and 11 and in several recent reviews [12,40,41]. This chapter highlights drug discovery efforts focusing on H$_3$ receptor antagonists as antiobesity agents and further evidence for the central role of H$_3$ receptors in the regulation of feeding behavior and weight homeostasis will be described in the context of these compounds later.

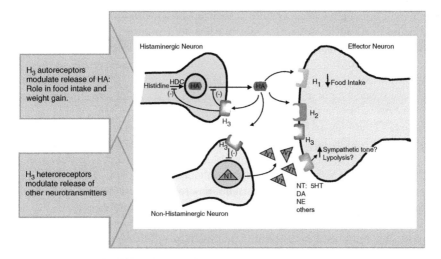

FIGURE 9.1 Schematic representation of histaminergic receptor function. Stimulation of presynaptic H$_3$ autoreceptors on histaminergic neurons by histamine (HA) inhibits the synthesis of histamine (through HDC) and also inhibits the release of HA from the neuron. Postsynaptically, HA activates H$_1$ receptors to decrease feeding. Stimulation of presynaptic H$_3$ heteroreceptors on nonhistaminergic neurons inhibits the release of a number of neurotransmitters (NT) including serotonin (5HT), dopamine (DA), norepinephrine (NE), and others that can then activate their respective target receptors postsynaptically to evoke homeostatic responses.

In addition to the central localization of H_3 receptors, there is evidence of H_3 receptor mRNA expression in brown adipose tissue (BAT) in developing and adult rats [42,43]. In rodents, BAT expresses mitochondrial uncoupling protein 1 (UCP-1) [44] and plays an important role in regulating heat production although the presence of BAT in humans is uncertain [45]. Thus, it has been postulated that the H_3 receptors could regulate BAT thermogenic function peripherally [42], but to date, no direct evidence for a peripheral H_3 receptor-mediated effect in BAT has been shown. Instead, most findings to date that have examined the role of the histaminergic system on BAT thermoregulation have shown enhanced BAT sympathetic nerve activity following administration of intraperitoneal histidine or intracerebroventricular histamine with an associated increase in the level of BAT UCP-1 after histamine infusion [46–48]. Thioperamide, an H_3 receptor antagonist (imidazole-based H receptor antagonists), administered intracerebroventricularly also activated sympathetic nerve activity and lipolysis in adipose tissue, suggesting a central role for H_3 receptors in this response [46]. Paradoxically, UCPs are upregulated in adipose tissue upon the central administration of histamine [13] but downregulated in H_3 receptor knockout mice [49], illustrating the difficulties of differentiating peripheral from central sites of action for H_3 receptor regulation of feeding and weight.

HISTAMINERGIC GENETIC MODIFICATIONS AND WEIGHT REGULATION

Modification of genes related to histaminergic function, in particular, ablation of histaminergic receptors and enzymes associated with the biosynthesis of histamine, have helped inform researchers about the potential role of histamine and H_1 and H_3 receptors in the regulation of food consumption and weight. Knockout of the HDC (the final enzyme in the histamine synthetic pathway) gene results in mice that exhibit increased body weight on both standard and high-fat diets with an increase in adipose tissue weight and decrease in *ob* mRNA expression on a high-fat diet as compared to wild-types [50]. Knockout of the HDC gene in mice results in large increases in leptin levels and decreased glucose tolerance associated with a phenotype characterized by late-onset obesity [22]. These findings suggest a fundamental role for histamine in mediating central leptin signaling; indeed, it has been shown that systemic administration of leptin can enhance hypothalamic histamine release [51], and thus, knockout of the HDC gene may reflect the disruption of the leptin-histamine pathway and subsequent hyperleptinemia and obese phenotype.

In studies investigating the role of the histamine receptor targets in weight homeostasis, it has been demonstrated that the targeted disruption of the histamine H_1 receptor gene in mice presents a phenotype of decreased energy expenditure and late-onset obesity [52]. In addition, the feeding cycle was disrupted before the onset of obesity in H_1 receptor knockout mice [52]. Feeding a high-fat diet to H_1 receptor knockout mice results in obesity and associated fat deposits, increased *ob* gene expression, blunting of leptin-mediated appetite suppression, and increased expression of UCP mRNA [52]. In addition, the effects of leptin were reduced, and the H_3 antagonist thioperamide did not suppress feeding in H_1 receptor knockout mice [53]. Similar to what was seen in the HDC knockout mice, leptin appeared to be less effective in mediating its effects since the anorectic activity of centrally administered leptin was greatly reduced in these mice [54], suggesting a fundamental role of H_1 receptors in the leptin–histamine-signaling pathway (Table 9.1).

The metabolic and homeostatic roles of the H_3 receptor have also been extensively explored by Takahashi et al. [49] *in vivo* in mice in which the gene has been disrupted resulting in complete ablation of H_3 receptor mRNA and protein expression and as well as no changes in gene expression of H_1 or H_2 as a result of the loss of the H_3 receptor. Relative to their wild-type littermates, these H_3 receptor knockout mice showed enhanced histamine release as determined by *tele*-methylhistamine levels in multiple brain areas including hypothalamus, hippocampus, and forebrain [49]. Both the male and the female H_3 receptor knockout mice exhibited enhanced weight gain along with increased food consumption and decreased energy expenditure, likely contributing to the obese phenotype [3]. Interestingly, these H_3 receptor knockout mice also display lower expression of the energy regulatory UCPs in BAT (UCP-1) and brown and white adipose tissues as well as skeletal muscle (UCP-3), perhaps due to resistance to leptin and accounting for the decreased level of energy expenditure by these animals [49]. Additionally, these late-onset obesity in H_3 knockout mice displayed hallmark signs of human obesity, notably increased blood levels of insulin and leptin. Although the plasma glucose levels of the H_3 knockout mice were comparable to their wild-type littermates under normal conditions, these mice displayed signs of insulin resistance since they exhibited impaired responses in insulin tolerance tests [3,49].

The obese phenotype seen with the HDC and H_1 receptor knockout mice makes intuitive sense, given the direct role of histamine in activating H_1 receptor-mediated anorectic effects. However, the obese phenotype seen with the H_3 receptor knockout mice described by Takahashi et al. [49] seems paradoxical, given that increased histamine levels are seen in these animals. Although the laboratory of Tokita has, to date, provided the most detailed description of the weight gain/metabolic phenotype of their obese H_3 knockout mice [3,49], other groups have also provided some limited information concerning the feeding and weight behaviors of H_3 knockout mice that do not appear to display significant changes in weight. In contrast to the previously described H_3 receptor knockout mice, the H_3 receptor knockout mice reported by Toyota et al. [58] display a slightly, although not significant, decreased body weight than their wild-type littermates, and a later report showed no significant differences between H_3 receptor knockout mice and control mice when comparing body weight gain, food intake, and fat mass for mice on either control and high-fat diets [60]. Additionally, the H_3 receptor knockout mice used by Hancock et al. [61] were only slightly heavier than their wild-type counterparts. These apparently different H_3 receptor knockout mice metabolic/weight phenotypes from a slight decrease to marginal to significant increases in body weight illustrate the potential importance of the background strain, diet, and perhaps other factors when using these transgenic animals in determining the role of the H_3 receptor as well as the efficacy of H_3 receptor ligands in feeding, weight gain, and metabolic homeostasis. These ideas will be further expanded in the following section.

TABLE 9.1

Metabolic Phenotypes of Mice with Ablated Histaminergic-Associated Genes

Receptor	Physical Phenotype	Blood Biochemistry	References
$H_1^{-/-}$	Normal weight at birth; feeding cycle disruption, mature-onset obesity, increase in WAT mass at 48 weeks of age (epididymal, mesenteric, and retroperitoneal fat); elevated triglycerides in liver and skeletal muscle at 48 weeks; increased expression of *ob* mRNA in epididymal WAT; decreased expression of UCP-1 mRNA in BAT at 48 weeks; anorectic activity of ICV-administered leptin is significantly attenuated	Increased fasting serum concentrations of insulin and FFAs; increased concentration of serum leptin; no significant changes in glucose levels	52,54
	Decreased levels of hypocretin-1 and -2 (orexin A and B) in the brain		55
	Increased concentrations of dopamine, DOPAC, and HVA in cortex; turnover rates of 5-HT significantly increased in all brain regions; increased 5-HT release		56,57
Agouti yellow $H_1^{-/-}$	Targeted disruption of H_1 gene attenuates histamine-induced reduction in food intake and histamine-induced increase in BAT UCP-1 mRNA observed in A^y/a mice		29
$H_3^{-/-}$	Fertile and viable, possess slightly increased body weights at birth; exhibit mild hyperphagia and late-onset obesity; increased adiposity and decreased energy expenditure; reduced expression of UCP-1 and UCP-3 in adipose tissues; increased levels of *tele*-methylhistamine in hypothalamic/thalamic sections; normal levels of H_1R and H_2R mRNA; decreased H_1R binding activity in the brain	Hyperinsulinemia and hyperleptinemia; retain normal levels of glucose, T4, FFA, cholesterol, and TG; display impaired ITT and GTT	3,49
	Normal levels of hypocretin-1 and -2 (orexin A and B)		55
	Possess slightly lower body weights; have normal brain levels of dopamine, norepinephrine and serotonin, but decreased levels of histamine		58
$HDC^{-/-}$	Fertile, increased body weight at 12 weeks; less reactive when handled	No difference in plasma leptin concentration between diets	59
	Increased body weight on both standard and high-fat diets as compared to controls; increased adipose tissue weight on HFD; decrease in *ob* mRNA expression on HFD (compared to STD)		50
	Normal body weights at birth, late-onset obesity, increased epididymal WAT, increased interscapular BAT fat pads; no hyperphagia; impaired ability to metabolize energy stores decreased mRNA levels of full-length leptin receptor isoform	Increased serum leptin levels, impaired glucose tolerance, hyperinsulinemia; slightly elevated levels of plasma corticosterone; normal levels of serum triglyceride, cholesterol, and HDL	21,22

Note: WAT, white adipose tissue; ICV, intracerebroventricular; DOPAC, 3,4–dihydroxyphenylacetic acid; HVA, homovanillic acid; FFA, free fatty acid; ITT, Insulin tolerance test; GTT, glucose tolerance test; HFD, high fat diet; STD, standard diet.

PRECLINICAL ANTIOBESITY EFFECTS OF H₃ RECEPTOR ANTAGONISTS

Given the role of histamine in homeostatic mechanisms regulating feeding and weight gain and the central localization of H_3 receptors and their modulatory role on neurotransmission in brain regions associated with these regulatory pathways, this receptor offers an attractive drug target for antiobesity agents. A number of pharmaceutical companies have been actively conducting drug discovery efforts in designing effective H_3 receptor antagonists with druglike properties to optimize antiobesity properties in preclinical models of feeding and diet-induced obesity. These will be discussed in the following sections, where findings from earlier imidazole-based H_3 antagonists and the currently pursued nonimidazole-based H_3 antagonists will be highlighted (Table 9.2). Several comprehensive reviews on the potential of H_3 receptor antagonists for the treatment of obesity have also been recently published [1–3].

IMIDAZOLE-BASED H₃ RECEPTOR ANTAGONISTS

Thioperamide (Figure 9.2), a prototypic imidazole-based histamine H_3 receptor antagonist, was shown early on in studies investigating the role of H_3 receptors in acute feeding behavior to reduce rat food intake upon central injection [62]. This effect would presumably occur through both the enhancement of histamine synthesis and the release resulting from H_3 receptor blockade and the subsequent activation of postsynaptic histamine H_1 receptors (see Figure 9.1) as described earlier. Subsequent work with thioperamide by this laboratory [46,63] and others [1,53,64–67] provided additional evidence supporting the concept of H_3 receptor blockade and regulation of feeding and appetite. In particular, thioperamide revealed that H_3 receptors were involved in the regulation of food consumption in rats by neuropeptides such as cholecystokinin [64–66].

Additional studies with thioperamide utilizing rodent strains predisposed to weight gain or in which histamine receptors have been knocked out have further revealed the potential of H_3 antagonists in the regulating feeding behavior. In our laboratories, food consumption in both Sprague–Dawley rats and *fa/fa* rats was attenuated by thioperamide [1]. Thioperamide has also been shown to block snacking behavior (eating of a palatable high-carbohydrate or high-fat meals) in obese Zucker rats [68]. Further work examining the effects of thioperamide on acute feeding in transgenic animals showed that this compound failed to suppress feeding in H_1 receptor knockout mice [53], implicating the central role of histamine in H_3 receptor antagonist effects. Additionally, in H_3 receptor knockout mice, thioperamide did not reduce acute feeding responses, again demonstrating that the expression of H_3 receptors is necessary to reveal the effects of H_3 antagonists such as thioperamide on feeding and weight regulation [49].

Ciproxifan (Figure 9.2) is another well-characterized H_3 antagonist for which there is evidence of antiobesity properties, although this compound has been much less extensively profiled than thioperamide in feeding models. When administered peripherally, this compound elevates hypothalamic histamine levels and blocks acute food intake in rats trained to respond to a 3-h feeding regime [69]. Ciproxifan (30 mg/kg/day) also decreased weight gain in a mouse model of diet-induced obesity

TABLE 9.2

Antiobesity Effects of H₃ Receptor Antagonists

Compound	Species	Effect	References
Thioperamide	Nonobese rats and mice	Decrease in food intake	1,53,62–64
	Nonobese rats	ICV administration accelerates lipolysis in the epididymal adipose tissue	46
		Increase in histamine contents in brain and stomach. Potentiation of the CCK-8-induced inhibition of food intake	64
		No effect on food intake in sated rats. Decreased feeding responses induced by NPY but not by dynorphin A1-17 or pancreatic polypeptide. Pretreatment with thioperamide suppresses water intake in the NPY treatment group. Does not suppress food intake induced by fasting	65,66
		Blocks effects of imetit on bombesin-induced suppression of food intake	67
	Obese Zucker *fa/fa* rats	Decrease in food intake	1
		Blocks snacking behavior	68
	H₁ KO mice	Complete ablation of the anorexic effect	53
	H₃ KO mice	Loss of anorexigenic activity in response to NPY-induced feeding behavior	49
Ciproxifan	Sprague–Dawley rats	Decrease in food intake increase in hypothalamic histamine	69
	Diet–induced obese mice	Decreased body weight gain	70
	Mice	Blocks (R)-α-MeHA- induced dipsogenia	71
GT2394	Sprague–Dawley rats	Decrease in food intake. Decrease in body weight. No effect on water intake following acute administration	72–75

GT2016	24-h fasted rats	Decrease in food intake	76
A-331440	DIO mice	Significant decrease in body weight, decrease in epididymal fat pad weights, food consumption, and leptin levels	77
	ob/ob mice	Decreased the rate of weight gain; reduced epididymal fat pad weight; reduced plasma ghrelin levels	61,78
	H3 KO mice	No effect on body weight or food intake	1
A-417022	DIO mice	Weight loss	79
A-423579	DIO mice and rats	Weight loss, reduced fat content, reduction in plasma leptin levels, decreased triglyceride levels. No change in behavioral satiety sequence	79
NNC 38-1049	Old and DIO rats	Decrease in food intake and body weight; no acute changes in behavioral satiety sequence or pica behavior	80
NNC 38-1202	Normal rats	Decrease in food intake after acute dosing	81
	DIO rats	Decrease in food intake and body weight following chronic dosing. Reduced plasma triglycerides, increased plasma-free fatty acids and beta-hydroxybutyrate levels. No change in energy expenditure, whole-body lipid oxidation significantly increased	81
	Pigs and rhesus monkeys	Decrease in food intake following intragastric (pigs) and acute s.c. (monkeys) administration	82

Note: NPY, neuropeptide Y; CCK, cholecystokinin; MeHA, methyl histamine; DIO, diet induced obesity.

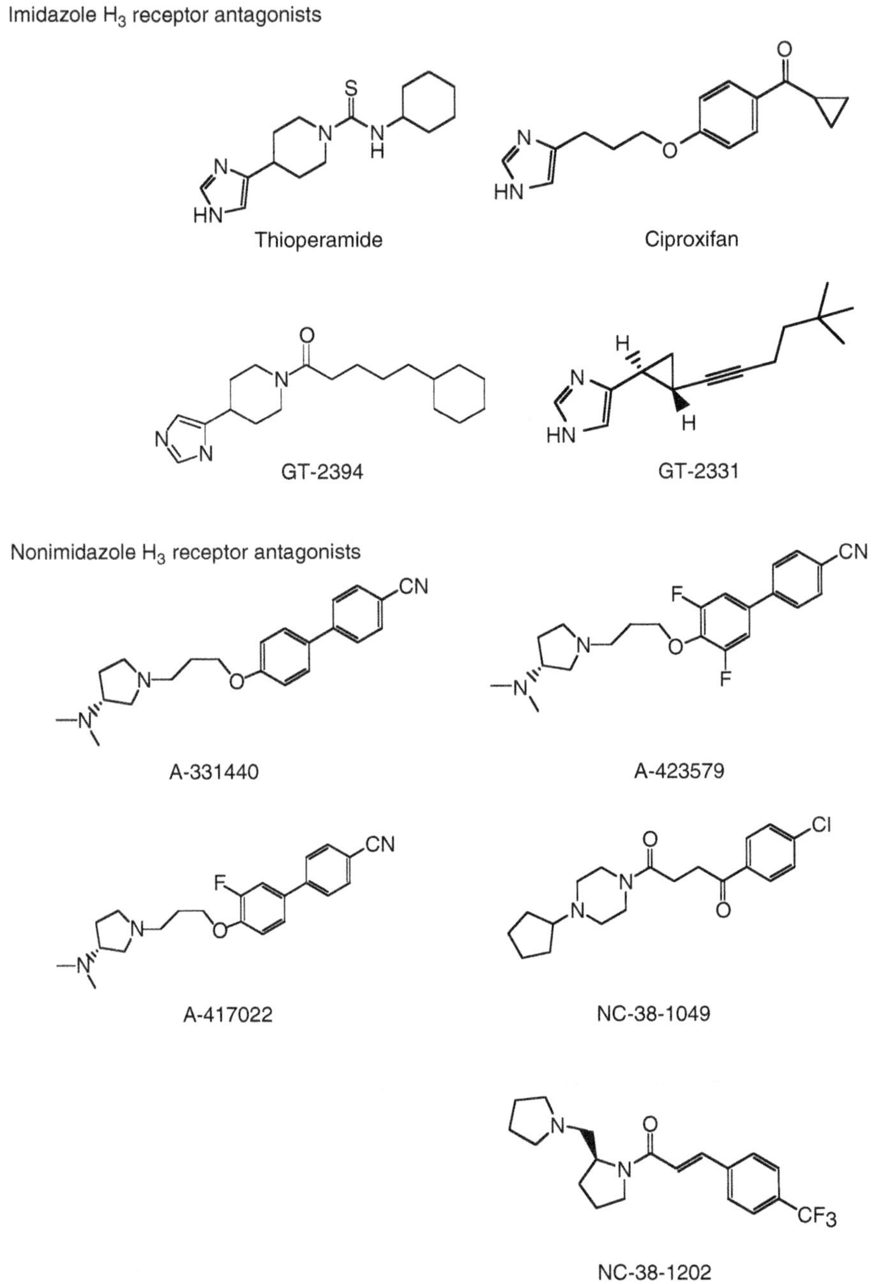

Imidazole H$_3$ receptor antagonists

Thioperamide

Ciproxifan

GT-2394

GT-2331

Nonimidazole H$_3$ receptor antagonists

A-331440

A-423579

A-417022

NC-38-1049

NC-38-1202

FIGURE 9.2 Chemical structures of imidazole-based (top panel) and nonimidazole-based (bottom panel) H$_3$ receptor antagonists with demonstrated preclinical antiobesity effects.

that was associated with increased c-fos activation in the hypothalamic paraventricular nucleus [70]. This compound has also been shown to inhibit R-α-methylhistamine-induced dipsogenia in mice [71].

GT-2394 [((1R,2R)-*trans*-2-imidazol-4ylcyclo-propyl)(cyclohexyl-methoxy) carboxamide] (Figure 9.2) is another imidazole-based H$_3$ antagonist with inverse agonist activity capable of reducing food intake and weight gain in rats [72,73]. Gliatech patent applications revealed that GT-2394 (10 mg/kg i.p.) decreased food consumption measured in rats over a 24-h time period [74,75]. GT-2394 (3–10 mg/kg, p.o.) was also shown to reduce body weight gain from 2–5% and decrease cumulative food consumption by 3–6%. Interestingly, no rebound increase in food consumption was induced by this compound when dosing was stopped [74]. In another Gliatech patent application, GT-2016 (5-cyclohexyl-1-[4-(3H-imidazol-4-yl)-piperidin-1yl]-pentan-1-one) was also shown to decrease food consumption dose dependently (3–30 mg/kg, i.p.) in 24-h fasted rats [76].

Although these early imidazole-based H$_3$ antagonists were important tool compounds in helping to determine the potential role of H$_3$ receptors in homeostatic mechanisms involved in feeding and weight gain, as a class, they suffer from a number of drawbacks that make them less than optimum as potential clinical drug candidates. These drawbacks include the finding that many imidazole-based H$_3$ receptor antagonists exhibit lower potency at human versus rodent H$_3$ receptors [83–86]; however, some nonimidazole-based H$_3$ antagonists also exhibit this characteristic [87]. As a class, imidazole-based H$_3$ antagonists also exhibit relatively high affinity, and thus lower selectivity, versus other potential target sites including the histamine H$_4$, α_{2a}- and α_{2c}-adrenergic, and serotonin 5HT$_3$ receptors [87–89]. Another potential liability of imidazole-based H$_3$ antagonists is that the imidazole moiety is known to interact with CYP isoenzymes and potentially inhibits the metabolism of other drugs [90–92]. Additionally, there exist many examples of imidazoles that have limited ability to cross the blood–brain barrier [93], and H$_3$ antagonists such as clobenpropit display a decreased ability to penetrate the central compartment [94]. These disadvantages have led toward a concerted effort among academic and pharmaceutical laboratories to discover nonimidazole H$_3$ antagonists, which may be less prone to the aforementioned liabilities of imidazole-based compounds. These will be described in the next section.

NONIMIDAZOLE-BASED H$_3$ RECEPTOR ANTAGONISTS

More recent reports are now being published demonstrating that novel H$_3$ antagonists that lack the imidazole moiety are efficacious in suppressing feeding and reducing weight in various animal models of obesity. Many highly potent and selective nonimidazole-based H$_3$ receptor antagonists have been discovered and characterized by numerous academic and industrial research teams (for recent reviews see Refs 40, 41, 95, and 96). These compounds are expected to avoid the well-known imidazole-based CYP and drug–drug interactions and have also been shown to exhibit high potency and selectivity for the H$_3$ receptor with minimized pharmacological differences across species with demonstrated good CNS penetration [86,89,97–99], thus offering the potential for more druglike characteristics. Although many of these novel nonimidazole-based H_3 antagonists are targeting various cognitive deficits associated with CNS disorders such as ADHD, Alzheimer's disease, and schizophrenia, a number of reports have illustrated the antiobesity properties of these compounds in multiple animal models across species.

A-331440 {4'-[3-(3(R)-(dimethylamino)-pyrrolidinyl-1-yl)-propoxy]-biphenyl-4-carbonitrile} (Figure 9.2) has been an extensively profiled compound from Abbott Laboratories [77,100], demonstrating high potency and selectivity as an H_3 antagonist (respective K_i values of 3 and 6 nM for recombinant human and rat H_3 receptors) in addition to potent inverse agonist properties [77]. It has demonstrated efficacy in several rodent models of obesity and has been compared to reference compounds that induce weight loss in rodents [77]. In two rodent models, diet-induced obesity in mice and *ob/ob* mice, A-331440 was efficacious in dose-dependently producing significant weight loss and preventing weight gain, respectively. The degree of efficacy was comparable or superior to the reference standards, dexfenfluramine or BRL-37344, a β_3-adrenoceptor agonist [77,78,101]. In the high-fat diet-induced obese mouse model, A-331440 (5 mg/kg, p.o., twice daily) induced a comparable weight loss to that seen with dexfenfluramine [77]. In contrast to the rapid weight loss and subsequent plateau in weight gain seen with dexfenfluramine, A-331440 exhibited a more gradual weight loss that was equivalent to that with dexfenfluramine by the end of 4 weeks and at a higher dose (15 mg/kg, p.o., twice daily); the animals had lost all of the weight gained while on the high-fat diet, and their body weights were equivalent to those seen in lean control animals. Interestingly, the weight loss induced by A-331440 appeared to be specifically attributable to the loss of body fat as determined by magnetic resonance imaging techniques or epididymal fat pad weights (Figure 9.3), suggesting that white adipose tissue may also be a target for the weight loss [77]. Additionally, after 4 weeks of dosing, A-331440 decreased food consumption and normalized leptin and insulin levels to those seen in lean controls at the highest tested dose (15 mg/kg, p.o., twice daily) [77].

In *ob/ob* mice, A-331440 reduced epididymal fat pad weights like the β_3 receptor agonist BRL-37344 but did not stimulate respiration nor elevate oxygen consumption, in contrast to BRL-37344 [78]. A-331440 also decreased plasma ghrelin levels in *ob/ob* mice, possibly contributing to the decreased food consumption also seen in these animals [78]. Interestingly, in H_3 receptor knockout animals, A-331440 had no effect on body weight or on food consumption, suggesting that the compound lacked nonspecific effects (such as taste aversion) that might influence body weight and that the compound mediates its effects through H_3 receptor-regulated effects on body weight. Further safety profiling of this compound however revealed that it had a structurally dependent genotoxic effect that precluded further advancement of this compound [102].

A-417022 [4'-{3-[(3R)-3-(dimethylamino)-1-pyrrol-idinyl]propoxy}-3'-fluoro-1,1'-biphenyl-4-carbonitrile] and A-423579 [4'-{3-[(3R)-3-(dimethylamino)-1-pyrrolidi-nyl]-propoxy}-3',5'-difluoro-1,1'-biphenyl-4-carbonitrile] (Figure 9.2) are analogs of A-331440, discovered as part of an effort at Abbott Laboratories to find compounds with equal potency and selectivity for the H_3 receptor as the parent compound, but lack the genotoxic effect [102]. Both of these fluorinated analogs of A-331440 exhibit comparable antagonist/inverse agonist properties as the parent as detailed in an

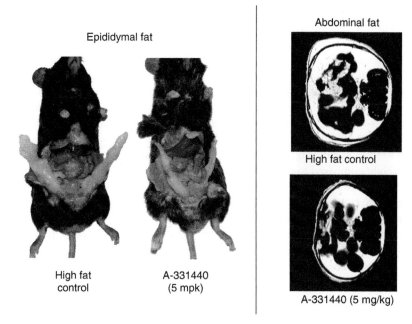

FIGURE 9.3 Effects of A-331440 on mouse epididymal (left panel) and abdominal (right panel) fat content. Mice (C57BL/6J) on a high-fat diet were administered either A-331440 (5 mg/kg, p.o., twice daily) or vehicle for 28 days, and the effect on fat content was determined. The left panel shows the effects of A-331440 on epididymal fat in comparison with the high-fat control animal. The right panels depict MRI images across the abdomen at the kidney level and illustrate the decrease in both abdominal and subcutaneous fat accumulation in A-331440-treated animals (right bottom panel) in comparison with high-fat control mice (right top panel).

article that describes the structure–activity relationships of these and related analogs [102]. A-417022 produced gradual weight loss, although a bit less than A-331440, over a period of 4 weeks in the diet-induced obese mouse model with a maximal weight loss comparable to that seen with sibutramine [102]. A-423579 decreased weight gain in both diet-induced obese mice and rats maintained on high-fat diets [79]. A-423579 was found to decrease body fat content and plasma leptin levels, as was also seen with A-331440, but in addition also reduced triglyceride levels [79]. This compound also caused a small, but sustained, decrease in total food consumed over the 4 week study but did not affect oxygen consumption [79]. In another measure of feeding behavior, A-423579 did not disrupt a behavioral satiety sequence test. The efficacious weight loss, especially in adipose tissues combined with the beneficial effects on triglyceride levels, suggests that H_3 antagonists may have utility in diabetes and a number of other metabolic diseases.

NNC 38-1049 [1-(4-chloro-phenyl)-4-(4-cyclopentyl-piperazin-1-yl)-butane-1, 4-dione] (Figure 9.2) was the first extensively profiled H_3 antagonist profiled for antiobesity effects from Novo-Nordisc [80]. This compound competitively blocks both human and rat H_3 receptor binding and function ($\leq$10 nM). Following single oral doses (15–60 mg/kg) in rats, NNC 38-1049 was detected in both the plasma and the brain, and when tested at a single 20 mg/kg (i.p.) dose, hypothalamic histamine release was enhanced. No acute changes in behavioral satiety sequence nor pica behavior were noted at the 20 mg/kg dose, and repeated administration of NNC 38-1049 for 7 days did not induce a conditioned taste aversion response. NNC 39-1049 caused a dose-dependent reduction in food intake in rats and tended to decrease the respiratory quotient at higher doses, perhaps indicating increased lipid oxidation, while not changing energy expenditure. In old and diet-induced obese rats, NNC 38-1049 at 20 mg/kg given twice daily for 2 weeks caused a sustained reduction in food intake throughout the study period and caused a significant decrease in body weight compared to controls.

NNC 38-1202 [(E)-1-((S)-2-pyrrolidin-1-ylmethyl-pyrrolidin-1-yl)-3-(4-trifluoro-methyl-phenyl)-propenone] (Figure 9.2) [81,103] is the most recently described H_3 antagonist from the Novo-Nordisc group. NNC 38-1202 competitively blocks both human and rat H_3 receptor binding (5 and 60 nM, respectively), is highly H_3 selective, and is an inverse agonist (EC_{50} of 2.1 nM) [103]. This compound, like NNC 38-1049, penetrates the brain, increasing rat hypothalamic paraventricular nuclear histamine when given as single 15 and 30 mg/kg oral doses and significantly reducing food intake at the same doses. On repeated daily dosing of 5 mg/kg for 22 days in diet-induced obese rats, NNC 38-1202 decreased food consumption and caused a loss in body weight compared with rats receiving vehicle that continued to gain weight. NNC 38-1202 also favorably altered the lipid profiles of the animals, reducing plasma triglycerides although increasing plasma-free fatty acids and beta-hydroxybutyrate levels. There were no changes in energy expenditure associated with these changes in food intake and body weight but whole-body lipid oxidation was increased. These effects are unlikely related to nonspecific, nonhomeostatic mechanisms since no effects were seen on a behavioral satiety sequence, on pica behavior, or taste aversion.

In the first description of the preclinical utility of H_3 antagonists to antiobesity effects in higher species, the effects of NNC 38-1202 on caloric intake in pigs and rhesus monkeys were examined [82]. NNC 38-1202 was shown to be potent (<20 nM) at porcine and monkey H_3 receptors. This compound, when given intragastrically (15 mg/kg) to normal pigs, significantly reduced caloric intake compared with vehicle control animals. NNC 38-1202 (0.1 and 1 mg/kg, s.c.) decreased average calorie intakes by 40 and 75%, respectively, in obese rhesus monkeys, demonstrating that H_3 receptor blockade reduces caloric intake in higher mammalian species.

CHALLENGES AND PROMISES OF CLINICAL UTILITY OF H_3 RECEPTOR ANTAGONISTS FOR THE TREATMENT OF OBESITY

As described earlier, the promising preclinical findings with H_3 antagonists in animal models of obesity suggest potential clinical utility. The H_3 receptor itself certainly exhibits many attributes that make it an attractive drug development target. However, the degree of potential for H_3 receptor antagonists to provide improved treatment of human obesity and associated metabolic disorders compared to current pharmacotherapies is unknown due to the absence of clinical validation and some confounding preclinical data. Some challenges, perhaps inherent with the molecular target itself and others maybe associated with the chemical structures of H_3 antagonists, as is typical of preclinical programs in general, confront drug discovery scientists in the quest to develop viable H_3 antagonist clinical candidates for the treatment of obesity as will be described later.

Although the vast majority of studies support appetite-suppressant or weight loss effects of H_3 antagonists, there have been several reports using thioperamide, an imidazole-based H_3 receptor antagonist that has proven to be a useful tool in the evaluation of the role of H_3 receptors in appetite, feeding, and weight regulation as described earlier, that do not support this contention. This compound has been shown to enhance food consumption in a rat model of diazepam-induced hyperphagia [104]. In addition, a recent study by Yoshimoto et al. [105] showed that thioperamide increased feeding and weight gain in diet-induced obese mice. Additionally, a study [106] examining the effects of thioperamide, administered both orally and i.p., demonstrated confounding results with respect to its effects on feeding and metabolic parameters. The CNS H_3 receptor occupancy, *tele*-methylhistamine levels (an assessment of histamine turnover), and pharmacokinetic profiles were found to be comparable whether thioperamide was given orally or i.p. However, thioperamide suppressed acute food consumption, energy expenditure, and respiratory quotient when given i.p., not orally. The researchers also found that thioperamide caused conditioned taste aversion when dosed at 30 mg/kg i.p. [106], and the decreased food consumption seen with i.p. dosing was attributed to either visceral illness or irritation at the injection site, raising doubt about the role of H_3 antagonists in reducing acute food consumption and rate of weight gain. However, it should be noted that thioperamide reduced food consumption in a histaminergic-dependent manner when administered intracerebroventricularly [62]. In addition, A-331440, an H_3 antagonist that decreases body weight in rodent models of obesity, as described previously, does not appear to have taste aversion-like properties since it does not affect body weight or food consumption in H_3 receptor knockout mice [1]. It is therefore important to consider the route of administration, experimental paradigm, and the animal strain/species when interpreting the antiobesity effects of H_3 antagonists such as thioperamide.

In addition to the data reported on the efficacy of thioperamide, another topic concerning the antiobesity activity of H_3 receptor antagonists encompassing structurally diverse imidazole- and nonimidazole-based compounds is the observation that several H_3 antagonists do not display any effect on food consumption or weight gain despite high affinity and selectivity for H_3 receptors, favorable pharmacokinetic properties, and demonstrable efficacy *in vivo* in other H_3 receptor-mediated effects in cognition and sleep models. Among imidazole-based H_3 receptor antagonists, GT-2227 [4-(6-cyclohex-*cis*-3-enyl)imidazole] and GT-2331 [(1*S*,2*S*,)-*trans*-4-(2-(5,5-dimethylhex-1-ynyl)cyclopropyl)imidazole] did not decrease food consumption [74,75] despite demonstrable cognitive efficacy of GT-2331 in the five-trial inhibitory avoidance model in SHR pups [107]. Among nonimidazole H_3 receptor antagonists, the enantiomers A-631972 [4-{2-[2-(2*S*-methyl-pyrrolidin-1-yl)-ethyl]-benzofuran-5-yl}-benzonitrile] and ABT-239 [4-{2-[2-(2*R*-methyl-pyrrolidin-1-yl)-ethyl]-benzofuran-5-yl}-benzonitrile] are potent and selective H_3 receptor antagonist/inverse agonists that exhibit activity in various cognitive behavioral models [1,89,108,109]. However, both A-631972 (0.5–1.5 mg/kg/day) and ABT-239 (3–30 mg/kg/day) are ineffective in decreasing food consumption or weight gain in diet-induced obese mice [1,70] at doses that elicit beneficial effects in preclinical models of learning and memory. Additionally, some other nonimidazole H_3 receptor antagonists representing other distinct structural classes also fail to demonstrate antiobesity properties in rodents at doses comparable to those effective in CNS behavioral models. One such compound is JNJ-5207852 {1-[4[(3-piperidin-1-yl-propoxy)-benzyl}-piperidine}, a potent diamine-based H_3 receptor antagonist with acute wake-promoting properties [110]. JNJ-5207852 (10 mg/kg/day i.p. for 4 weeks) did not lower body weight in *ob/ob* or C57BL/6 mice. Given the ability of all three of these nonimidazole H_3 receptor antagonists to penetrate the brain and elicit centrally mediated effects on cognition and sleep behaviors, the absence of any antiobesity effects are not due simply to the inability of the compounds to induce CNS pharmacological effects. It has been postulated that perhaps cognition-enhancing H_3 receptor antagonists such as ABT-239 that lack antiobesity activity differentially activate c-fos in the brain in comparison with antiobesity H_3 antagonists such as A-331440. Indeed, at doses of A-331440 that elicit weight loss in mice with diet-induced obesity, c-fos is activated in the hypothalamic paraventricular nucleus, whereas ABT-239 does not activate c-fos in this area at the doses tested [70]. However, ABT-239 activates c-fos in cingulate cortex and hippocampal regions at doses (1 mg/kg) that elicit cognitive effects, whereas A-331440 and other antiobesity H_3 antagonists do not. However, whether these observations generalize to other chemical classes of H_3 antagonists remains to be determined.

Another challenge to the role of H_3 receptor antagonists as antiobesity agents is the appearance of an obese phenotype in H_3 receptor knockout mice if one assumes that with the absence of these presynaptic receptors (analogous to H_3 receptor blockade by antagonists), there would be no tonic inhibition of histamine release and synthesis with the resultant increase in postsynaptic histamine H_1 receptors activation and subsequent decreases in food consumption and body weight. Indeed, Takahashi et al. [49] have shown that hypothalamic histamine levels are increased in H_3 knockout mice displaying an obese phenotype. This group has indicated that the etiology of the obese phenotype in these animals remains to be determined [3], suggesting that perhaps neural circuitry is affected during development in the absence of H_3 receptors. This group has also proposed that elevated levels of histamine release could desensitize postsynaptic H_1 histamine receptors, reducing histaminergic tone resulting in increased feeding and weight gain [3,49]. This hypothesis is supported by the finding that the amount of H_1 receptor binding in H_3 receptor knockout mice is lower than in wild-type mice despite comparable levels of H_1 mRNA [3]. However, it should be noted that this perhaps paradoxical phenotype in H_3 receptor knockout mice is with precedence where the knockout of other hypothalamic body weight modulators results in phenotypes that would not be as predicted [111]. In any event, the varied phenotypes that have been observed for H_3 receptor knockout animals, from a slight decrease in weight to an obese phenotype, suggest that investigators need to provide detailed descriptions of the experimental protocols, so that data can be put into the proper context to interpret basal physiological parameters as well as the effects of H_3 receptor ligands in these animals and the associated wild-type animals. Further development of H_3 receptor knockout mice on a background strain that may be more conducive to develop an obese phenotype may also be helpful in further deciphering the role of H_3 receptors in feeding behavior and regulation of body weight.

An additional challenge to the rationale for antiobesity activity of H_3 receptor antagonists comes from findings that H_3 receptor agonists have appetite suppressant and weight loss effects in rodent models. These findings appear, in some instances, to be more consistent with the aforementioned obese phenotype observed in some H_3 receptor knockout mice, assuming the effects are H_3 receptor-mechanism-based and not due to general effects on taste-aversion-induced antifeeding responses. In a previously described study examining diazepam-induced hyperphagia in rats, when the selective H_3 receptor agonist, R-α-methylhistamine, was administered i.c.v., food intake was decreased [104]. More recently, Yoshimoto et al. [105] examined the effects of H_3 receptor agonists and antagonists on feeding behavior and regulation of body weight in both H_3 receptor knockout and wild-type mice. In this report, these researchers demonstrated that in diet-induced obese wild-type mice, thioperamide increased, but the H_3 receptor agonist imetit decreased both food consumption and body weight. Interestingly, imetit decreased liver triglycerides, plasma leptin and insulin levels, and adipose mass in diet-induced obese wild-type mice but not in H_3 receptor knockout mice. Although these effects of imetit on feeding behavior, weight gain, and associated metabolic profiles were associated with a decrease in histamine release, it was noted that reduction of histamine release by α-fluoromethylhistamine, an inhibitor of histamine synthesis, resulted in an increase in food consumption. The authors concluded that the effects of imetit on weight gain and food consumption may be independent from the modulation of histamine release and may be dependent on the modulation of the release of other neurotransmitters such as norepinephrine, serotonin, dopamine, and others [105]. Additionally, this group showed that the effects of imetit were independent of the melanocortin system by showing that imetit could still reduce food consumption in melanocortin receptor knockout mice. These researchers have proposed that H_3 receptor agonists may have a potential therapeutic role in treating obesity and metabolic disorders such as diabetes perhaps through the modulation of neurotransmitters other than histamine [105].

Overall, however, it must be recognized that there is a significant body of preclinical data to date finding that H_3 antagonists have antiobesity effects. The overall antiobesity profile (benefits on lipid profiles and triglyceride levels) may provide clinical advantages over historical or currently available antiobesity drugs, despite the aforementioned unanswered questions raised by some reports. Other examples of distinct therapeutic potential include minimal risk of abuse liability, as supported by a lack of behavioral sensitization [112] and stimulant-like behavior [78,109] seen in rodents following the administration of H_3 antagonists that appears to differentiate these compounds from stimulants. Additionally, nonimidazole H_3 antagonists demonstrate minimal stimulant-like effects on EEG waveforms [109], in contrast to amphetamine. These may be distinct advantages for H_3 antagonists, given the potential addiction and abuse liability of stimulants such as amphetamine used for the treatment of obesity [109]. Another potential advantage to their profile as antiobesity agents is supported by the observations that H_3 antagonists tend to display a rather small and continuously gradual suppression of food consumption with a consequent gradual decrease in body weight in diet-induced obese rodents, as described earlier. This is in marked contrast to some antiobesity drugs such as dexfenfluramine that cause very rapid and profound decreases in food consumption and weight but with an efficacy that declines over time. Whether the more gradual effect of H_3 receptor antagonists on decreasing food consumption and weight seen in obese rodents would translate to better efficacy long term in the clinic remains to be seen, but there is the potential for longer-term maintenance of weight loss.

CONCLUSIONS

When examining the histaminergic system and its important role in regulating feeding and weight homeostasis, central H_3 receptors seem to provide the best histaminergic target for obesity intervention, given its fundamental role in augmenting histamine synthesis and release. The resultant decrease in appetite, feeding, and weight gain, presumably through H_1 receptors, and the concomitant effects on circulating leptin and triglyceride levels and fat storage offer the potential for beneficial treatment of obesity, diabetes, and other metabolic diseases. Recent advances in the understanding of the molecular, pharmacological, and physiological properties of the H_3 receptor have led to an increased interest in developing H_3 antagonists to act at this attractive CNS target for multiple indications including obesity and associated metabolic disorders, where considerable progress has been made in our understanding of H_3 receptor modulation of weight homeostasis. Academic and pharmaceutical laboratories have synthesized large numbers of highly potent and selective H_3 receptor antagonists, including A-423579 and NNC-38 1202, with encouraging efficacy in various preclinical models of obesity in rodents, pigs, and primates. However, despite the enthusiasm generated from these preclinical studies, questions and challenges remain unanswered, reflecting the complex biology of the histaminergic system, as well as compound-related issues common to all drug discovery efforts including pharmaceutics, pharmacokinetics, ADME, and safety/toxicology properties that confront drug discovery scientists in developing an effective antiobesity H_3 receptor antagonist. Thus, at this early stage, there is as yet no human clinical demonstration for *proof-of-concept* for H_3 receptor antagonist efficacy in treating obesity. Efforts are certain to continue to further our understanding of the complex biology of the weight-regulating systems modulated by this important CNS histaminergic receptor in order to develop novel therapeutic agents for the treatment of obesity.

ACKNOWLEDGMENTS

The authors thank the Abbott members of the extended H_3 Receptor Antagonist Project team for their considerable contributions to the work presented in this chapter that flowed from their collaborative effort. We also acknowledge Marlon D. Cowart, Gerard B. Fox, and Kaitlin Browman for the discussions and ideas that have ensued through the years and have contributed to this chapter, and Isabel Lopez for formatting and designing the figures. Finally, we dedicate this chapter in the memory of the late Arthur A. Hancock, PhD, who was the primary advocate for examining the antiobesity properties of Abbott H_3 receptor antagonists, and whose leadership, insight, and friendship are remembered fondly.

REFERENCES

1. Hancock, A.A. and Brune, M.E., 2005. Assessment of pharmacology and potential anti-obesity properties of H_3 receptor antagonists/inverse agonists. *Expert Opin. Investig. Drugs* 14(3): 223–241.
2. Malmlof, K., Hohlweg, R., and Rimvall, K., 2006. Targeting of the central histaminergic system for treatment of obesity and associated metabolic disorders. *Drug Dev. Res.* 67: 651–665.
3. Tokita, S., Takahashi, K., and Kotani, H., 2006. Recent advances in molecular pharmacology of the histamine systems: physiology and pharmacology of histamine H_3 receptor: roles in feeding regulation and therapeutic potential for metabolic disorders. *J. Pharmacol. Sci.* 101(1): 12–18.
4. Masaki, T. and Yoshimatsu, H., 2006. The hypothalamic H_1 receptor: a novel therapeutic target for disrupting diurnal feeding rhythm and obesity. *Trends Pharmacol. Sci.* 27(5): 279–284.
5. Halford, J.C., Obesity drugs in clinical development. *Curr. Opin. Invest. Drugs* 7(4): 312–318.
6. Stein, C.J. and Colditz, G.A., 2004. The epidemic of obesity. *J. Clin. Endocrinol. Metab.* 89(6): 2522–2525.
7. Schwartz, J.C., Arrang, J.M., Garbarg, M., Pollard, H., and Ruat, M., 1991. Histaminergic transmission in the mammalian brain. *Physiol. Rev.* 71(1): 1–51.
8. Brown, R.E., Stevens, D.R., and Haas, H.L., 2001. The physiology of brain histamine. *Prog. Neurobiol.* 63(6): 637–672.
9. Onodera, K., Yamatodani, A., Watanabe, T., and Wada, H., 1994. Neuropharmacology of the histaminergic neuron system in the brain and its relationship with behavioral disorders. *Prog. Neurobiol.* 42(6): 685–702.
10. Kukko-Lukjanov, T.K. and Panula, P., 2003. Subcellular distribution of histamine, GABA and galanin in tuberomamillary neurons in vitro. *J. Chem. Neuroanat.* 25(4): 279–292.
11. Blandina, P., Bacciottini, L., Giovannini, M.G., and Mannaioni, P.F., 1998. H_3 receptor modulation of the release of neurotransmitters in vivo. In: *The Histamine H_3 Receptor*, eds. Timmerman, H., Leurs, R., pp. 27–40, Elsevier: Amsterdam.
12. Passani, M.B., Lin, J.S., Hancock, A., Crochet, S., and Blandina, P., 2004. The histamine H_3 receptor as a novel therapeutic target for cognitive and sleep disorders. *Trends Pharmacol. Sci.* 25(12): 618–625.
13. Masaki, T., Yoshimatsu, H., Chiba, S., Watanabe, T., and Sakata, T., 2001. Central infusion of histamine reduces fat accumulation and upregulates UCP family in leptin-resistant obese mice. *Diabetes* 50(2): 376–384.
14. Vaziri, P., Dang, K., and Anderson, G.H., 1997. Evidence for histamine involvement in the effect of histidine loads on food and water intake in rats. *J. Nutr.* 127(8): 1519–1526.
15. Yoshimatsu, H., Chiba, S., Tajima, D., Akehi, Y., and Sakata, T., 2002. Histidine suppresses food intake through its conversion into neuronal histamine. *Exp. Biol. Med.* 227(1): 63–68.
16. Sakata, T., Yoshimatsu, H., Masaki, T., and Tsuda, K., Anti-obesity actions of mastication driven by histamine neurons in rats. *Exp. Biol. Med.* 228(10): 1106–1110.
17. Yamanaka, A., Tsujino, N., Funahashi, H., Honda, K., Guan, J.L., Wang, Q.P., Tominaga, M., Goto, K., Shioda, S., and Sakurai, T., Orexins activate histaminergic neurons via the orexin 2 receptor. *Biochem. Biophys. Res. Commun.* 290(4): 1237–1245.

18. Schlicker, E. and Kathmann, M., 1998. Modulation of in vitro neurotransmission in the CNS and in the retina via H_3 heteroreceptors. In: *The Histamine H_3 Receptor*, eds. Timmerman, H., Leurs, R., pp. 13–26, Elsevier: Amsterdam.

19. Nishino, S., Fujiki, N., Ripley, B., Sakurai, E., Kato, M., Watanabe, T., Mignot, E., and Yanai, K., 2001. Decreased brain histamine content in hypocretin/orexin receptor-2 mutated narcoleptic dogs. *Neurosci. Lett.* 313(3): 125–128.

20. Kok, S.W., Overeem, S., Visscher, T.L., Lammers, G.J., Seidell, J.C., Pijl, H., and Meinders, A.E., 2003. Hypocretin deficiency in narcoleptic humans is associated with abdominal obesity. *Obes. Res.* 11(9): 1147–1154.

21. Hegyi, K., Fulop, K.A., Kovacs, K.J., Falus, A., and Toth, S., 2004. High leptin level is accompanied with decreased long leptin receptor transcript in histamine deficient transgenic mice. *Immunol. Lett.* 92(1–2): 193–197.

22. Fulop, A.K., Foldes, A., Buzas, E., Hegyi, K., Miklos, I.H., Romics, L., Kleiber, M., Nagy, A., Falus, A., and Kovacs, K.J., 2003. Hyperleptinemia, visceral adiposity, and decreased glucose tolerance in mice with a targeted disruption of the histidine decarboxylase gene. *Endocrinology* 144(10): 4306–4314.

23. Itateyama, E., Chiba, S., Sakata, T., and Yoshimatsu, H., 2003. Hypothalamic neuronal histamine in genetically obese animals: its implication of leptin action in the brain. *Exp. Biol. Med.* 228(10): 1132–1137.

24. Morimoto, T., Yamamoto, Y., Mobarakeh, J.I., Yanai, K., Watanabe, T., and Yamatodani, A., 1999. Involvement of the histaminergic system in leptin-induced suppression of food intake. *Physiol. Behav.* 67(5): 679–683.

25. Hough, L.B., 2001. Genomics meets histamine receptors: new subtypes, new receptors. *Mol. Pharmacol.* 59(3): 415–419.

26. Yanai, K. and Tashiro, M., 2007. The physiological and pathophysiological roles of neuronal histamine: an insight from human positron emission tomography studies. *Pharmacol. Ther.* 113(1): 1–15.

27. Sakata, T., Yoshimatsu, H., and Kurokawa, M., 1997. Hypothalamic neuronal histamine: implications of its homeostatic control of energy metabolism. *Nutrition* 13(5): 403–411.

28. Mollet, A., Meier, S., Riediger, T., and Lutz, T.A., 2003. Histamine H_1 receptors in the ventromedial hypothalamus mediate the anorectic action of the pancreatic hormone amylin. *Peptides* 24(1): 155–158.

29. Masaki, T., Chiba, S., Yoshimichi, G., Yasuda, T., Noguchi, H., Kakuma, T., Sakata, T., and Yoshimatsu, H., 2003. Neuronal histamine regulates food intake, adiposity, and uncoupling protein expression in agouti yellow (A(y)/a) obese mice. *Endocrinology* 144(6): 2741–2748.

30. McIntyre, R.S., Mancini, D.A., and Basile, V.S., 2001. Mechanisms of antipsychotic-induced weight gain. *J. Clin. Psychiatry* 62(Suppl 23): 23–29.

31. Kroeze, W.K., Hufeisen, S.J., Popadak, B.A., Renock, S.M., Steinberg, S., Ernsberger, P., Jayathilake, K., Meltzer, H.Y., and Roth, B.L., 2003. H_1-histamine receptor affinity predicts short-term weight gain for typical and atypical antipsychotic drugs. *Neuropsychopharmacology* 28(3): 519–526.

32. Kim, S.F., Huang, A.S., Snowman, A.M., Teuscher, C., and Snyder, S.H., 2007. Antipsychotic drug-induced weight gain mediated by histamine H_1 receptor-linked activation of hypothalamic AMP-kinase. *Proc. Natl Acad. Sci. U.S.A.* 104(9): 3456–3459.

33. Basile, V.S., Masellis, M., McIntyre, R.S., Meltzer, H.Y., Lieberman, J.A., and Kennedy, J.L., 2001. Genetic dissection of atypical antipsychotic-induced weight gain: novel preliminary data on the pharmacogenetic puzzle. *J. Clin. Psychiatry* 62(Suppl 23): 45–66.

34. Lacour, M. and Sterkers, O., 2001. Histamine and betahistine in the treatment of vertigo: elucidation of mechanisms of action. *CNS Drugs* 15(11): 853–870.

35. Szelag, A., Trocha, M., and Merwid-Lad, A., 2001. Betahistine inhibits food intake in rats. *Pol. J. Pharmacol.* 53(6): 701–707.
36. Rossi, R., Del Prete, E., and Scharrer, E., 1999. Effect of the H_1-histamine receptor agonist betahistine on drinking and eating behavior in pygmy goats. *Physiol. Behav.* 66(3): 517–521.
37. Poyurovsky, M., Pashinian, A., Levi, A., Weizman, R., and Weizman, A., 2005. The effect of betahistine, a histamine H_1 receptor agonist/H_3 antagonist, on olanzapine-induced weight gain in first-episode schizophrenia patients. *Int. Clin. Psychopharmacol.* 20(2): 101–103.
38. Pillot, C., Heron, A., Cochois, V., Tardivel-Lacombe, J., Ligneau, X., Schwartz, J.C., and Arrang, J.M., 2002. A detailed mapping of the histamine H_3 receptor and its gene transcripts in rat brain. *Neuroscience* 114(1): 173–193.
39. Anichtchik, O.V., Peitsaro, N., Rinne, J.O., Kalimo, H., and Panula, P., 2001. Distribution and modulation of histamine H_3 receptors in basal ganglia and frontal cortex of healthy controls and patients with Parkinson's disease. *Neurobiol. Dis.* 8(4): 707–716.
40. Esbenshade, T.A., Fox, G.B., and Cowart, M.D., 2006. Histamine H_3 receptor antagonists: preclinical promise for treating obesity and cognitive disorders. *Mol. Interv.* 6(2): 77–88, 59.
41. Celanire, S., Wijtmans, M., Talaga, P., Leurs, R., and de Esch, I.J., 2005. Keynote review: histamine H_3 receptor antagonists reach out for the clinic. *Drug Discov. Today* 10(23–24): 1613–1627.
42. Karlstedt, K., Ahman, M.J., Anichtchik, O.V., Soinila, S., and Panula, P., 2003. Expression of the H_3 receptor in the developing CNS and brown fat suggests novel roles for histamine. *Mol. Cell. Neurosci.* 24(3): 614–622.
43. Karlstedt, K.A., Ahman, M.J., and Panula, P., 2001. Histamine H_3 receptor expression during rat development and in adult rat peripheral tissues. *Soc. Neurosci. Abstr.* 27: 378.9.
44. Unami, A., Shinohara, Y., Kajimoto, K., and Baba, Y., 2004. Comparison of gene expression profiles between white and brown adipose tissues of rat by microarray analysis. *Biochem. Pharmacol.* 67(3): 555–564.
45. Collins, S., Cao, W., and Robidoux, J., 2004. Learning new tricks from old dogs: beta-adrenergic receptors teach new lessons on firing up adipose tissue metabolism. *Mol. Endocrinol.* 18(9): 2123–2131.
46. Tsuda, K., Yoshimatsu, H., Niijima, A., Chiba, S., Okeda, T., and Sakata, T., 2002. Hypothalamic histamine neurons activate lipolysis in rat adipose tissue. *Exp. Biol. Med.* 227(3): 208–213.
47. Yasuda, T., Masaki, T., Chiba, S., Kakuma, T., Sakata, T., and Yoshimatsu, H., 2004. L-histidine stimulates sympathetic nerve activity to brown adipose tissue in rats. *Neurosci. Lett.* 362(2): 71–74.
48. Yasuda, T., Masaki, T., Sakata, T., and Yoshimatsu, H., 2004. Hypothalamic neuronal histamine regulates sympathetic nerve activity and expression of uncoupling protein 1 mRNA in brown adipose tissue in rats. *Neuroscience* 125(3): 535–540.
49. Takahashi, K., Suwa, H., Ishikawa, T., and Kotani, H., 2002. Targeted disruption of H_3 receptors results in changes in brain histamine tone leading to an obese phenotype. *J. Clin. Invest.* 110(12): 1791–1799.
50. Jorgensen, E.A., Vogelsang, T.W., Knigge, U., Watanabe, T., Warberg, J., and Kjaer, A., 2006. Increased susceptibility to diet-induced obesity in histamine-deficient mice. *Neuroendocrinology* 83(5–6): 289–294.
51. Morimoto, T., Yamamoto, Y., and Yamatodani, A., 2001. Brain histamine and feeding behavior. *Behav. Brain Res.* 124(2): 145–150.
52. Masaki, T., Chiba, S., Yasuda, T., Noguchi, H., Kakuma, T., Watanabe, T., Sakata, T., and Yoshimatsu, H., 2004. Involvement of hypothalamic histamine H_1 receptor in the regulation of feeding rhythm and obesity. *Diabetes* 53(9): 2250–2260.

53. Mollet, A., Lutz, T.A., Meier, S., Riediger, T., Rushing, P.A., and Scharrer, E., 2001. Histamine H_1 receptors mediate the anorectic action of the pancreatic hormone amylin. *Am. J. Physiol. Regul. Integr. Comp. Physiol.* 281(5): R1442–R1448.

54. Masaki, T., Yoshimatsu, H., Chiba, S., Watanabe, T., and Sakata, T., 2001. Targeted disruption of histamine H_1 receptor attenuates regulatory effects of leptin on feeding, adiposity, and UCP family in mice. *Diabetes* 50(2): 385–391.

55. Lin, L., Wisor, J., Shiba, T., Taheri, S., Yanai, K., Wurts, S., Lin, X., Vitaterna, M., Takahashi, J., Lovenberg, T.W., Koehl, M., Uhl, G., Nishino, S., and Mignot, E., 2002. Measurement of hypocretin/orexin content in the mouse brain using an enzyme immunoassay: the effect of circadian time, age and genetic background. *Peptides* 23(12): 2203–2211.

56. Yanai, K., Son, L.Z., Endou, M., Sakurai, E., Nakagawasai, O., Tadano, T., Kisara, K., Inoue, I., Watanabe, T., and Watanabe, T., 1998. Behavioural characterization and amounts of brain monoamines and their metabolites in mice lacking histamine H_1 receptors. *Neuroscience* 87(2): 479–487.

57. Yanai, K., Son, L.Z., Endou, M., Sakurai, E., and Watanabe, T., 1998. Targeting disruption of histamine H_1 receptors in mice: behavioral and neurochemical characterization. *Life Sci.* 62(17–18): 1607–1610.

58. Toyota, H., Dugovic, C., Koehl, M., Laposky, A.D., Weber, C., Ngo, K., Wu, Y., Lee, D.H., Yanai, K., Sakurai, E., Watanabe, T., Liu, C., Chen, J., Barbier, A.J., Turek, F.W., Fung-Leung, W.P., and Lovenberg, T.W., 2002. Behavioral characterization of mice lacking histamine H_3 receptors. *Mol. Pharmacol.* 62(2): 389–397.

59. Parmentier, R., Ohtsu, H., Djebbara-Hannas, Z., Valatx, J.L., Watanabe, T., and Lin, J.S., 2002. Anatomical, physiological, and pharmacological characteristics of histidine decarboxylase knock-out mice: evidence for the role of brain histamine in behavioral and sleep-wake control. *J. Neurosci.* 22(17): 7695–7711.

60. Pudiak, C.M., Chen, X., Barbier, A.J., Demarest, K.T., and Lovenberg, T.W., 2005. The effect of a high-fat diet on body weight and food intake in H_3 -/- mutant and control mice. *Soc. Neurosci. Abstr.* 532: 4.

61. Hancock, A.A., Bush, E.N., Jacobson, P.B., Faghih, R., and Esbenshade, T.A., 2004. Histamine H_3 antagonists in models of obesity. *Inflamm. Res.* 53(Suppl 1): S47–S48.

62. Sakata, T., Ookuma, K., Fujimoto, K., Fukagawa, K., and Yoshimatsu, H., 1991. Histaminergic control of energy balance in rats. *Brain. Res. Bull.* 27(3–4): 371–375.

63. Ookuma, K., Sakata, T., Fukagawa, K., Yoshimatsu, H., Kurokawa, M., Machidori, H., and Fujimoto, K., 1993. Neuronal histamine in the hypothalamus suppresses food intake in rats. *Brain. Res.* 628(1–2): 235–242.

64. Attoub, S., Moizo, L., Sobhani, I., Laigneau, J.P., Lewin, M.J., and Bado, A., 2001. The H_3 receptor is involved in cholecystokinin inhibition of food intake in rats. *Life Sci.* 69(4): 469–478.

65. Itoh, E., Fujimiya, M., and Inui, A., 1998. Thioperamide, a histamine H_3 receptor antagonist, suppresses NPY-but not dynorphin A-induced feeding in rats. *Regul. Pept.* 75–76: 373–376.

66. Itoh, E., Fujimiya, M., and Inui, A., 1999. Thioperamide, a histamine H_3 receptor antagonist, powerfully suppresses peptide YY-induced food intake in rats. *Biol. Psychiatry* 45(4): 475–481.

67. Merali, Z. and Banks, K., 1994. Does the histaminergic system mediate bombesin/GRP-induced suppression of food intake? *Am. J. Physiol.* 267(6 Pt 2): R1589–R1595.

68. Bjenning, C., Liu, W., and Rimvall, K., 2000. Peripherally administered histamine H_3 antagonist potently reduces snacking behavior in the obese Zucker rat. *Int. Sendai Histamine Meet. Abstr.* 40: 145.

69. Bjenning, C., Johanesson, U., Juul, A.G., Lange, K.Z., and Rimvall, K., 2000. Peripherally administered ciproxifan elevates hypothalamic histamine levels and potently reduces food intake in the Sprague Dawley rat. *Int. Sendai Histamine Meet. Abstr.* 40: 144.

70. Hancock, A.A., Bitner, R.S., Krueger, K.M., Otte, S., Nikkel, A.L., Fey, T.A., Bush, E.N., Dickinson, R.W., Shapiro, R., Knourek-Segel, V., Droz, B.A., Brune, M.E., Jacobson, P.B., Cowart, M.D., and Esbenshade, T.A., 2006. Distinctions and contradistinctions between antiobesity histamine H_3 receptor (H_3R) antagonists compared to cognition-enhancing H_3 receptor antagonists. *Inflamm. Res.* 55(Suppl 1): S42–S44.

71. Fox, G.B., Pan, J.B., Esbenshade, T.A., Bitner, R.S., Nikkel, A.L., Miller, T., Kang, C.H., Bennani, Y.L., Black, L.A., Faghih, R., Hancock, A.A., and Decker, M.W., 2002. Differential in vivo effects of H_3 receptor ligands in a new mouse dipsogenia model. *Pharmacol. Biochem. Behav.* 72(3): 741–750.

72. Yates, S.L., Pawlowski, G.P., Antal, J.M., Ali, S.M., Jiang, J., and Brunden, K.R., 2000. Effects of a novel histamine H_3 receptor antagonist, GT-2394 on food intake and weight gain in Sprague–Dawley rats. *Soc. Neurosci. Abstr.* 26: 102.10.

73. Yates, S.L., Pawlowski, G., Babu, J.S., Rajagopalan, R., Wawro, W.J., and Tedford, C.E., 2003. Inverse agonists of the histamine-H_3 receptor as appetite suppressants. *Am. Chem. Soc. Abstr.* 225 MEDI: 2.

74. Yates, S.L., Tedford, C.E., and Brunden, K.R., 2003. Use of histamine H_3 receptor inverse agonists for the control of appetite and treatment of obesity. US0069295A1.

75. Yates, S.L., Tedford, C.E., and Brunden, K.R., 2002. The use of histamine H_3 receptor inverse agonists for the control of appetite and treatment of obesity. WO158905A1.

76. Durant, G.J., Kahn, A.M., and Tedford, C.E., 1996. Histamine H_3 receptor antagonists and therapeutic uses thereof. US5486526.

77. Hancock, A.A., Bennani, Y.L., Bush, E.N., Esbenshade, T.A., Faghih, R., Fox, G.B., Jacobson, P., Knourek-Segel, V., Krueger, K.M., Nuss, M.E., Pan, J.B., Shapiro, R., Witte, D.G., and Yao, B.B., 2004. Antiobesity effects of A-331440, a novel non-imidazole histamine H_3 receptor antagonist. *Eur. J. Pharmacol.* 487(1–3): 183–197.

78. Bush, E., Dickinson, R.W., Shapiro, R., Adler, A.L., Droz, B., Faghih, R., Hancock, A.A., Brune, M.E., and Jacobson, P.B., 2003. Effects of histamine H_3 receptor antagonist A-331440, triiodothyronine (T_3) and β_3-adrenergic agonist BRL-37344 (BRL) on body weight, food intake and metabolic rate in obese (ob/ob) mice. *FASEB J.* 17: 3763.

79. Hancock, A.A., Diehl, M.S., Fey, T.A., Bush, E.N., Faghih, R., Miller, T.R., Krueger, K.M., Pratt, J.K., Cowart, M.D., Dickinson, R.W., Shapiro, R., Knourek-Segel, V.E., Droz, B.A., McDowell, C.A., Krishna, G., Brune, M.E., Esbenshade, T.A., and Jacobson, P.B., 2005. Antiobesity evaluation of histamine H_3 receptor (H_3R) antagonist analogs of A-331440 with improved safety and efficacy. *Inflamm. Res.* 54(Suppl 1): S27–S29.

80. Malmlof, K., Zaragoza, F., Golozoubova, V., Refsgaard, H.H., Cremers, T., Raun, K., Wulff, B.S., Johansen, P.B., Westerink, B., and Rimvall, K., 2005. Influence of a selective histamine H_3 receptor antagonist on hypothalamic neural activity, food intake and body weight. *Int. J. Obes.* 29(12): 1402–1412.

81. Malmlof, K., Golozoubova, V., Peschke, B., Wulff, B.S., Refsgaard, H.H., Johansen, P.B., Cremers, T., and Rimvall, K., 2006. Increase of neuronal histamine in obese rats is associated with decreases in body weight and plasma triglycerides. *Obesity* 14(12): 2154–2162.

82. Malmlof, K., Hastrup, S., Wulff, B.S., Hansen, B.C., Peschke, B., Jeppesen, C.B., Hohlweg, R., and Rimvall, K., 2007. Antagonistic targeting of the histamine H_3 receptor decreases caloric intake in higher mammalian species. *Biochem. Pharmacol.* 73(8): 1237–1242.

83. Hancock, A.A., Esbenshade, T.A., Krueger, K.M., and Yao, B.B., 2003. Genetic aspects to pharmacological heterogeneity of histamine H_3 receptors. *Life Sci.* 73: 3043–3072.

84. Ligneau, X., Morisset, S., Tardivel-Lacombe, J., Gbahou, F., Ganellin, C.R., Stark, H., Schunack, W., Schwartz, J.C., and Arrang, J.M., 2000. Distinct pharmacology of rat and human histamine H_3 receptors: role of two amino acids in the third transmembrane domain. *Br. J. Pharmacol.* 131(7): 1247–1250.

85. Yao, B.B., Sharma, R., Cassar, S., Esbenshade, T.A., and Hancock, A.A., 2003. Cloning and pharmacological characterization of the monkey histamine H_3 receptor. *Eur. J. Pharmacol.* 482(1–3): 49–60.

86. Hancock, A.A., 2006. The challenge of drug discovery of a GPCR target: analysis of preclinical pharmacology of histamine H_3 antagonists/inverse agonists. *Biochem. Pharmacol.* 71(8): 1103–1113.

87. Esbenshade, T.A., Krueger, K.M., Miller, T.R., Kang, C.H., Denny, L.I., Witte, D.G., Yao, B.B., Fox, G.B., Faghih, R., Bennani, Y.L., Williams, M., and Hancock, A.A., 2003. Two novel and selective nonimidazole histamine H_3 receptor antagonists A-304121 and A-317920: I. In vitro pharmacological effects. *J. Pharmacol. Exp. Ther.* 305(3): 887–896.

88. Esbenshade, T.A., Fox, G.B., Krueger, K.M., Baranowski, J.L., Miller, T.R., Kang, C.H., Denny, L.I., Witte, D.G., Yao, B.B., Pan, J.B., Faghih, R., Bennani, Y.L., Williams, M., and Hancock, A.A., 2004. Pharmacological and behavioral properties of A-349821, a selective and potent human histamine H_3 receptor antagonist. *Biochem. Pharmacol.* 68(5): 933–945.

89. Esbenshade, T.A., Fox, G.B., Krueger, K.M., Miller, T.R., Kang, C.H., Denny, L.I., Witte, D.G., Yao, B.B., Pan, L., Wetter, J., Marsh, K., Bennani, Y.L., Cowart, M.D., Sullivan, J.P., and Hancock, A.A., 2005. Pharmacological properties of ABT-239 [4-(2-{2-[(2R)-2-Methylpyrrolidinyl]ethyl}-benzofuran-5-yl)benzonitrile]: I. Potent and selective histamine H_3 receptor antagonist with drug-like properties. *J. Pharmacol. Exp. Ther.* 313(1): 165–175.

90. Liedtke, S., Flau, K., Kathmann, M., Schlicker, E., Stark, H., Meier, G., and Schunack, W., 2003. Replacement of imidazole by a piperidine moiety differentially affects the potency of histamine H_3 receptor antagonists. *Naunyn Schmiedebergs Arch. Pharmacol.* 367(1): 43–50.

91. Lin, J.H. and Lu, A.Y., 1998. Inhibition and induction of cytochrome P450 and the clinical implications. *Clin. Pharmacokinet.* 35(5): 361–390.

92. Yang, R., Hey, J.A., Aslanian, R., and Rizzo, C.A., 2002. Coordination of histamine H3 receptor antagonists with human adrenal cytochrome P450 enzymes. *Pharmacology* 66(3): 128–135.

93. Silva, C., Mor, M., Bordi, F., Rivara, S., Caretta, A., Ballabeni, V., Barocelli, E., and Plazzi, P.V., 1997. Plasma concentration and brain penetration of the H_3 receptor antagonist thioperamide in rats. *Farmaco.* 52(6–7): 457–462.

94. Mochizuki, T., Jansen, F.P., Leurs, R., Windhorst, A.D., Yamatodani, A., Maeyama, K., and Timmerman, H., 1996. Brain penetration of the histamine H_3 receptor antagonists thioperamide and clobenpropit in rat and mouse, determined with ex vivo [^{125}I]iodophenpropit binding. *Brain Res.* 743(1–2): 178–183.

95. Stark, H., 2003. Recent advances in histamine H_{-3}/H_{-4} receptor ligands. *Exp. Opin. Therap. Pat.* 13(6): 851–865.

96. Cowart, M.D., Altenbach, R.A., Black, L.A., Faghih, R., Zhao, C., and Hancock, A.A., 2004. Medicinal chemistry and biological properties of non-imidazole histamine H_3 antagonists. *Mini-Rev. in Med. Chem.* 4: 997–1010.

97. Ligneau, X., Perrin, D., Landais, L., Camelin, J.C., Calmels, T.P., Berrebi-Bertrand, I., Lecomte, J.M., Parmentier, R., Anaclet, C., Lin, J.S., Bertaina-Anglade, V., la Rochelle, C.D., d'Aniello, F., Rouleau, A., Gbahou, F., Arrang, J.M., Ganellin, C.R., Stark, H., Schunack, W., and Schwartz, J.C., 2007. BF2.649 [1-{3-[3-(4-Chlorophenyl)propoxy] propyl}piperidine, hydrochloride], a nonimidazole inverse agonist/antagonist at the human histamine H_3 receptor: Preclinical pharmacology. *J. Pharmacol. Exp. Ther.* 320(1): 365–375.

98. Medhurst, A.D., Atkins, A.R., Beresford, I.J., Brackenborough, K., Briggs, M.A., Calver, A.R., Cilia, J., Cluderay, J.E., Crook, B., Davis, J.B., Davis, R.K., Davis, R.P., Dawson, L.A., Foley, A.G., Gartlon, J., Gonzalez, M.I., Heslop, T., Hirst, W.D., Jennings, C., Jones, D.N., Lacroix, L.P., Martyn, A., Ociepka, S., Ray, A., Regan, C.M., Roberts, J.C., Schogger, J., Southam, E., Stean, T.O., Trail, B.K., Upton, N., Wadsworth, G., Wald, J.A., White, T., Witherington, J., Woolley, M.L., Worby, A., and Wilson, D.M., 2007. GSK189254, a novel H_3 receptor antagonist that binds to histamine H_3 receptors in Alzheimer's Disease brain and improves cognitive performance in preclinical models. *J. Pharmacol. Exp. Ther.* 321(3): 1032–1045.

99. Bonaventure, P., Letavic, M., Dugovic, C., Wilson, S., Aluisio, L., Pudiak, C., Lord, B., Mazur, C., Kamme, F., Nishino, S., Carruthers, N., and Lovenberg, T., 2007. Histamine H_3 receptor antagonists: from target identification to drug leads. *Biochem. Pharmacol.* 73(8): 1084–1096.

100. Faghih, R., Esbenshade, T.A., Krueger, K.M., Yao, B.B., Witte, D.G., Miller, T.M., Kang, C.H., Fox, G.B., Cowart, M., Bennani, Y.L., and Hancock, A.A., 2004. Structure–activity relationships of A-331440: a new histamine-3 antagonist with antiobesity properties. *Inflamm. Res.* 53(Suppl 1): S79–S80.

101. Bush, E.N., Shapiro, R., Nuss, M., Knourek-Segel, V., Wilcox, D., Droz, B., Faghih, R., Bennani, Y., Esbenshade, T., Jacobson, P.B., and Hancock, A.A., 2002. The histamine H_3 receptor antagonist A-331440 decreases body weight in male C57BL/6J mice with high fat diet-induced obesity. *Am. Diab. Assoc. Abstr.* 1715 P.

102. Hancock, A.A., Diehl, M.S., Faghih, R., Bush, E.N., Krueger, K.M., Krishna, G., Miller, T.R., Wilcox, D.M., Nguyen, P., Pratt, J.K., Cowart, M.D., Esbenshade, T.A., and Jacobson, P.B., 2004. In vitro optimization of structure activity relationships of analogues of A-331440 combining radioligand receptor binding assays and micronucleus assays of potential antiobesity histamine H_3 receptor antagonists. *Basic Clin. Pharmacol. Toxicol.* 95(3): 144–152.

103. Peschke, B., Bak, S., Hohlweg, R., Pettersson, I., Refsgaard, H.H., Viuff, D., and Rimvall, K., 2004. Cinnamic amides of (S)-2-(aminomethyl)pyrrolidines are potent H_3 antagonists. *Bioorg. Med. Chem.* 12(10): 2603–2616.

104. Naruse, T. and Ishii, R., 1995. Relationship between histamine receptors in the brain and diazepam-induced hyperphagia in rats. *Pharmacol. Biochem. Behav.* 51(4): 923–927.

105. Yoshimoto, R., Miyamoto, Y., Shimamura, K., Ishihara, A., Takahashi, K., Kotani, H., Chen, A.S., Chen, H.Y., Macneil, D.J., Kanatani, A., and Tokita, S., 2006. Therapeutic potential of histamine H_3 receptor agonist for the treatment of obesity and diabetes mellitus. *Proc. Natl Acad. Sci. U.S.A.* 103(37): 13866–13871.

106. Sindelar, D.K., Shepperd, M.L., Pickard, R.T., Alexander-Chacko, J., Dill, M.J., Cramer, J.W., Smith, D.P., and Gadski, R., 2004. Central H_3R activation by thioperamide does not affect energy balance. *Pharmacol. Biochem. Behav.* 78(2): 275–283.

107. Fox, G.B., Pan, J.B., Esbenshade, T.A., Bennani, Y.L., Black, L.A., Faghih, R., Hancock, A.A., and Decker, M.W., 2002. Effects of histamine H_3 receptor ligands GT-2331 and ciproxifan in a repeated acquisition avoidance response in the spontaneously hypertensive rat pup. *Behav. Brain Res.* 131(1–2): 151–161.

108. Cowart, M., Faghih, R., Curtis, M.P., Gfesser, G.A., Bennani, Y.L., Black, L.A., Pan, L., Marsh, K.C., Sullivan, J.P., Esbenshade, T.A., Fox, G.B., and Hancock, A.A., 2005. 4-(2-[2-(2(R)-methylpyrrolidin-1-yl)ethyl]benzofuran-5-yl)benzonitrile and related 2-aminoethylbenzofuran H_3 receptor antagonists potently enhance cognition and attention. *J. Med. Chem.* 48(1): 38–55.

109. Fox, G.B., Esbenshade, T.A., Pan, J.B., Radek, R.J., Krueger, K.M., Yao, B.B., Browman, K.E., Buckley, M.J., Ballard, M.E., Komater, V.A., Miner, H., Zhang, M., Faghih, R., Rueter, L.E., Bitner, R.S., Drescher, K.U., Wetter, J., Marsh, K., Lemaire, M., Porsolt, R.D., Bennani, Y.L., Sullivan, J.P., Cowart, M.D., Decker, M.W., and Hancock, A.A., 2005. Pharmacological properties of ABT-239 [4-(2-{2-[(2R)-2-Methyl pyrrolidinyl]ethyl}-benzofuran-5-yl)benzonitrile]: II. Neurophysiological characterization and broad preclinical efficacy in cognition and schizophrenia of a potent and selective histamine H_3 receptor antagonist. *J. Pharmacol. Exp. Ther.* 313(1): 176–190.

110. Barbier, A.J., Berridge, C., Dugovic, C., Laposky, A.D., Wilson, S.J., Boggs, J., Aluisio, L., Lord, B., Mazur, C., Pudiak, C.M., Langlois, X., Xiao, W., Apodaca, R., Carruthers, N.I., and Lovenberg, T.W., 2004. Acute wake-promoting actions of JNJ-5207852, a novel, diamine-based H_3 antagonist. *Br. J. Pharmacol.* 143(5): 649–661.

111. Van den Pol, A.N., 2003. Weighing the role of hypothalamic feeding neurotransmitters. *Neuron* 40(6): 1059–1061.

112. Komater, V.A., Browman, K.E., Curzon, P., Hancock, A.A., Decker, M.W., and Fox, G.B., 2003. H_3 receptor blockade by thioperamide enhances cognition in rats without inducing locomotor sensitization. *Psychopharmacology* 167(4): 363–372.

113. Bray, G.A., 2000. A concise review on the therapeutics of obesity. *Nutrition* 16(10): 953–960.

10 Epilepsy

Divya Vohora and Krishna K. Pillai

CONTENTS

Introduction...305
Histaminergic Agents and Seizures..306
    Evidence Linking H_1 Receptor...306
    Controversies Surrounding H_2..312
    H_3 Receptor Antagonists as Potential Anticonvulsants 312
Efficacy against Different Seizure Models..312
    Electroshock- and Chemoshock-Induced Seizures........................312
    Chronic Models (Kindling)...313
    Genetic Models...314
    Kainic Acid-Induced Seizures and Neuronal Damage 315
Relationship of Histamine with Convulsants and Antiepileptic Drugs.................315
Possible Mechanisms 317
Clinical Studies..319
Evidence as an Endogenous Anticonvulsant 319
Therapeutic Advantage 320
    Central Localization...320
    Procognitive Effects 320
    Provigilant Effects..321
    Antidepressant and Anxiolytic Effects 321
Conclusion..322
References...322

INTRODUCTION

Research into the pathophysiology of epileptic seizures has largely focused on various neurotransmitter and neuropeptide systems although mainly on inhibition of glutamatergic (excitatory) or potentiation of GABAergic (inhibitory) system. It is only in recent years that a concerted effort is made to provide more rationally designed and selective drugs for the treatment of this disorder. Although currently available drugs are able to prevent seizures in majority of the patients, ~30% of the patients are uncontrolled [1,2], even those controlled experience a lot of adverse effects and interactions with other drugs. There remains a clear unmet need for novel targets/drugs. Histaminergic mechanisms appear to be one such target. The first indication for the histamine hypothesis of epilepsy was derived from clinical observations, where classically used antihistaminics (H_1 antagonists) occasionally produced convulsions in epileptic patients [3] and also in younger children [4]. Later on, various experimental studies were carried out that suggested histamine to be a potential target around which further experiments could be carried out.

Earlier, we have reviewed the role of histamine as an inhibitory anticonvulsant neurotransmitter. Many developments have taken place since then, and various possible mechanisms for the effect of histaminergic agents and H_3 receptor modulators on seizures have been evaluated. One of the H_3 receptor antagonists was also evaluated recently in epileptic patients with encouraging results [5]. Regardless of all these efforts, no compound has yet been approved for clinical use in epilepsy. The aim of this chapter is to provide an overview of the available information on the role of histamine in epileptic seizures and to evaluate the present status of H_3 receptor antagonists as future antiepileptic drugs (AEDs).

HISTAMINERGIC AGENTS AND SEIZURES

Various drugs that modulate brain histamine affect experimental seizures. Drugs that enhance brain histamine, for example, histamine precursor (L-histidine), histamine N-methyl transferase (HNMT) inhibitors (HNMT being an enzyme solely responsible for the termination of neurotransmitter action of histamine in brain), and histamine itself (when given intracerebroventricularly), exhibit potent anticonvulsant effects not only in electroshock- and chemoshock-induced seizure models but also in kindling and, more recently, genetic models of epilepsy (for details, see Table 10.1). However, drugs such as α-fluoromethylhistidine (FMH) and brocresine, both of which are histidine decarboxylase (HDC) inhibitors and deplete brain histamine, exhibit proconvulsant effects in the aforementioned models (see Table 10.1). Indeed, it has been reported that in patients with higher brain histamine content (the so-called histidinemic patients), the incidence of convulsions during childhood is much lower than normal children [6].

EVIDENCE LINKING H_1 RECEPTOR

Consistent with the earliest clinical observation on classically used antihistaminics, various experimental studies reported a proconvulsant effect with H_1 receptor antagonists and an anticonvulsant effect with H_1 receptor agonists. The anticonvulsant effects of histaminergic drugs, whether it is histamine or histamine precursors, HNMT inhibitors and H_1 agonists were shown to be reversed by centrally acting H_1 antagonists but not by central administration of peripherally as well as centrally acting H_2 antagonists (see Table 10.1), thus indicating a role of H_1, and not H_2, in the inhibition of seizures in rodents. This was later confirmed by a study on both H_1 receptor and HDC gene knockout mice, where pentylenetetrazole (PTZ)-induced seizures [29] and amygdala-kindled seizures [30] were greatly accelerated in animals with very low brain histamine content. A binding potential of H_1 receptors has also been shown to increase in amygdala-kindled rats [31]. In addition, an increase in H_1 receptor density has been reported in the temporal cortex of patients with complex partial seizures (CPS) [32] and in brain regions of rats with absence

TABLE 10.1

Effect of Histaminergic Agents on Experimental Convulsions

Histaminergic Agents	Animals Tested	Effective Doses/Dose Range and Route of Administration	Electroshock Seizures	PTZ	PTX	PTZ Kindling	Amygdala Kindling	Genetic	Kainic Acid	References
1	2	3	4	5	6	7	8	9	10	11
Drugs enhancing brain histamine										
Histamine	Mice	12.5–200 μg/mouse i.c.v.	—	No effect	—	—	—	—	—	7
	Mice	20–40 μg/mouse i.c.v.	—	No effect	Protection[a]	—	—	—	—	8
	GEPRs (audiogenic)	30–300 ng/mouse i.c.v.	Protection[a,b,c,d]	No effect	—	—	—	—	—	9
		40–60 nmol i.c.	—	—	—	—	—	Protection	—	10
L-Histidine (histamine precursor)	Mice	500 mg/kg i.p. 3 times	—	No effect	—	—	—	—	—	7
	Mice	200 mg/kg i.p.	—	↑Threshold	—	—	—	—	—	11
	Mice	800 mg/kg i.p.	Protection[b,c] (clonic but not tonic)	—	—	—	—	—	—	12
	Rats	1000–1500 mg/kg i.p.	—	—	—	—	Inhibition[a,b,c,e] retarded the development	—	—	13
	Rats	500 and 1000 mg/kg i.p.	—	—	—	Inhibition and retarded the development[a,f,g]	—	—	—	14
	EL mice (vestibular)	1000 mg/kg i.p.	—	↑Threshold[e]	—	—	—	Protection[e]	—	15
Metoprine (N-methyltransferase inhibitor)	Mice	5 mg/kg i.p.	Protection[a]	↑Threshold[e]	—	—	—	—	—	11
	Rats	1.25–20 mg/kg i.p.	—	—	—	—	—	—	—	11

(continued)

TABLE 10.1 (Continued)

Histaminergic Agents	Animals Tested	Effective Doses/Dose Range and Route of Administration	Electroshock Seizures	PTZ	PTX	PTZ Kindling	Amygdala Kindling	Genetic	Kainic Acid	References
1	2	3	4	5	6	7	8	9	10	11
	Mice	20–40 mg/kg s.c.	—	Protection (latency to onset but not duration)	Protection	—	—	—	—	8
	Mice	2.5–10 mg/kg i.p.	Protection[a]	—	—	—	Inhibition[a,c] (protection)	—	—	12
	Rats	10–20 mg/kg i.p.		—	—	—		—	—	13
	EL mice	20 mg/kg i.p.		—	—	—		Protection[c]	—	15
Drugs depleting brain histamine (HDC inhibitors)										
α-FMH	Mice	25–100 mg/kg i.p.		Proconvulsant (clonic but not tonic phase)						12
Brocresine	Mice	200–300 mg/kg i.p.		Proconvulsant (clonic) biphasic effect (tonic)						7
Drugs acting at H₁ receptors										
Agonists										
2-Thiazolylethylamine	Mice	300–1000 ng/mouse i.c.v.	Protection[a]	Protection[a]						9
Antagonists										
Cyclizine	Mice	25 mg/kg i.p.	—	Proconvulsant (clonic) and ↓ incidence (tonic)						7
Diphenhydramine, pyrilamine, tripelennamine, chlorpheniramine	Mice	20 mg/kg i.p.	—	Proconvulsant (clonic) and ↓ incidence (tonic)						7

Drug	Species	Dose							Ref.
Dexbrompheniramine	Mice	60 mg/kg i.p.	—	Proconvulsant (clonic) and ↓ incidence (tonic)	—	—	—	—	7
Phenindamine	Mice	20 mg/kg i.p.	—	Protection (tonic)	—	—	—	—	7
Chlorcyclizine and pyrathiazine	Mice	20 mg/kg i.p.	—	No effect	—	—	—	—	7
Diphenhydramine, pyrilamine	Rats	10–20 mg/kg i.v.	Epileptic signs in EEG	Proconvulsant (clonic)	—	—	—	—	16
pyrilamine	Rats	i.p.	—	—	—	—	Proconvulsant	—	17
Dimethindene	Mice	0.03–0.12 mg/kg	No effect	↓ Threshold	—	—	—	—	11
Promethazine	Mice	0.1–0.4 mg/kg	No effect	↓ Threshold	—	—	—	—	11
Acrivastine	Mice	1–5 µg/mouse i.c.v.	—	—	Proconvulsant (clonic)	—	—	—	8
Loratidine, cetrizine	Rats	40 mg/kg i.p.	—	—	—	—	No effect	—	17
Astemizole	Mice	2 mg/kg i.p.	Proconvulsant	—	—	—	—	—	18
Diphenhydramine	EL mice	15 mg/kg i.p.	—	—	—	—	—	—	15
Antazoline	Mice	0.5 mg/kg	↓ Threshold	—	—	—	—	—	19
Ketotifen	Mice	8 mg/kg	↓ Threshold	—	—	—	—	—	19
Drugs acting at H₂ receptors									
Agonists									
4-Methylhistamine	Mice	40 µg/mouse i.c.v.	—	No effect	—	—	—	—	16
Dimaprit	Mice	100 ng/mouse i.c.v.	No effect	No effect	—	—	—	—	20
Antagonists									
Burimamide	Mice	100 mg/kg i.p.	—	No effect	—	—	—	—	7
Metiamide	Mice	100–200 mg/kg i.p.	—	Proconvulsant (tonic) no effect (clonic)	—	—	—	—	7
Oxmetidine	Mice	0.5–2 mg/kg	No effect	No effect	—	—	—	—	11
Ranitidine	Mice	1–4 mg/kg	No effect	No effect	—	—	—	—	11
	Mice	10–25 µg/mouse i.c.v.	—	—	No effect	—	—	—	8
	Mice	477–954 nmol i.c.v.	Proconvulsant[i]	—	—	—	—	—	21

(continued)

TABLE 10.1 (Continued)

Histaminergic Agents	Animals Tested	Effective Doses/Dose Range and Route of Administration	Electroshock Seizures	PTZ	PTX	PTZ Kindling	Amygdala Kindling	Genetic	Kainic Acid	References
1	2	3	4	5	6	7	8	9	10	
Zolantidine	Mice	0.25–8 mg/kg	No effect	No effect	—	—	—	—	—	11
		20 mg/kg						No effect[h]	—	15
	Mice	721–1236 nmol i.c.v.	Proconvulsant[i] (without any model used)[j]							21
	Mice	7.4–44 nmol i.c.v.	Proconvulsant[i]							21
	Mice	226–603 nmol i.c.v.	Proconvulsant[i]							21
Drugs acting at H₃ receptors										
Agonists										
R (α)methyl-histamine (RAMH)	Mice	10–40 mg/kg i.p.	No effect	No effect	—	—	No effect	—	—	11
	Mice	10–20 µg/mouse i.c.v.	—	—	—	—	No effect	—	—	22
	Mice	100–1000 ng/mouse i.c.v.	No effect	—	—	—	—	—	—	20
Imetit	Mice	100–1000ng/mouse i.c.v.	No effect	—	—	—	—	—	—	20
Antagonists										
Thioperamide	Mice	2–10 mg/kg i.p.	No effect	No effect	—	—	—	—	—	11
	Mice	3.75–15 mg/kg i.p.	Protection[a,b,c,j]							23
	Mice	10–50 µg/ mouse i.c.v.					Inhibition[a,b,c,e,j] (protection)			22
	Mice	5–10 mg/kg i.p.					Inhibition[a,b,c,e,j] (protection)			22
	Mice	7.5–15 mg/kg i.p.		Protection[a,j]						24
	EL mice	25 mg/kg i.p.						Protection[e]		15
	Rats	20 mg/kg i.p.					No effect			25

Compound	Species	Dose							Ref.
Clobenpropit	Mice	5–10 mg/kg i.p.	Protection[b,c,e,j]	—	—	—	—	—	20
	Mice	20 and 40 mg/kg i.p.	Protection[a,g,j]	No effect	—	—	—	—	26
	Rats	i.c.v. and i.p.	—	—	—	—	Inhibition[a,b,c,j,k]	—	27
	Rats	1–3 mg/kg i.p.	—	—	Retarded the development[b,c,f,j]	—	—	—	14
	Rats	10–20 μg/mouse i.c.v.	—	—	—	—	—	—	
AQ0145	Rats	i.c.v. and i.p.	—	—	—	—	Inhibition[a,b,c,j,k]	—	27
	Rats	21 mg/kg i.p.	—	—	—	—	Inhibition[a]	—	28
Iodophenpropit	Rats	2.57 mg/kg i.p.	Protection	—	—	—	Inhibition[a]	—	28
Tiprolisant	Mice	100 mg/kg p.o.	—	—	—	—	—	Protection in EEG	5
(BF 2.649)	Mice	5–20 mg/kg i.p.	No effect	—	—	—	—	—	5
	Rats (GAERs)	10–20 mg/kg i.p.	—	—	—	—	—	Protection in EEG	5

Note: GEPRs, genetically epilepsy prone rats; HDC, histidine decarboxylase; i.c., inferior colliculus; i.c.v., intracerebroventricular; PTX, picrotoxin; PTZ, pentylenetetrazole; GAERs, genetically absence epilepsy rats of Strasbourg.

a Dose-dependent effect.
b Effect antagonized by H_1 blocker(s).
c Effect not antagonized by H_2 blocker(s).
d Effect not antagonized by peripherally acting H_1 blocker(s).
e Effects substantiated by measuring brain levels of histamine/HDC activity.
f Effect antagonized by α-FMH.
g ↑ Anticonvulsant efficacy of carbamazepine and valproate.
h Effects contradicted by measuring HDC.
i Tonic (but not clonic) convulsions suppressed by GABAergic or glutamatergic anticonvulsant.
j Effect antagonized by H_3 agonist(s).
k GABAmimetics potentiate and bicuculline antagonizes.

Source: Updated from Vohora, D., Pal, S. N., Pillai, K. K. Curr. Neuropharmacol. 2, 421–423, 2004. With permission.

epilepsy [33]. All these observations confirm a suppressive role of histamine in seizure generation through H_1 receptors.

CONTROVERSIES SURROUNDING H_2

Majority of the studies rule out the involvement of H_2 receptors in seizures as neither the antagonists of these receptors reverses the anticonvulsant effects of histaminergic drugs nor the central administration of agonists has any effect (Table 10.1). Even zolantidine, an H_2 receptor antagonist that readily enters the central nervous system (CNS), does not affect the seizure threshold in rodents [11,15]. However, there are a few reports that indicate otherwise. For example, in a study by Shimokawa et al. [21], proconvulsant effects were observed with some H_2 receptor antagonists administered intracerebrally to rodents and were not controlled by standard AEDs, suggesting mechanisms different from those of well-known convulsants. In another study, H_2 receptor antagonists reduced the amount of convulsants needed to provoke chemically induced seizures [3]. In addition to these experimental reports, an isolated clinical evidence of a 65-year-old woman developing generalized seizures when treated with famotidine is available [34].

H_3 RECEPTOR ANTAGONISTS AS POTENTIAL ANTICONVULSANTS

Like H_1, H_3 receptors are known to be involved in the inhibition of seizures. Antagonists and inverse agonists of H_3 receptors have been shown to protect against experimental seizures by various workers. The effects are further shown to be reversed by selective H_3 receptor agonists and H_1 antagonists but not H_2 antagonist (see Table 10.1). It has been suggested that released histamine, by blocking the autoinhibitory H_3 receptors, interacts with H_1 receptors on the postsynaptic neurons to produce anticonvulsant effect. H_3 receptor antagonists were shown to have protective effects against both electroshock [20,23] and chemoshock [24] models as well as against chronic models such as PTZ [35] and amygdala kindling [22,28] in rodents and more recently against genetic models of epilepsy [5,15]. However, as seen in Table 10.1, a few workers found thioperamide (THP), a selective H_3 receptor antagonist, to have no effect against electroshock [11] as well as amygdala-kindled seizures in rodents [25]. A few other H_3 receptor antagonists including clobenpropit [26] and BF 2.649 [5] were reported not to protect against PTZ-induced seizures. Although the reason for these discrepancies is not clear, the lack of effect could be due to species differences, doses employed, or the experimental procedure used.

EFFICACY AGAINST DIFFERENT SEIZURE MODELS

ELECTROSHOCK- AND CHEMOSHOCK-INDUCED SEIZURES

The effect of various histaminergic agents on electrically and chemically induced seizures have been summarized in Table 10.1. The i.c.v. administration of histamine and i.p. administration of drugs enhancing brain histamine are generally protective in maximal electroshock (MES) and PTZ-induced convulsions [9,11,12]. A few studies also reported a protective action against picrotoxin (PTX)-induced seizures [8]. However, there were a lot of discrepancies/contradictions among various studies. For instance, histamine administered i.c.v. protected against PTZ-induced seizures in one study [9] but not in the other study [8]. Neither i.c.v. histamine nor i.p. L-histidine could protect mice against PTZ-induced seizures [7]. Furthermore, H_3 receptor antagonists were protective against PTZ-induced seizures and kindling in a number of studies [24,35] but were without any effect in a number of other studies [11,25, 26]. A study also reported THP and another H_3 antagonist burimamide to increase the severity of PTX-induced clonic convulsions in mice [36]. The dual effects of these compounds could be due to their nonspecificity. For instance, burimamide has also H_2 antagonistic activity, whereas THP is an inverse agonist of H_3 receptor. In contrast to this study, both THP and clobenpropit were generally found to be effective and were more efficacious against clonic phase of electroconvulsions as compared to the tonic phase [20,23]. This was further supported by the fact that both HDC inhibitors and H_1 antagonists exhibited proconvulsant effect in the clonic but not tonic phase [7,12], suggesting that histaminergic drugs may have a potential against generalized absence type of seizures. Furthermore, studies indicate histaminergic agents to be more efficacious against chemoconvulsions in contrast to electroconvulsions. It was suggested that PTZ first stimulates the most sensitive structures in the brain stem and then proceeds to the telencephalon and other brain structures, whereas in case of electroconvulsions, the whole brain is stimulated within 0.2 s, leaving no time for the inhibitory action of histamine [11]. However, Harada et al. [28] reported a reduction of tonic seizures induced by MES following THP, clobenpropit, iodophenpropit, and some other H_3 receptor antagonists (VUF5514, VUF5515, and VUF4929) without any effect on the clonic phase, and a potential of these ligands in secondary generalized and tonic-clonic seizures was suggested.

CHRONIC MODELS (KINDLING)

Electrically or chemically induced seizure models represent models of seizure states rather than epilepsy, a chronic disorder [37]. The term *kindling* refers to a phenomenon whereby repeated administration of an initially subconvulsive stimulus results in progressive intensification of seizures, culminating in a generalized seizure [38]. Kindling is a model of epilepsy that has the advantages of both an epileptogenic and a spontaneous seizure model [39], and thus, it resembles human epilepsy. Amygdala, being a sensitive structure, drugs modulating brain histamine has been widely investigated against amygdala kindling. Furthermore, high densities of H_3 receptors in amygdaloid complex in central, lateral, and basolateral nuclei have been reported [40]. A few studies have also evaluated the effects of histaminergic agents on PTZ kindling. Both i.c.v. histamine and L-histidine have been shown to protect against amygdala-kindled seizures. L-Histidine, in addition, also retarded the development of PTZ kindling. Indeed, the development of amygdaloid kindling was greatly accelerated in HDC and H_1 receptor-deficient mice. H_1 antagonists including diphenhydramine, pyrilamine, and ketotifen, but not loratidine and cetirizine, however, elicited epileptogenic activity in amygdala-kindled rats [17]. Carnosine (β-alanyl L-histidine), a naturally occurring dipeptide, was reported to exhibit anticonvulsant effects in amygdaloid and PTZ-kindled rats [41] and against PTZ-induced seizures in wild-type mice [42]; the effects being mediated through histaminergic mechanisms by its conversion into histidine and further into histamine in the brain.

H_3 receptor antagonists including THP, clobenpropit, AQ 0145, and iodophen-propit have all been demonstrated to retard the development and to protect against amygdala-kindled seizures. Clobenpropit, in addition, has been studied on PTZ-induced kindling and inhibited kindled seizures [17]. Harada et al. [28,43] recently compared the effects of THP, clobenpropit, AQ 0145, and iodophenpropit on amyg-daloid-kindled seizures and found a dose-dependent inhibition of both seizure-stage and afterdischarge duration by all the drugs and more potent inhibition by iodophen-propit (an iodinated derivative of clobenpropit) when compared with THP. Yoshida et al. [25], however, reported no protection of amygdaloid-kindled seizures following THP, L-histidine, and betahistine, a nonselective mixed H_3 antagonist/H_1 agonist in rats. Furthermore, Wada et al. [44] reported a facilitation of kindling following L-histidine. Thus, the dual effects of histaminergic agents have been reported following kindling as well. Haas and coworkers reported an increase in burst activity of pyra-midal cells in CA3 region [45] and potentiation of N-methyl-D-aspartate (NMDA) responses in hippocampal neurons following histamine [46]. Whether these effects contribute to excitation and proconvulsive effects reported with histaminergic agents in some models including kindling remains to be determined.

It is well known that kindled seizures are associated with an increase in gamma amino butyric acid (GABA) release. THP has been shown to increase the release of GABA from the rat hypothalamus [47]. A similar mechanism could be possible for anticonvulsant effects of clobenpropit and iodophenpropit as well. Indeed, combina-tion of clobenpropit with some GABAmimetic drugs such as diazepam, muscimol, and sodium valproate, at their subeffective doses, resulted in a significant inhibition of amygdala-kindled seizures [48]. Furthermore, the protective action of clobenpro-pit was antagonized by bicuculline, $GABA_A$ antagonist. Thus, available evidence indicates that histaminergic mechanisms play an important role in suppressing amygdala-kindled seizures through H_1 receptors and GABA. Moreover, there is a close relationship between GABA and histamine. Neurons of the histaminergic tuberomamillary nucleus (TMN) contain GABA, and the GABA content of ICR mice was reduced to 85% following α-FMH [49].

GENETIC MODELS

Animals with chronically recurring spontaneous seizures represent ideal models for human epilepsy, but the major drawback of these models is that naturally occurring seizures cannot be elicited by an investigator. In some species, however, stimulation (auditory, photic, etc.) results in seizures (semispontaneous models). For example, genetically epilepsy prone rats (GEPRs) exhibit audiogenic seizures. Genetic strains also have a very low threshold to a number of epileptogenic agents. Onodera et al. [50] reported significantly lower levels of histamine in many brain regions of GEPRs as compared to those in epilepsy-resistant Wistar rats. To our knowledge, only a few studies have investigated the effect of histaminergic drugs on genetic models of epi-lepsy. The inferior colliculus is an important midbrain nucleus for processing audi-tory information and plays an important role in the initiation of audiogenic seizures in GEPRs. Histamine, injected into inferior colliculus, was reported to significantly inhibit audiogenic seizures in GEPRs [10]. Recently, Yawata et al. [15] studied the effect of L-histidine, metoprine, and THP on the development of seizures in EL mouse following vestibular stimulation. EL mouse is an established genetic model of human temporal lobe epilepsy/CPS and exhibits seizures in response to vestibular stimulation by repeated tosses into the air or by altering the equilibrium of the mice. All the three drugs, L-histidine, metoprine, and THP, elevated brain histamine levels and retarded the time of onset of seizure episodes. THP also increased brain HDC activity. However, H_1 antagonist diphenhydramine accelerated the initiation of seizure episode.

Recently, Schwartz and Lecomte [5] patented a nonimidazole H_3 receptor antagonist BF 2.649 for the treatment of epilepsy. In addition to other models, the compound was also evaluated on a genetic strain of rats termed *genetic absence epilepsy rats of Strasbourg* (GAERs). These rats exhibited spontaneous generalized nonconvulsive seizures resembling human absence seizures. BF 2.649 reduced both the number and the cumulated durations of spike and wave discharges in Electroencephalogram (EEG) in GAERs.

KAINIC ACID-INDUCED SEIZURES AND NEURONAL DAMAGE

Kainic acid (KA) is an analog of glutamate, an excitatory amino acid (EAA) neurotransmitter. Systemic or central administration of KA has toxic effects on hippocampus causing cell injury, whereas in lower doses seizures are induced [51]. KA-induced seizures resemble the behavioral and EEG characteristics of human temporal lobe epilepsy. KA model is useful for studying not only the development of temporal lobe epilepsy but also the state of status epilepticus (SE) and compensatory mechanisms as the brain damage and subsequent spontaneous seizures last for a longer time [52]. The role for histamine and H_3 receptors in convulsive SE induced by KA was also recently suggested [53]. A highly increased histamine concentrations and fiber densities were detected in the areas of neuronal damage in this model and in convulsive SE in hippocampus, piriform, and amygdala [53]. Jin et al. [52] studied the modulation of H_1 and H_3 receptors in the thalamus of rats following KA-induced SE and suggested neuroprotective and compensatory mechanisms through H_3 receptor activation during KA-induced seizures. In another study, histaminergic neurons were shown to protect the pyramidal CA3a/b neurons from KA-induced neuronal damage in the developing hippocampus, the protective effect being mediated through H_1 and H_3 receptors [54]. The possible interaction of KA on the kinetics of histamine synthesis in various brain regions is discussed in Chapter 4. Recently, Schwartz and Lecomte [5] studied the effects of BF 2.649 (tiprolisant) on kainate-induced hippocampal seizures in mice and found a reduced duration and number of hippocampal discharges in the EEG. It is noteworthy that all other AEDs tested in this model (phenytoin [PHT], carbamazepine [CBZ], valproate, and levetiracetam) except benzodiazepines were ineffective. Thus, histamine may play a role in temporal lobe epilepsy, a pharmacoresistant form of epilepsy in humans.

RELATIONSHIP OF HISTAMINE WITH CONVULSANTS AND ANTIEPILEPTIC DRUGS

Although a large amount of data point toward a role of drugs modulating brain histamine on seizures, there are relatively fewer studies examining the role of drugs modulating seizures on brain histamine. To clarify any such role, we investigated the modulation of brain histamine levels following common convulsants and AEDs [55]. A reduction of histamine levels in cerebral cortex, hypothalamus, brain stem, and cerebellum was observed following PTZ-induced clonic convulsions in mice. Kamei et al. [13] have also reported a similar reduction of histamine content in amygdala and hypothalamus following kindling model. A seizure-induced rapid removal and depletion of histamine may partially explain the reduction in histamine levels. A seizure-induced increase of neuronal histamine release may then occur causing inhibitory effect on the subsequent seizure-reflecting activation of protective histaminergic mechanisms [56]. In fact, we also reported an elevation of brain-stem histamine following MES [55]. Since brain stem and a number of other brain stem structures have been implicated in seizure arrest [57], an elevation following MES could reflect protective physiological mechanisms, supporting the concept of histamine as an endogenous anticonvulsant. On the contrary, it was reported that depolarization induced by potassium stimulated the release of histamine from brain slices, whereas barbiturates reduced the rate of endogenous histamine synthesis in the brain [7].

Another convulsant that may possibly act through histaminergic mechanisms is methionine-sulfoximine (MSO). The latter is known to increase the activity of HNMT, an enzyme responsible for catabolism of histamine [58]. Our unpublished data on THP and R(α)-methylhistamine (RAMH) did not reveal any modulation of MSO-induced convulsions in mice. Thus, the convulsant action of MSO does not appear to be mediated through histaminergic mechanism and may be attributed to its well-known effects on GABA synthesis (unpublished observation).

In addition to the effect of well-known convulsive agents on brain histamine, some AEDs were also investigated for the modulation of histamine levels in different brain areas. Although PHT and gabapentin were reported to increase cortical and brain stem histamine, sodium valproate reduced hypothalamic histamine content [55]. Thus, a role for histamine exists not only in seizure mechanisms but also in its management by AEDs. Furthermore, H_3 receptor antagonists were effectively combined with low doses of AEDs in rodents for therapeutic advantage: additive/synergistic effects on anticonvulsant efficacy and reduced risk of dose-related toxicities [26,55]. In addition to H_3 receptor antagonists, L-histidine also augmented the protective effects of PHT and CBZ against electroconvulsions in mice [59]. In another study, antazoline, an H_1 receptor antagonist, reduced the protective efficacy of PHT and CBZ against MES, whereas ketotifen reduced the protection offered by CBZ and increased the adverse motor and cognitive effects of AEDs, suggesting that H_1 antagonists should be used with caution in epileptic patients [19].

The well-known proconvulsant effects of theophylline were studied in a developing mouse on electrically induced seizures. Although the proconvulsive effects were inhibited in the presence of phenobarbital, other well-established AEDs failed to reverse such effects and were countered by an H_3 receptor antagonist [60]. Contrary to the aforementioned reports, BF 2.649 failed to modify/enhance the anticonvulsant activity of a series of AEDs including CBZ, sodium valproate, PHT, diazepam, and phenobarbital in the PTZ model [5]. In fact, the compound showed encouraging results in the pharmacoresistant model of epilepsy in which most of these AEDs were ineffective.

POSSIBLE MECHANISMS*

Various workers substantiated the anticonvulsant effects of histaminergic agents by measuring brain histamine content. A good linear correlation was demonstrated between histamine concentrations in brain and protection from seizures. Such a correlation was evident for drugs such as L-histidine and metoprine, both of which enhanced brain histamine levels and provided protection against seizures [11,62]. It was suggested that the histaminergic pathway projecting into the telencephalon through the medial forebrain bundle was implicated in the inhibition of generalized epileptic discharge [11]. α-FMH, however, depleted brain histamine and exhibited proconvulsant effect. Such effects of α-FMH were reported to be independent of its effects on Norepinephrine (NE), Dopamine (DA), and 5-hydroxytryptamine (5-HT) concentrations in the brain [12]. Interestingly, all the three drugs (metoprine, L-histidine, and α-FMH) affected histamine levels in similar regions of rodent brain including cerebral cortex, diencephalon, and midbrain; the regions in which histaminergic neuronal pathways are localized. Histamine H_1 receptors are especially dense in the cerebral cortex of rodents, a region considered relevant for epilepsy. Furthermore, histamine has been shown to have marked effects on cortical and hippocampal neurons, structures involved in different types of epilepsies [62]. Similar correlation has been reported between the anticonvulsant effects of H_3 receptor antagonists and an increase in HDC activity in the brain [20]. Contrary to all these reports, a study by Skaper et al. [63] indicated otherwise. According to their study, under Mg^{2+} free conditions, histamine could enhance the sensitivity of hippocampal neurons to synaptically mediated excitotoxicity involving NMDA receptors causing local acidification. This may have important implications for the conditions of enhanced glutamatergic transmission with tissue acidification such as cerebral ischemia and epilepsy. However, the authors also reported a depressant action of histamine when alkaline transients occur during normal synaptic release of glutamate conferring neuroprotection. In fact, more recently, it was demonstrated that depending on the concentration, histamine either depressed excitatory synaptic transmission in the basolateral amygdaloid nucleus through presynaptic H_3 receptors or facilitated the same by some unknown mechanism [64].

A study by Yokoyama et al. [65] suggested that histamine may have a role in inhibiting seizures at a younger age to compensate for the immaturity of other protective systems such as GABA. Some speculated the role of cAMP in the anticonvulsant effects of histamine as histamine stimulates adenylate cyclase (AC) and raises cAMP, which has been postulated to have anticonvulsant effects [62]. Some workers demonstrated the role of Ca-calmodulin-dependent protein kinase-II activation pathway in histamine-induced inhibition of seizures [66].

H_3 receptor activation, however, is known to inhibit AC and to reduce intracellular cAMP levels with subsequent reduction of protein kinase A activity. H_3 receptor antagonists including THP, clobenpropit, and ciproxyfan, being inverse agonists, reverse this inhibition of AC and thus increase cAMP [67]. However, even the involvement

---

* Portions of the text have been taken from our review in *Current Neuropharmacology* [61], with permission.

of cAMP in epileptic seizures is controversial. Although it was reported to have anti-convulsant effect by some workers [62], others have shown an increase after discharge generation in rat hippocampal slices following activation of AC and cAMP-dependent protein kinases [68]. Besides the effects of H_3 receptors on inhibiting AC and activation of PLA2 through $G\alpha_{i/o}$ proteins, $G\beta\gamma$ subunits are known to activate mitogen-activated protein kinase (MAPK) pathway [67]. Activation of H_3 receptors leads to phosphorylation of MAPK. The latter is known to be involved in cell growth, differentiation, neuronal plasticity, and memory processes [67]. Increase in MAPK activation in neurons can cause excessive neuronal excitability. Activation of MAPK and their transcription factors is involved in convulsive SE [53]. Activation of MAPK has also been reported in the hippocampus following KA and electrically induced seizures [69]. In fact, agents that inhibit phosphorylation or kinase activation of MAPK cascade have been claimed to have antiepileptic potential [70]. In addition to MAPK, H_3 receptors also activate protein kinase B/serine-threonine kinase (Akt)/glycogen synthase kinase 3β (GSK-3β) axis, which can be reversed by H_3 receptor inverse agonists such as THP [67]. GSK-3β axis is known to play a role in neuronal apoptosis and is altered in neurological disorders including epilepsy and following KA-induced seizures [67,71]. The mechanisms of differential regulation of the H_3 receptor isoforms in experimental seizures has been discussed by Professor Haas in Chapter 3.

Presynaptic H_3 receptors occur both on histaminergic neurons of the CNS (autoreceptors) and on nonhistaminergic neurons of the CNS and autonomic nervous system [72]. Thus, they regulate the release of not only histamine but also other important transmitters such as norepinephrine (NE) [73], dopamine (DA) [74], 5-hydroxytryptamine (5-HT)[75], acetylcholine (Ach)[76] and gamma amino butyric acid (GABA) [47] through heteroreceptors in the CNS. Such effects of H_3 heteroreceptors have been most thoroughly investigated in the mouse brain cortex where they cause inhibition of NE release [77] and in the guinea pig small intestine causing inhibition of ACh release [78]. H_3 receptor antagonists have been demonstrated to enhance whereas histamine and H_3 receptor agonists have been shown to reduce the release of these transmitters in *in vitro* studies. All these transmitters are related in some or the other way to epilepsy and epileptic seizures [57]. Although THP, an H_3 receptor antagonist, was found to increase the release of GABA from the rat hypothalamus [47], RAMH, a selective agonist, inhibited the release [79]. It is needless to emphasize the importance of GABA in seizures and epilepsy. The effect of these ligands on GABA release correlates well with their effects on modulation of seizure activity. A study by Arrang et al. [80], however, demonstrated no inhibition of ACh release from rat entorhinal cortex synaptosomes following H_3 receptor activation. H_3 receptor antagonists also provided protection against amygdala kindling in rats [22]. A reduction in DA and NE content occurs following amygdala kindling [13]. Thus, it is possible that the protection afforded by these agents involve an indirect action through the enhancement of release of these neurotransmitters in brain. However, the dose of THP employed in the study provided protection but did not affect the brain levels of DA, 3,4-dihydroxyphenylacetic acid, 5-HT, and 5-hydoxyindoleacetic acid [23]; thus, ruling out the possibility of involvement of these neurotransmitters in the protective effect. The role for NE, however, may not be overlooked, as H_3 receptors regulating the release of NE are located in the catecholaminergic nerve terminals. However, the modulation of even catecholaminergic tone was also not confirmed by *in vivo* studies [61]. In view of all these observations, the heteroreceptor function seems to play a minor role in contrast with the modulation of histamine release by these receptors [81].

In addition to the aforementioned proposed mechanisms, we have recently reported a neuroprotective potential of THP due to its ability to cause concentration-dependent reduction of intracellular calcium in mouse brain synaptosomes [82]. The latter could be a major mechanism for the antiepileptic and procognitive effects of H_3 receptor antagonists and has implications for various other clinical conditions associated with intracellular calcium accumulation such as cerebral ischemia. Our study was also recently supported by other workers demonstrating a reversal of NMDA-induced excitotoxicity by clobenpropit by increasing GABA release and reducing the intracellular calcium levels in cocultured cortical neurons [83].

CLINICAL STUDIES

The first clinical study on epileptic patients was performed with compound BF 2.649 on pharmacoresistant epilepsy and on photosensitive seizures [5]. For pharmacoresistant epilepsy, patients suffering from high frequency seizures (>10 seizures per month) despite AED treatment were selected. BF 2.649 was administered in doses between 20 and 40 mg/kg for 3 months. Surprisingly, seizure frequency was reduced by 50% in a significant number of patients. In another study on 12 epileptic patients prone to photosensitive seizures, single doses ranging from 20 to 60 mg were studied in patients who were already on AED therapy with uncontrolled photosensitive seizures. BF 2.649 dose dependently suppressed partial or total photo paroxysmal response (PPR). In addition to antiepileptic efficacy, the drug was very well tolerated in both the studies. Thus, BF 2.649 appears to be a promising candidate as an add-on therapy with other AEDs. However, long-term (chronic) toxicological evaluation with specific effects on liver and kidney functions as well as clinical efficacy in a larger group of patients would only determine its fate as a future AED.

EVIDENCE AS AN ENDOGENOUS ANTICONVULSANT

Immediately after a seizure, there is a relative resistance to the induction of further seizure, a state called postictal seizure protection (PSP) or postictal refractory period (PIRP), which possibly is involved in seizure termination. It is possible that the spontaneous arrest of seizures and the PSP/PIRP are due to the activation of endogenous anticonvulsant mechanisms [57]. The TMN located in the PH is the only locus of histaminergic neurons in the brain and sends projections to almost all parts of the brain. Among its five subregions, E2 region contains highest density of histaminergic neurons. Recently, it was reported that a lesion in the E2 region of TMN significantly attenuated PSP in rats in intermittent MES model mediated by lesion-induced reduction of histaminergic activity. Thus, histamine in the TMN may be responsible for the initiation of a postictal refractory state in epileptics [56] and thus can be regarded as an endogenous anticonvulsant substance (EAS). As per criteria laid down for an EAS [57,84], the exogenous administration of histamine produces anticonvulsant action; seizure activity produces changes in the levels of histamine; and the substance is endogenously present, released upon seizures, and is involved in termination of seizure activity.

Interestingly, deep brain stimulation of the TMN in the posterior hypothalamus activated the histaminergic neuronal system to exert antiepileptic effect in PTZ-induced convulsions in rat. TMN stimulation reduced the PTZ-induced seizure duration, prolonged latency and EEG desynchronization. There was a massive release of histamine in the frontal cortex after TMN stimulation. The antiepileptic effect of deep brain stimulation in the TMN was blocked by H_1 antagonist [85].

THERAPEUTIC ADVANTAGE

CENTRAL LOCALIZATION

Brain histamine is found in mast cells or neurons. All histaminergic cell bodies are located in the TMN of the posterior hypothalamus and send projections to all regions of brain and down the spinal cord [86,87]. H_1 and H_3 receptors are especially densed in regions considered relevant for epilepsy, that is, amygdala, cerebral cortex, hippocampus, thalamus, olfactory bulb, and hypothalamus. A highly localized CNS distribution of H_3 receptors is certainly an advantage with less likelihood of peripheral adverse effects.

PROCOGNITIVE EFFECTS

A significant proportion of epileptic patients experience memory disturbances. This is well documented, and several reports are available on the subject [88–90]. Although the underlying brain pathology, type, frequency, and severity of seizures and psychosocial factors play an important role, paradoxically the therapy used (AEDs) also adds to the problem.

Concept of an Inverse Relationship between Seizure Control and Cognitive Function: Is It Unavoidable?

A close look at the scientific data available on the subject suggests an inverse relationship between cellular mechanisms underlying seizure control and cognitive function. Both epilepsy and cognitive function have been linked to abnormalities in the EAA neurotransmission, long-term potentiation (LTP), and GABAergic inhibition in an opposite manner. Furthermore, epilepsy and memory are reported to share the same anatomical loci in the brain in such a way that the regions of brain, considered important for memory, may provoke a seizure [89,90]. Such biological/pharmacological antagonism (e.g., cognitive deficits by AEDs) has been responsible for compromises in the therapeutic approach toward drug therapy and the management of epilepsy for decades.

Histamine and drugs enhancing histaminergic neurotransmission as well as H_3 receptor antagonists appear to have a beneficial role in both seizures and learning/memory processes [91–93]. Several experimental studies confirm a role for H_3 receptor antagonists in improving cognitive functions in various tasks. The details of these ligands in cognitive functions and in specific models of Alzheimer's disease as well as in clinical trials have been discussed in detail in Chapter 7. Their effect on cognitive functions is exciting as majority of the AEDs impair cognition [90,94]. Recently, H_3 receptor antagonists including THP and JNJ-5207852 were found to ameliorate PTZ-kindling-induced learning and mnemonic deficits in social discrimination, acoustic fear conditioning, and passive avoidance test in weanling mice, suggesting a potential of H_3 antagonists in treating cognitive impairment in epileptics [95].

Provigilant Effects

Histamine is considered to be a *waking amine*. Pharmacological blockade of pre-synaptic H_3 receptors promote wakefulness, and its stimulation induces sedation through their action on H_1 receptors [96], and unlike currently available drugs, they are devoid of addictive liability [97]. H_3 receptor stimulation and blockade, thus, holds a lot of promise in the treatment of sleep disorders such as narcolepsy and to promote wakefulness in vigilance deficits. Their potential in treatment of narcolepsy, sleep apnea, and other sleep disorders has been discussed in detail in Chapter 8. Since sedation is a significant problem associated with both classical and newer AEDs [98], the arousal and provigilant effects make them stand apart from other AEDs where sedation and vigilance problems have greatly compromised the quality of life.

Antidepressant and Anxiolytic Effects

A significant percentage of epileptic patients are depressed [99]. Tricyclic antidepressants are well known for their proconvulsant potential [100]. Even selective serotonin reuptake inhibitors (SSRIs) have been reported to have dual effects on seizures, and their use in epileptic patients is controversial [101]. Although there is no direct correlation between histamine and depression, there are indirect evidences such as reduced H_1 receptor binding in depressed patients [102] and that most symptoms observed in depressed patients, such as disturbance of sleep and appetite, are directly associated with functions of the histaminergic neuron system [103]. Interestingly, histamine, L-histidine, and THP have been reported to significantly ameliorate seizures induced by imipramine in amygdala-kindled rats [104]. Since imipramine has H_1 antagonistic effects, histaminergic mechanisms possibly contribute to its proconvulsant effects. There are a very few studies reporting antidepressant potential of H_3 receptor antagonist in animal models of depression [105,106]. However, not many reports are available, and whether an H_3 receptor antagonist would be effective in epileptic patients who are depressed is yet to be investigated. Interestingly, Johnson & Johnson recently combined H_3 blockade with selective serotonin reuptake inhibitors (SSRIs); however, not for antidepressant efficacy but for combating fatigue of SSRIs.

Although there is some literature available regarding their role in anxiety as well, generally the reports do not point toward a significant role of these ligands in anxiety (see Chapter 12). Our studies on THP and RAMH did not reveal any modulation of anxiety in elevated plus maze and Vogel's conflict test in mice [107].

CONCLUSION

The potential of histamine H_3 receptor ligands in epileptic seizures highlights an important role of histaminergic mechanisms in the pathophysiology of epilepsy and thus identifies histamine as yet another novel molecular target that can be exploited for AED development. Although the roles of neuronal histamine and H_3 receptor ligands have been extensively investigated in animal models of epilepsy, a very few human studies are available. BF 2.649 is the only H_3 receptor antagonist that has reached phase II in clinical trials on epileptic patients. In view of a lot of advantages that H_3 receptor antagonists promise to offer over the present AEDs (as discussed previously) coupled with efficacy in pharmacoresistant model of epilepsy in rodents and epileptic patients, it becomes exciting to evaluate other nonimidazole H_3 receptor antagonists in human studies also warranting detailed toxicological evaluation, drug–drug interactions, and teratogenic potential that are the drawbacks of the available AEDs. Only time will tell if we will see yet another class of novel AEDs.

REFERENCES

1. Kwan, P. and Brodie, M. J. 2000. Early identification of refractory epilepsy. *N. Engl. J. Med.* 342: 314–319.
2. Brodie, M. J. 2005. Diagnosing and predicting early refractory epilepsy. *Acta Neurol. Scand. Suppl.* 181: 36–39.
3. Churchill, J. A. and Gammon, G. D. 1949. The effect of antihistaminic drugs on convulsive seizures. *JAMA* 141: 18–21.
4. Wyngarden, J. B. and Seevers, M. H. 1951. The toxic effects of antihistaminic drugs. *JAMA* 145: 277–283.
5. Schwartz, J. C. and Lecomte, J. 2006. Treatment of epilepsy with non-imidazole alkylamine histamine H_3 receptor ligands, WO2006103537A2.
6. Yokoyama, H. 2001. The role of central histaminergic neuron system as an anticonvulsive mechanism in the developing brain. *Brain Dev.* 23: 542–547.
7. Gerald, M. C. and Richter, N. A. 1976. Studies on the effects of histaminergic agents on seizure susceptibility in mice. *Psychopharmacologia* 46: 277–282.
8. Sturman, G. and Freeman, P. 1992. Histaminergic modulation and chemically-induced seizures in mice. *Agents Actions* C358–C360.
9. Yokoyama, H., Onodera, K., Iinuma, K. and Watanabe T. 1994. 2-Thiazolylethylamine, a selective histamine H_1-agonist, decreases seizure susceptibility in mice. *Pharmacol. Biochem. Behav.* 47: 503–507.
10. Feng, H. and Faingold, C. L. 2000. Modulation of audiogenic seizures by histamine and adenosine receptors in the inferior colliculus. *Exp. Neurol.* 163: 264–270.
11. Scherkl, R., Hashem, A. and Frey, H. H. 1991. Histamine in brain: its role in regulation of seizure susceptibility. *Epilepsy Res.* 10: 111–118.
12. Yokoyama, H., Onodera, K., Maeyama, K., Yanai, K., Iinuma, K., Tuomisto, L. and Watanabe, T. 1992. Histamine levels and clonic convulsions of electrically induced seizures in mice: the effects of α-fluoromethylhistidine and metoprine. *Naunyn-Schmiedeberg's Arch. Pharmacol.* 346: 40–45.
13. Kamei, C., Ishizawa, K., Kakinoki, H. and Fakunaga, M. 1998. Histaminergic mechanisms in amygdaloid kindled seizures in rats. *Epilepsy Res.* 30: 187–194.
14. Zhang, L. S., Chen, Z., Huang, Y. W., Hu, W. W., Wei, E. Q. and Yanai, K. 2003. Effects of endogenous histamine on seizure development of pentylenetetrazole induced kindling in rats. *Pharmacology* 69: 27–32.

15. Yawata, I., Tanaka, K., Nakagawa, Y., Watanabe, Y., Murashima, Y. L. and Nakano, K. 2004. Role of histaminergic neurons in development of epileptic seizures in EL mice. *Mol. Brain Res.* 132: 13–17.

16. Tasaka, K., Kamei, C., Katayama, S., Kitazumi, K., Akahuri, H. and Hokonohara, T. 1986. Comparative study of various H1-blockers on neuropharmacological and behavioral effects including 1-(2-ethoxyethyl)-2-)4-methyl-1-homopiperazinyl) benzimidazole difumarate (KB-2413), a new antiallergic agent. *Arch. Int. Pharmacodyn. Ther.* 280: 275–291.

17. Fujii, Y., Tanaka, T., Harada, C., Hirai, T. and Kamei, C. 2003. Epileptogenic activity induced by histamine H_1 antagonists in amygdala-kindled rats. *Brain Res.* 991: 258–261.

18. Swaider, M., Wielsoz, M. and Czuczwar, S. J. 2003. Interaction of astemizole, an H_1 receptor antagonist, with conventional antiepileptic drugs in mice. *Pharmacol. Biochem. Behav.* 76: 169–178.

19. Swaider, M., Weilosz, M. and Czuczwar, S. J. 2004. Influence of antazoline and ketotifen on the anticonvulsant activity of conventional antiepileptics against maximal electroshock in mice. *Eur. Neuropsychopharmacol.* 14: 307–318.

20. Yokoyama, H., Onodera, K., Maeyama, K., Sakurai, E., Iinuma, K., Leurs, R., Timmerman, H. and Watanabe, T. 1994. Clobenpropit (VUF-9153), a new histamine H_3 receptor antagonist, inhibits electrically induced convulsions in mice. *Eur. J. Pharmacol.* 260: 23–28.

21. Shimokawa, M., Yamamoto, K., Kawakami, J., Sawada, Y. and Iga, T. 1996. Neurotoxic convulsions induced by histamine H_2 receptor antagonists in mice. *Toxicol. Appl. Pharmacol.* 136: 317–323.

22. Kakinoki, H., Ishizawa, K., Fakunaga, M., Fujie, Y. and Kamei, C. 1998. The effects of histamine H_3 receptor antagonists on amygdaloid kindled seizures in rats. *Brain Res. Bull.* 46: 461–465.

23. Yokoyama, H., Onodera, K., Iinuma, K. and Watanabe, T. 1993. Effects of thioperamide, a histamine H_3 receptor antagonist, on electrically-induced convulsions in mice. *Eur. J. Pharmacol.* 234: 129–133.

24. Vohora, D., Pal, S. N. and Pillai, K. K. 2000. Thioperamide, a selective H_3 receptor antagonist, protects against PTZ induced seizures in mice. *Life Sci.* 66: 297–301.

25. Yoshida, M., Noguchi, E. and Tsuru, N. 2000. Lack of substantial effect of the H_3 antagonist thioperamide and of the non-selective mixed H_3-antagonist/H_1-agonist betahistine on amygdaloid kindled seizures. *Epilepsy Res.* 40: 141–145.

26. Fischer, W. and van der Goot, H. 1998. Effect of clobenpropit, a centrally acting histamine H_3 receptor antagonist, on electroshock and pentylenetetrazole induced seizures in mice. *J. Neural. Transm.* 105: 587–599.

27. Kamei, C. and Okuma, C. 2001. Role of central histamine in amygdaloid kindled seizures. *Nippon Yakurigaku Zasshi* 117: 329–334.

28. Harada, C., Fujii, Y., Hirai, T., Shinomiya, K. and Kamei, C. 2004. Inhibitory effect of iodophenpropit, a selective H_3 antagonist, on amygdaloid kindled seizures. *Brain Res. Bull.* 63: 143–146.

29. Chen, Z., Li, Z., Sakuai, E., Izadi Mobarakeh, J., Ohtsu, H., Watanabe, T., Iinuma, K. and Yanai, K. 2003. Chemical kindling induced by PTZ in histamine H_1 receptor gene knock out mice (H(1)KO), histidine decarboxylase deficient mice (HDC (-1-)) and mast cell deficient w/w(v) mice. *Brain Res.* 968: 162–166.

30. Hirai, T., Okuma, C., Harada, C., Mio, M., Ohtsu, H., Watanabe, T. and Kamei, C. 2004. Development of amygdaloid kindling in histidine decarboxylase deficient and histamine H_1 receptor deficient mice. *Epilepsia* 45: 309–313.

31. Toyota, H., Ito, C., Yanai, K., Sato, M. and Watanabe, T. 1999. Histamine H_1 receptor binding capacities in the amygdalas of amygdaloid kindled rat. *J. Neurochem.* 72: 2177–2180.

32. Iinuma, K., Yokoyama, H., Otsuki, T., Yanai, K., Watanabe, T. and Itoh, M. 1993. Histamine H_1 receptors in complex partial seizures. *Lancet* 341: 238.
33. Midzyanovskaya, I. S. and Tuomisto, L. 2003. Increased density of H_1 histamine receptors in brain regions of rats with absence epilepsy. *Inflammatory Res.* 52(Suppl 1): S29–S30.
34. VonEinsidel, R. W., Roesch-Ely, D., Diebold, D., Sartor, K., Mundt, C. and Bergemann, N. 2002. Histamine H_2 antagonist (famotidine) induced adverse CNS reactions with long standing secondary mania and epileptic seizures. *Pharmacopsychiatry* 35: 152–154.
35. Zhang, L., Chen, Z., Ren, K., Leurs, R., Chen, J., Zhang, W., Ye, B., Wei, E. and Timmerman, H. 2003. Effects of clobenpropit on pentylenetetrazole-kindled seizures in rats. *Eur. J. Pharmacol.* 482: 169–175.
36. Sturman, G., Freeman, P., Meade, H. M. and Seelay, N. A. 1994. Modulation of intracellular and H_3 histamine receptors on chemically induced seizures in mice. *Agents Actions* 41(special conference issue): C68–C69.
37. Loscher, W. and Schmidt, D. 1988. Which animal models should be used in the search for new antiepileptic drugs? A proposal based on experimental and clinical considerations. *Epilepsy Res.* 2: 145–181.
38. McNamara, J. O. 1984. Kindling: an animal model of complex partial epilepsy. *Ann. Neurol.* 16: S72–S76.
39. McNamara, J. O. 1988. Pursuit of the mechanisms of kindling. *Trends Neurosci.* 11: 32–36.
40. Schwartz, J. C., Arrang, J. M., Garbarg, M. and Pollard, H. 1991. The third histamine receptor. In: *Histaminergic Neurons: Morphology and Function*, eds. T. Watanabe and H. Wada, pp. 85–104, CRC Press, Boca Raton, FL.
41. Zhu, Y., Zhu-Ge, Z.-B., Wu, D., Wang, S., Liu, L., Ohtsu, H. and Zhong, C. 2007. Carnosine inhibits pentylenetetrazol-induced seizures by histaminergic mechanisms in histidine decarboxylase knock-out mice. *Neurosci. Lett.* 416: 211–216.
42. Wu, X., Ding, M., Zhu-Ge, Z.-B., Zhu, Y., Jin, C. and Zhong, C. 2006. Carnosine, a precursor of histidine, ameliorates pentylenetetrazole-induced kindled seizures in rat. *Neurosci. Lett.* 400: 146–149.
43. Harada, C., Hirai, T., Fujii, Y., Harusawa, S., Kurihara, T. and Kamei, C. 2004. Intracerebroventricular administration of histamine H_3 receptor antagonists decreases seizures in rat models of epilepsy. *Methods Find. Exp. Clin. Pharmacol.* 26: 263–270.
44. Wada, Y., Shiraishi, J., Nakamura, M. and Koshino, Y. 1996. Biphasic action of the histamine precursor ʟ-histidine in the rat kindling model of epilepsy. *Neurosci. Lett.* 204: 205–208.
45. Yanovsky, Y. and Haas, H. L. 1998. Histamine increases the bursting activity of pyramidal cells in the CA3 region of the mouse hippocampus. *Neurosci. Lett.* 240: 110–112.
46. Vorobjev, V. S., Sharonova, I. N., Walsh, I. V. and Haas, H. L. 1993. Histamine potentiates NMDA responses in acutely isolated hippocampal neurons. *Neuron* 11: 837–844.
47. Yamamoto, Y., Mochizuki, T., Okakura-Mochizuki, K., Uno, A. and Yamamatodani, A. 1997. Thioperamide, a histamine H_3 receptor antagonist, increases GABA release from the rat hypothalamus. *Methods Find. Exp. Clin. Pharmacol.* 19: 289–298.
48. Ishizawa, K., Chen, Z., Okuma, C., Sugimoto, Y., Fujii, Y. and Kamei, C. 2000. Participation of GABAergic and histaminergic systems in inhibiting amygdaloid kindled seizures. *Jpn. J. Pharmacol.* 82: 48–53.
49. Sakai, N., Sakurai, E., Onodera, K., Sakurai, E., Asada, H., Miura, Y. and Watanabe, T. 1996. Long-term depletion of brain histamine induced by α-FMH increases feeding-associated locomotor activity in mice with a modulation of brain amino acid levels. *Behav. Brain Res.* 72: 83–88.
50. Onodera, K., Tuomisto, L., Tacke, U. and Airaksinen, M. 1992. Strain differences in regional brain histamine levels between genetically epilepsy prone and resistant rats. *Methods Find. Exp. Clin. Pharmacol.* 14: 13–16.

51. Gupta, Y. K., Malhotra, J., George, B. and Kulkarni, S. K. 1999. Methods and considerations for experimental evaluation of antiepileptic drugs. *Indian J. Physiol. Pharmacol.* 43: 25–43.

52. Jin, C., Lintunen, M. and Panula, P. 2005. Histamine H_1 and H_3 receptors in the rat thalamus and their modulation after systemic kainic acid administration. *Exp. Neurol.* 194: 43–56.

53. Lintunen, M., Sallmen, T., Karlstedt, K. and Panula, P. 2005. Transient changes in the limbic histaminergic system after Kainic acid induced seizures. *Neurobiol. Dis.* 20: 155–169.

54. Kukko-Lukjanov, T., Soini, S., Taira, T., Michelsen, K. A., Panula, P. and Holopainen, I. E. 2006. Histaminergic neurons protect the developing hippocampus from kainic acid-induced neuronal damage in an organotypic coculture system. *Neurobiol. Dis.* 26: 1088–1097.

55. Vohora, D., Pal, S. N. and Pillai, K. K. 2001. Histamine and selective H_3 receptor ligands: a possible role in the mechanism and management of epilepsy. *Pharmacol. Biochem. Behav.* 68: 735–741.

56. Jin, C., Zhuge, Z., Wu, D., Zhu, Y., Wang, S., Luo, J. and Chen, Z. 2007. Lesion of the tuberomamillary nucleus E2-region attenuates post-ictal seizure protection in rats. *Epilepsy Res.* 73: 250–258.

57. Dragunow, M. 1986. Endogenous anticonvulsant substances. *Neurosci. Biobehav. Rev.* 10: 229–244.

58. Schatz, R. A. and Sellinger, O. Z. 1975. The elevation of cerebral histamine-N- and catechol-o-methyl transferase activities by l-methionine-dl-sulfoximine. *J. Neurochem.* 25: 73–78.

59. Kaminski, R. M., Zolkowska, D., Kozicka, M., Kleinrok Z. and Czuczwar, S. J. 2004. l-histidine is a beneficial adjuvant for antiepileptic drugs against maximal electroshock induced seizures in mice. *Amino Acids* 26: 85–89.

60. Yokoyama, H., Onodera, K., Yaqi, T. and Iinuma, K. 1997. Therapeutic doses of theophylline exert proconvulsant effect in developing mice. *Brain Dev.* 19: 403–407.

61. Vohora, D., Pal, S. N. and Pillai, K. K. 2004. Histamine as an anticonvulsant inhibitory neurotransmitter. *Curr. Neuropharmacol.* 2: 419–425.

62. Tuomisto, L. and Tacke, U. 1986. Is histamine an anticonvulsive inhibitory transmitter? *Neuropharmacol.* 25: 955–958.

63. Skaper, S. D., Facci, L., Kee, W. J. and Strijbos, P. J. L. M. 2001. Potentiation by histamine of synaptically mediated excitotoxicity in cultured hippocampal neurons: a possible role for mast cells. *J. Neurochem.* 76: 47–55.

64. Jiang, X., Chen, A. and Li, H. 2005. Histaminergic modulation of excitatory synaptic transmission in the rat basolateral amygdala. *Neuroscience* 131: 691–703.

65. Yokoyama, H., Onodera, K., Iinuma, K. and Watanabe, T. 1993. Proconvulsive effects of histamine H_1 antagonists on electrically induced seizures in developing mice. *Psychopharmacologia* 112: 199–203.

66. Okuma, C., Hirai, T. and Kamei, C. 2001. Mechanism of inhibitory effect of histamine on amygdaloid kindled seizures on rats. *Epilepsia* 42: 1494–1500.

67. Bongers, G., Bakker, R. A. and Leurs, R. 2007. Molecular aspects of the histamine H_3 receptor. *Biochem. Pharmacol.* 73: 1195–1204.

68. Higashima, M., Ohno, K. and Koshino, Y. 2002. Cyclic AMP-mediated modulation of epileptiform afterdischarge generation in rat hippocampal slices. *Brain Res.* 949: 157–161.

69. Jeon, S. H., Kim, Y. S., Bae, C. and Park, J. 2000. Activation of JNK and p38 in rat hippocampus after kainic acid induced seizure. *Exp. Mol. Med.* 32: 227–230.

70. Sweatt, D. J. and Anderson, A. E. 2002. Methods for treating seizure disorders by inhibiting MAPK pathway activation with nitriles. WO2002/002097.

71. Crespo-Biel, N., Canudas, A. M., Camins, A. and Pallas, M. 2007. Kainate induces AKT, ERK and cdk5/GSK3β pathway deregulation, phosphorylates tau protein in mouse hippocampus. *Neurochem. Int.* 50: 435–442.

72. Schlicker, E., Kathmann, M., Bitschnau, H. et al. 1996. Potencies of antagonists chemically related to iodoproxyfan at histamine H_3 receptors in mouse brain cortex and guinea pig ileum: evidence for H_3 receptor heterogeneity. *Naunyn-Scheimedeberg's Arch. Pharmacol.* 353: 482–488.

73. Schlicker, E., Fink, K., Hinterthaner, M. and Gothert, M. 1989. Inhibition of noradrenaline release in the rat brain cortex by presynaptic H_3 receptors. *Naunyn-Schemiedeberg's Arch. Pharmacol.* 340: 633–638.

74. Schlicker, E., Fink, K., Detzner, M. and Gothert, M. 1993. Histamine inhibits dopamine release in the mouse striatum via presynaptic H_3 receptors. *J. Neural. Transm.* 93: 1–10.

75. Schlicker, E., Betz, R. and Gothert, M. 1988. Histamine H_3 receptor mediated inhibition of serotonergic release in the rat brain cortex. *Naunyn-Schmiedeberg's Arch. Pharmacol.* 337: 588–590.

76. Blandina, P., Giorgetti, M., Bartoline, L., Cecchi, M., Timmerman, H., Leurs, R., Pepea, G. and Giovannini, M. G. 1996. Inhibition of cortical acetylcholine release and cognitive performance by histamine H_3 receptor activation in rats. *Br. J. Pharmacol.* 119: 1656–1664.

77. Schlicker, E., Behling, A., Lummen, G. and Gothert, M. 1992. Histamine H_{3A}-receptor mediated inhibition of noradrenaline release in the mouse brain cortex. *Naunyn-Schmiedeberg's Arch. Pharmacol.* 345: 489–493.

78. Hew, R. W. S., Hodgkinson, C. R. and Hill, S. J. 1990. Characterization of histamine H_3 receptors in guinea pig ileum with H_3 selective ligands. *Br. J. Pharmacol.* 101: 621–624.

79. Jang, I. S., Rhee, J. S., Watanabe, T. and Akaike, N. 2001. Histaminergic modulation of GABAergic transmission in rat ventromedial hypothalamic neurons. *J. Physiol.* 534: 791–803.

80. Arrang, J. M., Drutel, G. and Schwartz, J. C. 1995. Characterization of histamine H_3 receptors regulating ACh release in rat entorhinal cortex. *Br. J. Pharmacol.* 114: 1518–1522.

81. Oishi, R., Nishibori, M., Itoh, Y., Shishido, S. and Saeki, K 1990. Is monoamine turnover in the brain regulated by histamine H_3 receptor? *Eur. J. Pharmacol.* 184: 135–142.

82. Vohora, D., Pal, S. N. and Pillai, K. K. 2007. Thioperamide reduces intracellular calcium in mouse brain synaptosomes. *Eur. Neuropsychopharmacol.* 17: 375–376.

83. Dai, H., Fu, Q., Shen, Y., Hu, W., Zhang, Z., Timmerman, H., Leurs, R. and Chen, Z. 2007. The histamine H_3 receptor antagonist clobenpropit enhances GABA release to protect against NMDA-induced excitotoxicity through the cAMP/ protein kinase A pathway in cultured cortical neurons. *Eur. J. Pharmacol.* 563: 117–123.

84. Gupta, Y. K. and Malhotra, J. 1997. Adenosinergic system as an endogenous anticonvulsant mechanism. *Indian J. Physiol. Pharmacol.* 41: 329–343.

85. Nishida, N., Huang, Z., Mikuni, N., Miura, Y., Urade, Y. and Hashimoto, N. 2007. Deep brain stimulation of the posterior hypothalamus activates the histaminergic system to exert antiepileptic effect in rat pentylenetetrazole model. *Exp. Neurol.* 205: 132–144.

86. Lipinski, J. F., Schaumburg, H. H. and Baldessarini, R. J. 1973. Regional distribution of histamine in human brain. *Brain Res.* 52: 403–408

87. Wada, H., Inagaki, N., Yamatodani, A. and Watanabe, T. 1991. Is the histaminergic neuron system a regulatory center for whole brain activity? *Trends Neurol. Sci.* 14: 415–418.

88. Thompson, P. J. 1991. Memory function in patients with epilepsy. *Adv. Neurol.* 55: 369–384.

89. Halgren, E., Stapleton, J., Domalski, P., Swartz, B. E., Delgado-Escueta, A. V., Walsh, G. O., Mandelkern, M., Blahd, W. and Ropchan, J. 1991. Memory dysfunction in epilepsy patients as a derangement of normal physiology. *Adv. Neurol.* 55: 385–410.

90. Smith, D. B. 1991. Cognitive effects of antiepileptic drugs. *Adv. Neurol.* 55: 197–212.

91. Vohora, D. 2005. Histamine, selective H_3 receptor ligands and cognitive functions: an overview. *IDrugs* 7: 667–673.

92. Medhurst, A. D., Atkins, A. R., Beresford, I. J. et al. 2007. GSK 189254, a novel H_3 receptor antagonist that binds to histamine H_3 receptors in Alzheimer's disease brain and improves cognitive performance in preclinical models. *J. Pharmacol. Exp. Ther.* 321: 1032–1045.

93. Witkin, J. M. and Nelson, D. L. 2004. Selective histamine H_3 receptor antagonists for treatment of cognitive deficiencies and other disorders of the central nervous system. *Pharmacol. Ther.* 103: 1–20.

94. Aldencamp, A. P., DeKrom, M. and Reijs, R. 2003. Newer antiepileptic drugs and cognitive issues. *Epilepsia* 44(Suppl 4): 21–29.

95. Jia, F., Kato, M., Dai, H., Xu, A., Okuda, T., Sakurai, E., Okamura, M., Lovenberg, T. W., Barbier, A., Carruthers, N. I., Iinuma, K. and Yanai, K. 2006. Effects of histamine H_3 receptor antagonists and donepezil on learning and mnemonic deficits induced by PTZ kindling in weanling mice. *Neuropharmacology* 50: 404–411.

96. Huang, Z. L., Mochizuki, T., Qu, W. M. et al. 2006. Altered sleep–wake characteristics and lack of arousal response to H_3 receptor antagonist in H_1 receptor knock-out mice. *Proc. Natl Acad. Sci. U.S.A.* 103: 4687–4692.

97. Komater, V. A., Browman, K. E., Curzon, P., Hancock, A. A., Decker, M. W. and Fox, G. B. 2003. H_3 receptor blockade by thioperamide enhances cognition in rats without inducing locomotor sensitization. *Psychopharmacologia* 167: 363–372.

98. Roks, G., Deckers, C. L. P., Meinardi, H., Dirkson, R., Egmond, J. V. and Rijn, C. M. 1999. Effects of polytherapy combined with monotherapy in antiepileptic drugs: an animal study. *J. Pharmacol. Exp. Ther.* 288: 472–477.

99. Attarian, H., Vahle, V., Cartar, J., Hykes, E. and Gilliam, F. 2003. Relationship between depression and intractability of seizures. *Epilepsy Behav.* 4: 298–301.

100 Preskorn, S. H. and Fast, G. A. 1992. Tricyclic antidepressant-induced seizures and plasma drug concentration. *J. Clin. Psychiatry* 53: 160–162.

101. Marwah, R., Pal, S. N. and Pillai, K. K. 1999. Effect of fluoxetine on increasing current electroshock seizures (ICES) in mice. *Indian J. Pharmacol.* 31: 350–353.

102. Kano, M., Fukudo, S., Tashiro, A., Utsumi, A., Tamura, D., Itoh, M., Iwata, R., Tashiro, M., Mochizuki, H., Funaki, Y., Kato, M., Hongo, M. and Yanai, K. 2004. Decrease histamine H_1 receptor binding in the brain of depressed patients. *Eur. J. Neurosci.* 20: 803–810.

103. Yanai, K. and Tashiro, M. 2007. The physiological and pathophysiological roles of neuronal histamine: an insight from human positron emission tomography studies. *Pharmacol. Ther.* 113: 1–15.

104. Ago, J., Ishikawa, T., Matsumoto, M., Rahman, M. A. and Kamei, C. 2004. Mechanism of imipramine-induced seizures in amygdala kindled rats. *Epilepsy Res.* 72: 1–9.

105. Akhtar, M., Pillai, K. K. and Vohora, D. 2005. Effect of thioperamide on modified forced swimming test-induced oxidative stress in mice. *Basic Clin. Pharmacol. Toxicol.* 97: 218–221.

106. Perez-Garcia, C., Morales, L., Cano, M. V., Sancho, I. and Alguacil, L. F. 1999. Effects of histamine H_3 receptor ligands in experimental models of anxiety and depression. *Psychopharmacologia* 142: 215–220.

107. Akhtar, M. 2008. Selective histamine H_3 receptor ligands as modulators of CNS functions. PhD Thesis, Jamia Hamdard, New Delhi.

11 Schizophrenia

Kaitlin E. Browman, Min Zhang, Gerard B. Fox, and Lynne E. Rueter

CONTENTS

Introduction 330
Disease State 330
Therapeutic Options and Considerations 331
    Current Therapies 331
    Unmet Medical Need 332
Theories of the Disease Basis 333
    Dopamine Hypothesis 334
    Glutamate Hypothesis 334
    Neurodevelopmental Hypothesis 334
Rationale for H_3 Receptor Antagonist Efficacy in Schizophrenia 335
    Neuroanatomical Rationale 335
    Neurochemical and Functional Rationale 337
Experimental Disease Models 338
    Animal Models of Schizophrenia 338
        Dopaminergic Hypothesis 338
        Glutamatergic Hypothesis 340
        Sensorimotor Gating 340
        Side-Effect Liabilities 341
    Preclinical Profiling of H_3 Receptor Antagonists/Inverse Agonists 342
        Psychomotor Stimulant-Induced Hyperactivity 342
        Apomorphine-Induced Climbing Behavior 342
        Potential Mechanisms Underlying the Antagonistic Interactions
            between H_3 Receptor Antagonists and Dopamine
            Agonists 342
        MK-801-Induced Hyperlocomotion 344
        Sensorimotor Gating: Prepulse Inhibition 344
        Sensorimotor Gating: N40 Gating 344
        Cataleptic Potential 345
Potential Future Directions 345
Conclusions 346
References 347

INTRODUCTION

Schizophrenia is a devastating chronic mental illness that impacts all aspects of life function. As a heterogeneous disorder, it comprises classical symptoms such as positive (e.g., delusions and hallucinations) and negative symptoms (e.g., blunted affect and social withdrawal) as well as cognitive deficits (e.g., impaired attention, memory, and executive function). More than 50 years ago, the first antipsychotic, chlorpromazine, was discovered, and the treatment of schizophrenia was radically changed as it became possible to significantly reduce positive symptoms. However, although many antipsychotics have subsequently been developed, it has become apparent that current therapies are not sufficient. Namely, these medications show limited efficacy against negative symptoms and cognitive deficits associated with schizophrenia. The current desire in drug development is to discover medications that would more broadly treat the symptoms of schizophrenia and adjunctive medications with significant efficacy against negative symptoms or cognitive deficits.

Although the predominant theories of the neuropathology of schizophrenia implicate neurodevelopmental processes and the dopaminergic and glutamatergic systems, there has been an increasing interest in the potential role of the histaminergic system in the pathology and treatment of the disorder. As evidence, there are reports of alterations in the functioning of the histaminergic system in schizophrenic patients. Additionally, histamine receptor subtypes such as the histamine H_3 receptor exhibit receptor localization and neuroanatomical connectivity that suggest a potential role in the treatment of schizophrenia. This chapter explores the disease state and disease basis of schizophrenia, summarizes experimental disease models of the disorder, and focuses largely on the putative role of H_3 receptor antagonists/inverse agonists as potential therapies.

DISEASE STATE

Schizophrenia is a complex, heterogeneous psychiatric disorder that affects between 0.5 and 1.5% of the worldwide population [1,2]. With a typical differential diagnosis in the late teens or twenties, it is a lifelong illness with worsening life function and poorer prognosis as the disease progresses. In addition to personal suffering of both the individuals with the schizophrenia and their families, the social burden of the disorder is substantial including sizeable health care costs as well as high levels of lost productivity [1]. Finally, schizophrenia is associated with significantly increased mortality, attributable to varying factors such as suicide and increased rates of cardiovascular disease [3]. There is no single defining symptom and, to date, a diagnosis of schizophrenia requires the observation and recognition of a constellation of positive (e.g., delusions, hallucinations) or negative symptoms (e.g., affective flattening, poverty of speech) [4] (Table 11.1).

In addition to the central symptom clusters, there are well-described cognitive deficits associated with schizophrenia. These include impaired attention, poor executive functioning, and deficits in working memory [5] (Table 11.1).

TABLE 11.1

Overview of the Symptom Clusters of Schizophrenia, Ability of Currently Available Antipsychotic Medication to Alleviate the Symptom Clusters, and Predominate Theories for Neurochemical Disturbances Underlying Each Cluster

Symptom Cluster	Typical Symptoms	Addressed by Antipsychotic Medication	Predominant Theories
Positive symptoms	Delusions Hallucinations Disorganized speech Grossly disorganized or catatonic behavior	Adequately, although relapse can occur	Dopamine hyperactivity
Negative symptoms	Affective flattening Alogia Avolition Anhedonia [6]	Poorly	Dopamine hypofunction NMDA hypofunction
Associated cognitive deficits[a] [5]	Attention/vigilance Executive function/ reasoning and problem solving Working memory Social cognition Verbal learning and memory Speed of processing Visual learning and memory	Poorly	Dopamine hypofunction Cholinergic hypofunction Serotonergic imbalance Glutamatergic imbalance Histaminergic imbalance

[a] From the NIMH initiative titled Measurement and Treatment Research to Improve Cognition in Schizophrenia (MATRICS) program.

THERAPEUTIC OPTIONS AND CONSIDERATIONS

CURRENT THERAPIES

There are currently a substantial number of antipsychotic medications available. These are typically divided into conventional or first-generation antipsychotics (FGAs) and atypical or second-generation antipsychotics (SGAs). The distinction between FGAs and SGAs is made based on relative affinities of the drugs for dopamine (DA) versus serotonin (5-HT) receptors and the relative rates of induction of side effects such as extrapyramidal symptoms (EPS). Thus, FGAs are predominately preferential DA D_2 antagonists, whereas SGAs have a more balanced affinity profile between DA D_2 and 5-HT$_{2A}$ receptors [7]. This distinction is simplistic to a degree since SGAs, as well as FGAs, have affinity for other receptors beyond D_2 and 5-HT$_{2A}$, and since the affinity profiles of individual drugs within the SGA class can be quite

TABLE 11.2

Overview of Currently Available Antipsychotic Medications

	Examples of Available Medications: Drug Name (Trade Name)	Primary Receptor Affinities	Primary Side-Effect Profile
FGA	Haloperidol (Haldol™), Chlorpromazine (Thorazine™) Perphenazine (Minitran™, Trilafon™) Thioridazine (Melleril™)	D_2	High incidence of EPS and prolactin elevation, sedation
SGA	Clozapine (Clozaril™) Risperidone (Risperdal™) Olanzapine (Zyprexa™) Aripiprazole (Abilify™) Quetiapine (Seroquel™) Ziprasidone (Geodon™)	D_2, 5-HT_{2A} Differential affinities for 5-HT_{1A}, α_1 adrenergic, H_1 histaminergic, M_1 muscarinic	Decreased incidence of EPS and prolactin elevation For some antipsychotics, increased incidence of weight gain/dyslipidemia/diabetes

distinct from each other (Table 11.2); however, it has proved to be a useful heuristic in the classification of antipsychotic medications [7]. The second classical distinction between FGAs and SGAs is the differential risk of D_2-mediated side effects such as EPS and prolactin elevation. Again, the distinction is somewhat simplistic as many SGAs can also induce these side effects at higher doses. However, there is typically a greater therapeutic window between an efficacious dose and a dose that induces EPS for SGAs, an increased safety window that is attributed to additional antipsychotic activity being mediated through affinities at receptors such as the 5-HT_{2A} and 5-HT_{1A} receptor and blockade of side-effect induction through affinities at receptors such as the 5-HT_{1A} receptor [7,8].

Although EPS induction and prolactin elevation are a significant problem for FGAs and can be a problem for high doses of some SGAs such as risperidone (Risperdal) [9], there are other side effects that are worth noting. Most antipsychotic medications induce sedation [10]. SGAs such as clozapine and olanzapine can induce significant weight gain and have been associated with the onset of dyslipidemia and diabetes [10] (see Table 11.2 for summary) and may have the potential for exacerbating the higher prevalence of metabolic syndrome risk factors present in patients with schizophrenia [11]. Thus, future compounds that can positively impact weight gain or the metabolic syndrome should be beneficial to treating this disorder.

UNMET MEDICAL NEED

Despite the number of antipsychotic medications available, there remains a significant unmet need in the treatment of schizophrenia. Some patients do not respond to the medications, whereas others show only a partial response [7]. In particular, although these medications attenuate positive symptoms in most patients, they often have a minimal effect on negative symptoms or cognitive deficits. It has become increasingly apparent that the presence of these residual negative and cognitive symptoms is highly predictive of acute symptom relapse, low social and life functioning, and a poor lifetime prognosis [12].

Cognitive deficits are estimated to occur in 75–80% of patients diagnosed with schizophrenia [13]. Indeed, cognitive deficits of schizophrenia, including impairments in areas such as memory, attention, and executive function, often precede the onset of clinical symptoms in patients [13] and are a major determinant and predictor of long-term disability in schizophrenia. For example, although nearly all patients with schizophrenia receive pharmacological treatment, according to the 2004 NOP World study of schizophrenia, nearly 80% remain unemployed. In addition, the suicide rate in this population is very high, underlining the need for treatments that improve the functional outcome for the patients.

For some time, it has been postulated that SGAs such as olanzapine, ziprasidone, and risperidone are more effective at treating negative symptoms and cognitive deficits associated with schizophrenia [14]. However, recent evidence from the Clinical Antipsychotic Trials in Intervention Effectiveness (CATIE) suggests that although SGAs and low dose administration of FGAs share a modest but significant ability to attenuate negative symptoms, this modest efficacy is not sufficient to return patients to normal levels of psychosocial function or to significantly improve their quality of life [15].

No drugs are currently indicated for the treatment of cognitive deficits associated with schizophrenia although there is an ongoing collaboration among NIMH, industry, and the FDA (measurement and treatment research to improve cognition in schizophrenia [MATRICS], www.matrics.ucla.edu) designed to elucidate a pathway to evaluate compounds for this indication. Although atypical antipsychotics are the mainstay of treating the psychotic symptoms of schizophrenia and some have offered some benefit in treating cognitive symptoms [16], they are not expected to compete with novel agents developed to treat this subset of symptoms. Rather, the use of atypical antipsychotics in combination with agents designed to improve cognitive function is likely to be the next step in effectively treating cognitive disorders association with schizophrenia.

THEORIES OF THE DISEASE BASIS

To understand the proposed role of the histaminergic system in the etiology of schizophrenia and the potential capacity of H_3 receptor antagonists to treat aspects of the disorder, it is first important to review the most widely accepted theories on the neurological bases of schizophrenia. Although many mechanisms, receptors, and neurotransmitters have been proposed to play a role in the development and expression of schizophrenia, three theories predominate. They are the DA hypothesis, glutamate hypothesis, and neurodevelopmental hypothesis. Although they are often presented as competing or mutually exclusive theories, it is likely that a synthesis of these and other theories are the true reflection of the heterogeneous disorder schizophrenia.

DOPAMINE HYPOTHESIS

In its basic form, the DA hypothesis states that positive symptoms are a consequence of dopaminergic hyperactivity in the limbic areas, whereas dopaminergic hypoactivity in cortical areas may underlie negative symptoms and cognitive deficits. The hypothesis is based, first and foremost, on the finding that all currently available antipsychotic medications are D_2 ligands. Indeed, antipsychotic activity is positively correlated with the degree of D_2 binding, that is, the optimal response for most antipsychotic medications is seen with 60–65% blockade of the D_2 receptor [17]. The theory is further supported by clinical observations and genetic association studies. For example, chronic use of drugs of abuse that increase extracellular levels of DA, such as cocaine and the amphetamines, can induce a psychotic syndrome that bears a significant resemblance to the positive symptoms of schizophrenia and can exacerbate symptoms in schizophrenic patients (DSMIV-TR, 2000 [18]). Furthermore, one of the genes that is more consistently implicated in conveying increased risk for schizophrenia is catechol-*o*-methyl transferase (COMT), an enzyme that catalyses monoamines such as DA, thus serving a role in controlling the extracellular levels of DA in some areas of the brain [19].

GLUTAMATE HYPOTHESIS

In recent years, the glutamate hypothesis has gained increased support among investigators. It originated in clinical observations of phencyclidine (PCP) users who showed both positive-like symptoms such as paranoid delusions and auditory hallucinations as well as negative-like symptoms such as withdrawal and blunted effect and cognitive impairments such as deficits in attention and deficits in concrete thought [20,21]. Similar to the psychostimulants listed earlier, noncompetitive N-methyl-D-aspartic acid (NMDA) antagonists such as PCP and ketamine not only induce schizophrenic-like symptoms in a nonpsychiatric population but also exacerbate symptoms in patients with schizophrenia [20]. The glutamate theory is further supported by postmortem findings, genetic association studies, and clinical investigations. For example, postmortem studies of schizophrenia patients reveal changes in multiple glutamatergic receptors including the kainate and alpha-amino-3-hydroxy-5-methyl-4-isoxazolepropionic acid (AMPA) receptors [21]. Furthermore, genetic association studies have shown that an increased risk of schizophrenia is associated with variability in the metabotropic glutamate receptor, mGluR3, and G72 and D-amino acid oxidase (DAAO). Although increasingly controversial, variability in the alleles that regulate DAAO could potentially lead to changes in the activation of glutamate receptors since DAAO metabolizes D-serine, an essential cotransmitter at the NMDA glutamate receptor complex [19]. Finally, clinical studies have investigated the adjunctive use of agonists at the glycine modulatory site on the NMDA glutamate receptor complex such as glycine and D-serine. In patients stabilized on an antipsychotic, these compounds significantly reduce negative symptoms and often induce small improvements in positive symptoms and cognitive functioning [21].

NEURODEVELOPMENTAL HYPOTHESIS

The neurodevelopmental hypothesis states that "schizophrenia is the behavioral outcome of an aberration in neurodevelopmental processes that begins long before the onset of clinical symptoms and is caused by a combination of environmental and genetic factors" [22]. It has been postulated that these aberrations in neurodevelopment result in inappropriate connections between key brain regions such as the striatum, nucleus accumbens, and frontal cortex [23]. Evidence in support of the theory comes from various sources. First, there is a typical progression of the disorder itself from a prodromal phase in childhood and the early teen years to a typical progressive worsening of both symptoms and prognosis across the life of the disorder [12]. Second, there is a significant genetic component to the risk of developing schizophrenia, for example, while there is about 1% prevalence in the general population, the risk increases to 10–15% if a first-order relative is diagnosed with schizophrenia and to 30–65% if an identical twin is diagnosed [2]. Genetic association studies further support this as susceptibility genes such as neuregulin 1 and dysbindin play roles in neural development and neuronal connectivity [19]. Third, various pre- and perinatal risk factors have been identified including prenatal infections, famine during pregnancy, and obstetric complications [2]. Finally, brain morphology is often altered in schizophrenia patients, with increases in the volume of the lateral ventricle being one of the most common changes described [22].

RATIONALE FOR H_3 RECEPTOR ANTAGONIST EFFICACY IN SCHIZOPHRENIA

Impaired dopaminergic and glutamatergic neurotransmission are widely implicated in the pathophysiology of schizophrenia. However, in recent years, increased attention has been focused on the role of the histaminergic system, particularly with respect to histamine H_3 receptors. This is largely due to publication of findings in animal models predictive of efficacy as stand-alone or add-on therapies in schizophrenia (see section Experimental Disease Models) and the realization that current treatments fall short of allowing schizophrenic patients to resume normal function. In addition, histaminergic H_3 receptors are found in high abundance in brain regions implicated in schizophrenia, and recent data have demonstrated functional relationships between histaminergic, dopaminergic, and glutamatergic systems that suggest a role in the pathophysiology of the disease and in the action of current antipsychotics. Thus, a review of our current knowledge of neuroanatomical, neurochemical, and functional roles for H_3 receptors and targeted ligands is warranted.

NEUROANATOMICAL RATIONALE

Histaminergic neurons in the brain originate in the tuberomammillary nucleus of the posterior hypothalamus and project extensively to multiple brain regions including striatum, thalamus, basal ganglia, amygdala, hippocampus, and all areas of the cortex. A description of this system was first made by two laboratories working independently of each other [24,25] although the biological actions of histamine and the existence of two distinct pharmacologies (H_1, H_2 receptors) were known long before this [26,27]. It is now known that histamine also exerts biological activity through at least two additional receptor subtypes, H_3 (first described [28]) and H_4 [29]. Following its recent cloning and expression [30], multiple splice variants of the H_3 receptor have also been described, some of which may be differentially distributed in the brain and across species, utilize different signal transduction mechanisms, and exhibit dimerization (for recent reviews of this literature, see Refs 31 and 32).

H_3 receptors were first identified as autoreceptors on presynaptic terminals of the histaminergic system, controlling the release of histamine itself [28]. Interestingly, H_3 receptors are also known to function as heteroreceptors and are located on the presynaptic terminals of neurons across other neurotransmitter systems, regulating the release of neurotransmitters such as DA, glutamate, GABA, acetylcholine, norepinephrine, and 5-HT [33–37]. Although widely distributed throughout the brain, the highest densities of H_3 receptors are found in the striatum, frontal cortex, and substantia nigra, with lower densities observed in the amygdala, hippocampus, and multiple cortical regions as determined with autoradiography using various agonist or inverse agonist ligands [24,38–40]. This distribution is consistent across many mammalian species, including rodent and human, and lends support for a functional role for H_3 receptors in sensory processing and cognition.

It is important to note that in some regions (e.g., hippocampus, amygdala), H_3 receptor distribution is largely consistent with the distribution of histaminergic nerve terminals, and it is likely that much of this population represents autoreceptors [41,42] (Chapter 1), although heteroreceptors regulating the release of norepinephrine may be present [43]. In the hippocampus, expression of H_3 receptors appears restricted to the dendritic field of the granule cells in the dentate and neurons in the CA1 pyramidal cell layer [44], similar to binding patters observed for H_1 and H_2 receptors. Since it is long recognized that these hippocampal cell types play an important function in cognition and neural plasticity [45], it is possible that histamine receptors play a regulatory role. However, in many other brain regions, the majority of H_3 receptors are likely heteroreceptors. One observation suggests that most H_3 receptors expressed in the striatum are present on GABAergic neurons, whereas other observations suggest H_3 receptors are also found on cholinergic inputs or on glutamatergic or dopaminergic projections [44,46]. One notable difference between rat and human is the relatively high expression of H_3 receptors in the outer layers of the human cortex, which do receive dense histaminergic innervation [47].

Further detailed mapping of the expression of H_3 receptors and gene transcripts indicate a considerable overlap in terms of anatomical localization with the dopaminergic system in regions such as the striatum and frontal cortex, and recent work has identified coexpression of H_3 receptors with D1 and D2 receptors [44]. Furthermore, recent work from the laboratories of Jean-Michel Arrang indicates that H_3 and D2 receptors in the striatum may act in an additive manner, generating schizophrenic symptoms [48]. As a result, the clinical implication of modulating H_3 receptors in neuropsychiatric diseases is an area receiving significant attention since antipsychotic-like efficacy may result by blocking H_3 receptors. However, despite this knowledge, the precise nature of interactions between the histaminergic system and other neurotransmitter systems known to be involved in schizophrenia is still not clear. Moreover, since the localization of many presumed H_3 autoreceptors does not parallel histaminergic innervation, it is important to investigate how these receptors are activated and functioned.

NEUROCHEMICAL AND FUNCTIONAL RATIONALE

Early attempts at understanding the neurochemical basis for blockade of H_3 receptors in schizophrenia and other neurological disorders utilized *in vitro* evoked release in cortical slices or *in vivo* microdialysis techniques. Recently, following treatment with the selective H_3 receptor inverse agonists, ABT-239, GSK189254, or BF2.649, increased acetylcholine, DA, or norepinephrine levels were observed in prefrontal cortex [40,49,50] of freely moving rats, whereas DA levels remained unchanged in the striatum of the same rats [49,50]. These effects were interpreted in each case as providing evidence for potentially overcoming dopaminergic hypofrontality observed in schizophrenia while avoiding exacerbation of extrapyramidal-like side effects common with present treatments. That is, hypofrontality is implicated in negative symptoms, so an increase in DA in this region might be associated with an increased risk for negative symptoms/cognitive deficits. Increased activation of DA D2 receptors in the striatum is associated with EPS. In effect, blockade of H_3 receptors could beneficially alter levels of at least two neurotransmitters implicated in the pathophysiology of schizophrenia and potentially address an unmet need of improving cognitive functioning. There is also evidence from additional studies that histamine plays a modulatory role on dopaminergic neurotransmission [51]. Similar modulatory effects of H_3 receptors have been observed for glutamatergic neurotransmission following PCP [52,53] and MK-801 [53] administration. Finally, this H_3-heteroreceptor-mediated regulation of dopaminergic and glutamatergic neurotransmission is reflected in the modulation of behavior, consistent with antipsychotic-like efficacy in preclinical studies modeling aspects of schizophrenia [49,50]. In this regard, improved sensorimotor gating and cognition in other animal models (see section Experimental Disease Models) following H_3 receptor blockade has been attributed to improved dopaminergic and cholinergic function over impairment naturally occurring in the animals used in these studies [49,50,54]. However, the apparent disconnect between histaminergic innervation and the differential densities of H_3 receptor expression patterns gives rise to a fundamental question: How are many of these presumed autoreceptors activated?

To address this question, one must consider recent work describing recombinant or native H_3 receptors as being constitutively active in rat [55,56] or human [56]. Thus, H_3 receptors can regulate release of neurotransmitters in the absence of a specific ligand. Because of this, and the differential nature of G-protein coupling among splice variants [57–59] (see also Refs 31 and 32), specific H_3 receptor ligands can act as protean agonists, exhibiting a range of pharmacological activities from inverse agonist or neutral antagonist to full inverse agonist. The development of new tool compounds and greater understanding of the interactions of native autoreceptors *in vivo* with other neurotransmitter systems will open many opportunities for modulating systems implicated in schizophrenia and offers advantages over other approaches.

The histaminergic system in the human brain has also been implicated in the pathophysiology of schizophrenia. Levels of *tele*-methylhistamine, a metabolite of histamine, are significantly increased in the cerebrospinal fluid of schizophrenic patients when compared with healthy controls [60]. Overdose of central nervous system (CNS)-penetrating H_1 receptor antagonists was reported to induce toxic psychoses with hallucinations resembling schizophrenia, resulting in these drugs being abused [61]. In addition, a downregulation of H_1 receptors is evident in the frontal cortex of patients with chronic schizophrenia in postmortem binding studies [62] and in positron emission tomography (PET) imaging studies [63]. Quantification of H_1 receptor density using PET showed a significant reduction in the frontal, prefrontal, and cingulate cortices of schizophrenic patients compared with age-matched healthy subjects [63]. Successful demonstration of selective PET [64,65] or single photon emission computed tomography (SPECT) [66,67] radioligands for H_3 receptors has remained elusive. In the end, clinical proof of efficacy for H_3 antagonists/ inverse agonists, given alone or as adjunctive treatment with neuroleptics, will drive further research in this promising field.

EXPERIMENTAL DISEASE MODELS

ANIMAL MODELS OF SCHIZOPHRENIA

As described earlier, schizophrenia is a clinically heterogeneous neuropsychiatric disorder with symptomatic components of positive symptoms, negative symptoms, and cognitive deficits. There is no definitive animal model of schizophrenia, but individual behavioral symptoms can be assessed in laboratory animals. There are many advantages in developing appropriate animal models of any disorder: a simpler system may be easier to interpret than the complex clinical syndrome, potential treatment groups are genetically homogeneous, and testing environments can be tightly controlled.

Ideally, animal models should closely resemble the clinical disorder in as many ways as possible including etiology, pathophysiology, behavioral phenotype, and response to pharmacotherapies that are clinically effective. Thus, in evaluating animals models, it is useful to consider (1) the model is based on a valid etiological theory such as a proposed pathophysiology or genetic mutation (also known as construct validity), (2) behavioral deficits in the model closely resemble those commonly observed in the clinic (also known as face validity), and (3) the model can selectively predict efficacy of known and unknown therapeutics or underlying aspects of the disorder (commonly referred to as predictive validity). Several of the more standard animal models that have been used to profile H_3 receptor antagonists are reviewed here.

Dopaminergic Hypothesis

As mentioned earlier, one of the prominent theories describing positive symptoms of schizophrenia is the DA hypothesis. The administration of psychomotor stimulants to patients with schizophrenia can exacerbate symptoms in schizophrenic patients [18]. Psychomotor stimulant abuse in humans can induce psychosis and other behavioral manifestations similar to those observed in paranoid schizophrenia [68]. In nonhuman primates, the chronic continuous administration of psychomotor stimulants elicits behaviors that approximate the visual or auditory hallucinations observed in psychomotor stimulant psychosis as well as in patients with schizophrenia [69]. This dosing regimen, however, induces neural toxicity in regions that are not implicated in the neuropathology of schizophrenia. Animal models of schizophrenia testing the DA hypothesis therefore tend to rely on either the acute administration of psychomotor stimulants/DA agonists, or on the repeated, intermittent administration of psychomotor stimulants.

Psychomotor Stimulant-Induced Hyperactivity

Given that chronic use of psychomotor stimulants can induce psychotic symptoms in humans [70,71] and can exacerbate symptoms in schizophrenic patients, psychomotor stimulant-induced alterations in behavior have been used in preclinical experiments designed to model aspects of the disorder. The acute administration of methamphetamine results in a robust increase in locomotor activity, and efficacious antipsychotics are able to reverse this hyperactivity. Methamphetamine increases the extracellular levels of DA, and activation of the mesolimbic dopaminergic system may be involved in the pathophysiology of schizophrenia [72]. Methamphetamine-induced hyperactivity therefore has some construct validity related to positive symptoms of schizophrenia. The face validity of psychomotor-induced hyperactivity is less clear, as it is not clear specifically how hyperactivity relates to positive symptoms of schizophrenia such as hallucinations. One of the appealing aspects of methamphetamine-induced hyperactivity assay is predictive validity. Therapies efficacious in treating positive symptoms in schizophrenics are efficacious in inhibiting methamphetamine-induced hyperactivity, and therefore, the predictive validity of this assay is high.

Apomorphine-Induced Climbing Behavior

In addition to inducing locomotor hyperactivity, as described for methamphetamine-induced hyperactivity earlier, DA agonists (including apomorphine) induce stereotypes. Stereotyped behavior can be characterized as the continuous and repeated manifestation of a given behavior (sniffing, rearing, or other focused behaviors). In mice, the administration of apomorphine induces a climbing behavior that is not observed in naïve mice [73]. The climbing behavior activated by apomorphine is due to the stimulation of DA receptors in the striatum [73], which is consistent with some of the underlying neuropathology of schizophrenia. As with methamphetamine-induced hyperactivity, it is not clear how the climbing behavior specifically reflects positive symptoms of schizophrenia in humans. Clinically used antipsychotic medications are effective in reducing apomorphine-induced climbing behavior in mice [74], and as such, this assay is considered to be predictive of antipsychotic potential.

Behavioral Sensitization

Some people who repeatedly use stimulant drugs, such as amphetamine, develop an amphetamine-induced psychosis that is similar to paranoid schizophrenia. Chronic amphetamine exposure can produce different syndromes that have been proposed as animal models of psychosis (for a review see Ref. 68). By maintaining elevated brain concentrations of amphetamine for prolonged periods of time, neurotoxicity occurs and is characterized by behavior that has been described as reflecting hallucinatory behavior. The repeated administration of low doses of psychomotor stimulants such as amphetamine results in long-term behavioral changes that are similar to both the negative (psychomotor depression) and the positive (hallucination-like) symptoms of schizophrenia [68,75]. Behavioral sensitization is characterized by a progressive and enduring enhancement in many amphetamine-induced behaviors and is not accompanied by brain damage. It is argued that the changes in the brain and behavior associated with the phenomenon of behavioral sensitization provide a better preclinical model of psychosis than those associated with neurotoxicity.

Glutamatergic Hypothesis

The DA hypothesis of schizophrenia is the principal explanatory model of antipsychotic drug action. Recent discoveries extend our understanding of the neurochemistry of schizophrenia, with increasing evidence of dysfunction in glutamate and GABA as well as DA systems. NMDA/glutamate-receptor antagonists such as PCP can induce schizophrenic-like symptoms in humans and exacerbate symptoms in patients with schizophrenia [18]. Data are accumulating, providing support for hypofunction in the glutamatergic as a viable hypothesis for neuropathological effects in schizophrenia.

MK-801-Induced Hyperlocomotion
Low doses of NMDA-receptor antagonists such as ketamine replicate in normal volunteers positive, negative, and cognitive symptoms of schizophrenia. Similar to effects on positive symptoms observed in humans, the administration of the NMDA antagonist dizocilpine (MK-801) [76] generates behavioral abnormalities in animals, such as hyperactivity [77]. Genetic studies indicate risk genes for schizophrenia that affect NMDA-receptor function or glutamatergic neurotransmission [78]. Although it is not clear how the increase in locomotor activity parallels positive symptoms in humans, compounds that are efficacious in treating positive symptoms in patients with schizophrenia (e.g., haloperidol and clozapine) are efficacious in ameliorating MK-801-induced hyperactivity in rodents [79], providing predictive validity of this animal model.

Sensorimotor Gating

Schizophrenic patients show impairments in sensorimotor gating [80–82], probably a reflection of the disrupted information-filtering mechanism contributing to overloading irrelevant stimuli in the brain [83]. Sensory gating is an automatic mechanism for filtering redundant inputs and has been proposed to be an early component of attention sometimes described as *preattention*.

Prepulse Inhibition
One way to assess sensorimotor gating is to measure prepulse inhibition (PPI) of the startle reflex, an operational measure of sensorimotor gating in which the involuntary startle reflex is reduced when a startling stimulus is preceded by a weak acoustic stimulus. Consistent with DA-, glutamate-, and serotonin-based hypotheses of schizophrenia, PPI in rodents can be disrupted by direct or indirect DA agonists, NMDA-receptor blockers, and 5-HT2A agonists [84–89]. The reversal of these pharmacologically induced PPI deficits has been considered to indicate antipsychotic potential. In addition to the pharmacological models, it was recently suggested that the increase of PPI of startle reflex in DBA/2 mice displaying naturally occurring

low PPI response compared to other mouse strains may represent an attractive animal model for assessing novel antipsychotic mechanisms [90]. To support the predictive validity of the model, it has been demonstrated that clinically effective antipsychotics such as haloperidol, risperidone, and clozapine are effective in enhancing PPI of startle reflex in DBA mice [90,91].

N40 Gating

Normally, the evoked potentials of P50 or N40 waves elicited by the second or test stimulus (T) are smaller in amplitude than the potentials evoked by the first or conditioning stimulus (C). The difference between the two evoked potential amplitudes or the T:C ratio is considered to indicate sensory gating function [92]. The N40 rodent model is analogous to the P50 auditory-evoked response in humans. Schizophrenic patients and about 50% of their first relatives display decreased P50 suppression (reflected by higher T:C ratios) compared with nonschizophrenic individuals [92–94], suggesting a deficient inhibitory auditory processing. Similarly, a decreased N40 suppression relative to other mouse strains has been observed in the DBA mouse strain. In the DBA/2 mouse, the phenotype of deficient sensory gating corresponds with lowered $\alpha7$ receptor levels in the hippocampus [95]. The naturally occurring auditory gating deficits observed in the DBA/2 mouse can be attenuated by the atypical antipsychotic, clozapine, but not by the typical antipsychotic, haloperidol [96]. The data in animals are consistent with clinical reports, suggesting that typical antipsychotics such as clozapine, risperidone, and olanzapine, but not typical antipsychotics, improved P50 suppression in schizophrenic patients. Thus, this preclinical model has some predictive as well as face validity. Interestingly, although both clozapine and haloperidol attenuates positive symptoms in schizophrenics (e.g., hallucinations), only clozapine has efficacy against the cognitive deficits, although these effects, like those in DBA/2 mice, are modest. Additionally, nicotine, which has been shown to enhance cognition in schizophrenia patients, also improves auditory gating in humans [97,98].

Side-Effect Liabilities

It is well known that antipsychotics, especially typical antipsychotics, have liabilities of extrapyramidal side effects (EPS) [99], resembling the symptoms of Parkinson's disease. These debilitating motor side effects are hypothesized to be mediated by antagonism of DA D2 receptors in the basal ganglia [100–102].

Catalepsy

Typical antipsychotics produce a number of side effects including EPS (e.g., akathesias, acute dystonia, and tardive dyskinesia). Although a number of behavioral paradigms have been developed in rodents to predict EPS liability, catalepsy in rodents has been considered as an animal model predictive of EPS liability [102]. Catalepsy can be simply defined as the inability to correct an unusual posture [103], and typically consists of placing an animal into an unusual posture and recording the time taken to correct this posture. This time is regarded as an index of the intensity of catalepsy. Most drugs effective in treating schizophrenia produce EPS in humans and catalepsy in rodents, with clozapine a notable exception. Clozapine induces negligible

EPS in humans and does not produce catalepsy in rodents. Owing to the face and predictive validity of this assay, catalepsy has been proposed as a critical screening model for predicting EPS liabilities in humans, especially when separation between efficacious doses and those producing catalepsy are compared [104].

PRECLINICAL PROFILING OF H_3 RECEPTOR ANTAGONISTS/INVERSE AGONISTS

Psychomotor Stimulant-Induced Hyperactivity

As mentioned previously, preclinical and clinical evidences have implicated dopaminergic hyperfunction as an important contributor to psychosis. Reversal of DA agonist-induced hyperactivity in rodents has been routinely used to assess antipsychotic potentials of a compound, given that clinically used antipsychotics are effective in these models. We and other laboratories have demonstrated that blockade of H_3 receptor with ciproxifan, thioperamide, ABT-239, and BF2.649 attenuates amphetamine- or methamphetamine-induced hyperactivity [50,51,105–107], an effect that can be reversed by the H_3 receptor agonist (R)-α-methylhistamine (RAMH) [106], suggesting the observed effects are mediated by H_3 receptor. Furthermore, unlike antipsychotics whose efficacies are often accompanied by sedative effects on their own, H_3 antagonists/inverse agonists are devoid of hypolocomotion at efficacious doses (Table 11.3 for a summary of preclinical findings with H_3 receptor antogonists in models of psychosis.).

Apomorphine-Induced Climbing Behavior

Recently, Akhtar et al. [105] reported that thioperamide-attenuated apomorphine-induced climbing behavior in mice, an effect that can be partially reversed in the presence of RAMH. The climbing behavior induced by apomorphine, a direct DA agonist, is known to be mediated by DA receptor activation in the striatum [108] and can be antagonized by antipsychotics [73]. The mechanisms underlying these effects are not well understood.

Potential Mechanisms Underlying the Antagonistic Interactions between H_3 Receptor Antagonists and Dopamine Agonists

It has been suggested that brain histamine has an inhibitory role in the behavioral effects of DA agonists. Enhancing brain histamine by systemic administration of L-histidine or inhibition of histamine metabolism through applying a histamine-N-methyltransferase inhibitor decreases methamphetamine-induced effects on hyperactivity or stereotypy [109–111]. Repeated exposure to amphetamine or methamphetamine is well known to produce behavioral sensitization, characterized by an augmented response to a subsequent challenge injection. Interestingly, L-histadine inhibits the development of methamphetamine-induced behavioral sensitization [109]. The putative antagonistic interaction between brain histamine and methamphetamine has been further implicated by the finding of enhanced sensitivity to methamphetamine-induced hyperactivity and behavioral sensitization in histidine decarboxylase gene knockout mice that are deficient of histamine [112]. A compensatory role of histamine has been speculated in a study showing a delayed increase of

TABLE 11.3

Summary of Preclinical Findings with H_3 Antagonists/Inverse Agonists in Psychosis Models

Compounds	Animal Models	Effective Doses	Results	References
Ciproxifan	METH-induced hyperactivity	3 mg/kg, i.p.	Attenuation	51
	MK-801-induced hyperactivity	1 mg/kg, i.p.	Attenuation	53
	PPI in DBA mice	1 and 10 mg/kg, i.p.	Increase of PPI	54
	Catalepsy	1.5 mg/kg, i.p.	Augmentation when administered with haloperidol	117
		3 mg/kg, i.p.	Augmentation when administered with haloperidol or risperidone	118
Thioperamide	AMPH-induced hyperactivity	2 mg/kg, i.p., or 10 and 20 ug, i.c.v.	Attenuation	106
		3.75 and 7.5 mg/kg, i.p.	Attenuation	105
	APO-induced climbing	15 mg/kg, i.p.	Attenuation	105
	PPI in DBA mice	30 mg/kg	Increase of PPI	54
	Catalepsy	3.75 and 7.5 mg/kg, i.p.	Augmentation when administered with haloperidol	105
		3.2 mg/kg	Augmentation when administered with risperidone	118
ABT-239	METH-induced hyperactivity	1 mg/kg, i.p.	Attenuation	107
	PPI in DBA mice	3 mg/kg, i.p.	Increase of PPI	107
	N40 gating	1 and 3 mg/kg, i.p.	Reduce of T:C ratio	107
	Catalepsy	1.5 and 3 mg/kg, i.p.	No augmentation when administered with haloperidol or risperidone	118
BF2.649	METH-induced hyperactivity	2.649 mg/kg, i.p.	Attenuation	50
	MK-801-induced hyperactivity	5 mg/kg, i.p.	Attenuation	50
	APO-induced PPI disruption	3 mg/kg, i.p.	Attenuation	50

Note: METH, methamphetamine; AMPH, amphetamine; APO, apomorphine.

histamine activity in methamphetamine-treated rats [51] as well as in a clinical study demonstrating that schizophrenic patients may have increased histamine activity [60]. Taken together, it is reasonable to speculate that facilitatory effects of H_3 receptor antagonists/inverse agonists on histamine release may underline their effects on antagonizing methamphamine or amphetamine-induced behavioral changes. However, the potential H_3 and DA interactions may involve more than elevation of brain histamine. For example, blockade of H_3 receptor results in an increase of ACh release [107], which may subsequently have an inhibitory control on dopaminergic systems, given the suggestion that agents enhancing ACh activation may have antipsychotic-like profiles in preclinical and clinical studies [113–115]. In consideration of the complicated neurochemical effects of H_3 receptor antagonists/inverse agonists, complex neurobiological interactions may be involved in H_3 receptor effects in DA-based models. What neurotransmission systems are activated by H_3 receptor antagonism, to what degree, in what brain regions, and how to interact with DA may determine the behavioral outcome.

MK-801-Induced Hyperlocomotion

In addition to dopaminergic hypothesis of psychosis, a hypofunction of NMDA receptors has also been implicated as mentioned previously. NMDA antagonist-induced behavioral changes have served as preclinical animal models of psychosis, whose predictive validities are supported by the efficacies of antipsychotics in these models. Recently, Faucard et al. showed ciproxifan-attenuated MK-801-induced hyperlocomotion at a dose that did not affect spontaneous activity [53]. A similar finding was reported with BF2.649 [50]. Interestingly, it has been reported that the administration of MK-801 and PCP increases histaminergic activity, suggesting a compensatory mechanism leading to an increase of histaminergic activity in response to psychotomimetic drugs, and this compensatory reaction would be facilitated by drugs such as H_3 receptor antagonists or inverse agonists that promote histamine release [53].

Sensorimotor Gating: Prepulse Inhibition

Intriguingly, we found that blockade of H_3 receptors with thioperamide, ciproxifan, and ABT-239 can enhance PPI in DBA/2 mice to the same degree as can antipsychotics [54,107]. Unlike antipsychotics that often suppress startle response while enhancing PPI of startle reflex [54,116], H_3 receptor antagonism does not appear to result in startle suppression at PPI-enhancing doses [54]. Recently, Ligneau et al. [50] reported that BF2.649 attenuated apomorphine-induced disruptive effects on PPI in Swiss mice.

Sensorimotor Gating: N40 Gating

We also investigated ABT-239 in another gating model, N40 in DBA/2 mice assessing hippocampal-evoked potentials in response to pairs of auditory clicks. In our studies, ABT-239 treatment significantly normalized N40 suppression to a similar degree of the effects induced by nicotine in these mice [107]. Given the importance of hippocampal cholinergic systems in inhibitory auditory processing [95,96], it is likely that ABT-239 may normalize auditory gating through cholinergic action, given that ABT-239 increases acetylcholine levels in hippocampus and prefrontal cortex [107]. Our data in N40 gating model and PPI of startle response suggest that the H_3 antagonists/inverse agonists may have potential in treating sensory gating deficits in schizophrenia.

Cataleptic Potential

Unlike cataleptogenic effects frequently observed with antipsychotics, H_3 antagonists/inverse agonists do not induce catalepsy [105,117,118]. We and other laboratories have reported that imidazole-based H_3 antagonists/inverse agonists such as ciproxifan and thioperamide augment cataleptogenic effects of antipsychotics [105,118,119]. However, we did not find catalepsy-enhancing effects when nonimidazole H_3 receptor antagonists/inverse agonists, ABT-239 and A-431404, were coadministered with haloperidol or risperidone [118]. Given that ciproxifan and thioperamide are inhibitors of cytochrome P450 enzymes, responsible for metabolizing risperidone and haloperidol, we further investigated the possibility that augmentation of antipsychotics by imidazoles may result from drug–drug interactions and found that ciproxifan, but not ABT-239, potently inhibited the metabolism of haloperidol and risperidone [118]. Our studies suggest that the potentiation of antipsychotic-induced catalepsy by imidazole H_3 receptor antagonists/inverse agonists may, at least partly, result from pharmacokinetic drug–drug interactions and that H_3 receptor blockade does not necessarily potentiate the cataleptogenic effects of antipsychotics in rats or predict exacerbation of EPS in patients.

POTENTIAL FUTURE DIRECTIONS

Although the role of histaminergic neurons in schizophrenia has perhaps been less well validated than the role of other neurotransmitter systems, evidence indicates there is an increase in histaminergic activity in patients with schizophrenia. Evidence from clinical studies has implicated the histamine H_1 receptor in schizophrenia; broader evidence has implicated the histaminergic system in general (see Ref. 120 for a review). Of the known histamine receptors, recent preclinical evidence supports a role for the H_3 receptor, and in particular antagonism/inverse agonism at this receptor, as having putative efficacy in rodent assays of schizophrenia. In addition, H_3 receptor antagonists/inverse agonists have demonstrated efficacy in some preclinical models of schizophrenia. Thus, H_3 receptor antagonists may have the capability of meeting some of the significant unmet medical need in this devastating disorder, although the exact neurochemical mechanisms underlying these observed preclinical effects are not clear. One of the interesting observations in our testing of H_3 receptor antagonists/inverse agonists is that the dose required for efficacy in models of psychosis tends to be higher than that required for efficacy in assays of cognition [49]. It is not clear why this potential disconnect in doses is observed, and the results of ongoing clinical trials should be informative in understanding observed preclinical results and the relationship to aspects of this disorder (see Table 11.4 for a summary of some H_3 receptor antagonists/inverse agonists reportedly in development). Given the available evidence, H_3 receptor antagonists/inverse agonists show efficacy as cognitive enhancers, may therefore be

TABLE 11.4

Summary of H₃ Antagonists/Inverse Agonists in Development

Name	Company	Status	General Information
Thioperamide	INSERM and Bioproject	Discontinued	Potent activity *in vivo*, with high doses required enhancing histamine release in the brain. It was originally considered for the treatment of psychiatric and cognitive disorders
Ciproxifan	INSERM	Discovery	Indications include schizophrenia, epilepsy, Alzheimer's disease, and dementia
Cipralisant (GT-2331)	Gliatech/Merck	Discontinued	Eating disorder, Alzheimer's disease, sleep disorder, attention-deficit hyperactivity disorder
GT-2016	Gliatech/Merck	Discontinued	Alzheimer's disease, obesity, sleep disorder
BF2.649 Ciproxidine	Bioprojet and Ferrer	Clinical development	Alzheimer's disease Attention deficit hyperactivity disorder
JNJ-5207852	Johnson & Johnson	Discovery	Cognitive disorder, narcolepsy
SCH-79687	Schering-Plough	Discovery	Cognitive disorder, sleep disorder, allergy, epilepsy
GSK-189254A	GSK	Phase 1	Efficacious in preclinical models of cognition. Is reportedly in development for schizophrenia, Alzheimer's disease, and narcolepsy. Reportedly in Phase 2 for narcolepsy
VUF-5000 VUF-5182	Vrije Universiteit van Amsterdam	Research tool	Synthesized as a potential new ligand to be used with PET imaging to study disorders such as epilepsy, Alzheimer's disease, Schizophrenia

Source: Derwent Discovery Information Ltd., IDdb, March 15, 2007.

efficacious in treating the cognitive deficits associated with schizophrenia, and has efficacy in some preclinical assays of positive symptomology.

CONCLUSIONS

In conclusion, it is clear that we have come a long way in more than 50 years since chlorpromazine was discovered and used to treat schizophrenia. In addition to the typical antipsychotics, we now have a new generation of antipsychotics with reduced side-effect liability and perhaps, in some cases, greater efficacy. We now have a clear idea of schizophrenia as a disorder including positive, negative, and cognitive symptoms, and we have interesting animal paradigms to model aspects of schizophrenia. H₃ receptor antagonists/inverse agonists are currently being tested in the clinic as putative therapies for the treatment of a number of CNS disorders including schizophrenia, and the results of these clinical trials will be interesting in light of the preclinical data discussed in this chapter.

REFERENCES

1. Rossler, W., H.J. Salize, J. van OS, and A. Riecher-Rossler, 2005, Size of burden of schizophrenia and psychotic disorders. *Eur Neuropsychopharmacol* 15: 399–409.
2. Maki, P., J. Veijola, P.B. Jones et al., 2005, Predictors of schizophrenia—a review. *Br Med Bull* 73–74: 1–15.
3. Auquier, P., C. Lancon, F. Rouillon, M. Lader, and C. Holmes, 2006, Mortality in schizophrenia. *Pharmacoepidemiol Drug Saf* 15: 873–879.
4. American Psychiatric Association, 2000, *Diagnostic and Statistical Manual of Mental Disorders* Fourth Edition. Text Revision. APA, Washington.
5. Nuechterlein, K.H., T.W. Robbins, and H. Einat, 2005, Distinguishing separable domains of cognition in human and animal studies: what separations are optimal for targeting interventions? A summary of recommendations from breakout group 2 at the measurement and treatment research to improve cognition in schizophrenia new approaches conference. *Schizophr Bull* 31: 870–874.
6. Andreasen, N.C., 1982, Negative symptoms in schizophrenia. Definition and reliability. *Arch Gen Psychiatry* 39: 784–788.
7. Krebs, M., K. Leopold, A. Hinzpeter, and M. Schaefer, 2006, Current schizophrenia drugs: efficacy and side effects. *Expert Opin Pharmacother* 7: 1005–1016.
8. Kleven, M.S., C. Barret-Grevoz, L. Bruins Slot, and A. Newman-Tancredi, 2005, Novel antipsychotic agents with 5-HT(1A) agonist properties: role of 5-HT(1A) receptor activation in attenuation of catalepsy induction in rats. *Neuropharmacology* 49: 135–143.
9. American Psychiatric Association, 2002, *Practice Guidelines for the Treatment of Psychiatric Disorders*. Compendium. APA, Washington.
10. Lublin, H., J. Eberhard, and S. Levander, 2005, Current therapy issues and unmet clinical needs in the treatment of schizophrenia: a review of the new generation antipsychotics. *Int Clin Psychopharmacol* 20: 183–198.
11. Newcomer, J.W., 2006, Medical risk in patients with bipolar disorder and schizophrenia. *J Clin Psychiatry* 67(Suppl 9): 25–30; discussion 36–42.
12. Lieberman, J.A., D. Perkins, A. Belger et al., 2001, The early stages of schizophrenia: speculations on pathogenesis, pathophysiology, and therapeutic approaches. *Biol Psychiatry* 50: 884–897.
13. Reichenberg, A., M. Weiser, A. Caspi et al., 2006, Premorbid intellectual functioning and risk of schizophrenia and spectrum disorders. *J Clin Exp Neuropsychol* 28: 193–207.
14. Meltzer, H.Y., 1999, The role of serotonin in antipsychotic drug action. *Neuropsychopharmacology* 21(Suppl 2): 106S–115S.
15. Swartz, M.S., D.O. Perkins, T.S. Stroup et al., 2007, Effects of antipsychotic medications on psychosocial functioning in patients with chronic schizophrenia: findings from the NIMH CATIE study. *Am J Psychiatry* 164: 428–436.
16. Woodward, N.D., S.E. Purdon, H.Y. Meltzer, and D.H. Zald, 2005, A meta-analysis of neuropsychological change to clozapine, olanzapine, quetiapine, and risperidone in schizophrenia. *Int J Neuropsychopharmacol* 8: 457–472.
17. Kapur, S. and D. Mamo, 2003, Half a century of antipsychotics and still a central role for dopamine D2 receptors. *Prog Neuropsychopharmacol Biol Psychiatry* 27: 1081–1090.
18. Yui, K., K. Goto, S. Ikemoto et al., 1999, Neurobiological basis of relapse prediction in stimulant-induced psychosis and schizophrenia: the role of sensitization. *Mol Psychiatry* 4: 512–523.

19. Harrison, P.J. and D.R. Weinberger, 2005, Schizophrenia genes, gene expression, and neuropathology: on the matter of their convergence. *Mol Psychiatry* 10: 40–68; image 5.

20. Krebs, M.O., 1995, Glutamatergic hypothesis of schizophrenia: psychoses induced by phencyclidine and cortical-subcortical imbalance. *Encephale* 21: 581–588.

21. Tsai, G. and J.T. Coyle, 2002, Glutamatergic mechanisms in schizophrenia. *Annu Rev Pharmacol Toxicol* 42: 165–179.

22. Rapoport, J.L., A.M. Addington, S. Frangou, and M.R. Psych, 2005, The neurodevelopmental model of schizophrenia: update 2005. *Mol Psychiatry* 10: 434–449.

23. Lipska, B.K., 2004, Using animal models to test a neurodevelopmental hypothesis of schizophrenia. *J Psychiatry Neurosci* 29: 282–286.

24. Panula, P., H.Y. Yang, and E. Costa, 1984, Histamine-containing neurons in the rat hypothalamus. *Proc Natl Acad Sci USA* 81: 2572–2576.

25. Watanabe, T., Y. Taguchi, H. Hayashi et al., 1983, Evidence for the presence of a histaminergic neuron system in the rat brain: an immunohistochemical analysis. *Neurosci Lett* 39: 249–254.

26. Ash, A.S. and H.O. Schild, 1966, Receptors mediating some actions of histamine. *Br J Pharmacol Chemother* 27: 427–439.

27. Dale, H.H. and P.P. Laidlaw, 1910, The physiological action of beta-iminazolylethylamine. *J Physiol* 41: 318–344.

28. Arrang, J.M., M. Garbarg, and J.C. Schwartz, 1983, Auto-inhibition of brain histamine release mediated by a novel class (H_3) of histamine receptor. *Nature* 302: 832–837.

29. Oda, T., N. Morikawa, Y. Saito, Y. Masuho, and S. Matsumoto, 2000, Molecular cloning and characterization of a novel type of histamine receptor preferentially expressed in leukocytes. *J Biol Chem* 275: 36781–36786.

30. Lovenberg, T.W., B.L. Roland, S.J. Wilson et al., 1999, Cloning and functional expression of the human histamine H_3 receptor. *Mol Pharmacol* 55: 1101–1107.

31. Bongers, G., R.A. Bakker, and R. Leurs, 2007, Molecular aspects of the histamine H_3 receptor. *Biochem Pharmacol* 73: 1195–1204.

32. Passani, M.B., J.S. Lin, A. Hancock, S. Crochet, and P. Blandina, 2004, The histamine H_3 receptor as a novel therapeutic target for cognitive and sleep disorders. *Trends Pharmacol Sci* 25: 618–625.

33. Blandina, P., M. Giorgetti, L. Bartolini et al., 1996, Inhibition of cortical acetylcholine release and cognitive performance by histamine H_3 receptor activation in rats. *Br J Pharmacol* 119: 1656–1664.

34. Schlicker, E., B. Malinowska, M. Kathmann, and M. Gothert, 1994, Modulation of neurotransmitter release via histamine H_3 heteroreceptors. *Fundam Clin Pharmacol* 8: 128–137.

35. Brown, R.E. and H.L. Haas, 1999, On the mechanism of histaminergic inhibition of glutamate release in the rat dentate gyrus. *J Physiol* 515 (Pt 3): 777–786.

36. Brown, R.E., D.R. Stevens, and H.L. Haas, 2001, The physiology of brain histamine. *Prog Neurobiol* 63: 637–672.

37. Garduno-Torres, B., M. Trevino, R. Gutierrez, and J.A. Arias-Montano, 2007, Presynaptic histamine H_3 receptors regulate glutamate, but not GABA release in rat thalamus. *Neuropharmacology* 52: 527–535.

38. Jin, C.Y., H. Kalimo, and P. Panula, 2002, The histaminergic system in human thalamus: correlation of innervation to receptor expression. *Eur J Neurosci* 15: 1125–1138.

39. Drutel, G., N. Peitsaro, K. Karlstedt et al., 2001, Identification of rat H_3 receptor isoforms with different brain expression and signaling properties. *Mol Pharmacol* 59: 1–8.

40. Medhurst, A.D., A.R. Atkins, I.J. Beresford et al., 2007, GSK189254, a novel H_3 receptor antagonist that binds to histamine H_3 receptors in Alzheimer's disease brain and improves cognitive performance in preclinical models. *J Pharmacol Exp Ther* 321: 1032–1045.

41. Arrang, J.M., M. Garbarg, and J.C. Schwartz, 1985, Autoregulation of histamine release in brain by presynaptic H₃ receptors. *Neuroscience* 15: 553–562.
42. Arrang, J.M., M. Garbarg, and J.C. Schwartz, 1987, Autoinhibition of histamine synthesis mediated by presynaptic H₃ receptors. *Neuroscience* 23: 149–157.
43. Alves-Rodrigues, A., H. Timmerman, E. Willems et al., 1998, Pharmacological characterisation of the histamine H₃ receptor in the rat hippocampus. *Brain Res* 788(1–2): 179–186.
44. Pillot, C., A. Heron, V. Cochois et al., 2002, A detailed mapping of the histamine H(3) receptor and its gene transcripts in rat brain. *Neuroscience* 114: 173–193.
45. Regan, C.M. and G.B. Fox, 1995, Polysialylation as a regulator of neural plasticity in rodent learning and aging. *Neurochem Res* 20: 593–598.
46. Chazot, P.L. and V. Hann, 2001, Overview: H₃ histamine receptor isoforms: new therapeutic targets in the CNS? *Curr Opin Investig Drugs* 2: 1428–1431.
47. Panula, P., M.S. Airaksinen, U. Pirvola, and E. Kotilainen, 1990, A histamine-containing neuronal system in human brain. *Neuroscience* 34: 127–132.
48. Humbert-Claude, M., S. Morisset, F. Gbahou, and J.M. Arrang, 2007, Histamine H₃ and dopamine D2 receptor-mediated [35S]GTPgamma[S] binding in rat striatum: evidence for additive effects but lack of interactions. *Biochem Pharmacol* 73: 1172–1181.
49. Fox, G.B., T.A. Esbenshade, J.B. Pan et al., 2005, Pharmacological properties of ABT-239 [4-(2-{2-[(2R)-2-Methylpyrrolidinyl]ethyl}-benzofuran-5-yl)benzonitrile]: II. Neurophysiological characterization and broad preclinical efficacy in cognition and schizophrenia of a potent and selective histamine H₃ receptor antagonist. *J Pharmacol Exp Ther* 313: 176–190.
50. Ligneau, X., L. Landais, D. Perrin et al., 2007, Brain histamine and schizophrenia: potential therapeutic applications of H(3)-receptor inverse agonists studied with BF2.649. *Biochem Pharmacol* 73: 1215–1224.
51. Morisset, S., C. Pilon, J. Tardivel-Lacombe et al., 2002, Acute and chronic effects of methamphetamine on tele-methylhistamine levels in mouse brain: selective involvement of the D(2) and not D(3) receptor. *J Pharmacol Exp Ther* 300: 621–628.
52. Itoh, Y., R. Oishi, M. Nishibori, and K. Saeki, 1985, Phencyclidine and the dynamics of mouse brain histamine. *J Pharmacol Exp Ther* 235: 788–792.
53. Faucard, R., V. Armand, A. Heron et al., 2006, N-methyl-D-aspartate receptor antagonists enhance histamine neuron activity in rodent brain. *J Neurochem* 98: 1487–1496.
54. Browman, K.E., V.A. Komater, P. Curzon et al., 2004, Enhancement of prepulse inhibition of startle in mice by the H₃ receptor antagonists thioperamide and ciproxifan. *Behav Brain Res* 153: 69–76.
55. Morisset, S., A. Rouleau, X. Ligneau et al., 2000, High constitutive activity of native H₃ receptors regulates histamine neurons in brain. *Nature* 408: 860–864.
56. Rouleau, A., X. Ligneau, J. Tardivel-Lacombe et al., 2002, Histamine H₃ receptor-mediated [35S]GTP gamma[S] binding: evidence for constitutive activity of the recombinant and native rat and human H₃ receptors. *Br J Pharmacol* 135: 383–392.
57. Krueger, K.M., D.G. Witte, L. Ireland-Denny et al., 2005, G protein-dependent pharmacology of histamine H₃ receptor ligands: evidence for heterogeneous active state receptor conformations. *J Pharmacol Exp Ther* 314: 271–281.
58. Witte, D.G., B.B. Yao, T.R. Miller et al., 2006, Detection of multiple H₃ receptor affinity states utilizing [3H]A-349821, a novel, selective, non-imidazole histamine H₃ receptor inverse agonist radioligand. *Br J Pharmacol* 148: 657–670.
59. Yao, B.B., D.G. Witte, T.R. Miller et al., 2006, Use of an inverse agonist radioligand [3H]A-317920 reveals distinct pharmacological profiles of the rat histamine H₃ receptor. *Neuropharmacology* 50: 468–478.

60. Prell, G.D., J.P. Green, C.A. Kaufmann et al., 1995, Histamine metabolites in cerebro-spinal fluid of patients with chronic schizophrenia: their relationships to levels of other aminergic transmitters and ratings of symptoms. *Schizophr Res* 14: 93–104.

61. Sangalli, B.C., 1997, Role of the central histaminergic neuronal system in the CNS toxic-ity of the first generation H_1-antagonists. *Prog Neurobiol* 52: 145–157.

62. Nakai, T., N. Kitamura, T. Hashimoto et al., 1991, Decreased histamine H_1 receptors in the frontal cortex of brains from patients with chronic schizophrenia. *Biol Psychiatry* 30: 349–356.

63. Iwabuchi, K., C. Ito, M. Tashiro et al., 2005, Histamine H_1 receptors in schizophrenic patients measured by positron emission tomography. *Eur Neuropsychopharmacol* 15: 185–191.

64. Airaksinen, A.J., J.A. Jablonowski, M. van der Mey et al., 2006, Radiosynthesis and biodistribution of a histamine H_3 receptor antagonist 4-[3-(4-piperidin-1-yl-but-1-ynyl)-[11C]benzyl]-morpholine: evaluation of a potential PET ligand. *Nucl Med Biol* 33: 801–810.

65. Yanai, K. and M. Tashiro, 2007, The physiological and pathophysiological roles of neuro-nal histamine: an insight from human positron emission tomography studies. *Pharmacol Ther* 113: 1–15.

66. Windhorst, A.D., H. Timmerman, R.P. Klok et al., 1999, Radiosynthesis and biodistribu-tion of 123I-labeled antagonists of the histamine H_3 receptor as potential SPECT ligands. *Nucl Med Biol* 26: 651–659.

67. Sasse, A., X. Ligneau, B. Sadek et al., 2001, Benzophenone derivatives and related com-pounds as potent histamine H_3 receptor antagonists and potential PET/SPECT ligands. *Arch Pharm* 334: 45–52.

68. Robinson, T.E. and J.B. Becker, 1986, Enduring changes in brain and behavior produced by chronic amphetamine administration: a review and evaluation of animal models of amphetamine psychosis. *Brain Res* 396: 157–198.

69. Ellinwood, E.H., Jr., A. Sudilovsky, and L.M. Nelson, 1973, Evolving behavior in the clinical and experimental amphetamine (model) psychosis. *Am J Psychiatry* 130: 1088–1093.

70. Ellinwood, E.H. and S. Cohen, 1971, Amphetamine abuse. *Science* 171: 420–421.

71. Sato, M., C.C. Chen, K. Akiyama, and S. Otsuki, 1983, Acute exacerbation of paranoid psychotic state after long-term abstinence in patients with previous methamphetamine psychosis. *Biol Psychiatry* 18: 429–440.

72. Carlsson, A., 1978, Antipsychotic drugs, neurotransmitters, and schizophrenia. *Am J Psychiatry* 135: 165–173.

73. Costall, B., R.J. Naylor, and V. Nohria, 1978, Climbing behaviour induced by apomor-phine in mice: a potential model for the detection of neuroleptic activity. *Eur J Pharma-col* 50: 39–50.

74. Bardin, L., M.S. Kleven, C. Barret-Grevoz, R. Depoortere, and A. Newman-Tancredi, 2006, Antipsychotic-like vs cataleptogenic actions in mice of novel antipsychotics having D2 antagonist and 5-HT1A agonist properties. *Neuropsychopharmacology* 31: 1869–1879.

75. Castner, S.A. and P.S. Goldman-Rakic, 1999, Long-lasting psychotomimetic conse-quences of repeated low-dose amphetamine exposure in rhesus monkeys. *Neuropsycho-pharmacology* 20: 10–28.

76. Wong, E.H., J.A. Kemp, T. Priestley et al., 1986, The anticonvulsant MK-801 is a potent N-methyl-D-aspartate antagonist. *Proc Natl Acad Sci USA* 83: 7104–7108.

77. Jentsch, J.D. and R.H. Roth, 1999, The neuropsychopharmacology of phencyclidine: from NMDA receptor hypofunction to the dopamine hypothesis of schizophrenia. *Neuropsychopharmacology* 20: 201–225.

78. Coyle, J.T., 2006, Glutamate and schizophrenia: beyond the dopamine hypothesis. *Cell Mol Neurobiol* 26: 365–384.
79. Leriche, L., J.C. Schwartz, and P. Sokoloff, 2003, The dopamine D3 receptor mediates locomotor hyperactivity induced by NMDA receptor blockade. *Neuropharmacology* 45: 174–181.
80. Braff, D., C. Stone, E. Callaway et al., 1978, Prestimulus effects on human startle reflex in normals and schizophrenics. *Psychophysiology* 15: 339–343.
81. Braff, D.L., C. Grillon, and M.A. Geyer, 1992, Gating and habituation of the startle reflex in schizophrenic patients. *Arch Gen Psychiatry* 49: 206–215.
82. Braff, D.L., M.A. Geyer, G.A. Light et al., 2001, Impact of prepulse characteristics on the detection of sensorimotor gating deficits in schizophrenia. *Schizophr Res* 49: 171–178.
83. McGhie, A. and J. Chapman, 1961, Disorders of attention and perception in early schizophrenia. *Br J Med Psychol* 34: 103–116.
84. Varty, G.B. and G.A. Higgins, 1998, Dopamine agonist-induced hypothermia and disruption of prepulse inhibition: evidence for a role of D3 receptors? *Behav Pharmacol* 9: 445–455.
85. Swerdlow, N.R., S.B. Caine, and M.A. Geyer, 1991, Opiate-dopamine interactions in the neural substrates of acoustic startle gating in the rat. *Prog Neuropsychopharmacol Biol Psychiatry* 15: 415–426.
86. Swerdlow, N.R. and M.A. Geyer, 1993, Clozapine and haloperidol in an animal model of sensorimotor gating deficits in schizophrenia. *Pharmacol Biochem Behav* 44: 741–744.
87. Sipes, T.A. and M.A. Geyer, 1994, Multiple serotonin receptor subtypes modulate prepulse inhibition of the startle response in rats. *Neuropharmacology* 33: 441–448.
88. Mansbach, R.S., D.L. Braff, and M.A. Geyer, 1989, Prepulse inhibition of the acoustic startle response is disrupted by N-ethyl-3,4-methylenedioxyamphetamine (MDEA) in the rat. *Eur J Pharmacol* 167: 49–55.
89. Mansbach, R.S. and M.A. Geyer, 1988, Blockade of potentiated startle responding in rats by 5-hydroxytryptamine1A receptor ligands. *Eur J Pharmacol* 156: 375–383.
90. Olivier, B., C. Leahy, T. Mullen et al., 2001, The DBA/2J strain and prepulse inhibition of startle: a model system to test antipsychotics? *Psychopharmacology* 156: 284–290.
91. McCaughran, J., Jr., E. Mahjubi, E. Decena, and R. Hitzemann, 1997, Genetics, haloperidol-induced catalepsy and haloperidol-induced changes in acoustic startle and prepulse inhibition. *Psychopharmacology* 134: 131–139.
92. Freedman, R., L.E. Adler, M. Myles-Worsley et al., 1996, Inhibitory gating of an evoked response to repeated auditory stimuli in schizophrenic and normal subjects. Human recordings, computer simulation, and an animal model. *Arch Gen Psychiatry* 53: 1114–1121.
93. Boutros, N.N., G. Zouridakis, and J. Overall, 1991, Replication and extension of P50 findings in schizophrenia. *Clin Electroencephalogr* 22: 40–45.
94. Freedman, R., L.E. Adler, M.C. Waldo, E. Pachtman, and R.D. Franks, 1983, Neurophysiological evidence for a defect in inhibitory pathways in schizophrenia: comparison of medicated and drug-free patients. *Biol Psychiatry* 18: 537–551.
95. Stevens, K.E., W.R. Kem, V.M. Mahnir, and R. Freedman, 1998, Selective alpha7-nicotinic agonists normalize inhibition of auditory response in DBA mice. *Psychopharmacology* 136: 320–327.
96. Simosky, J.K., K.E. Stevens, L.E. Adler, and R. Freedman, 2003, Clozapine improves deficient inhibitory auditory processing in DBA/2 mice, via a nicotinic cholinergic mechanism. *Psychopharmacology* 165: 386–396.
97. Adler, L.E., L.D. Hoffer, A. Wiser, and R. Freedman, 1993, Normalization of auditory physiology by cigarette smoking in schizophrenic patients. *Am J Psychiatry* 150: 1856–1861.

98. Domino, E.F. and T. Kishimoto, 1999, Short and middle latency auditory evoked potentials in non-smokers and tobacco smokers. *Electroencephalogr Clin Neurophysiol Suppl* 49: 36–40.

99. Leucht, S., G. Pitschel-Walz, D. Abraham, and W. Kissling, 1999, Efficacy and extrapyramidal side-effects of the new antipsychotics olanzapine, quetiapine, risperidone, and sertindole compared to conventional antipsychotics and placebo. A meta-analysis of randomized controlled trials. *Schizophr Res* 35: 51–68.

100. Casey, D.E., 1991, Extrapyramidal syndromes in nonhuman primates: typical and atypical neuroleptics. *Psychopharmacol Bull* 27: 47–50.

101. Crocker, A.D. and K.M. Hemsley, 2001, An animal model of extrapyramidal side effects induced by antipsychotic drugs: relationship with D2 dopamine receptor occupancy. *Prog Neuropsychopharmacol Biol Psychiatry* 25: 573–90.

102. Wadenberg, M.L., A. Soliman, S.C. VanderSpek, and S. Kapur, 2001, Dopamine D(2) receptor occupancy is a common mechanism underlying animal models of antipsychotics and their clinical effects. *Neuropsychopharmacology* 25: 633–641.

103. Sanberg, P.R., M.D. Bunsey, M. Giordano, and A.B. Norman, 1988, The catalepsy test: its ups and downs. *Behav Neurosci* 102: 748–759.

104. Hoffman, D.C. and H. Donovan, 1995, Catalepsy as a rodent model for detecting antipsychotic drugs with extrapyramidal side effect liability. *Psychopharmacology* 120: 128–133.

105. Akhtar, M., P. Uma Devi, A. Ali, K.K. Pillai, and D. Vohora, 2006, Antipsychotic-like profile of thioperamide, a selective H₃ receptor antagonist in mice. *Fundam Clin Pharmacol* 20: 373–378.

106. Clapham, J. and G.J. Kilpatrick, 1994, Thioperamide, the selective histamine H₃ receptor antagonist, attenuates stimulant-induced locomotor activity in the mouse. *Eur J Pharmacol* 259: 107–114.

107. Fox, G.B., T.A. Esbenshade, J.B. Pan et al., 2005, Selective H₃ receptor (H3R) blockade: broad efficacy in cognition and schizophrenia. *Inflamm Res* 54(Suppl 1): S23–S24.

108. Protais, P., J. Costentin, and J.C. Schwartz, 1976, Climbing behavior induced by apomorphine in mice: a simple test for the study of dopamine receptors in striatum. *Psychopharmacology* 50: 1–6.

109. Ito, C., K. Onodera, T. Watanabe, and M. Sato, 1997, Effects of histamine agents on methamphetamine-induced stereotyped behavior and behavioral sensitization in rats. *Psychopharmacology* 130: 362–367.

110. Itoh, Y., M. Nishibori, R. Oishi, and K. Saeki, 1984, Neuronal histamine inhibits methamphetamine-induced locomotor hyperactivity in mice. *Neurosci Lett* 48: 305–309.

111. Onodera, K., C. Itoh, M. Sato, and T. Watanabe, 1998, Motor behavioural function for histamine-dopamine interaction in brain. *Inflamm Res* 47(Suppl 1): S30–S31.

112. Kubota, Y., C. Ito, E. Sakurai, T. Watanabe, and H. Ohtsu, 2002, Increased methamphetamine-induced locomotor activity and behavioral sensitization in histamine-deficient mice. *J Neurochem* 83: 837–845.

113. Bodick, N.C., W.W. Offen, A.I. Levey et al., 1997, Effects of xanomeline, a selective muscarinic receptor agonist, on cognitive function and behavioral symptoms in Alzheimer disease. *Arch Neurol* 54: 465–473.

114. Stanhope, K.J., N.R. Mirza, M.J. Bickerdike et al., 2001, The muscarinic receptor agonist xanomeline has an antipsychotic-like profile in the rat. *J Pharmacol Exp Ther* 299: 782–792.

115. Kaufer, D., 1998, Beyond the cholinergic hypothesis: the effect of metrifonate and other cholinesterase inhibitors on neuropsychiatric symptoms in Alzheimer's disease. *Dement Geriatr Cogn Disord* 9(Suppl 2): 8–14.

116. Zhang, M., M.E. Ballard, K.L. Kohlhaas et al., 2006, Effect of dopamine D3 antago-
     nists on PPI in DBA/2J mice or PPI deficit induced by neonatal ventral hippocampal
     lesions in rats. *Neuropsychopharmacology* 31: 1382–1392.
117. Pillot, C., J. Ortiz, A. Heron et al., 2002, Ciproxifan, a histamine H_3 receptor antago-
     nist/inverse agonist, potentiates neurochemical and behavioral effects of haloperidol in
     the rat. *J Neurosci* 22: 7272–7280.
118. Zhang, M., M.E. Ballard, L. Pan et al., 2005, Lack of cataleptogenic potentiation
     with non-imidazole H_3 receptor antagonists reveals potential drug–drug interactions
     between imidazole-based H_3 receptor antagonists and antipsychotic drugs. *Brain Res*
     1045: 142–149.
119. Pillot, C., A. Heron, J.C. Schwartz, and J.M. Arrang, 2003, Ciproxifan, a histamine
     H_3 receptor antagonist/inverse agonist, modulates the effects of methamphetamine on
     neuropeptide mRNA expression in rat striatum. *Eur J Neurosci* 17: 307–314.
120. Arrang, J.M., 2007. Histamine and schizophrenia. *Int Rev Neurobiol* 78: 247–287.

12 Other Central Nervous System Diseases and Disorders

Paul L. Chazot and Fiona C. Shenton

CONTENTS

Introduction...355
Locomotion and Movement Disorders 356
    Parkinson's Disease and Huntington's Disease...........................357
Stress, Anxiety, and Depression 359
Nociceptive Pathway and Pain..360
Other Forms of Pain 363
    Migraine 363
Neuroprotection and Cerebral Ischemia..364
References...365

INTRODUCTION

Histamine is a chemical messenger that is released by neuronal and nonneuronal sources [1]. Histamine can act at four known types of histamine receptors, including H_3 receptors (H_3Rs) [1,2]. Although H_3Rs were originally reported to be presynaptic inhibitory autoreceptors [3,4], lesion studies have revealed that a large fraction of brain H_3Rs exist as postsynaptic inhibitory heteroreceptors [5]. Subsequently, pre- and postsynaptic expression of H_3Rs has been detected throughout the central nervous system (CNS). The central histaminergic system has gained increasing significance over the past decade, with topographical definition of histaminergic neuronal pathways and the identification of four histamine receptor subtypes in the human CNS. The focus of this chapter lies in the H_3R subtype that has grown in importance as a therapeutic target in a wide array of central clinical indications.

On the basis of the physiological role of histamine and the histaminergic system, the anatomical distribution of the H_3R and its modulation of key transmitter systems, as discussed in previous chapters, the H_3R represents a potential therapeutic target in a very broad range of CNS diseases and disorders. This chapter focuses on the role and potential of the H_3R in a range of CNS dysfunctions, including movement disorders, anxiety/fear-related disorders, hyperalgesia, and brain ischemia.

LOCOMOTION AND MOVEMENT DISORDERS

The basal ganglia play central roles in the control of voluntary movement. Although present understanding of the neurochemical and cellular anatomy of the basal ganglia is incomplete, neuromodulators such as histamine are key players. Furthermore, there is anatomical evidence for high levels of H_3R in the striatum and substantia nigra (SN) both in rodents [6–9] and in humans [10] (Figure 12.1). The substantia nigra pars reticulata (SNr) is a key basal ganglia output nucleus, with inhibitory outputs encoded in spike frequency and patterns of the respective SNr projection neurons. SNr output intensity and pattern are often aberrant in movement disorders of basal ganglia origin. Using whole cell patch-clamp recordings, histamine increases SNr inhibitory projection neuron firing frequency and thus inhibitory output, through histamine H_1Rs and H_2Rs that induce inward currents and depolarization. In contrast, histamine H_3R activation hyperpolarizes and inhibits SNr inhibitory projection

(a)

(b)

FIGURE 12.1 (See color insert following page 148.) High expression of the histamine H_3R in the mammalian SN. Immunohistochemical labeling of the H_3 histamine receptor in the SN using a selective anti-H_3 349-358 histamine receptor antibody [6]. (a) Wild-type mouse; (b) $H_3(-/-)$ mouse. (Image produced by Dr. Keri Cannon in the laboratories of Dr. Frank Rice and Professor Lindsay Hough, Albany, NY.)

neurons, thus decreasing the intensity of basal ganglia output. H_3R activation also increases the irregularity of the interspike intervals or alters the pattern of SNr inhibitory neuron firing [11]. These results suggest that H_1Rs/H_2Rs and H_3R exert opposite effects on SNr inhibitory projection neurons, presumably based on their post- and presynaptic location, respectively. The functional balance of the different histamine receptors may contribute to the appropriate intensity and pattern of basal ganglia output and, as a consequence, are likely to exert important effects on motor control. Therefore, any imbalance in their function would have potentially deleterious implications on mobility.

Activation of H_3Rs leads to the selective inhibition of the component of depolarization-induced [^3H] GABA release in SNR slices, which are dependent on D_1-receptor activation. This appears to be largely an action at the terminals of the striatonigral GABA projection neurons, which may be enhanced by a partial inhibition of dendritic [^3H] dopamine release [12]. On the basis of fast-scan cyclic voltammetry and immunohistochemistry, it has also been shown that H_3R regulate 5-HT release in the SNR [13]. Furthermore, H_3R activation regulates dopamine synthesis/release (input nigrostriatal dopaminergic neurons), acetylcholine release (interneurons), and glutamate release (input corticostriatal glutamatergic) neurons in the rat striatum [14–17]. These findings provide further evidence for the importance of the H_3 heteroreceptor in basal ganglia function.

PARKINSON'S DISEASE AND HUNTINGTON'S DISEASE

Parkinson's disease (PD) is a progressive nervous disease occurring most often after the age of 50, associated with the destruction of brain cells within the SN that produce the neurotransmitter, dopamine. PD is characterized by slowing of movement (bradykinesia), muscular tremor, partial facial paralysis, peculiarity of gait and posture, and weakness. It is also known as *paralysis agitans* or shaking palsy. In the later stages of the disease, dementia, psychiatric, and autonomic problems often occur. To date, the most effective therapy utilized for PD is L-3,4-dihydroxyphenylalanine (L-dopa/levodopa), which is a precursor to dopamine. However, long-term use of this drug eventually leads to debilitating dyskinesias. New strategies are currently needed to combat dyskinesias, which are particularly prevalent in younger PD sufferers. Huntington's disease (HD) is an inherited condition characterized by abnormal body movements, dementia, and psychiatric problems. It is a progressive disorder involving atrophy of caudate structures within the striatum. It is caused by multiple copies of a single faulty gene, *huntingtin*, located on human chromosome number 4.

In a well-characterized animal model of PD, whereby dopaminergic lesions are elicited by the injection of 6-hydroxydopamine (6-OHDA) into the striatum, the numbers of H_3R-binding sites have been shown to be differentially regulated in key brain areas, when comparing the 6-OHDA-lesioned side with the sham operated hemisphere [18]. H_3Rs were upregulated by ~1.7- and 1.2-fold in the SN and striatum, respectively. In addition, histaminergic innervation in the SN was elevated in 6-OHDA-lesioned rats [19].

In human studies, the role of the histaminergic system is less clear. The distribution of histaminergic fibers in the SN in postmortem brain samples from patients suffering from PD and normal controls was examined with a specific immunohistochemical method. The presence of histaminergic innervation of the human substantia nigra pars compacta (SNc) and SNr was demonstrated. Interestingly, the density of histaminergic fibers and levels of histamine in the middle portion of SNc and SNr were increased in brains with PD. In PD, the morphology of histaminergic fibers was distinctly different, being thinner than in controls and displaying enlarged varicosities [20,21]. The apparent increase in histaminergic innervation may reflect compensatory mechanisms in the brain due to dopamine deficiency. This may reflect primary or secondary events [20].

H_3R-binding sites were detected using N-alpha-methylhistamine (NAMH) autoradiography in the human basal ganglia and cortex, being most abundant in the SN and striatum [20]. Modulation of the histamine H_3R in PD was seen at the level of the mRNA expression in the striatum and receptor density in the SN, but the receptor activity, based on GTPgS-binding studies, appeared unchanged [20]. In contrast, in another study, no difference in [^3H] RAMH binding was seen in many areas of brains from PD sufferers [22], whereas H_3R binding was significantly lower in the caudate putamen and globus pallidus of HD cases. HD is characterized by degeneration of the medium-sized spiny projection neurons, whereas the striatal interneurons are largely spared. This suggests that H_3Rs are present on the striatonigral projection neurons of the direct and indirect movement pathways, whereby they could provide histaminergic control over both routes [22]. It should be noted that Chazot et al. [6] reported immunoreactivity and the possible presence of presynaptic H_3R on cholinergic interneuron terminals, suggesting that the H_3R may not be found exclusively on projection neurons. Detailed characterization of striatal H_3Rs and their part in signaling within this brain region may lead to novel remedies, both in respect of the loss of motor control and with regard to the cognitive deficits manifest in these complex diseases.

Within the basal ganglia, abnormalities in different nondopaminergic components of the circuitry have been investigated in levo-dopa-induced dyskinesias (LID). In particular, a role for enhanced inhibition of basal ganglia outputs by the GABAergic direct pathway has been suggested as a basic mechanism underpinning LID.

Rats, lesioned neonatally with 6-OHDA and primed with a dopamine receptor agonist, initiate the appearance of vacuous chewing movements in humans with tardive dyskinesia, but also the onset of motor LIDs in PD patients. *In vivo* microdialysis established that neither imetit nor thioperamide altered extraneuronal levels of dopamine and its metabolites in the striatum of 6-OHDA-lesioned rats, but H_3R agonists increased dyskinesias induced by dopamine receptor agonists [23].

Some promising results have recently been reported using H_3R antagonists to reduce LIDs in a nonhuman primate model of PD [24]. Interestingly, when dyskinesias were separately rated as chorea and dystonia, coadministration of L-dopa with the H_3 agonists, immepip or imetit (both 10 mg/kg), significantly reduced chorea, but had no effect on dystonia symptoms. The antidyskinetic actions of the H_3 agonists were not accompanied by alteration in the antiparkinsonian actions of L-dopa. *In vivo* microdialysis established that neither imetit nor thioperamide altered extraneuronal levels of dopamine and its metabolites in the striatum of 6-OHDA-lesioned rats. This latter observation indicates that the histaminergic systems may reduce dyskinesias induced by dopamine receptor agonists, independent of direct actions on dopaminergic neurons [23].

STRESS, ANXIETY, AND DEPRESSION

Anxiety and fear are normal human emotional states seen throughout the animal kingdom. Emotions are central to the quality of everyday human experience and represent complex physiological states involving the assessment of the value of environmental stimuli, which refers to an organism's ability to sense whether events in its environment are more or less desirable. In this regard, fear and anxiety serve an adaptive function, since survival across species depends critically on the ability to perceive, assess, learn about, and appropriately respond to cues and contexts that predict or signal danger. However, excessive fear and anxiety are hallmarks of various disabling disorders (anxiety disorders) that affect millions of people throughout the world. A substantial proportion of patients do not respond to either pharmacotherapy or psychotherapy, and treatments combining both are not associated with greater overall efficacy than that achieved with either treatment alone [25]. Clearly, new anxiolytic agents are needed, and preclinical tests representing single or complex traits of human anxiety disorders (e.g., discriminating the emotional and cognitive components) and bearing vulnerability traits (e.g., genetically more anxious mice and gender) are needed to improve their predictability.

Histamine acting on the hypothalamus affects the release of many hormones from the pituitary gland [26]. The hypothalamic–pituitary–adrenal axis (HPA axis) constitutes a major part of the neuroendocrine system that controls reactions to stress and regulates various body processes including digestion, the immune system, mood and sexuality, and energy usage. Species from humans to the most ancient organisms share the major components of the HPA axis. It is the mechanism for a set of interactions among glands, hormones, and parts of the mid-brain that mediate a general adaptation syndrome. Since histamine has a key role in learning and memory as well as homeostasis during times of stress or threat, a persuasive case has been made for the physiological role of histamine and the histaminergic system as key player in the response to danger [27]. For example, the anti-dressant amitriptyline partially prevented the increase in plasma corticosterone and the concomitant decrease in [^{3}H]histamine-binding sites elicited by footshock-induced stress in rats [28,29]. The release of histamine in prefrontal cortex produced by handling was antagonized by intracortical administration of RAMH and potentiated by thioperamide [30]. The effects of other stress hormones (ACTH and prolactin) were also suppressed by the administration of H_3R agonists, an effect again abolished by thioperamide [31]. The facts that brain histamine levels are increased under some conditions of stress and that H_3 antagonists reduce histamine brain levels and enhance performance in a host of models of cognition are consistent with the proposal that a certain modest level of stress or arousal is beneficial for behavioral performance. However, histamine is augmented in brain with stress, and the putative benzodiazepine and $5\text{-}HT_{1A}$-receptor agonist anxiolytics decrease histamine turnover in rodents [32–34], suggesting that increases in central histamine with H_3 antagonists could push the system too far and exacerbate existing fear responses.

Little attention has been paid to the role of histaminergic neurons in anxiety, but several lines of evidence support their fundamental involvement. Brain histamine levels vary across different behavioral contexts associated with stress or anxiety and the response of 5-HT neurons to restraint-induced stress/anxiety depends on brain histamine. Orexin neurons, through their dense innervations, produce strong direct depolarization effects on histamine cells [26], and their important role in behavioral and emotional control during waking may suggest a function in anxiety. The role of histamine in anxiety, however, is still unclear due to the lack of validated animal models for anxiety. All models to date have measured fear-avoidance rather than anxiety responses *per se*.

The $H_3(-/-)$ mice displayed age-independent reduced measures of fear-avoidance in the elevated plus-maze and elevated zero-maze models [35]. In contrast, using a pharmacological approach, neither thioperamide nor RAMH significantly changed animal behavior in the elevated plus-maze [36]. These findings point to the H_3R as a potential new target for posttraumatic stress syndromes and perhaps anxiety disorders. Notably, recent unpublished data from our own laboratory would suggest that the H_3R does not play a major role in anxiety itself (Chazot and Ennaceur, submitted), using new validated animal tests which distinguish between anxiety and fear-avoidance [37].

H_3R antagonists may have efficacy as antidepressants. Analogous to the tricyclic antidepressants (TCAs), imipramine and amitriptyline, thioperamide has been reported to decrease immobility in the mouse forced swim test, a model of behavioral despair with some predictive validity for antidepressant efficacy in humans. The effects of thioperamide were prevented by RAMH [36], and recent studies have indicated that this effect may be mediated through serotonergic- or antioxidant-based mechanisms [38].

NOCICEPTIVE PATHWAY AND PAIN

A large number of studies have examined the role of the central histamine system in modulating the perception of pain (nociception). Although peripheral histamine is involved in the stimulation of nociceptive fibers, it appears that central histamine is important in antinociception [39,40]. Histamine when administered i.c.v. can elicit either antinociceptive or hypernociceptive effects, depending on the site of injection and the dose in a number of rodent models [41–46]. It has been speculated that these apparently paradoxical effects are due to the presence of pre- and postsynaptic receptors. However, since the advent of cloning and identification of distinct H_3R isoforms, and the recently identified H_4Rs, further explanations are possible. Increasing overall histamine concentrations, using various methods including application of the histamine precursor, L-histidine, the H_3R prototypical antagonist, thioperamide, and the catabolism inhibitor metoprine have all been shown to elicit antinociception (reviewed in Refs 40 and 47).

There is growing evidence to suggest a role for H_3Rs in nociception, with H_3R antagonists reported to elicit antinociceptive effects [46,48]. In these early studies, a role for histamine in pain elicited by mechanical, chemical, and thermal stimuli was demonstrated in mice and rats. Thioperamide produced small but significant antinociceptive effects through both parenteral and i.c.v. routes. Moreover, RAMH was hyperalgesic and also ablated the effects of thioperamide. Additional studies with the H_3R antagonists, impromidine and burimamide, showed limited antinociceptive efficacy [49].

Therefore, the role of H_3R in nociception is clearly complex. Neither RAMH nor thioperamide alone elicited any antinociceptive action using thermal or chemical tests. However, thioperamide reduced the effects of morphine in the tail-emersion model, whereas RAMH potentiated its effects in the hotplate test. This indicates the close association of the opioid and histaminergic systems in certain pain states [50]. Conversely, in the tail flick test, pretreatment with thioperamide attenuated the inhibition of the tail flick response induced by endorphin or U50, 4888H, but not morphine, administered i.t. [51].

RAMH, although clearly active both *in vitro* and *in vivo* in rodents, was found early on in development, to display comparatively low plasma concentrations in healthy volunteers in phase I trials. This was subsequently ascribed to the methylation of the imidazole ring with histamine-*N*-methyltransferase (HMT). BP 2-94 is a prodrug that overcomes this problem. It is an azomethane derivative of RAMH, optimized for hydrolysis rate, oral bioavailability, and resistance to HMT. BP 2-94 inhibited capsaicin-induced plasma protein extravasation in rat tissues (ED_{50} values 0.6–1.4 μmol/kg p.o.) and zymosan-induced paw swelling in mice (ED_{50} 1 μmol/kg p.o.). BP 2-94 also displayed potent activity in the phenylbenzoquinone-induced writhing or formalin test in mice (ED_{50} = 0.03 mol/kg p.o.), but not in the hot plate test [52].

$H_3R^{-/-}$ mice are refractory to the nociceptive effects of thioperamide [53,54]. Several functional studies have revealed that administration of H_3R agonists inhibits neuropeptide release from sensory fibers in the heart, lung, and skin, leading to the initial hypothesis that H_3Rs are located on peptidergic C fibers (reviewed in Ref. 54). Recent detailed immunohistochemical studies provide the anatomical framework for addressing this question [54]. This study strongly suggests that H_3Rs-containing perivascular fibers play an afferent role in nociceptive transmission as Aδ high-threshold mechanoreceptors (HTMs) [54] (Figure 12.2). Furthermore, a recent study has implied that acid-sensing ion-channel-3 (ASIC3)-containing fibers participate in mechanical nociceptive transmission [54]. The observations that activation of H_3Rs attenuates low-intensity mechanical pinch and that H_3Rs colocalize with ASIC3 on deep dermal perivascular (potentially Aδ HTM) fibers suggest that H_3R-containing, ASIC3-expressing, deep dermal fibers may be involved in mechanical nociceptive transmission.

In addition to an afferent role, H_3R-containing, deep dermal, peptidergic Aδ fibers may also play an efferent role. The close apposition of these fibers to the adventitial layers of arterioles suggests that they may also be involved in modulating blood flow [54], which may have significance in migraine as discussed later. Under normal, uninjured conditions, these fibers may be subjected to mechanical forces produced by dilating blood vessels. To maintain a stable microenvironment, these fibers may respond to these pressures by adjusting the flow of blood through the dermal vasculature. During injury, H_3R-containing, deep dermal, perivascular fibers could contribute to the pain and inflammation through two possible mechanisms. First, upon tissue damage, these deep dermal peptidergic fibers may cause vasodilation and plasma extravasation of the vasculature through the release of calcitonin gene-related peptide (CGRP) and substance P (SP) [54]. Vasodilation and plasma extravasation permit the infiltration of several inflammatory mediators, including

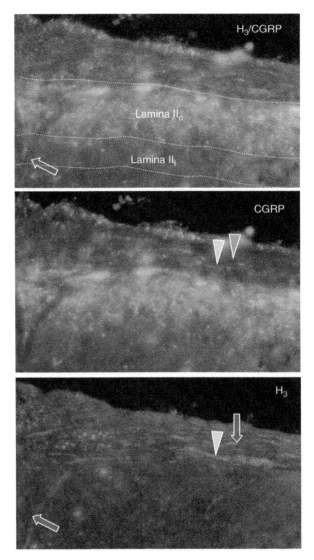

FIGURE 12.2 (See color insert following page 148.) The histamine H_3R is expressed on a subpopulation of $A\delta$ fibers in the spinal cord. Immunhistochemical double labeling of the H_3 histamine receptor (red) and CGRP (green) in the dorsal horn of the mouse spinal cord, showing CGRP-positive fibers with (yellow arrow) and without (red arrow) H_3R-LI ramified extensively in lamina II. These and other published data show that periarterial, peptidergic, and H_3R-containing $A\delta$ fibers may be sources of high-threshold mechanical nociception [54]. (Image produced by Dr. Keri Cannon in the laboratories of Dr. Frank Rice and Professor Lindsay Hough, Albany, NY.)

prostaglandins and cytokines, and initiate the onset of inflammation at the site of injury. Second, these fibers may promote the activation of mast cells through the release of CGRP and SP. Upon activation, mast cells release histamine into the surrounding tissue, which can activate H_1Rs located on nociceptive fibers and result in sensitization and pain hypersensitivity. Therefore, it is possible that activation of H_3Rs on the peripheral endings of deep dermal perivascular fibers could inhibit the release of CGRP and SP and result in the inhibition of pain and inflammation associated with tissue damage. However, further important studies are required to delineate the pathophysiological conditions under which H_1Rs and H_3Rs may be activated. A note of caution should be added here that the most recently discovered H_4R is also an important mediator of inflammatory responses. Since some of the drugs hitherto considered selective for the H_3R are now known to have at least some activity against this latest histamine receptor, findings of past studies may need to be reevaluated (see earlier chapters).

OTHER FORMS OF PAIN

MIGRAINE

Current drug treatment for migraine headaches includes nonsteroidal antiinflammatory drugs (NSAIDs) such as ibuprofen, the ergot dihydroergotamine (DHE) and the $5\text{-}HT_{1D}$ agonist, sumatriptan. NSAIDs inhibit prostaglandin synthesis and attenuate neurogenic inflammation in the trigeminovascular system. However, NSAIDs are ineffective for many migraine patients and are associated with the risk of dyspepsia and gastrointestinal hemorrhage. DHE is associated with nausea, vomiting, abdominal pain, diarrhea, and cerebral vasoconstriction. Side effects associated with sumatriptan are coronary vasospasm and chest heaviness (reviewed in Ref. 40). Furthermore, both DHE and sumatriptan are significantly less active in humans after oral administration. Newer $5\text{-}HT_{1D}$ agonists are available (e.g., Eletriptan and Almotriptan). These drugs are orally active and are more potent than sumatriptan; however, the pharmacology of these second-generation *sumatriptanlike drugs* does not exclude potential cardiovascular effects. In light of these therapeutic limitations, an antimigraine drug that demonstrates oral efficacy without the cardiovascular liability of current therapies is still required.

In the early 1990s, it was shown that plasma protein leakage within the dura mater in rats and guinea pigs could be blocked with H_3R agonists by prejunctional mechanisms [55]. Subsequently, in the late 1990s, a selective H_3R agonist, SCH 50971 (i.v. and p.o.) was shown to inhibit plasma protein extravasation in the dura mater of guinea pigs after electrical stimulation of the trigeminal ganglia. The minimum effective dose of SCH50971 was 3.0 mg/kg i.v. p.o., which produced a 40% decrease in plasma protein extravasation, respectively. The effects of SCH 50971 (3.0 mg/kg i.v.) were attenuated by the histamine H_3 antagonist thioperamide at an equivalent dose. The $5\text{-}HT_{1D}$ agonist, sumatriptan (0.3 mg/kg i.v.), and the prototypical histamine H_3R agonist, RAMH (0.3 mg/kg), also inhibited plasma extravasation by 40 and 46%, respectively [56].

In phase I and II trials, NAMH was tested as a potential migraine prophylactic treatment, through inhibition of the neurogenic edema response involved in migraine pathophysiology. In 30 healthy volunteers, the effects of the subcutaneous administration of NAMH and placebo were studied and found to have no undesirable symptomatic effects. In the phase-II trial, NAMH, at doses of 1–3 ng, significantly reduced the intensity, frequency, and duration of migraine attacks, as well as the requirement for rescue analgesics. However, it was noted that, at doses >3 ng, patients paradoxically experienced intense headache. Therefore, this study provided evidence of the safety and utility of NAMH applied subcutaneously at doses of 1–3 ng twice a week, but showed the potential problems at higher doses [57].

In a follow-up study, a controlled double-blind, placebo-controlled clinical trial for 12 weeks, 60 patients with migraine, who fit the criteria established by the International Headache Society, were selected. The efficacy of subcutaneous administration of NAMH (1–3 ng twice a week against placebo) was studied. Comparison between the groups treated with placebo ($n = 30$) and NAMH ($n = 30$), on data collected for the 4th, 8th, and 12th weeks of treatment, revealed that NAMH exerted a significant ($p < .0001$) reduction (compared to placebo) in intensity, frequency, and duration of migraine attacks, as well as on the use of analgesic intake. No significant ($p > .05$) adverse experiences or side effects developed in either group, offering a new therapeutic alternative and laying the clinical and pharmacological foundation for the use of histaminergic H_3 agonists in migraine prophylaxis, which may specifically inhibit the neurogenic edema response involved in migraine pathophysiology [58].

NEUROPROTECTION AND CEREBRAL ISCHEMIA

There is growing evidence for the involvement of histamine in brain ischemia. For example, middle cerebral artery occlusion in rat induces an increase in neuronal histamine release in the rat striatum by facilitation of histaminergic activity, which is both gradual and long-lasting [59]. Histamine depletion with α-fluoromethylhistidine (α-FMH) significantly increases the number of necrotic pyramidal cells in hippocampal CA1 region in rats subjected to cerebral ischemia [60]. However, postischemic loading with histidine decreases the amount of neuronal damage in the rat striatum [61]. Excessive glutamatergic neurotransmission, particularly when mediated by the N-methyl-D-aspartate (NMDA) subtype of glutamate receptor, is believed to underlie neuronal death in many common neurological disorders. Histamine has been reported to potentiate NMDA receptor-mediated excitotoxicity, which may have important implications for our understanding of conditions where enhanced glutamatergic neurotransmission is observed in conjunction with tissue acidification, such as cerebral ischemia and epilepsy.

First, central histamine receptor expression and ligand binding are altered in brain ischemia in distinct areas and may participate in neuroprotection or ischemia-associated neuronal damage [62]. H_3R mRNA expression was increased in the caudate putamen of the postischemic brain but was decreased in the globus pallidus and the thalamus; in association with this, H_3R-binding densities were increased in the cortex, caudate-putamen, globus pallidus, and hippocampus. The upregulation of H_3R ligand binding may be involved in the previously reported continuous neuronal histamine release in postischemic brain. Therefore, central H_3Rs may participate (together with H_1Rs) in endogenous neuroprotection.

In an organotypical coculture system, containing hippocampal neurons grown in the presence of hypothalamic histaminergic slice, thioperamide was shown to enhance the neuroprotective effects against kainate treatment endowed by the histaminergic slice [63]. Two further studies have shown that blockade of the H_3R

with clobenpropit- or thioperamide-attenuated NMDA-induced excitotoxicity in rat cortical cultured neurons in a calcium/GABA release-dependent mechanism [64].

Using a cyanide model to induce neurotoxic effects in rat brain homogenates, the neuroprotective properties of three H_3R antagonists, namely, clobenpropit, thioperamide, and impentamine, were examined and compared to aspirin, a known neuroprotective agent. Superoxide anion levels and malondialdehyde concentration were assessed using the nitroblue tetrazolium and lipid peroxidation assays. Both clobenpropit and thioperamide significantly reduced superoxide anion generation and lipid peroxidation. Impentamine reduced lipid peroxidation at all concentrations used, but only reduced superoxide anion generation at a high concentration of 1 mM. In the lipid peroxidation assay, all the drugs compared favorably to aspirin. This study demonstrates the potential of these agents as neuroprotectants by exerting antioxidant effects [65].

The SN is highly sensitive to histamine-derived neurotoxicity, where inflammatory processes mediated by histamine could be important in the pathological changes that lead to dopaminergic neuronal damage after histamine infusion [66]. No effects of histamine were noted on CHAT- or GAD-positive neurons, demonstrating the selectivity of action. In parallel, an acute inflammatory response was noted shown by a loss of glial fibrillary acidic protein-immunolabeled astrocytes and, in precisely the same loci, an activation of microglia. This may have implications for PD as well as ischemia (see section Locomotion and Movement Disorders).

The histidine-containing dipeptide, carnosine (beta-alanyl-L-histidine), has recently been shown to be a neuroprotective agent in an *in vitro* model of neurotoxicity induced by NMDA in differentiated PC12 cells [67,68]. Pretreatment with carnosine increased the viability and decreased the number of apoptotic and necrotic cells assessed by MTT and Hoechst 33342 and propidium iodide (PI) double-staining assays. The protection by carnosine was reversed by FMH, the selective and irreversible inhibitor of histidine decarboxylase (HDC). Furthermore, pyrilamine and thioperamide, selective central histamine H_1 and H_3R antagonists, respectively, also significantly reversed the protection of carnosine. The inhibition of glutamate release by carnosine was reversed by thioperamide. Therefore, the protective mechanism of carnosine may involve not only the carnosine–histidine–histamine pathway but also the H_1Rs and H_3Rs and the effective inhibition of glutamate release. This study indicates that carnosine may be an endogenous protective factor and calls for its further study as a new antiexcitotoxic structural template.

There is clearly considerable potential for H_3R-directed CNS therapies. The challenge is to meet this potential [69].

REFERENCES

1. Arrang, J.M., Garbarg, M., Schwart, J.C. 1983. Auto-inhibition of brain histamine release mediated by a novel class (H3) of histamine receptors. *Nature* 302: 832–837.
2. Arrang, J.M., Schwartz, J.C., Schunack, W. 1985. Stereoselectivity of the histamine H_3 presynaptic autoreceptor. *Eur. J. Pharmacol.* 117: 109–114.
3. Lovenberg, T.W., Roland, B.L., Wilson, S.J., Jiang, X., Pyati, J., Havar, A., Jackson, M.R., Erlander, M.G. 1999. Cloning and functional expression of the human H_3 receptor. *Mol. Pharmacol.* 55: 1101–1107.

4. Tardivel-Lacombe, J., Rouleau, A., Heron, A., Morisset, S., Pillot, C., Cochois, V., Schwartx, J.C., Arrang, J.M. 2000. Cloning and cerebral expression of the guinea pig histamine H_3 receptor: evidence for two isoforms. *NeuroReport* 11: 755–759.
5. Lovenberg, J.W., Pyati, J., Chang, H., Wilson, S.J., Erlander, M.G. 2000. Cloning of the rat histamine H_3 receptor reveals distinct species pharmacological profiles. *J. Parmacol. Exp. Ther.* 293: 771–778.
6. Chazot, P.L., Hann, V., Wilson, C., Lees, G., Thompson, C.L. 2001. Immunological identification of the mammalian H_3 histamine receptor in the mouse brain. *NeuroReport* 12: 259–262.
7. Drutel, G., Peitsaro, N., Karlstedt, K., Wieland, K., Smit, M.J., Timmerman, H., Panula, P., Leurs, R. 2000. Identification of rat H_3 receptor isoforms with different brain expression and signalling properties. *Mol. Pharmacol.* 59: 1–8.
8. Pollard, H., Moreau, J., Arrang, J.M., Schwartz, J.C. 1993. A detailed autoradiographic mapping of histamine H3 receptors in rat brain areas. *Neuroscience* 52: 169–189.
9. Pillot, C., Heron, A., Cochois, V., Tardivel-Lacombe, J., Ligneau, X., Schwartz, J.-C., Arrang, J.-M. 2002. A detailed mapping of the histamine H_3 receptor and its gene transcripts in rat brain. *Neuroscience* 114: 173–193.
10. Coge, F., Guenin, S.P., Audinot, V., Renouard-Try, A., Beauverger, P., Macia, C., Ouvry, C., Nagel, N., Rique, H., Boutin, J.A., Galizzi, J.P. 2001. Genomic organisation and characterisation of splice variants of human histamine H_3 receptor. *Biochem. J.* 355: 279–288.
11. Zhou, F.W., Xu, J.J., Zhao, Y., LeDoux, M.S., Zhou, F.M. 2006. Opposite functions of histamine H1 and H2 receptors and H3 receptor in substantia nigra pars reticulate. *Neurophysiology* 96: 1581–1591.
12. Garcia, M., Floran, B., Arias-Montano, J.A., Young, J.M., Aceves, J. 1997. Histamine H3 receptor activation selectively inhibits dopamine D1 receptor-dependent 3H.GABA release from depolarization-stimulated slices of rat substantia nigra pars reticulata. *Neuroscience* 80: 241–249.
13. Threlfell, S., Cragg, S.J., Kallo, I., Turi, G.F., Coen, C.W., Greenfield, S.A. 2004. Histamine H3 receptors inhibit serotonin release in substantia nigra pars reticulata. *J. Neurosci.* 24: 8704–8710.
14. Prast, H., Tran, M.H., Fischer, H., Kraus, M., Lamberti, C., Grass, K., Philippu, A. 1999. Histaminergic neurons modulate acetylcholine release in the ventral striatum: role of H_3 histamine receptors. *Naunyn Schmiedebergs Arch. Pharmacol.* 360: 558–564.
15. Schlicker, E., Fink, K., Detzner, M., Gothert, M. 1993. Histamine inhibits dopamine release in the mouse striatum via presynaptic H_3 receptors. *J. Neural. Trans.* 93: 1–10.
16. Doreulee, N., Yanovsky, Y., Flagmeyer, I., Stephens, D.R., Haas, H., Brown, R.E. 2001. Histamine H_3 receptors depress synaptic transmission in the corticostriatal pathway. *Neuropharmacology* 40: 106–113.
17. Molina-Hernandez, A., Nunez, A., Arias-Montano, J.A. 2000. Histamine H_3 receptor activation inhibits dopamine synthesis in rat striatum. *NeuroReport* 11: 163–166.
18. Ryu, J.H., Yanai, K., Watanabe, T. 1994. Marked increase in histamine H3 receptors in the striatum and substantia nigra after 6-hydroxydopamine-induced denervation of dopaminergic neurons: an autoradiographic study. *Neurosci. Lett.* 178: 19–22.
19. Anichtchik, O.V., Rinne, J.O., Kalimo, H., Panula, P. 2000. An altered histaminergic innervation of the substantia nigra in Parkinson's disease. *Exp. Neurol.* 163: 20–30.
20. Anichtchik, O.V. 2001. Distribution and modulation of histamine H(3) receptors in basal ganglia and frontal cortex of healthy controls and patients with Parkinson's disease. *Neurobiol. Dis.* 8: 707–716.
21. Rinne, J.O., Anichtchik, O.V., Eriksson, K.S., Kaslin, J., Tuomisto, L., Kalimo, H., Roytta, M., Panula, P. 2002. Increased brain histamine levels in Parkinson's disease but not in multiple system atrophy. *J. Neurochem.* 81: 954–960.

22. Goodchild, R.E., Court, J.A., Hobson, I., Piggott, M.A., Perry, R.H., Ince, P., Jaros, E., Perry, E.K. 1999. Distribution of histamine H3-receptor binding in the normal human basal ganglia: comparison with Huntington's and Parkinson's disease cases. *Eur. J. Neurosci.* 11: 449–456.

23. Nowak, P., Dabrowska, J., Bortel, A., Biedka, I., Szczerbak, G., Slomian, G., Kostrzewa, R.M., Brus, R. 2006. Histamine H3 receptor agonist- and antagonist-evoked vacuous chewing movements in 6-OHDA-lesioned rats occurs in an absence of change in microdialysate dopamine levels. *Eur. J. Pharmacol.* 552: 46–54.

24. Gomez-Ramirez, J., Johnston, T.H., Visanji, N.P., Fox, S.H., Brotchie, J.M. 2006. Histamine H3 receptor agonists reduce l-dopa-induced chorea, but not dystonia, in the MPTP-lesioned nonhuman primate model of Parkinson's disease. *Mov. Disord.* 21: 839–846.

25. Garakani, A., Mathew, S.J., Charney, D.S. 2006. Neurobiology of anxiety disorders and implications for treatment. *Mt. Sinai J. Med.* 73: 941–949.

26. Eriksson, K.S., Sergeeva, O., Brown, R.E., Haas, H. 2001. Orexin/hypocretin excites the histaminergic neurons of the tuberomammillary nucleus. *J. Neurosci.* 21: 9273–9279.

27. Brown, R.E., Stevens, D.R., Haas, H.L. 2002. The physiology of brain histamine. *Prog. Neurobiol.* 63: 637–672.

28. Ghi, P., Ferretti, C., Blengio, M. 1995. Effects of different types of stress on histamine-H3 receptors in the rat cortex. *Brain Res.* 690: 104–107.

29. Ghi, P., Ferretti, C., Blengio, M., Portaleone, P. 1995. Stress-induced changes in histaminergic system: effects of diazepam and amitriptyline. *Pharmacol. Biochem. Behav.* 51: 65–68.

30. Westernik, B.H., Cremers, T.I., De Vries, J.B., Liefers, H., Tran, N., De Boer, P. 2002. Evidence for activation of histamine H3 autoreceptors during handling stress in the prefrontal cortex of the rat. *Synapse* 43: 238–243.

31. Knigge, U., Soe-Jensen, P., Jorgensen, H., Kjaer, A., Moller, M., Warberg, J. 1999. Stress-induced release of anterior pituitary hormones: effect of H3 receptor-mediated inhibition of histaminergic activity or posterior hypothalamic lesion. *Neuroendocrinology* 69: 44–53.

32. Oishi, R., Nishibori, M., Itoh, Y., Saeki, K. Diazepam-induced decrease in histamine turnover in mouse brain. *Eur. J. Pharmacol.* 124: 337–342.

33. Oishi, R., Itoh, Y., Saeki, K. 1992. Inhibition of histamine turnover by 8-OH-DPAT, buspirone and 5-hydroxytryptophan in the mouse and rat brain. *Naunyn Schmiedebergs Arch. Pharmacol.* 345: 495–499.

34. Chikai, T., Oishi, R., Saeki, K. 1993. Microdialysis study of the effects of sedative drugs on extracellular histamine in the striatum of freely moving rats. *J. Pharmacol. Exp. Ther.* 266: 1277–1281.

35. Toyota, H., Dugovic, C., Koehl, M., Laposky, A.D., Weber, C., Ngo, K., Wu, Y., Lee, D.H., Yanai, K., Sakurai, E., Watanabe, T., Liu, C., Chen, J., Barbier, A.J., Turek, F.W., Fung-Leung, W.P., Lovenberg, T.W. 2002. Behavioral characterization of mice lacking histamine H_3 receptors. *Mol. Pharmacol.* 62: 389–397.

36. Perez-Garcia, C., Morales, L., Cano, M.V., Sancho, I., Alguacil, L.F. 1999. Effects of histamine H3 receptor ligands in experimental models of anxiety and depression. *Psychopharmacology* 142: 215–220.

37. Ennaceur, A., Michalikova, S., van Rensburg, R., Chazot, P.L. 2006. Models of anxiety: Responses of mice to novelty and open spaces in a 3D maze. *Behav. Brain Res.* 174: 9–38.

38. Akhtar, M., Pillai, K.K., Vohora, D. 2005. Effect of thioperamide on modified forced swimming test-induced oxidative stress in mice. *Basic Clin. Pharmacol. Toxicol.* 97: 218–221.

39. Hough, L. 1988. Cellular localization and possible functions for brain histamine: recent progress. *Prog. Neurobiol.* 30: 469–505

40. Chazot, P.L. 2005. Histamine H₃ receptors and analgesia. *Curr. Anaesthesia. Crit. Care* 16: 94–98.
41. Rumore, M.M., Schlichting, D.A. 1985. Analgesic effects of antihistaminics. *Life Sci.* 36: 403–416.
42. Millan, M.J. 1999. The induction of pain: an integrative review. *Prog. Neurobiol.* 57: 1–164.
43. Yanai, K. 2003. Roles of histamine receptors in pain perception: a study using receptors gene knockout mice. *Nippon Yakurigaku Zasshi.* 122: 391–399.
44. Chung, Y.H., Miyake, H., Kamei, C., Tasaka, K. 1984. Analgesic effect of histamine induced by intracerebral injection in mice. *Agents Actions* 15: 137–142.
45. Glick, S.D., Crane, L.A. 1978. Opiate-like and abstinence-like effects of itracerebral histamine administration in rats. *Nature* 273: 547–549.
46. Malmberg-Aiello, P., Lamberti, C., Ghelardini, C., Gotti, A., Bartolini, A. 1994. A role of histamine in rodent antinociception. *Br. J. Pharmacol.* 111: 1269–1279.
47. Chazot, P.L., Hann, V. 2001. Central H₃ histamine receptors: potential novel therapeutic targets. *Curr. Opin. Investig. Drugs* 2: 1428–1431.
48. Malmberg-Aiello, P., Lamberti, C., Ipponi, A., Hanninen, J., Ghelardini, C., Bartolini, A. 1997. Effects of two histamine-N-methyltransferase inhibitors, SKF 91488 and BW 301 U, in rodent antinociception. *Naunyn Schmiedebergs Arch. Pharmacol.* 355: 354–360.
49. Lamberti, C., Bartolini, A., Ghelardini, C., Malmberg-Aiello, P. 1996. Investigation into the role of histamine receptors in rodent antinociception. *Pharmacol. Biochem. Behav.* 53: 567–574.
50. Owen, S.M., Sturman, G., Freeman, P. 1994. Modulation of morphine-induced antinociception in mice by histamine H3-receptor ligands. *Agents Actions* 41: C62–C63.
51. Suh, H.W., Chung, K.M., Kim, Y.H., Huh, S.O., Song, D.K. 1999. Effects of histamine receptor antagonists injected intrathecally on antinociception induced by opioids administered intracerebroventricularly in the mouse. *Neuropeptides* 33: 121–129.
52. Rouleau, A., Stark, H., Schunack, W., Schwartz, J.C. 2000. Anti-inflammatory and antinociceptive properties of BP 2-94, a histamine H(3)-receptor agonist prodrug. *J. Pharmacol. Exp. Ther.* 295: 219–225.
53. Cannon, K.E., Malwark, J.W., Stadel, R., Ge, P., Lawsan, D., Silos-Santiago, I., Hough, L.B. 2003. Activation of spinal histamine H3 receptors inhibits mechanical-induced nociception. *Eur. J. Pharmacol.* 470: 139–147.
54. Cannon, K.E., Chazot, P.L., Hann, V., Shenton, F.C., Hough, L.B., Rice, F.L. 2007. Immunohistochemical localization of histamine H3 receptors in rodent skin, dorsal root ganglia, superior cervical ganglia, and spinal cord: potential antinociceptive targets. *Pain* 129: 76–92.
55. Matsubara, T., Moskowitz, M.A., Huang, Z. 1992. UK-14,304, R(-)-alpha-methyl-histamine and SMS 201-995 block plasma protein leakage within dura mater by prejunctional mechanisms. *Eur. J. Pharmacol.* 224: 145–150.
56. McLeod, R.L., Aslanian, R., del Prado, M., Duffy, R., Egan, R.W., Kreutner, W., McQuade, R., Hey, J.A. 1998. SCH 50971, an orally active histamine H₃ receptor agonist, inhibits central neurogenic vascular inflammation and produces sedation in the guinea pig. *J. Pharmacol. Exp. Ther.* 287: 43–50.
57. Millan-Guerrero, R.O., Pineda-Lucatero, A.G., Hernandez-Benjamin, T., Tene, C.E., Pacheco, M.F. 2003. Nalpha-methylhistamine safety and efficacy in migraine prophylaxis: phase I and phase II studies. *Headache* 43: 389–394.
58. Millan-Guerrero, R.O., Isais-Millan, R., Benjamin, T.H., Tene, C.E. 2006. Nalpha-methyl histamine safety and efficacy in migraine prophylaxis: phase III study. *Can. J. Neurol. Sci.* 33: 195–199.

59. Adachi, N., Itoh, Y., Oishi, R., Saeki, K. 1992. Direct evidence for increased continuous histamine release in the striatum of conscious freely moving rats produced by middle cerebral artery occlusion. *J. Cereb. Blood Flow Metab.* 12: 477–483.

60. Adachi, N., Oishi, R., Itano, Y., Yamada, T., Hirakawa, M., Saeki, K. 1993. Aggravation of ischemic neuronal damage in the rat hippocampus by impairment of histaminergic neurotransmission. *Brain Res.* 602: 165–168.

61. Adachi, N., Liu, K., Arai, T. 2004. Alleviation of ischemic neuronal damage by postischemic loading with histidine in the rat striatum. *Brain Res.* 998: 136–138.

62. Lozada, A., Munyao, N., Sallmen, T., Lintunen, M., Leurs, R., Lindsberg, P.J., Panula, P. 2005. Postischemic regulation of central histamine receptors. *Neuroscience* 136: 371–379.

63. Kukko-Lukjanov, T.K., Soini, S., Taira, T., Michelsen, K.A., Panula, P., Holopainen, I.E. 2006. Histaminergic neurons protect the developing hippocampus from kainic acid-induced neuronal damage in an organotypic coculture system. *J. Neurosci.* 26: 1088–1097.

64. Dai, H., Zhang, Z., Zhu, Y., Shen, Y., Hu, W., Huang, Y., Luo, J., Timmerman, H., Leurs, R., Chen, Z. 2006. Histamine protects against NMDA-induced necrosis in cultured cortical neurons through H receptor/cyclic AMP/protein kinase A and H receptor/GABA release pathways. *J. Neurochem.* 96: 1390–1400.

65. Badenhorst, H.E., Maharaj, D.S., Malan, S.F., Daya, S., van Dyk, S. 2005. Histamine-3 receptor antagonists reduce superoxide anion generation and lipid peroxidation in rat brain homogenates. *J. Pharm. Pharmacol.* 57: 781–785.

66. Vizuete, M.L., Merino, M., Venero, J.L., Santiago, M., Cano, J., Machado, A. 2000. Histamine infusion induces a selective dopaminergic neuronal death along with an inflammatory reaction in rat substantia nigra. *J. Neurochem.* 75: 540–552.

67. Shen, Y., Fan, Y., Dai, H., Fu, Q., Hu, W., Chen, Z. 2007. Neuroprotective effect of carnosine on necrotic cell death in PC12 cells. *Neurosci. Lett.* 414: 145–149.

68. Shen, Y., Hu, W.W., Fan, Y.Y., Dai, H.B., Fu, Q.L., Wei, E.Q., Luo, J.H., Chen, Z. 2007. Carnosine protects against NMDA-induced neurotoxicity in differentiated rat PC12 cells through carnosine-histidine-histamine pathway and H(1)/H(3) receptors. *Biochem. Pharmacol.* 73: 709–717.

69. Hancock, A.A. 2006. The challenge of drug discovery of a GPCR target: analysis of preclinical pharmacology of histamine H3 antagonists/inverse agonists. *Biochem. Pharmacol.* 71: 1103–1113.

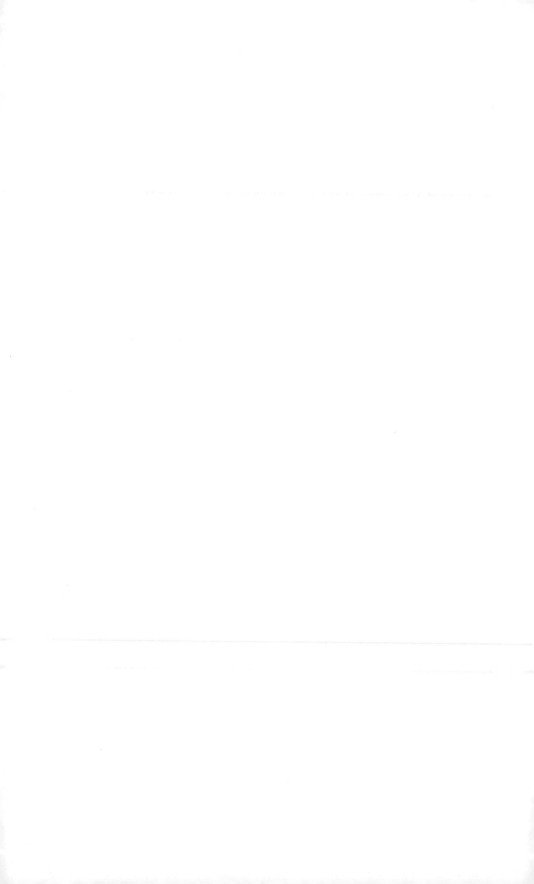

Index

A

Abbott Laboratories, 116–121, 150
Acetylcholine (Ach)
    attention-deficit hyperactivity disorder
        (ADHD), 217–218, 223–224
    drug development, 147
    epilepsy, 318
    histamine neurons, 39
    histamine research, 7, 14
    locomotion and movement disorders, 357
    obesity, 279, 281
    in peripheral tissues, 169, 172, 175–176
    schizophrenia, 337, 345
    sleep/wake cycle, 246–247, 249–252
Ach. *See* Acetylcholine (Ach)
AD. *See* Alzheimer's disease (AD)
Addiction-related behavior, 95–96
ADHD. *See* Attention-deficit hyperactivity
        disorder (ADHD)
Adipose tissue. *See* Obesity
AEDs. *See* Antiepileptic drugs (AEDs)
Agonists, HR3
    imidazole-based H3R modulators,
        108–109
    R-alpha-methylhistamine (RAMH)
        discovery, 6–8
        as drug development candidate, 18
        spatial memory and, 58
    sleep induction and promotion, 251
Alcohol-related behavior, 95–96
Allergic rhinitis, drugs targeting, 125
Allergies, 186–189
Alpha-fluoromethylhistidine, 96
Alpha-amino-3-hydroxy-5-methyl-4-
        isoxazolepropionic acid (AMPA),
        38–42
Alzheimer's disease (AD), 213–214, 222–230
    amyloid cascade hypothesis, 225
    cholinergic hypothesis, 223
    disease state, 222–223
    experimental disease models, 227–230
    future directions, 230
    H3/M2 antagonist, 11
    preclinical data, 227–230
    rationale for H3R antagonist efficacy, 7,
        225–227
    theories of disease basis, 224–225
    therapeutic options and considerations,
        223–224
Alzheimer's Disease Facts and Figures, 223
Amine synthesis, 167

AMPA. *See* Alpha-amino-hydroxy-methyl-
        isoxazolepropionic acid (AMPA)
Amyloid cascade hypothesis, Alzheimer's
        disease (AD), 225
Anabolic hormones, 51
Animal research
    attention-deficit hyperactivity disorder
        (ADHD), 218–220, 228
    hibernation, 93–94
    knockout (KO) mice
        cognitive functioning research, 57,
            218–219, 227
        histaminergic neurons, 38, 41, 46, 48
        obesity research, 284, 286–287
        sleep research, 41, 55, 57, 249, 256–260,
            264
        tiprolisant, 23–25
    primate research
        cognitive functioning, 229–230
        drug discovery, 118, 130
    schizophrenia, models of, 338–342
        catalepsy, 341–342
        dopaminergic hypothesis, 338–340
            apomorphine-induced climbing
                behavior, 339
            behavioral sensitization, 339–340
            psychomotor stimulant-induced
                hyperactivity, 339
        glutamatergic hypothesis, 340
        H3 antagonists/inverse agonists, 10
        MK-801-induced hyperlocomotion, 340
        N40 gating, 341
        prepulse inhibition (PPI), 27,
            340–341, 344
        sensorimotor gating, 340–341
        side-effect liabilities, 341–342
Antagonists, HR3
    Alzheimer's disease (AD) treatment, 225–227
    attention-deficit hyperactivity disorder
        (ADHD) treatment, 217–218
    epilepsy and epileptic seizure treatment,
        10, 312
    imidazole-based
        drug discovery and design, 109–111
        preclinical antiobesity effects of, 285–289
    nonimidazole-based, 116–121
        discovery of, 6
        drug discovery and design, 111–133
            Alzheimer's disease (AD), 145, 150
            antiobesity agents, 126–127, 150,
                289–292
            chemical class pioneers, 111–112

Antagonists, HR3 (*contd.*)
  drug design of novel cognitive
    enhancers, 116–121
  fluorescent H3 ligands, 116–121
  nonimidazole-based H3R
    antagonists, 121–127
  obesity, 126–127, 150, 289–292
  orally active H3 antagonist, 150
  by pharmaceutical companies, 112–133
  schizophrenia, 150
  targeting provigilant drugs, 112–116
drug discovery research, 111–133
obesity
  preclinical data, 285–292
  treatment, 7, 292–296
preclinical data
  antiobesity agents, 285–292
  schizophrenia, 342–345
research history, 20–21
schizophrenia
  animal models of, 10
  preclinical data, 342–345
in silico 3-D models, 135–143
sleep/wake cycle
  disorders, 261–267
  idiopathic hypersomnia, 267
  narcolepsy, 262–265
  serotonin reuptake inhibitors, 258–261
  sleep apnea, 265–267
  as wake-promoting agents, 251–254
thioperamide, 6, 18
Anticonvulsants, 10, 312, 319–320
Antidepressants, 316, 321
Antidiuretic hormone (ADH), 50
Antiepileptic drugs (AEDs), 10
Antihistamines
  excessive daytime sleepiness (EDS), 22–23
  H1R, 46
  and schizophrenia, 26
  as waking substance, 32
Antihypertensives, attention-deficit
    hyperactivity disorder
    (ADHD), 316
Antinarcoleptic efficacy of tiprolisant, 23–24
Antiobesity agents, medical chemistry program
    targeting, 126–127
Anxiety, 359–360
Apomorphine-induced climbing behavior, 339,
    342, 343
Apoptosis, 95
Appetite control. *See* Obesity
Arena Pharmaceuticals, 133
Attention-deficit hyperactivity disorder
    (ADHD), 213–222
  animal models, 218–220, 228
  disease state, 214–216
  experimental disease models, 218–222
  future directions, 230

H3R antagonists, rationale for efficacy, 7,
    24–25, 217–218
  H3R inverse agonists for, 25
  introduction, 213
  preclinical data, 218–222
  theories of disease basis, 217
  therapeutic options and considerations, 216–217
  tiprolisant use, 24–25
  utility of H3R ligands in, 8
Attention-deficit hyperactivity disorder ADHD,
    213–222
Autoradiography, receptor-binding, 93
Autoreceptors, histamine, discovery of, 14–16

B

Banyu Pharmaceutical, 132–133
Basal ganglia
  histaminergic actions, 51–52
  human brain, phylogeny of, 91–92
Behavior
  addiction-related behavior, 95–96
  alcohol-related behavior, 95–96
  climbing behavior, apomorphine-induced,
    339, 342, 343
  drinking behavior, 50
  feeding behavior, 50, 278–282 (*See also*
    Obesity)
  histamine as neurotransmitter, 54–58
    learning and memory, 57–58
    obesity, 56
    sleep/wake regulation, 54–56
    thermoregulation, 56
  hyperactive (*See* Attention-deficit
    hyperactivity disorder (ADHD))
  schizophrenia, 336, 339–340
Behavioral sensitization, animal models of
    schizophrenia, 339–340
Bioprojet, research at, 16–19
Blood vessels in cardiovascular system, 181–183
Body temperature, 50
Body weight regulation and histamine, 279–282.
    See also Obesity
Brain. *See* Human brain, phylogeny of
Brainstem, 48–50
Brain trauma, 95

C

Carcinogenesis, 189
Cardiovascular system
  heart, 178–181
  peripheral tissues, actions and therapeutic
    potential in, 178–183
  postsynaptic H3R, 181–183
  presynaptic H3R, 181–183

signal-transducing pathways, 178–181
vessels, 181–183
Catalepsy and schizophrenia
   animal models of, 341–342
   experimental disease models of, 345
Catecholamine
   epilepsy, 318–319
   histamine neurons, 32, 39–40
   histamine research, 14
   sleep/wake cycle, 248
Central nervous system (CNS) diseases and
         disorders
   Alzheimer's disease (AD), 213–214, 222–230
   attention-deficit hyperactivity disorder
         (ADHD), 213–222
   cerebral ischemia, 364–365
   drug discovery, 103–165
   epilepsy and epileptic seizures, 305–327
   locomotion and movement disorders,
         356–359
   obesity, 277–304
   pain
      migraine, 363–364
      perception of (nociception), 360–363
   peripheral tissues, actions and therapeutic
         potential in, 167–209
      allergy, 186–189
      carcinogenesis, 189
      cardiovascular system, 178–183
      gastrointestinal tract, 168–178
      immunity, 186–189
      inflammation, 186–189
      other peripheral locations and functions,
         189–191
      respiratory system, 184–186
   schizophrenia, 329–353
   sleep disorders, 241–275
   stress, anxiety and depression, 359–360
Cephalon, 146
Cerebral ischemia, 364–365
Chemoshock-induced seizures, epilepsy
         research, 307–311, 312–313
Chlorpromazine, 16
Cholinergic hypothesis for Alzheimer's disease
         (AD), 223
Ciproxifan, 20, 285–289
Circadian rhythms, 242, 245–246, 256, 262
Climbing behavior, apomorphine-induced,
         339, 342, 343
Cloned receptors, 6–8
Cloning of human H3R, 6
CNS. *See* Central nervous system (CNS)
         diseases and disorders
Cognitive functioning
   Alzheimer's disease (AD), 213–214, 222–230
      disease state, 222–223
      experimental disease models, 227–230
      H3/M2 antagonist, 11

rationale for H3R antagonist efficacy, 7,
         225–227
   theories of disease basis, 224–225
   therapeutic options and considerations,
         223–224
attention-deficit hyperactivity disorder
         (ADHD), 213–222
   animal models, 218–220, 228
   disease state, 214–216
   experimental disease models, 218–222
   future directions, 230
   H3R antagonists, rationale for efficacy, 7,
         24–25, 217–218
   H3R inverse agonists for, 25
   introduction, 213
   preclinical data, 218–222
   theories of disease basis, 217
   therapeutic options and considerations,
         216–217
   tiprolisant use, 24–25
enhancement
   Abbott Laboratories, 116–121
   novel cognitive enhancers, 116–121
   wakefulness, 22–23
schizophrenia, H3R antagonists/inverse
         agonists treatment, 4
Cortex, brain
   enthorhinal cortex, 91–92
   histaminergic actions, 53
   prefrontal cortex, 89
   temporal cortex, 89
Corticotrophin-releasing hormone (CRH), 41
CRH. *See* Corticotrophin-releasing hormone
         (CRH)

D

DA. *See* Dopamine (DA)
DAO. *See* Diamine oxidase (DAO)
Dementia. *See also* Alzheimer's disease (AD)
   drugs targeting, 7, 121–125
   as issue, 4, 7, 23
Depression
   antidepressants, 316, 321
   clinical, 258–261
   as CNS disorder, 359–360
   long-term depression (LTD), 53–54
Developmental expression, 88–89
*Diagnostic and Statistical Manual of Mental
         Disorders,* Fourth Edition, Text
         Revision (DSM-IV TR), 214–216
Diamine oxidase (DAO), 33
Digestive system. *See* Gastrointestinal tract
Dopamine (DA)
   alcohol-related behavior, 96
   attention-deficit hyperactivity disorder
         (ADHD), 217–218, 220

Dopamine (DA) (*contd.*)
  drug discovery, 120, 138
  histamine neurons and metabolism, 39–40, 42, 49, 51–52, 58
  histamine research, 14, 17, 21, 24–27
  locomotion and movement disorders, 357–358, 365
  obesity, 278, 281, 295
  schizophrenia, 330–331, 338–340, 342–344
  sleep/wake cycle, 94, 246, 249–250, 252, 254, 256, 260, 264–265
Dopaminergic hypothesis of schizophrenia, 338–340
Dream state, conscious, 39
Drinking behavior, 50
Drug discovery and design, 103–165
  clinical studies of H3R drug candidates, 149–151
  computer-aided drug design, 133–143
  fluorescent H3R ligands, 143–146
  future perspectives, 151–152
  highly competitive target H3R, 104–105
  H3R ligands, 105–108, 116–121, 135–143
  imidazole-based H3R
    antagonists, 109–111
    modulators, 108–111
  multitarget-oriented, 146–149
    clinical studies, 149–151
    drug combinations, 146
    hybrid combinations, 146–149
    preclinical data, 149–151
  natural products as potent H3R ligands, 105–108
  nonimidazole-based H3R antagonist, 111–133
    Alzheimer's disease (AD), 145, 150
    antiobesity agents, 126–127, 150, 289–292
    chemical class pioneers, 111–112
    drug design of novel cognitive enhancers, 116–121
    fluorescent H3 ligands, 116–121
    nonimidazole-based H3R antagonists, 121–127
    obesity, 126–127, 150, 289–292
    orally active H3 antagonist, 150
    by pharmaceutical companies, 112–133
    schizophrenia, 150
    targeting provigilant drugs, 112–116
  pharmaceutical companies
    Abbott Laboratories, 116–121, 150
    Arena Pharmaceuticals, 133
    Banyu Pharmaceutical, 132–133
    drug discovery programs, 112–133
    Eli Lilly & Co, 128–132
    GlaxoSmithKline (GSK), 121–127, 145, 150
    Hoffman-La Roche, 130–131
    Johnson & Johnson PRD, 112–116, 150
    Laboratoires Servier, 129–130
    Neurogen, 132–133
    new chemical entities, 132–133
    Novo-Nordisk, 126–127
    Pfizer, 131–132
  preclinical data, 149–151
  radiolabeled H3R ligands, 4, 143–146
  in silico 3-D models, 135–143
DSM-IV TR (*Diagnostic and Statistical Manual of Mental Disorders, Fourth Edition, Text Revision*), 214–216

E

EDS. *See* Excessive daytime sleepiness (EDS)
EEG. *See* Electroencephalogram (EEG)
Electroencephalogram (EEG)
  epilepsy, 25–26, 315, 320
  polysomnography, 242–243, 253, 257, 260
  sleep/wake studies, 22–23, 37, 55, 115, 242–264, 254–256
Electroshock-induced seizures, epilepsy research, 307–311, 312–313
Eli Lilly & Co, 128–132
Energy metabolism. *See* Obesity
Enkephalinase inhibitor, 16
Enthorhinal cortex, brain, 91–92
Epilepsy and epileptic seizures, 305–327
  anticonvulsants, 10, 312, 319–320
  antiepileptic drugs, 315–316
  chronic models (kindling), 313–314
  clinical studies, 319
  convulsants, 315–316
  genetic models, 314–315
  histaminergic agents and seizures, 306–312, 315–316
  H1R, evidence linking, 306–312
  H2R, controversies surrounding, 312
  H3R, in pathophysiology of, 4
  H3R antagonists, as anticonvulsants, 10, 312
  H3R inverse agonists, 10, 25–26
  induced seizures
    chemoshock-induced seizures, 307–311, 312–313
    electroshock-induced seizures, 307–311, 312–313
    kainic acid (KA)-induced seizures, 94–95, 307–311, 315
    PTX-induced seizures, 307–311, 312–313
  possible mechanisms, 317–319
  seizure models, 312–315
  therapeutic advantage, 320–321
    antidepressant, 321
    anxiolytic effects, 321
    central localization, 320
    procognitive effects, 320–321
    provigilant effects, 321

Excessive daytime sleepiness (EDS)
    antihistamines, 22–23
    treatment of
        H3R antagonists, 7, 261–262
        H3R inverse agonists, 22, 24
Experimental disease model of schizophrenia,
            338–342
    apomorphine-induced climbing behavior, 336
    cataleptic potential, 345
    dopamine agonists, H3R antagonistic
            interactions with, 342–344
    H3R antagonistic interactions with
            dopamine agonists, 342–344
    hyperactivity, psychomotor stimulant-
            induced, 342
    MK-801-induced hyperlocomotion, 344
    N40 gating, 344–345
    preclinical data, 342–345
    prepulse inhibition (PPI), 27, 340–341, 344
    psychomotor stimulant-induced
            hyperactivity, 342
    sensorimotor gating, 344–345

F

Feeding behavior, 50, 278–282. *See also* Obesity
First histamine receptor. *See* H1R
5HT. *See* Serotonin (5HT)
Fluid percussion model, 95
Fluorescent H3R ligands, 143–146
α-Fluoromethylhistidine, 96
Fourth histamine receptor. *See* H4R
French National Institute of Health and Medical
            Research (INSERM), research
            at, 14–17

G

GABA and GABAergic system
    alcohol sensitivity, 96
    cerebral ischema, 365
    epilepsy, 305, 311, 314, 316–320
    histamine neurons and metabolism, 33, 35,
            38–41
    histaminergic actions, 49–55
    locomotion and movement disorders, 357
    schizophrenia, 336, 340
    sleep/wake, 247–250, 265
GAERs. *See* Genetic absence epilepsy rats of
            Strasbourg (GAERs)
Galanin
    histamine neurons, 35, 40–41
    sleep/wake cycle, 247–248
Gastric acid secretion, 169–173
    gastrointestinal tract, 169–173
    Helicobacter pylori (Hp), 171–173

Gastric mucosal defense, 173–174
Gastrointestinal motility, 174–177
Gastrointestinal tract
    gastric acid secretion, 169–173
    gastric mucosal defense, 173–174
    gastrointestinal motility, 174–177
    Helicobacter pylori (Hp), 171–173
    heterogeneity of H3R, 175–177
    intestinal mucosal defense, 177–178
    intestinal secretion, 177
    peripheral tissues, actions and therapeutic
            potential in, 168–178
    visceral pain, 177–178
Gating and schizophrenia
    N40, 344–345
    sensorimotor, 27, 340–341, 344–345
Genes, knockout (KO) mice
    cognitive functioning research, 57,
            218–219, 227
    histaminergic neurons, 38, 41, 46, 48
    obesity research, 284, 286–287
    sleep research, 41, 55, 57, 249, 256–260, 264
    tiprolisant, 23–25
Gene structure and expression, 84–96
    in brain, 89–92
    developmental, 88–89
    isoforms, 84–87
    regulation, 92–96
    in vertebrate tissues, 87–88
Genetic absence epilepsy rats of Strasbourg
            (GAERs), 315
Genetically epilepsy prone rats (GEPRs),
            314–315
GEPRs. *See* Genetically epilepsy prone rats
            (GEPRs)
GHRH. *See* Growth hormone-releasing
            hormone (GHRH)
GlaxoSmithKline (GSK), 121–127, 145, 150
Glia, 54
Glutamate
    alcohol-related behavior
    drug discovery, 137
    epilepsy, 305, 315, 317
    histamine neurons and metabolism, 38–39,
            42, 47, 49–50, 52–54
    locomotion and movement disorders, 357,
            364–365
    obesity, 279
    schizophrenia, 26, 330–331,
            333–337, 340
Glutamatergic hypothesis of schizophrenia, 340
Glycine, 39
GnRH. *See* Gonadotrophin-releasing hormone
            (GnRH)
Gonadotrophin-releasing hormone (GnRH), 51
Growth hormone-releasing hormone
            (GHRH), 51
GSK. *See* GlaxoSmithKline (GSK)

H

HA. *See* Histamine (HA)
Hallucinations, 39
HDC. *See* Histidine-decarboxylase (HDC)
Headaches (migraine), 363–364
Heart, signal-transducing pathways in, 178–181.
         See also Cardiovascular system
Helicobacter pylori (Hp), 171–173
Hepatic encephalopathy, 56
Heterogeneity of H3R, gastrointestinal tract,
         175–177
H3 gene structure and expression, 84–96
Hibernation, 93–94
High-tech computer-aided drug design, 135–143
Hippocampus
    hibernation, 93–94
    hippocampal formation, 91–92
    histaminergic actions, 52–53
HIR. *See* Histamine metabotropic receptors (HIR)
Histamine (HA), as neurotransmitter
    behavior, 54–58
       learning and memory, 57–58
       obesity, 56
       sleep/wake regulation, 54–56
       thermoregulation, 56
    brain
       histamine metabolism, 32–34
       histaminergic actions, 48–54
    brainstem, 48–50
    discovery of, 31–32
    histamine neurons, 34–42
    histamine receptors, 43–48
    histaminergic actions, 48–54
       basal ganglia, 51–52
       cortex, 53
       epilepsy and seizures, 306–312
       glia, 54
       hippocampus, 52–53
       hypothalamus, 50–51
       synaptic plasticity, 53–54
       thalamus, 51
    histaminergic pathways, 42–43
    metabotropic receptors, 40, 43, 45–48
    pathophysiology and disease, 4, 58, 92–96
    regulation (*See* Histamine receptors)
    signal transduction, 84–85
    sleep/wake cycle, 54–56, 247–251
    in spinal cord, 48–50
Histamine autoreceptors, discovery of, 14–16
Histamine metabotropic receptors (HIR), 40,
         43, 45–48
Histamine neurons, 34–42, 38–42
    inputs, 38–42
    location, 34–35
    morphology, 34–35
    physiology, 35–38
Histamine *N*-methyltransferase (HNMT), 33

Histamine 3 receptor ligands. *See* H3R ligands
Histamine receptors
    histamine as neurotransmitter, 43–48
    histamine metabotropic receptors (HIR), 40,
       43, 45–48
    H1 receptors (*See* H1R)
    H2 receptors (*See* H2R)
    H3 receptors (*See* H3R)
    H4 receptors (*See* H4R)
    inotropic, 43
    metabotropic receptors, 40, 43, 45–48
    polyamine-binding site of NMDA receptors, 43
Histamine 1 receptors. *See* H1R
Histamine 2 receptors. *See* H2R
Histamine 3 receptors. *See* H3R
Histamine 4 receptors. *See* H4R
Histaminergic actions
    epilepsy and seizures, 306–312
    histamine as neurotransmitter, 48–54
       basal ganglia, 51–52
       cortex, 53
       glia, 54
       hippocampus, 52–53
       hypothalamus, 50–51
       synaptic plasticity, 53–54
       thalamus, 51
    histaminergic pathways, 42–43
Histidine-decarboxylase (HDC), 32–33, 39, 42,
         46, 54–55, 57
HNMT. *See* Histamine *N*-methyltransferase
         (HNMT)
Hoffman-La Roche, 130–131
Homeostatic mechanisms, sleep/wake cycle,
         245–246
Hormones
    anabolic hormones, 51
    antidiuretic hormone (ADH), 50
    catecholamine
       epilepsy, 318–319
       histamine neurons, 32, 39–40
       histamine research, 14
       sleep/wake cycle, 248
    corticotrophin-releasing hormone (CRH), 41
    gonadotrophin-releasing hormone (GnRH), 51
    growth hormone-releasing hormone
         (GHRH), 51
    leptin
       histamine neurons and metabolism, 41,
         56
       obesity, 278–279, 282–284, 290–291,
         295–296
       sleep/wake cycle, 245
    orexin (hypocretine)
       attention-deficit hyperactivity disorder
         (ADHD), 218
       histamine neurons and metabolism,
         23–24, 41, 51, 55–56
       obesity, 56, 278–279, 284

sleep/wake cycle, 247–249, 262–264
stress, 360
prolactin
  histamine neurons and metabolism, 51
  schizophrenia, 332
  sleep/wake cycle, 245
  stress, 359
prolactin-releasing hormone (PRH), 51
thyrotropine releasing-hormone (TRH), 35,
    41, 51–52, 56
Hp. See Helicobacter pylori (Hp)
HPA axis. *See* Hypothalamic–pituitary–adrenal
    axis (HPA axis)
H1R
  antihistamines, 46
  cloning, 7
  epilepsy and epileptic seizures, 306–312
  non-H1R, histamine autoreceptors as, 14–16
  obesity, 280
  overview, 45–46
H2R
  cloning, 7
  epilepsy and epileptic seizures, 312
  overview, 46–47
H4R
  overview, 48
  peripheral tissues, actions and therapeutic
      potential in, 191
H3R
  Alzheimer's disease (AD), 213–214, 222–230
  attention-deficit hyperactivity disorder
      (ADHD), 213–222
  cerebral ischemia, 364–365
  discovery of, 3–4, 8, 83–84
  drug discovery, 103–165
  epilepsy and epileptic seizures, 4, 305–327, 312
  gene expression, 84–96
  histamine autoreceptors, discovery of, 14–16
  identification of, 83–84
  imidazole-based modulators, 108–111
  locomotion and movement disorders, 356–359
  molecular identification, 84–85
  obesity, 277–304, 281–282
  overview, 47–48
  pain, 360–363, 363–364
  peripheral tissues, actions and therapeutic
      potential in, 167–209
  regulation of expression in physiological/
      pathophysiological conditions, 4,
      58, 92–96
  research experts, 3–16
  schizophrenia, 329–353
  sleep disorders, 241–275
  stress, anxiety and depression, 359–360
  as target, 13–29
H3R agonists
  imidazole-based H3R modulators, 108–109
  R-alpha-methylhistamine (RAMH)

discovery, 6, 7–8
as drug development candidate, 18
spatial memory and, 58
sleep induction and promotion, 251
H3R antagonists
  Alzheimer's disease (AD) treatment,
      225–227
  attention-deficit hyperactivity disorder
      (ADHD) treatment, 217–218
  epilepsy and epileptic seizure treatment,
      10, 312
  imidazole-based
    drug discovery and design, 109–111
    preclinical antiobesity effects of,
        285–289
  nonimidazole-based, 116–121
    discovery of, 6
    drug discovery and design, 111–133
      Alzheimer's disease (AD), 145, 150
      antiobesity agents, 126–127, 150,
          289–292
      chemical class pioneers, 111–112
      drug design of novel cognitive
          enhancers, 116–121
      fluorescent H3 ligands, 116–121
      nonimidazole-based H3R
          antagonists, 121–127
      obesity, 126–127, 150, 289–292
      orally active H3 antagonist, 150
      by pharmaceutical companies,
          112–133
      schizophrenia, 150
      targeting provigilant drugs, 112–116
    drug discovery research, 111–133
  obesity
    preclinical data, 285–292
    treatment, 7, 292–296
  preclinical data
    antiobesity agents, 285–292
    schizophrenia, 342–345
  research history, 20–21
  schizophrenia
    animal models of, 10
    preclinical data, 342–345
  in silico 3-D models, 135–143
  sleep/wake cycle
    disorders, 261–267
    idiopathic hypersomnia, 267
    narcolepsy, 262–265
    serotonin reuptake inhibitors, 258–261
    sleep apnea, 265–267
    as wake-promoting agents, 251–254
  thioperamide, 6, 18
H3R inverse agonists
  cognition enhancement, 22–23
  epilepsy and epileptic seizures, 10, 25–26
  nonimidazole-based, 116–121
  research history, 20–21

H3R inverse (*contd.*)
  schizophrenia
    animal models of, 10
    preclinical data, 342–345
  tiprolisant
    antiepileptic potential of, 26
    antinarcoleptic efficacy of, 23–24
    attention-deficit hyperactivity disorder
        (ADHD), 24–25
    clinical trials, 20
    schizophrenia and, 27
  wakefulness enhancement, 22–23
H3R ligands
  attention-deficit hyperactivity disorder
      (ADHD) utility, 8
  computer-aided drug design, 135–143
  drug discovery and research, 18–20,
      105–108, 116–121, 135–143
  fluorescent, 116–121, 143–146
  natural products as potent, 105–108
  radiolabeled, 4, 143–146
  schizophrenia, use in, 26–27
  in silico 3-D models, 135–143
  thioperamide, 6, 17–18, 22, 57
Human brain, phylogeny of, 89–92
  basal ganglia, 91–92
  brainstem, 48–50
  enthorhinal cortex, 91–92
  general expression patterns, 89
  hippocampal formation, 91–92
  histamine metabolism in, 32–34
  prefrontal cortex, 89
  spinal cord, 48–50
  synaptic plasticity, 53–54
  temporal cortex, 89
  thalamus, 90
  trauma, 95
Huntington's disease, 357–358
Hybrid combinations, multitarget-oriented H3R
      drug design, 146–149
Hyperactivity
  hyperactivity disorder (*See* Attention-deficit
      hyperactivity disorder (ADHD))
  psychomotor stimulant-induced,
      schizophrenia, 339, 342
Hyperlocomotion, MK-801-induced, 340, 344
Hypocretine (orexin)
  attention-deficit hyperactivity disorder
      (ADHD), 218
  histamine neurons and metabolism, 23–24,
      41, 51, 55–56
  obesity, 56, 278–279, 284
  sleep/wake cycle, 247–249, 262–264
  stress, 360
Hypothalamic–pituitary–adrenal axis (HPA
      axis), 359
Hypothalamus
  histaminergic actions, 50–51

sleep/wake cycle, 247
tuberomamillary nucleus (TMN), 32, 34–40
ventral lateral preoptic (VLPO) area,
      247–249
ventromedial hypothalamus (VMH), 51, 56

I

ICD-10 (*International Classification of Disease*
      manual), 215–216
Identification of, 83–84
Idiopathic hypersomnia, 267
Imidazole-based H3R agonists, 108–109
Imidazole-based H3R antagonists
  antiobesity preclinical data, 285–289
  drug discovery and design, 109–111
Imidazole-based H3R modulators, 110–111
Immunity, actions and therapeutic potential in,
      186–189
Inflammation
  actions and therapeutic potential in, 186–189
  drugs targeting, 125
Inotropic receptors, 43
Inputs to histamine neurons, 38–42
INSERM, research at, 14–17
in silico 3-D models, 135–143
International Classification of Disease manual
      (ICD-10), 215–216
Intestinal mucosal defense, 177–178
Intestinal secretion, 177
Intestinal tract. *See* Gastrointestinal tract
Inverse agonists, HR3
  cognition enhancement, 22–23
  epilepsy and epileptic seizures, 10, 25–26
  nonimidazole-based, 116–121
  research history, 20–21
  schizophrenia
    animal models of, 10
    preclinical data, 342–345
  tiprolisant
    antiepileptic potential of, 26
    antinarcoleptic efficacy of, 23–24
    attention-deficit hyperactivity disorder
        (ADHD), 24–25
    clinical trials, 20
    schizophrenia and, 27
  wakefulness enhancement, 22–23
Inverse docking, 140
Ionotropic purine receptors, 40
Ischemia, 94
Isoforms and gene structure, 84–87

J

J&J. *See* Johnson & Johnson PRD (J&J)
Johnson & Johnson PRD (J&J), 112–116, 150

K

KA-induced epilepsy. *See* Kainic acid (KA)
          induced epilepsy
Kainic acid (KA) -induced epilepsy, 94–95,
          307–311, 315
Kindling (chronic models), 313–314
Knockout (KO) mice
     cognitive functioning research, 57, 218–219,
          227
     histaminergic neurons, 38, 41, 46, 48
     obesity research, 284, 286–287
     sleep research, 41, 55, 57, 249, 256–260, 264
     tiprolisant, 23–25
KO mice. *See* Knockout (KO) mice

L

Laboratoires Servier, 129–130
Labyrinthectomy, brain studies, 96
Learning, and histamines, 57–58
Leptin
     histamine neurons and metabolism, 41, 56
     obesity, 278–279, 282–284, 290–291,
          295–296
     sleep/wake cycle, 245
Ligands
     development of first selective ligands for
          H3R, 16–18
     H3R
          attention-deficit hyperactivity disorder
               (ADHD) utility, 8
          computer-aided drug design, 135–143
          drug discovery and research, 18–20,
               105–108, 116–121, 135–143
          fluorescent, 116–121, 143–146
          natural products as potent, 105–108
          radiolabeled, 4, 143–146
          schizophrenia, use in, 26–27
          in silico models, 135–143
          thioperamide, 6, 17–18, 22, 57
     protean ligands, 20–21
Location of histamine neurons, 34–35
Locomotion
     disorders, 356–359
     hyperlocomotion, MK-801-induced, 340,
          344
Long-term depression (LTD), 53–54
LTD. *See* Long-term depression (LTD)

M

Medium spiny neurons (MSN), 52–53
Memory, 57–58. *See also* Alzheimer's
          disease (AD)
Mepyramine, 22

Messenger RNA (mRNA)
     gene structure and expression, 84–96
     as histamine neuron input, 39–40
     histaminergic actions, 49, 51
     obesity, 281–284, 294
     peripheral tissues and systems, 168, 175,
          184, 189
Metabolic syndrome, 27
Metabolism of histamine, in brain, 32–34
Metabotropic receptors, 40, 43, 45–48
Methamphetamine, 26
Tele-methylhistamine, 95–96
Mice, research with
     knockout (KO) genes
          cognitive functioning research, 57,
               218–219, 227
          histaminergic neurons, 38, 41, 46, 48
          obesity research, 284, 286–287
          sleep research, 41, 55, 57, 249, 256–260,
               264
          tiprolisant, 23–25
     other research with (*See specific topics*)
Migraine, 363–364
MK-801-induced hyperlocomotion,
          schizophrenia, 340, 344
Monkeys, research with
     cognitive functioning, 229–230
     drug discovery, 118, 130
Morphology of histamine neurons, 34–35
Motility, gastrointestinal, 174–177
Movement disorders, 356–358
MRNA. *See* Messenger RNA (mRNA)
MSN. *See* Medium spiny neurons (MSN)
Mucosal defense
     gastric, 173–174
     intestinal, 177–178
Multitarget-oriented H3R drug design, 146–149
     clinical studies, 149–151
     drug combinations, 146
     hybrid combinations, 146–149
     preclinical data, 149–151

N

NA. *See* Noradrenaline (NA)/norepinephrine (NE)
Narcolepsy
     antinarcoleptic efficacy of tiprolisant, 23–24
     drugs targeting, 121–125
     provigilant drugs, 10
     sleep/wake cycle, 262–265
     treatment, 4, 7, 10
Natural products as potent H3R ligands,
          105–108
Nature, 16, 18
NE. *See* Noradrenaline (NA)/norepinephrine
          (NE)
Neurogen, 132–133

Neurons
  damage to, and epileptic seizures, 315
  histamine, 34–42
    inputs, 38–42
    location, 34–35
    morphology, 34–35
    physiology, 35–38
  hypocretin-containing neurons, 41, 51
  medium spiny neurons (MSN), 52–53
  orexin-containing neurons, 23–24, 41, 51
  protection of, and cerebral ischemia,
       364–365
Neuropathic pain, 4, 7
Neurotransmitters
  acetylcholine (Ach)
    attention-deficit hyperactivity disorder
       (ADHD), 217–218, 223–224
    drug development, 147
    epilepsy, 318
    histamine neurons, 39
    histamine research, 7, 14
    locomotion and movement disorders, 357
    obesity, 279, 281
    in peripheral tissues, 169, 172, 175–176
    schizophrenia, 337, 345
    sleep/wake cycle, 246–247, 249–252
  dopamine (DA)
    alcohol-related behavior, 96
    attention-deficit hyperactivity disorder
       (ADHD), 217–218, 220
    drug discovery, 120, 138
    histamine neurons and metabolism,
       39–40, 42, 49, 51–52, 58
    histamine research, 14, 17, 21, 24–27
    locomotion and movement disorders,
       357–358, 365
    obesity, 278, 281, 295
    schizophrenia, 330–331, 338–340,
       342–344
    sleep/wake cycle, 94, 246, 249–250, 252,
       254, 256, 260, 264–265
  GABA and GABAergic system
    alcohol sensitivity, 96
    cerebral ischema, 365
    epilepsy, 305, 311, 314, 316–320
    histamine neurons and metabolism, 33,
       35, 38–41
    histaminergic actions, 49–55
    locomotion and movement
       disorders, 357
    schizophrenia, 336, 340
    sleep/wake, 247–250, 265
  glutamate
    alcohol-related behavior, 96
    drug discovery, 137
    epilepsy, 305, 315, 317
    histamine neurons and metabolism,
       38–39, 42, 47, 49, 50, 52–54

  locomotion and movement disorders,
       357, 364–365
  obesity, 279
  schizophrenia, 26, 330–331, 333–337,
       340
histamine (HA)
  behavior, 54–58
  brainstem, 48–50
  discovery of, 31–32
  histamine metabolism, 32–34
  histamine neurons, 34–42
  histamine receptors, 43–48
  histaminergic actions, 48–54
  histaminergic pathways, 42–43
  metabotropic receptors, 40, 43, 45–48
  pathophysiology and disease, 4, 58, 92–96
  in spinal cord, 48–50
noradrenaline (NA)/norepinephrine (NE)
  attention-deficit hyperactivity disorder
       (ADHD), 218
  drug discovery, 148
  epilepsy, 317–318
  histamine neurons and metabolism, 40,
       49, 52
  histamine research, 14, 23
  obesity, 278, 281, 295
  in peripheral tissues, 175–176, 178–180
  schizophrenia, 336–337
  sleep/wake cycle, 246–251, 254, 260,
       263, 265, 267
serotonin (5HT)
  attention-deficit hyperactivity disorder
       (ADHD), 217
  drug discovery, 130, 148
  epilepsy, 321
  histamine neurons and metabolism, 32,
       40, 49, 52
  histamine research, 23
  obesity, 278–279, 281, 289, 295
  schizophrenia, 331, 340
  sleep/wake cycle, 247, 249–251, 254,
       258–261, 265
N40 gating, schizophrenia, 341, 344–345
NMDA. *See* *N*-methyl-D-aspartate (NMDA)
       receptors
N-methyl-D-aspartate (NMDA) receptors, 26,
       39, 43–44
Nociceptin (orphanin FQ), 41
Nociception, 360–363
Non-H1R, histamine autoreceptors as, 14–16
Non-H2R, histamine autoreceptors as, 14–16
Nonimidazole-based H3R antagonists
  discovery of, 6
  drug discovery and design, 111–133
    Alzheimer's disease (AD), 145, 150
    antiobesity agents, 126–127, 150,
       289–292
    chemical class pioneers, 111–112

drug design of novel cognitive
        enhancers, 116–121
fluorescent H3 ligands, 116–121
nonimidazole-based H3R antagonists,
        121–127
obesity, 126–127, 150, 289–292
orally active H3 antagonist, 150
by pharmaceutical companies, 112–133
        Abbott Laboratories, 116–121, 150
        Arena Pharmaceuticals, 133
        Banyu Pharmaceutical, 132–133
        drug discovery programs, 112–133
        Eli Lilly & Co, 128–132
        GlaxoSmithKline (GSK), 121–127,
                145, 150
        Hoffman-La Roche, 130–131
        Johnson & Johnson PRD, 112–116, 150
        Laboratoires Servier, 129–130
        Neurogen, 132–133
        new chemical entities, 132–133
        Novo-Nordisk, 126–127
        Pfizer, 131–132
provigilant drugs, 112–116
schizophrenia, 150
targeting provigilant drugs, 112–116
Nonrapid eye movement (NREM) sleep,
        242–253, 257–261, 266
Nonsteroidal anti-inflammatory drugs
        (NSAIDs), 11
Nonstimulants, attention-deficit hyperactivity
        disorder (ADHD), 316
Noradrenaline (NA)/norepinephrine (NE)
attention-deficit hyperactivity disorder
        (ADHD), 218
drug discovery, 148
epilepsy, 317–318
histamine neurons and metabolism, 40, 49, 52
histamine research, 14, 23
obesity, 278, 281, 295
in peripheral tissues, 175–176, 178–180
schizophrenia, 336–337
sleep/wake cycle, 246–251, 254, 260, 263,
        265, 267
Novo-Nordisk, 126–127
NREM sleep. *See* Nonrapid eye movement
        (NREM) sleep
NSAIDs. *See* Nonsteroidal anti-inflammatory
        drugs (NSAIDs)

O

Obesity, 277–304
        current approaches to treatment of obesity,
                278
        drug discovery and design, antiobesity
                agents, 126–127, 150, 289–292
        feeding behavior, 50, 278–282

histamine, role in, 278–282
histaminergic genetic modifications and
        weight regulation, 282–284
H1R, 280
H3R, 281–282
H3R antagonists
        clinical utility of, 7, 292–296
        imidazole-based H3R antagonists,
                285–289
        nonimidazole-based H3R antagonists,
                289–292
        preclinical data, 285–292
Orexin
        attention-deficit hyperactivity disorder
                (ADHD), 218
        histamine neurons and metabolism, 23–24,
                41, 51, 55–56
        obesity, 56, 278–279, 284
        sleep/wake cycle, 247–249, 262–264
        stress, 360
Oxytocin, 50–51

P

Pain
        drugs targeting, 121–125
        migraine, 363–364
        neuropathic, 4, 7
        perception of (nociception), 360–363
        visceral, in gastrointestinal tract, 177–178
Paradoxical sleep, 22
Parkinson's disease, 357–358
Patent applications, drug, 104–105
PCP. *See* Phencyclidine (PCP)
Perception of pain (nociception), 360–363
Peripheral tissues, actions and therapeutic
        potential in, 167–209
        allergy, 186–189
        carcinogenesis, 189
        cardiovascular system, 178–183
        gastrointestinal tract, 168–178
        immunity, 186–189
        inflammation, 186–189
        other peripheral locations and functions,
                189–191
        respiratory system, 184–186
Pertussis toxin (PTX)
        epilepsy research, 307–308, 310–311,
                312–313
        H3R discovery, 84
        postsynaptic H3R receptors, 183
        signal transduction pathways, 181
Pfizer, 131–132
Pharmaceutical companies
        Abbott Laboratories, 116–121, 150
        Arena Pharmaceuticals, 133
        Banyu Pharmaceutical, 132–133

Pharmaceutical companies (*contd.*)
    drug discovery programs, 112–133
    Eli Lilly & Co, 128–132
    GlaxoSmithKline (GSK), 121–127, 145, 150
    Hoffman-La Roche, 130–131
    Johnson & Johnson PRD, 112–116, 150
    Laboratoires Servier, 129–130
    Neurogen, 132–133
    new chemical entities, 132–133
    Novo-Nordisk, 126–127
    Pfizer, 131–132
Pharmacophore model, 134–137, 140–142
Phencyclidine (PCP), 26
Phylogeny of human brain, 89–92
    basal ganglia, 91–92
    brainstem, 48–50
    enthorhinal cortex, 91–92
    general expression patterns, 89
    hippocampal formation, 91–92
    histamine metabolism in, 32–34
    prefrontal cortex, 89
    spinal cord, 48–50
    synaptic plasticity, 53–54
    temporal cortex, 89
    thalamus, 90
    trauma, 95
Physiology of histamine neurons, 35–38
PIH. *See* Prolactin-inhibiting hormone (PIH)
Plaques, Alzheimer's disease (AD), 225
Plasticity, synaptic, 53–54
Polyamine-binding site of NMDA receptors,
    43–44
Polysomnography, 242–243, 253, 257, 260
Postsynaptic histamine H3Rs, 181–183
PPI. *See* Prepulse inhibition (PPI)
Preclinical data
    Alzheimer's disease (AD), 227–230
    attention-deficit hyperactivity disorder
        (ADHD), 218–222
    drug discovery and design, 149–151
    obesity, 285–292
    schizophrenia, 342–345
Prefrontal cortex, brain, 89
Prepulse inhibition (PPI) and schizophrenia, 27,
    340–341, 344
Presynaptic histamine H3Rs, 181–183
PRH. *See* Prolactin-releasing hormone (PRH)
Primates, research with
    cognitive functioning, 229–230
    drug discovery, 118, 130
Prolactin
    histamine neurons and metabolism, 51
    schizophrenia, 332
    sleep/wake cycle, 245
    stress, 359
Prolactin-inhibiting hormone (PIH), 51
Prolactin-releasing hormone (PRH), 51
Protean ligands, 20–21

Provigilant drugs, 112–116
Psychiatric disorders
    anxiety, 359–360
    depression
        antidepressants, 321
        as CNS disorder, 359–360
        long-term depression (LTD), 53–54
    schizophrenia, 329–353
        animal models, 338–342
            catalepsy, 341–342
            dopaminergic hypothesis, 338–340
            glutamatergic hypothesis, 340
            H3 antagonists/inverse agonists, 10
            MK-801-induced hyperlocomotion,
                340
            N40 gating, 341
            prepulse inhibition (PPI), 27,
                340–341, 344
            sensorimotor gating, 340–341
            side-effect liabilities, 341–342
        apomorphine-induced climbing behavior,
            336, 339
        behavior, 336, 339–340
        current therapies, 331–332
        disease state, 330–331
        dopamine hypothesis, 334
        dopaminergic hypothesis of, 338–340
        experimental disease model, 338–342
            apomorphine-induced climbing
                behavior, 336
            cataleptic potential, 345
            dopamine agonists, H3R antagonistic
                interactions with, 342–344
            H3R antagonistic interactions with
                dopamine agonists, 342–344
            hyperactivity, psychomotor
                stimulant-induced, 342
            MK-801-induced hyperlocomotion,
                344
            N40 gating, 344–345
            preclinical data, 342–345
            prepulse inhibition (PPI), 27,
                340–341, 344
            psychomotor stimulant-induced
                hyperactivity, 342
            sensorimotor gating, 344–345
        future directions, 345–346
        glutamate hypothesis, 334
        H3R ligands use in, 26–27
        introduction, 330
        neuroanatomical rationale, 335–336
        neurochemical and functional rationale,
            337–338
        neurodevelopmental hypothesis, 334–335
        prepulse inhibition (PPI), 27, 340–341,
            344
        rationale for H3R antagonist efficacy in
            schizophrenia, 335–338

sensorimotor gating
　animal models, 340–341
　experimental disease models, 344–345
　introduction, 27
　N40 gating, 341, 344–345
　prepulse inhibition, 340–341, 344
theories of disease basis, 333–335
therapeutic options and considerations,
　331–333
unmet medical need, 332–333
Psychomotor stimulant-induced hyperactivity,
　339, 342
Psychostimulants, sleep/wake cycle, 254–256
PTX. See Pertussis toxin (PTX)
PTX-induced seizures, epilepsy research,
　307–311, 312–313
Purine receptors, metabotropic, 40

Q

Questionnaire to experts, 4, 6

R

Radiolabeled ligands, 4, 143–146
(R)-alpha-methylhistamine (RAMH)
　discovery, 6–8
　as drug development candidate, 18
　spatial memory and, 58
RAMH. See (R)-alpha-methylhistamine (RAMH)
Rapid eye movement (REM) sleep, 22, 242–265
Rats, research with. See Human brain,
　　　phylogeny of; specific research
Receptor-binding autoradiography, 93
Regulation of histamine. See Histamine receptors
REM sleep. See Rapid eye movement (REM)
　　　sleep
REM-sleep paralysis, 39
Research. See also specific topics
　Andrew D. Medhurst on, 6–7, 226
　at Bioprojet, 16–19
　drug design (See Drug discovery and design)
　expert opinion solicitation, 3–12
　at INSERM, 14–17
　Nicholas I. Carruthers, 7–8, 115–116
　questionnaire to, 4, 6
Respiratory system, actions and therapeutic
　　　potential in, 184–186

S

SAS. See Sleep apnea syndrome (SAS)
Schizophrenia, 329–353
　animal models, 338–342
　　catalepsy, 341–342
　　dopaminergic hypothesis, 338–340

glutamatergic hypothesis, 340
H3 antagonists/inverse agonists, 10
MK-801-induced hyperlocomotion, 340
N40 gating, 341
prepulse inhibition (PPI), 27, 340–341,
　344
sensorimotor gating, 340–341
side-effect liabilities, 341–342
apomorphine-induced climbing behavior,
　336, 339
behavior, 336, 339–340
current therapies, 331–332
disease state, 330–331
dopamine hypothesis, 334
dopaminergic hypothesis of, 338–340
experimental disease model, 338–342
　apomorphine-induced climbing behavior,
　　336
　cataleptic potential, 345
　dopamine agonists, H3R antagonistic
　　interactions with, 342–344
　H3R antagonistic interactions with
　　dopamine agonists, 342–344
　hyperactivity, psychomotor stimulant-
　　induced, 342
　MK-801-induced hyperlocomotion, 344
　N40 gating, 344–345
　preclinical data, 342–345
　prepulse inhibition (PPI), 27, 340–341,
　　344
　psychomotor stimulant-induced
　　hyperactivity, 342
　sensorimotor gating, 344–345
future directions, 345–346
glutamate hypothesis, 334
H3R ligands use in, 26–27
introduction, 330
neuroanatomical rationale, 335–336
neurochemical and functional rationale,
　337–338
neurodevelopmental hypothesis, 334–335
prepulse inhibition (PPI), 27,
　340–341, 344
rationale for H3R antagonist efficacy in
　schizophrenia, 335–338
sensorimotor gating
　animal models, 340–341
　experimental disease models, 344–345
　introduction, 27
　N40 gating, 341, 344–345
　prepulse inhibition, 340–341, 344
theories of disease basis, 333–335
therapeutic options and considerations,
　331–333
unmet medical need, 332–333
Schwartz, Jean-Charles, 3, 8, 250, 315
SCN. See Suprachiasmatic nucleus (SCN)
Second histamine receptor. See H2R

Secretion
    of gastric acid, 169–173
        gastrointestinal tract, 169–173
        Helicobacter pylori (Hp), 171–173
    intestinal, 177
Seizures, induced. *See also* Epilepsy and
        epileptic seizures
    chemoshock-induced seizures, 307–311,
        312–313
    electroshock-induced seizures, 307–311,
        312–313
    kainic acid (KA)-induced seizures, 94–95,
        307–311, 315
    PTX-induced seizures, 307–308, 307–311,
        310–311, 312–313
Selective serotonin reuptake inhibitors (SSRI),
    148, 259–260, 321
Sensorimotor gating and schizophrenia
    animal models, 340–341
    experimental disease models, 344–345
    introduction, 27
    N40 gating, 341, 344–345
    prepulse inhibition (PPI), 27, 340–341, 344
Serotonin (5HT)
    attention-deficit hyperactivity disorder
        (ADHD), 217
    drug discovery, 130, 148
    epilepsy, 321
    histamine neurons and metabolism, 32, 40,
        49, 52
    histamine research, 23
    obesity, 278–279, 281, 289, 295
    schizophrenia, 331, 340
    sleep/wake cycle, 247, 249–251, 254,
        258–261, 265
Serotonin 2CR, 40
Serotonin reuptake inhibitors, sleep/wake cycle,
    258–261
Side-effect liabilities, schizophrenia, 341–342
Signal transduction
    cardiac pathways, 178–181
    H3R-mediated, 84–85
Sleep apnea syndrome (SAS), 265–267
Sleep drunkenness, 267
Sleepologists, 22
Sleep/wake cycle, 241–275
    control, biochemical and physiological,
        246–247
    disorders, 261–267
        idiopathic hypersomnia, 267
        narcolepsy
            antinarcoleptic efficacy of tiprolisant,
                23–24
            drugs targeting, 121–125
            provigilant drugs, 10
            sleep/wake cycle, 262–265
            treatment, 4, 7, 10
    sleep apnea, 265–267

EEG spectral study, 254–256
function of, 244–245
hibernation, 93–94
histamine in regulation, 54–56, 247–251
H3R agonists and sleep induction/
    promotion, 251
H3R antagonist
    serotonin reuptake inhibitors, 258–261
    as wake-promoting agents, 251–254
nonrapid eye movement (NREM) sleep,
    242–253, 257–251, 266
polysomnography, 242–243, 253, 257, 260
rapid eye movement (REM) sleep, 22,
    242–265
regulation of, 54–56, 247–251
sleep apnea syndrome (SAS), 265–267
sleep induction and promotion, 251
sleep/wake cycle, 242–244
Spinal cord, histaminergic actions in, 48–50
SSRI. *See* Selective serotonin reuptake
    inhibitors (SSRI)
Stimulants
    attention-deficit hyperactivity disorder
        (ADHD), 316
    psychomotor stimulant-induced
        hyperactivity, 339, 342
    psychostimulants, sleep/wake cycle,
        254–256
Stimulants, sleep/wake cycle, 254–256
Stress, 359–360
Suprachiasmatic nucleus (SCN), 246
Synaptic plasticity, 53–54

T

Tangles, Alzheimer's disease (AD), 225
Tele-methylhistamine, 95–96
Temperature regulation, 56
Temporal cortex, 89
Temporal lobe epilepsy, 94
Thalamus
    histaminergic actions, 51
    human brain, phylogeny of, 90
Thermoregulation, 56
Thioperamide, 6, 17–18, 22, 57, 285–289
Third histamine receptor. *See* H3R
Thyroid-stimulating hormone (TSH), 51
Thyrotropine releasing-hormone (TRH), 35, 41,
    51–52, 56
Tiorfan, 16, 18
Tiprolisant
    antiepileptic potential of, 26
    antinarcoleptic efficacy of, 23–24
    attention-deficit hyperactivity disorder
        (ADHD), 24–25
    clinical trials, 20
    schizophrenia and, 27

Tissues
    carcinogenesis, 189
    expression in vertebrate, 87–88
    peripheral, actions and therapeutic potential
          in, 167–209
        allergy, 186–189
        carcinogenesis, 189
        cardiovascular system, 178–183
        gastrointestinal tract, 168–178
        immunity, 186–189
        inflammation, 186–189
        other peripheral locations and functions,
          189–191
        respiratory system, 184–186
TMN. *See* Tuberomamillary nucleus (TMN)
Transgenic models, sleep/wake regulation,
        256–258
TRH. *See* Thyrotropine releasing-hormone
        (TRH)
TSH. *See* Thyroid-stimulating
        hormone (TSH)
Tuberomamillary nucleus (TMN), in
        hypothalamus, 32, 34–40

U

Unilateral labyrinthectomy, brain studies, 96

V

Ventral lateral preoptic (VLPO) area, 247–249
Ventromedial hypothalamus (VMH), 51, 56
Vertebrate tissues, expression in, 87–88
Vessels in cardiovascular system, 181–183
Vestibular compensation, regulation of H3R
        expression, 96
Visceral pain in gastrointestinal tract, 177–178
VLPO area. *See* Ventral lateral preoptic (VLPO)
        area
VMH. *See* Ventromedial hypothalamus (VMH)

W

Waking substance, 32. *See also* Sleep/wake cycle
Weight regulation and histamine, 279–282.
        See also Obesity

Printed and bound by CPI Group (UK) Ltd, Croydon, CR0 4YY

23/10/2024

01778227-0017